The Gut-Brain Axis

The Gut-Brain Axis
Dietary, Probiotic, and Prebiotic Interventions on the Microbiota

Edited by

Niall Hyland
APC Microbiome Institute, and Department of
Pharmacology & Therapeutics
University College Cork, Ireland

Catherine Stanton
APC Microbiome Institute, and
Teagasc Moorepark Food Research Centre
Cork, Ireland

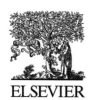

AMSTERDAM • BOSTON • HEIDELBERG • LONDON
NEW YORK • OXFORD • PARIS • SAN DIEGO
SAN FRANCISCO • SINGAPORE • SYDNEY • TOKYO

Academic Press is an imprint of Elsevier

ELSEVIER

Academic Press is an imprint of Elsevier
125 London Wall, London EC2Y 5AS, UK
525 B Street, Suite 1800, San Diego, CA 92101-4495, USA
50 Hampshire Street, 5th Floor, Cambridge, MA 02139, USA
The Boulevard, Langford Lane, Kidlington, Oxford OX5 1GB, UK

Notices
Knowledge and best practice in this field are constantly changing. As new research and experience broaden our understanding, changes in research methods, professional practices, or medical treatment may become necessary.

Practitioners and researchers must always rely on their own experience and knowledge in evaluating and using any information, methods, compounds, or experiments described herein. In using such information or methods they should be mindful of their own safety and the safety of others, including parties for whom they have a professional responsibility.

To the fullest extent of the law, neither the Publisher nor the authors, contributors, or editors, assume any liability for any injury and/or damage to persons or property as a matter of products liability, negligence or otherwise, or from any use or operation of any methods, products, instructions, or ideas contained in the material herein.

British Library Cataloguing-in-Publication Data
A catalogue record for this book is available from the British Library

Library of Congress Cataloging-in-Publication Data
A catalog record for this book is available from the Library of Congress

ISBN: 978-0-12-802304-4

For information on all Academic Press publications
visit our website at https://www.elsevier.com/

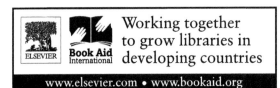

Working together
to grow libraries in
developing countries

www.elsevier.com • www.bookaid.org

Publisher: Nikki Levy
Acquisition Editor: Megan Ball
Editorial Project Manager: Billie Jean Fernandez
Production Project Manager: Caroline Johnson
Designer: Ines Cruz

Typeset by TNQ Books and Journals
www.tnq.co.in

10 9 8 7 6 5 4 3 2

Contents

CHAPTER 4   **Value of Microbial Genome Sequencing for Probiotic Strain Identification and Characterization: Promises and Pitfalls 45**

C.M. GUINANE, F. CRISPIE AND P.D. COTTER

CHAPTER 5   **Probiotics as Curators of a Healthy Gut Microbiota: Delivering the Solution 61**

A.B. MURPHY, T.G. DINAN, J.F. CRYAN, C. STANTON
AND R.P. ROSS

List of Contributors

A. Benítez-Páez
Institute of Agrochemistry and Food Technology, National Research Council (IATA-CSIC), Microbial Ecology, Nutrition & Health Research Group, Valencia, Spain

R.J. Brummer
Örebro University, Nutrition-Gut-Brain Interactions Research Centre, Faculty of Medicine and Health, Örebro, Sweden

M.L. Callegari
Università Cattolica del Sacro Cuore, Centro Ricerche Biotecnologiche, Cremona, Italy

G. Clarke
University College Cork, APC Microbiome Institute, Cork, Ireland; University College Cork, Department of Psychiatry and Neurobehavioural Science, Cork, Ireland

P.D. Cotter
Teagasc Food Research Centre, Fermoy, Cork, Ireland; University College Cork, APC Microbiome Institute, Cork, Ireland

F. Crispie
Teagasc Food Research Centre, Fermoy, Cork, Ireland; University College Cork, APC Microbiome Institute, Cork, Ireland

J.F. Cryan
University College Cork, APC Microbiome Institute, Cork, Ireland; University College Cork, Department of Anatomy and Neuroscience, Cork, Ireland

P. de Timary
Catholic University of Louvain, Institute of Neuroscience and Department of Adult Psychiatry, Brussels, Belgium; Saint Luc University Hospital, Department of Adult Psychiatry, Brussels, Belgium

W.M. de Vos
Wageningen University, Laboratory of Microbiology, Wageningen, The Netherlands; University of Helsinki, Haartman Institute, Department of Bacteriology and Immunology, Helsinki, Finland

J. Deane
Teagasc Food Research Centre, Cork, Ireland; University College Cork, Department of Medicine, Cork, Ireland

N.M. Delzenne
Catholic University of Louvain, Louvain Drug Research Institute, Metabolism and Nutrition Research Group, Brussels, Belgium

T.G. Dinan
University College Cork, APC Microbiome Institute, Cork, Ireland; University College Cork, Department of Psychiatry and Neurobehavioural Science, Cork, Ireland

S. Federici
Università Cattolica del Sacro Cuore, Centro Ricerche Biotecnologiche, Cremona, Italy

G. Fitzgerald
University College Cork, APC Microbiome Institute, Cork, Ireland; University College Cork, Department of Medicine and School of Microbiology, Cork, Ireland

F. Fouhy
Teagasc Food Research Centre, Fermoy, Cork, Ireland

M.G. Gareau
University of California Davis, Department of Anatomy, Davis, CA, United States

R.H. Ghomi
University of Washington, Seattle, WA, United States

E.M. Gómez Del Pulgar
Institute of Agrochemistry and Food Technology, National Research Council (IATA-CSIC), Microbial Ecology, Nutrition & Health Research Group, Valencia, Spain

C.M. Guinane
Teagasc Food Research Centre, Cork, Ireland

C.L. Hayes
McMaster University, Farncombe Family Digestive Health Research Institute, Division of Gastroenterology, Hamilton, ON, Canada

S. Holster
Örebro University, Nutrition-Gut-Brain Interactions Research Centre, Faculty of Medicine and Health, Örebro, Sweden

E.Y. Hsiao
California Institute of Technology, Pasadena, CA, United States

K. Huynh
University of California San Diego, Department of Medicine, La Jolla, CA, United States

F.N. Jacka
Deakin University, Geelong, VIC, Australia

A. Kirchgessner
Seton Hall University, School of Health and Medical Sciences, Department of Interprofessional Health Sciences and Health Administration, South Orange, NJ, United States

J. König
Örebro University, Nutrition-Gut-Brain Interactions Research Centre, Faculty of Medicine and Health, Örebro, Sweden

S. Leclercq
Catholic University of Louvain, Institute of Neuroscience and Department of Adult Psychiatry, Brussels, Belgium

P. Luczynski
University College Cork, APC Microbiome Institute, Cork, Ireland

M. Lyte
Iowa State University, Department of Veterinary Microbiology and Preventive Medicine, Ames, IA, United States

T.M. Marques
Örebro University, Nutrition-Gut-Brain Interactions Research Centre, Faculty of Medicine and Health, Örebro, Sweden

K.A. McVey Neufeld
University College Cork, APC Microbiome Institute, Cork, Ireland

L. Morelli
Università Cattolica del Sacro Cuore, Istituto di Microbiologia, Piacenza, Italy

K. Mungovan
McMaster University, Farncombe Family Digestive Health Research Institute, Department of Pediatrics, Hamilton, ON, Canada

A.B. Murphy
University College Cork, APC Microbiome Institute, Cork, Ireland; Teagasc Food Research Centre, Fermoy, Cork, Ireland; University College Cork, School of Microbiology, Cork, Ireland

K. Nemani
New York University School of Medicine, New York, NY, United States

M.C. Neto
University College Cork, School of Microbiology, Cork, Ireland

S.M. O' Mahony
University College Cork, Department of Anatomy and Neuroscience, Cork, Ireland; University College Cork, APC Microbiome Institute, Cork, Ireland

P.W. O'Toole
University College Cork, School of Microbiology, Cork, Ireland; University College Cork, APC Microbiome Institute, Cork, Ireland

B.J. Plant
University College Cork, Cork Cystic Fibrosis Centre, Cork University Hospital, Cork, Ireland; University College Cork, Department of Medicine, Cork, Ireland

K. Portune
Institute of Agrochemistry and Food Technology, National Research Council (IATA-CSIC), Microbial Ecology, Nutrition & Health Research Group, Valencia, Spain

E.M.M. Quigley
Houston Methodist Hospital and Weill Cornell Medical College, Division of Gastroenterology and Hepatology, Houston, TX, United States

E.M. Ratcliffe
McMaster University, Farncombe Family Digestive Health Research Institute, Department of Pediatrics, Hamilton, ON, Canada

M.C. Rea
Teagasc Food Research Centre, Fermoy, Cork, Ireland; University College Cork, APC Microbiome Institute, Cork, Ireland

G. Reid
Lawson Health Research Institute, Canadian Center for Human Microbiome and Probiotic Research, London, ON, Canada; Western University, Department of Microbiology and Immunology, Division of Urology, Department of Surgery, London, ON, Canada

R.P. Ross
University College Cork, APC Microbiome Institute, Cork, Ireland; University College Cork, College of Science, Engineering and Food Science, Cork, Ireland

P.M. Ryan
Teagasc Food Research Centre, Fermoy, Cork, Ireland; University College Cork, School of Microbiology, Cork, Ireland; University College Cork, APC Microbiome Institute, Cork, Ireland

Y. Sanz
Institute of Agrochemistry and Food Technology, National Research Council (IATA-CSIC), Microbial Ecology, Nutrition & Health Research Group, Valencia, Spain

M. Schneider
University of California San Diego, Department of Medicine, La Jolla, CA, United States

F. Shanahan
University College Cork, APC Microbiome Institute, Cork, Ireland; University College Cork, Department of Medicine, Cork, Ireland; University College Cork, School of Medicine, Cork, Ireland

C. Stanton
Teagasc Food Research Centre, Fermoy, Cork, Ireland; University College Cork, APC Microbiome Institute, Cork, Ireland

P. Stärkel
Saint Luc University Hospital, Department of Hepato-Gastroenterology, Brussels, Belgium; Catholic University of Louvain, Laboratory of Hepato-Gastroenterology, Institute of Experimental and Clinical Research (IREC), Brussels, Belgium

N. Sudo
Kyushu University, Department of Psychosomatic Medicine, Fukuoka, Japan

A. Thomas
Houston Methodist Hospital and Weill Cornell Medical College, Department of Medicine, Houston, TX, United States

E.F. Verdu
McMaster University, Farncombe Family Digestive Health Research Institute, Division of Gastroenterology, Hamilton, ON, Canada

R. Wall
Örebro University, Nutrition-Gut-Brain Interactions Research Centre, Faculty of Medicine and Health, Örebro, Sweden

J.M. Yano
California Institute of Technology, Pasadena, CA, United States

Preface

Given the ever-increasing body of evidence that the gut, and more particularly the enteric microbiota, can affect central nervous system (CNS) function, it is perhaps not unsurprising that alterations in the microbiome, in many instances also accompanied by gut dysfunction, have been associated with significant CNS disorders. Some of these have their focus intuitively in the gut, such as obesity (chapter: Gut Microbiota and Metabolism) and irritable bowel syndrome (chapter: Dietary Interventions and Irritable Bowel Syndrome), whereas others, until recently at least, may have been considered primarily disorders of the CNS. However, many common (pathophysiological) features are shared among these disorders, including, although not exclusively, alterations in gut permeability, microbiota diversity, and gut-brain signaling; the latter perhaps occurring consequent to alterations in the former. This of course represents a simplistic, albeit logical, explanation for the ensuing inflammation often associated with disorders of the microbiota-gut-brain axis, but nonetheless it establishes an attractive pathway for intervention. However, the temporal nature of the alterations in the microbiota, changes in gut barrier integrity and manifestation of pathology, and whether these represent predisposing factors or disease consequence remain unclear. Indeed both possibilities are plausible. To date, there has also been perhaps an underappreciation of the enteric nervous system (chapter: Influence of the Microbiota on the Development and Function of the "Second Brain"—The Enteric Nervous System), or "second brain," which is juxtaposed with the microbiota and represents an accessible window into the pathophysiology of CNS disorders. As our ability to study the complexity of the microbiota and microbiota–host interactions progresses, by harnessing the power of sequencing technologies and use of relevant animals models, such as germ-free or gnotobiotic species, our understanding of the interplay among the microbiota, gut, and brain continues to rapidly develop. This pace of discovery will undoubtedly help address the causality dilemma, but it requires coordinated efforts by multidisciplinary teams; the importance of such studies will only be truly demonstrated by translation to human populations.

In this book, we present evidence establishing a role for the microbiota in disorders of the gut-brain axis, and we have specifically invited commentary from our contributors on the potential for intervention by dietary, probiotic, or prebiotic means in their management. In this regard, advances in sequencing technology and metabolite analysis have provided insight into the identification of putative microbial-based interventions. However, this strategy is most likely to be further influenced by environmental factors in early life and by aging, diet, and exposure to antibiotics. These may well be viewed as confounding factors in experimental studies, but they are real, and variable, among populations and patients and are likely to influence and inform the success or failure of any given microbiota-targeted or dietary intervention. They may also be viewed as risk factors for gut-brain axis disorders. Here again, a common theme emerges throughout several chapters of this book, pointing toward critical periods in early life as key for establishing an appropriate microbiota profile for future well-being. This in turn raises questions about the optimum time for intervention and reversibility of established microbiota-associated alterations in the host (eg, "Can adverse microbiota-associated programming of the host in early life be later reversed to overcome CNS dysfunction?").

We also explore the characterization and optimal delivery of microbiota-targeted interventions. Strategies to restore the gut microbiota using probiotics are discussed, with examples of food- and nonfood-based probiotic carriers (chapter: Probiotics as Curators of a Healthy Gut Microbiota: Delivering the Solution) and the scientific basis for their use in a microbial endocrinology context and consideration as "drug delivery vehicles" (chapter: Microbial Endocrinology: Context and Considerations for Probiotic Selection). However, we also acknowledge the importance of diet as a possible and logical intervention given the global evidence-based literature for its impact on mental well-being. There is no doubt that diet must be considered as an intimate partner in the microbiota-gut-brain axis. However, the delivery of such therapeutic promise is not without its (regulatory) challenges, not least of which is how the field should define a probiotic that influences brain function (ie, a psychobiotic) and the need to demonstrate efficacy for the general population, excluding studies in disease subjects, validation of risk factors of developing a disease, and elucidating their mode of action. This of course applies more broadly and well beyond dietary probiotic and prebiotic interventions affecting the microbiota-gut-brain-axis. There are also global challenges to overcome, including how to ensure that populations in the developing world will benefit from microbial interventions on human health.

This book brings together a group of contributors, all experts in their respective fields, from those involved in brain-gut axis research to cross-cutting areas of technology, epidemiology, and regulation. With this in mind, the book is organized into four main areas. The first two provide background into the technologies, tools, and strategies used to explore the microbiome in health and disease and provide insight into the regulatory framework in which investigators will have to work to deliver the promise of microbial-based interventions to human populations. The third area explores the microbiome at the extremes of life and the importance of critical developmental periods that may provide opportunities for microbial-based interventions. We also introduce the importance and evidence for the role of diet in maintaining good mental health with a global perspective. The final area then addresses specific disorders of the gut-brain axis that may prove amenable to dietary interventions.

Niall Hyland and Catherine Stanton
Cork, Ireland
June 2016

Regulatory Considerations for the Use and Marketing of Probiotics and Functional Foods

L. Morelli

Università Cattolica del Sacro Cuore, Istituto di Microbiologia, Piacenza, Italy

M.L. Callegari, S. Federici

Università Cattolica del Sacro Cuore, Centro Ricerche Biotecnologiche, Cremona, Italy

REGULATORY IMPACT OF DEFINITIONS

Scientific research is the driving force of innovation in nearly all fields of human activity, including nutrition. In the context of nutrition science the management of enteric microbiota to achieve a "health effect" in a human host has enjoyed a long history. During his stay in the early 1900s at the Institute Pasteur, Elie Metchnikoff noticed the "…different susceptibilities of people to the harmful action of microbes and their products. Some can swallow without any evil result a quantity of microbes which in the case of other individuals would produce a fatal attack of cholera. Everything depends upon the resistance offered to the microbes by the invaded organism" (Metchnikoff, 1907). He focused on the sensitivity to low pH of pathogens most commonly isolated from the human gut at that time (*Enterobacteriaceae*); lactic acid-producing bacteria able to colonize the human gut seemed to Metchnikoff to constitute an ideal tool for inhibiting the growth of pathogens.

The following 50 years witnessed more efforts to develop Metchnikoff's ideas; for example, in Europe with *Escherichia coli* strain Nissle 1917 (Möllenbrink and Bruckschen, 1994) and in Japan with *Lactobacillus casei* Shirota (Morotomi, 1996). In the United States Nicholas Kopeloff studied *Lactobacillus acidophilus* (1926) (by lucky coincidence with the focus of this book, Kopeloff was an associate professor in bacteriology at the Psychiatric Institute of Ward's Island, New York), as did Rettger et al. (1935). However, the impact of these investigations on the market was limited, and these studies were ignored by regulatory agencies.

A breakthrough occurred with the appearance in the scientific literature of the term *probiotic*, which seems to have been coined during the 1950s (Hamilton-Miller et al., 2003) to identify substances able to support the growth of microorganisms; this term appears to have been chosen to oppose the concept of an antibiotic. However, the first

The Gut-Brain Axis. http://dx.doi.org/10.1016/B978-0-12-802304-4.00001-3

clear definition of the term *probiotic* in relation to beneficial bacteria emerged in the 1960s (Lilly and Stillwell, 1965). At that time research mainly focused on the selection and use of bacteria for use as feed additives. This peculiarity was made evident by Fuller (1989), who proposed to define probiotics as "a live microbial feed supplement which beneficially affects the host animal by improving its intestinal balance."

Probiotic use was extended to humans by Havenaar and Huis in't Veld (1992), who proposed the definition "a viable mono or mixed culture of bacteria which, when applied to animal or man, beneficially affects the host by improving the properties of the indigenous flora." The definition further evolved with the introduction of references to the quantity of viable cells necessary to exert probiotic action. For example, Guarner and Schaafsma (1998) suggested that probiotics be defined as "live microorganisms, which when consumed in adequate amounts, confer a health effect on the host." A further step was taken by the Food and Agricultural Organization (FAO)/World Health Organization (WHO) Joint Expert Consultation that redefined probiotics as "live microorganisms which when administered in adequate amounts confer a health benefit on the host" (FAO/WHO Joint Working Group, 2001). The verb *administered* was introduced instead of the word *consumed* to include beneficial bacteria in the urogenital tract or bacteria applied topically, according to studies published at the end of the last century that were the basis for products appearing on the market at the beginning of the 2000s (Ocaña et al., 1999; Parent et al., 1996). Further specification of the term *probiotic* was provided by the same expert group in 2002 (FAO/WHO Joint Working Group, 2002). Thus it is clear that definitions of the term *probiotic* have followed the advancement of scientific research, from the quest for substances with actions opposite to those of antibiotics to the selection of bacteria beneficial for humans (not only in the gut).

The two FAO/WHO documents strongly impacted not only science but also regulation, which is relevant for this chapter. Since 2002 these documents have been used as references by health and food-safety agencies all over the world. The European Food Safety Authority, the US Food and Drug Administration, and Health Canada have used them as templates for their own guidelines for probiotics, as have agencies in China, India, Brazil, Argentina, and other nations (Table 1.1). Thus these documents have clarified and improved the regulatory profile of probiotics.

At the time of this writing, the term *probiotic* has reached a consensus definition with two components: (1) viable bacteria (2) with documented (at the strain level) potential to confer health benefits in the host when administered in the necessary amount; this action could be independent of any effect on the composition of the host's gut microbiota. It is also assumed that a clear taxonomy has been assigned to the strains and that their intended use is safe. These considerations should be taken together with more general considerations about "active substances" from the regulatory point of view: (1) the need for accurate bacterial identifications, which imply precise definitions of the active substances; (2) the need to assess safety on the basis of a long history of safe use if the product is food or on the basis of specific testing if the product is pharmaceutical; and (3) the need to evaluate efficacy, which should be assessed in healthy people for food and in patients for drugs.

Table 1.1 List of Health and Food Safety Agencies Referring to Food and Agricultural Organization/World Health Organization Guidelines for Probiotic Definition and Evaluation

Regulatory Authority or Author (Country)	Document
US Food and Drug Administration (United States)	*Complementary and Alternative Medicine Products and Their Regulation by the Food and Drug Administration* (Food and Drug Administration, 2006).
US Pharmacopoeia (United States)	*Appendix XV: Microbial Food Cultures Including Probiotics* (US Pharmacopoeia, 2012).
Health Canada	*Guidance Document : The Use of Probiotic Microorganisms in Food* (Health Canada, 2009). The document "clarifies the acceptable use of health claims about probiotics, and provides guidance on the safety, stability and labeling aspects of food products containing probiotic microorganisms."
Administración Nacional de Medicamentos, Alimentos y Tecnología Médica (ANMAT; Argentina)	*Codigo Alimentario Argentino. Capitulo XVII: Alimentos de Regimen o Dietéticos* (A.N.M.A.T.).
Ministry of Health, China Food and Drug Administration (People's Republic of China)	*Regulatory for Probiotic Health Food Application and Examination* (interim; China Food and Drug Administration (CFDA), 2005). Most of the Food and Agricultural Organization/World Health Organization guidelines have been adopted. A list of 10 allowed probiotic species is furnished.
Indian Council of Medical Research-Department of Biotechnology (ICMR-DBT; India)	*ICMR-DBT Guidelines for Evaluation of Probiotics in Food* (Indian Council of Medical Research Task Force et al., 2011).
International Life Sciences Institute (ILSI)-India	*Guidelines and Criteria for Evaluation of Efficacy, Safety and Health Claim of Probiotic in Food Products in India* (ILSI–India, 2012).
Bureau of Food and Drugs, Department of Health (Philippines)	*Bureau Circular No. 16S 2004* (Bureau of Food and Drugs, 2004). Guidelines for definition and regulation of probiotics as food supplements in the Philippines. Bacterial groups different from Lactobacilli, Bifidobacteria, nonpathogenic Streptococci, *Bacillus clausii*, and *Saccharomyces boulardii* "shall be subject to demonstration of evidence of safe use as food supplement."
European Society for Paediatric Gastroenterology, Hepatology and Nutrition (ESPGHAN) working group (Poland, Italy, Croatia, Israel, Belgium)	*Use of Probiotics for Management of Acute Gastroenteritis* (Szajewska et al., 2014). Systematic review giving recommendation on the use of probiotics in previously healthy children with acute gastroenteritis. *Lactobacillus rhamnosus* GG and *S. boulardii* are strongly recommended as an adjunct to rehydratation therapy.

Continued

Table 1.1 List of Health and Food Safety Agencies Referring to Food and Agricultural Organization/World Health Organization Guidelines for Probiotic Definition and Evaluation—cont'd

Regulatory Authority or Author (Country)	Document
Nutrition and Metabolism Group of the Spanish Neonatology Society (Spain)	*Recommendations and Evidence for Dietary Supplementation with Probiotics in Very Low Birth Weight Infants* (Narbona López et al., 2014). It is associated with lower risk of enterocolitis and death, but protocols (dosage, strains, duration) are still not established.
World Allergy Organization	*Guidelines for Allergic Disease Prevention (GLAD-P): Probiotics* (Fiocchi et al., 2015). Recommendations for the use of probiotics in pregnant women or women breastfeeding otherwise healthy infants with risk of eczema, in which a likely net benefit is present, albeit with no clear evidence of a risk reduction of allergy. Clinical studies in this field present several methodological limitations.
World Gastroenterology Organisation	*World Gastroenterology Organisation Guideline: Probiotics and Prebiotics* (Guarner et al., 2012).
Institute of Food Technologists	*Health Benefits of Probiotics and Prebiotics* (Ohr, 2010). The global retail market for probiotic and prebiotic foods and drinks reached in 2008 approximately $15.4 billion (estimated by Packaged Facts); several probiotics approved by health claims are presented, such as oral probiotic gum prototype and herbal tea with probiotics.
Hoffmann DE, Fraser CM, Palumbo F, Ravel J, Rowthorn V, Schwartz J	*Federal Regulation of Probiotics: An Analysis of the Existing Regulatory Framework and Recommendations for Alternative Framework* (Hoffmann et al., 2012). Output resulting from a National Institutes of Health grant with the aim of examining the legal and regulatory issues raised by probiotics and to determine whether the current regulatory framework is a good fit for the range of probiotics that are on the market, under development, or that may be developed in the future.
Superior Health Council (Belgium)	*Publication of the Superior Health Council No. 8651, Probiotics and Their Implications for Belgian Public Health* (Publication of the superior health council no. 8651, 2012). The paper describes the importance of safety assessment of probiotics and bacterial identification by phenotypical and molecular approaches, with particular attention to the construction of a database.

Another fundamental regulatory issue must be addressed: the two FAO/WHO documents only deal with the use of probiotics in food, as clearly indicated with "the Consultation agreed that the scope of the meeting would include probiotics and prebiotics in food, and exclude reference to the term biotherapeutic agents, and beneficial microorganisms not used in food." The working group defined probiotics as "live microorganisms which when administered in adequate amounts confer a health benefit on the host" and restricted the scope of the discussion to this definition (FAO/WHO Joint Working Group, 2001). Therefore the working group appeared to focus on members of the genera *Lactobacillus* and *Bifidobacterium* and paid much less attention to beneficial microorganisms not used in food. This restriction has a strong regulatory impact because food legislation all over the world deals with products aimed to be provided to healthy people; substances aimed to treat, cure, and/or prevent pathological conditions are addressed under different legislation that covers drugs, medical devices, etc.

To underscore the relevance of this restricted area of applications, we refer to the second FAO/WHO document (2002), in which the expert working group provided a scheme (Fig. 1.1), entitled "Guidelines for the Evaluation of Probiotics for Food Use," in which actions, depicted as boxes, to be performed to grant probiotic status to a food

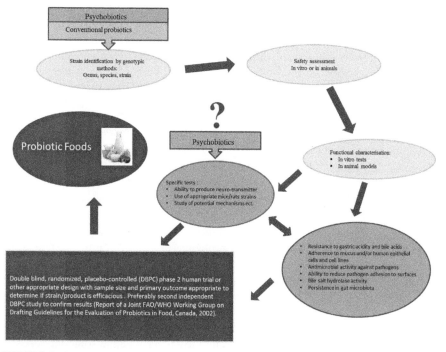

FIGURE 1.1

A possible evaluation scheme of psychobiotics compared to conventional probiotics for food use.

are listed in order and outlined by a row of arrows that connect each action to the next one. Not surprisingly the box containing the action "Phase 3, effectiveness trial is appropriate to compare probiotics with standard treatment of a specific condition" is not connected by an arrow to the final box granting probiotic food status. Therefore we infer that the word *probiotic* was proposed by the FAO/WHO to define bacteria with a beneficial action in pathological and healthy conditions, and that the word *probiotic* can be used for applications that are not related to food (e.g., vaginal or dermal administration). However, the scheme is to be used only for food applications—products targeted to healthy people. These observations are particularly relevant for the assessment of probiotic safety; the long history of safe use of *Lactobacillus* and *Bifidobacterium* provides a solid body of knowledge on their safety as food ingredients consumed by healthy people, but their use in pathological conditions remains unclear.

It is unfortunate that some members of the scientific and clinical worlds have paid little, if any, attention to this last point. Clinical trials have been conducted that did not pay enough attention to safety assessments of specific strains used in specific pathological settings. For example, there is little information about viable bacteria directly administered through a nasal tube into the intestine, which may result in a dose to the intestine that is higher than the dose that would be delivered via the usual oral route (Besselink et al., 2008). Obvious adverse effects were reported (Didari et al., 2014; Fijan, 2014; Kochan et al., 2011; Sanders et al., 2014; Shanahan, 2012; Urben et al., 2014) by some clinicians when probiotics were administered in clinical settings. It is less obvious whether the revision of safety guidelines for probiotics is being sought, although these guidelines are only applicable to healthy people. Use in pathological conditions is subject to safety-assessment procedures for drugs.

Because the probiotic definition is now very popular, not only in the scientific and clinical worlds (in the last 5 years three papers per day were uploaded to PubMed with the keyword *probiotics*) but also as a marketing tool, misuse of the term has boomed. For instance, it has been applied to cosmetic products such as shampoos and aftershave, for which no viability or efficacy of bacterial cells has ever been established. Moreover, in papers and meeting proceedings bacteria isolated from the gut are called *probiotics* even when characterization of their health effects is not provided.

These types of misuse of the term *probiotic* prompted the International Scientific Association for Probiotics and Prebiotics to publish a consensus statement on the appropriate use and scope of the term *probiotic* (Hill et al., 2014). This document categorizes the beneficial mechanisms of probiotics into three groups. The first group deals with mechanisms identified at the genus level, such as colonization resistance. The second group is related to species-specific effects, such as vitamin production in the gut. The third group addresses strain-specific effects; for the purposes of this book we include action on the gut–brain axis (neurological effects) in this group. The final recommendations of Hill et al. (2014) reinforce the concept that properly controlled studies supporting health effects are essential to properly define some microbes as probiotics. These studies may be conducted at the genus, species, or strain level according to the desired beneficial effect. This recommendation also implies that language any more specific than "contains probiotics" must be further substantiated.

Starter cultures may not be defined as probiotics when there is no evidence of health benefits, even if the cultures are traditionally associated with fermented foods. The same restriction applies to fecal microbiota transplants. It is interesting to note that an opportunity exists to define commensal microbes without a history of use in food as probiotics if they are well characterized and supported by adequate evidence of safety and efficacy. This strategy widens the potential for use of newly characterized gut-derived bacteria that exert beneficial actions. However, from the regulatory point of view it seems clear that this last group of probiotics will fall into the "pharma" category because they do not belong to the group of bacteria with a long history of safe use in food.

The scientific and regulatory histories of prebiotics are more recent than those of probiotics. The first definition of the term *prebiotic* appeared in 1995 when Gibson and Roberfroid introduced this neologism to identify a "non-digestible food ingredient that beneficially affects the host by selectively stimulating the growth and/or activity of one or a limited number of bacteria in the colon, and thus improves host health" (Gibson and Roberfroid, 1995). In 2004 the definition was slightly modified: "a prebiotic is a selectively fermented ingredient that allows specific changes, both in the composition and/or activity in the gastrointestinal microbiota that confers benefits upon host wellbeing and health" (Gibson et al., 2004). The second version lacked the phrase *non-digestible* while retaining the concept of fermentation by certain groups of bacteria. The definition proposed by the FAO was contained in the final report of a FAO Technical Meeting in 2007: "a prebiotic is a non-viable food component that confers a health benefit on the host associated with modulation of the microbiota" (FAO Technical Meeting on Prebiotics, 2007). This definition was recently challenged (Bindels et al., 2015) because it "does not require the prebiotic to be fermented or metabolized by the gut microbes, and therefore does not distinguish among substances that modulate gut microbiota composition solely through an inhibitory action. As a consequence, antibiotics would be prebiotics according to this definition." However, this remark does not account for the fact that antibiotics are pharmaceuticals and therefore cannot be defined as, or considered to be, food components.

A total of seven (Table 1.2) slightly different definitions of the term *prebiotic* were recently reviewed and discussed by Bindels et al. (2015), who also proposed a new definition. Five of the six available definitions refer to a specific/selective action of prebiotics on gut microbiota composition (Bindels et al., 2015); the only one that simply links the action of prebiotics to "modulation" is the FAO definition, as stated in the publication. It is important to note that it is not easy to establish a clear-cut differentiation between beneficial and detrimental members of communities of gut bacteria. Culture-independent, DNA-based approaches have determined that even the best-characterized prebiotics are not as specific as previously assumed.

From the regulatory point of view, the actions of probiotics and prebiotics are fundamentally different, as stated in their respective definitions; the former may directly exert their action whereas the latter may mediate changes in the composition of the gut microbiota. It may be simpler to assess the safety of probiotics than the safety of prebiotics. It is surprising to note that in contrast to the abundant literature on the

Table 1.2 Evolvement of Prebiotic Definition

References	Prebiotic Definition
Gibson and Roberfroid (1995)	"Nondigestible food ingredient that beneficially affects the host by selectively stimulating the growth and/or activity of one or a limited number of bacteria in the colon, and thus improves host health."
Reid et al. (2003)	"Nondigestible substances that provide a beneficial physiological effect on the host by selectively stimulating the favourable growth or activity of a limited number of indigenous bacteria."
Gibson et al. (2004)	"Selectively fermented ingredients that allow specific changes, both in the composition and/or activity in the gastrointestinal microflora that confer benefits upon host wellbeing and health."
Roberfroid (2007)	"Selectively fermented ingredient that allows specific changes, both in the composition and/or activity in the gastrointestinal microflora that confers benefits upon host wellbeing and health."
FAO Technical Meeting (2007)	"Nonviable food component that confers a health benefit on the host associated with modulation of the microbiota."
Gibson et al. (2010)	"Dietary prebiotic: a selectively fermented ingredient that results in specific changes in the composition and/or activity of the gastrointestinal microbiota, thus conferring benefit(s) upon host health."
Bindels et al. (2015)	"A nondigestible compound that, through its metabolization by microorganisms in the gut, modulates composition and/or activity of the gut microbiota, thus conferring a beneficial physiological effect on the host."

safety of probiotics (AlFaleh and Anabrees, 2013; Didari et al., 2014; Fijan, 2014; Kochan et al., 2011; Sanders et al., 2014; Shanahan, 2012; Urben et al., 2014), very little information is available for the assessment of the safety of prebiotics; most data are confined to prebiotic use in infant nutrition (López-Velázquez et al., 2013; Van den Nieuwboer et al., 2014, 2015a,b). Because "modern community-wide molecular approaches have revealed that even the established prebiotics are not as specific as previously assumed" (Bindels et al., 2015), it seems prudent to suggest that more data on the impact of prebiotics on the overall composition of the gut microbiota be pursued.

GUT–BRAIN AXIS: WHAT COULD BE RELEVANT FOR ESTABLISHING REGULATIONS?

We have established that the term *probiotic* is historically associated with the intestinal environment and functions such as the homeostasis or balance of gut microbiota. However, in the last 5 years the hypothesis that probiotics can influence brain functions and contribute to the amelioration or prevention of diseases such as depression, anxiety, and mood disorders has gained support from a growing body of evidence, which is reviewed in other chapters of this book. Because this research is opening new areas of applications that are currently not covered by existing regulations, we should expect new challenges from the regulatory point of view.

Should specific regulations be established for this class of probiotics? This question is pertinent because several studies have reported positive effects after probiotic administration in animal models, mostly germ-free or conventionally housed mice or rats. Fewer studies, which are often preclinical pilot trials, have been conducted in human subjects.

The first challenge is to refine or change the only available definition of probiotics that influence brain function. Dinan et al. (2013) proposed the term *psychobiotic* to mean "a live organism that, when ingested in adequate amounts, produces a health benefit in patients suffering from psychiatric illness." Note that this definition matches the definition of a drug; the reference to patients and illness clearly excludes the possibility of categorizing a psychobiotic as food. Moreover, Dinan et al. (2013) explained that the observed health benefit is related to strain-specific actions, such as the production and delivery of neuroactive substances such as gamma-aminobutyric acid (GABA) and serotonin. This example illustrates a "rare" probiotic effect (Hill et al., 2014), meaning that it is strain related and not widespread in all strains of a species. The claim of such an effect requires extensive trials in humans to be substantiated.

FAO/WHO guidelines (2001) and guidelines from the European Food Safety Authority (EFSA, 2009) recommend identification of bacteria at the levels of species and strain for several reasons, including safety, but mainly because it is important "to link a strain to a specific health effect as well as to enable accurate surveillance and epidemiological studies" (FAO/WHO Joint Working Group, 2001). This important aspect, which has been recognized for food-related probiotics, is a *conditio sine qua non* for psychobiotics (Fig. 1.1). For example, Barrett et al. (2012) reported that some strains of *Bifidobacterium* and *Lactobacillus* produced GABA when grown in the presence of monosodium glutamate. GABA is a neurotransmitter that regulates several psychological and physiological processes in the brain that contribute to depression and anxiety (Schousboe and Waagepetersen, 2007). To understand the prevalence of this microbial property in the bacteria of the same genus, Barrett et al. (2012) found that only one *Lactobacillus* strain and four strains of *Bifidobacterium* produced GABA out of 91 tested strains. This evaluation was performed using an in vitro test; when these strains were additionally evaluated in fecal fermentation medium, only *Lactobacillus brevis* DPC6108 produced GABA at high levels (Barrett et al., 2012). The authors concluded that this physiological property could be expressed in vivo and perhaps defined as "strain related and rarely present in lactobacilli and bifidobacteria" (Barrett et al., 2012). Therefore it seems clear that psychobiotics should be handled as pharmaceutical products and should be subject to pharmaceutical legislation.

Nonetheless, some studies indicate that probiotic bacteria play a role in the gut–brain axis in healthy people (Messaoudi et al., 2011a, b), which suggests that "food probiotics" may be exploited for management of the gut–brain axis. Here we only consider human studies (Benton et al., 2007; Rao et al., 2009; Steenbergen et al., 2015), although several studies reported positive effects after probiotic administration in animal models (Desbonnet et al., 2008, 2010). These animal models are often used to obtain insight into neurochemical changes induced by the modulation of intestinal microbiota via the administration of psychobiotic strains. Germ-free animal models are particularly useful for neurogastroenterology research, but animal data often cannot be translated to humans because they do not accurately reflect the physiology and environments of human populations.

Regulatory bodies require evidence obtained in humans. For example, in 2008 the European Union approved Commission Regulation (EC) No. 353/2008, which established and implemented rules for applications for the authorization of health claims. Article 5a of this regulation states that the scientific evidence to be provided to support the application for a health claim "shall consist primarily of studies in humans and, in the case of claims referring to children's development and health, from studies in children" (Commission Regulation (EC) No 353/2008).

Regarding the gut–brain axis in healthy subjects, in a pioneering study Marcos et al. (2014) monitored anxiety in young subjects under academic examination stress. Although fermented probiotic milk reduced the effect of stress on the immune system, there was no significant effect on anxiety (outcomes were similar in control and treatment groups; Marcos et al., 2014). A more recent investigation (Mohammadi et al., 2015) reported more promising results from a randomized, double-blind, placebo-controlled trial of 70 petrochemical workers who were healthy but under stress due to working conditions. Subjects were randomly assigned to receive 100 g/day probiotic yogurt plus one placebo capsule ($n=25$), one probiotic capsule daily plus 100 g/day conventional yogurt ($n=25$), or 100 g/day conventional yogurt plus one placebo capsule ($n=20$) for 6 weeks. Both probiotic-consuming groups received significantly improved scores on a general health questionnaire; stress-scale scores also improved. In contrast, no significant improvements were detected in the conventional yogurt group.

Another very recent study (Steenbergen et al., 2015) sought to assess whether a multispecies probiotic containing bifidobacteria, lactobacilli, and lactococci reduced cognitive reactivity in nondepressed individuals. In this triple-blind, placebo-controlled, randomized study, 20 healthy participants received a 4-week probiotic food supplement and 20 control participants received an inert placebo. A validated index of depression was used to evaluate cognitive reactivity to sad moods before and after the intervention. The treated group reported significant reductions in rumination and aggressive thoughts, leading to an overall reduced cognitive reactivity to sad mood versus participants who received the placebo intervention.

From the regulatory point of view, encouraging observations must be confirmed to enable food use that is supported by an approved health claim. A nonexhaustive list of example questions to be answered includes:

1. What is the rationale for using a seven-strain mixture in a particular probiotic?
2. What is the role of each bacterial component in the observed effect?
3. If the ratio of bacterial members in a marketed blend is different from that used in a clinical trial, will the results remain consistent?

We encourage prudence in drawing conclusions and recommend accounting for differences in approaches and needs between peer reviewers of scientific journals and examiners of regulatory administration.

CONCLUSIONS

If probiotics are to be used to manage human functions influenced by the gut–brain axis, then a clear definition of *psychobiotics* must be crafted. Results from animal trials must be confirmed in human trials in which healthy or unhealthy subjects are enrolled to support the development of food or pharmaceutical products.

As with conventional probiotics, it is important to identify the final target of individual psychobiotics, which will inform trial design. For healthy subjects, evaluation of probiotic/psychobiotic effectiveness should differ from evaluation in the context of illness. Trials should consist of randomized, double-blind placebo studies with rigorous definitions for measuring the effectiveness of psychobiotics, particularly for healthy people.

REFERENCES

AlFaleh, K., Anabrees, J., 2013. Efficacy and safety of probiotics in preterm infants. J. Neonatal Perinatal Med. 6, 1–9.

A.N.M.A.T., August 2013. Código Alimentario Argentino. Cap XVII: Alimentos de Régimen o Dietéticos. Resolución Conjunta SPReI N° 261/2011 y SAGyP N°22/2011, article no. 1389. Available online at: http://www.anmat.gov.ar/alimentos/codigoa/Capitulo_XVII.pdf.

Barrett, E., Ross, R.P., O'Toole, P.W., Fitzgerald, G.F., Stanton, C., 2012. γ-Aminobutyric acid production by culturable bacteria from the human intestine. J. Appl. Microbiol. 113, 411–417.

Benton, D., Williams, C., Brown, A., 2007. Impact of consuming a milk drink containing a probiotic on mood and cognition. Eur. J. Clin. Nutr. 61, 355–361.

Besselink, M.G., van Santvoort, H.C., Buskens, E., Boermeester, M.A., van Goor, H., Timmerman, H.M., Nieuwenhuijs, V.B., Bollen, T.L., van Ramshorst, B., Witteman, B.J., Rosman, C., Ploeg, R.J., Brink, M.A., Schaapherder, A.F., Dejong, C.H., Wahab, P.J., van Laarhoven, C.J., van der Harst, E., van Eijck, C.H., Cuesta, M.A., Akkermans, L.M., Gooszen, H.G., Dutch Acute Pancreatitis Study Group, 2008. Probiotic prophylaxis in predicted severe acute pancreatitis: a randomised, double-blind, placebo-controlled trial. Lancet 371, 651–659.

Bindels, L.B., Delzenne, N.M., Cani, P.D., Walter, J., 2015. Towards a more comprehensive concept for prebiotics. Nat. Rev. Gastroenterol. Hepatol. 12 (5), 303–310. http://dx.doi.org/10.1038/nrgastro.2015.47 [Published online 2015 March 31].

Bureau of Food and Drugs, Departement of Health, Republic of the Philippines, 2004. Guidelines on Probiotics. Bureau Circular No.16 S.2004.

Commission Regulation (EC) No 353/2008. Establishing Implementing Rules for Applications for Authorisation of Health Claims as provided for in Article 15 of Regulation (EC) No 1924/2006 of the European Parliament and of the Council. Available online at: http://eur-lex.europa.eu/legal-content/EN/TXT/?uri=CELEX:32008R0353#text (accessed on 02.05.15.).

China Food and Drug Administration (CFDA), 2005. Regulatory for Probiotic Health Food Application and Examination (Interim).

Desbonnet, L., Garrett, L., Clarke, G., Bienenstock, J., Dinan, T.G., 2008. The probiotic *Bifidobacteria infantis*: an assessment of potential antidepressant properties in the rat. J. Psychiatr. Res. 43, 164–174.

Desbonnet, L., Garrett, L., Clarke, G., Kiely, B., Cryan, J.F., Dinan, T.G., 2010. Effects of the probiotic *Bifidobacterium infantis* in the maternal separation model of depression. Neuroscience 170, 1179–1188.

Didari, T., Solki, S., Mozaffari, S., Nikfar, S., Abdollahi, M., 2014. A systematic review of the safety of probiotics. Expert opinion on drug safety. Informa Healthcare 13, 227–239.

Dinan, T.G., Stanton, C., Cryan, J.F., 2013. Psychobiotics: a novel class of psychotropic. Biol. Psychiatr. 74, 720–726.

EFSA, 2009. Scientific opinion on the substantiation of health claims related to non-characterised microorganisms pursuant to Article 13(1) of Regulation (EC) No 1924/20061. EFSA J. 7, 1247.

Fijan, S., 2014. Microorganisms with claimed probiotic properties: an overview of recent literature. Int. J. Environ. Res. Publ. Health 11, 4745–4767.

Joint FAO/WHO Expert Consultation on Evaluation of Health and Nutritional Properties of Probiotics in Food Including Powder Milk with Live Lactic Acid Bacteria, 2001. Available online at: ftp://ftp.fao.org/docrep/fao/009/a0512e/a0512e00.pdf (accessed on 02.05.15.).

Joint FAO/WHO Working Group Report on Drafting Guidelines for the Evaluation of Probiotics in Food, 2002. Available online at: ftp://ftp.fao.org/es/esn/food/wgreport2.pdf (accessed on 02.05.15.).

FAO Technical Meeting on Prebiotics, 2007. Available online at: http://www.aat-taa.eu/index/en/company/download/1262610500.html (accessed on 02.05.15.).

Fuller, R., 1989. Probiotics in man and animals. J. Appl. Bacteriol. 66, 365–378.

Food and Drug Administration, 2006. Guidance for Industry. Complementary and Alternative Medicine Products and Their Regulation by the Food and Drug Administration.

Fiocchi, A., Pawankar, R., Cuello-Garcia, C., Ahn, K., Al-Hammadi, S., Agarwal, A., Beyer, K., Burks, W., Canonica, G.W., Ebisawa, M., Gandhi, S., Kamenwa, R., Lee, B.W., Li, H., Prescott, S., Riva, J.J., Rosenwasser, L., Sampson, H., Spigler, M., Terracciano, L., Vereda-Ortiz, A., Waserman, S., Yepes-Nuñez, J.J., Brożek, J.L., Schünemann, H.J., 2015. World Allergy Organization-McMaster University guidelines for allergic disease prevention (GLAD-P): probiotics. World Allergy Organ. J. 8, 4.

Guarner, F., Schaafsma, G.J., 1998. Probiotics. Int. J. Food Microbiol. 39, 237–238.

Gibson, G.R., Probert, H.M., Loo, J.V., Rastall, R.A., Roberfroid, M.B., 2004. Dietary modulation of the human colonic microbiota: updating the concept of prebiotics. Nutr. Res. Rev. 17, 259–275.

Gibson, G.R., Roberfroid, M.B., 1995. Dietary modulation of the human colonic microbiota: introducing the concept of prebiotics. J. Nutr. 125, 1401–1412.

Guarner, F., Khan, A.G., Garisch, J., Eliakim, R., Gangl, A., Thomson, A., Krabshuis, J., Lemair, T., Kaufmann, P., de Paula, J.A., Fedorak, R., Shanahan, F., Sanders, M.E., Szajewska, H., Ramakrishna, B.S., Karakan, T., Kim, N., 2012. World gastroenterology organization guideline; probiotics and prebiotics. J. Clin. Gastroenterol. 48, 468–481.

Gibson, G.R., Scott, K.P., Rastall, R.A., Tuohy, K.M., Hotchkiss, A., Dubert-Ferrandon, A., Gareau, M., Murphy, E.F., Saulnier, D., Loh, G., Macfarlane, S., Delzenne, N., Ringel, Y., Kozianowski, G., Dickmann, R., Lenoir-Wijnkoop, I., Walker, C., Buddington, R., 2010. Dietary prebiotics: current status and new definition. Food Sci. Technol. Bull. Funct. Foods 7, 1–19.

Hamilton-Miller, J.M.T., Gibson, G.R., Bruck, W., 2003. Some insights into the derivation and early uses of the word 'probiotic'. Brit. J. Nutr. 90, 845.

Havenaar, R., Huis in't Veld, M.J.H., 1992. Probiotics: a general view. In: Wood, B.J.B. (Ed.), Lactic Acid Bacteria in Health and Disease. Elsevier Applied Science Publishers, Amsterdam, pp. 151–170.

Hill, C., Guarner, F., Reid, G., Gibson, G.R., Merenstein, D.J., Pot, B., Morelli, L., Canani, R.B., Flint, H.J., Salminen, S., Calder, P.C., Sanders, M.E., 2014. Expert consensus document. The international scientific association for probiotics and prebiotics consensus statement on the scope and appropriate use of the term probiotic. Nat. Rev. Gastroenterol. Hepatol. 11, 506–514.

Health Canada, 2009. Food Directorate, Health Products and Food Branch. Guidance Document – the Use of Probiotic Microrganisms in Food.

Hoffmann, D.E., Fraser, C.M., Palumbo, F., Ravel, J., Rowthorn, V., Schwartz, J., 2012. Federal Regulation of Probiotics: An Analysis of the Existing Regulatory Framework and Recommendations for Alternative Frameworks.

Indian Council of Medical Research Task Force, Co-ordinating Unit ICMR, Co-ordinating Unit DBT, 2011. ICMR-DBT guidelines for evaluation of probiotics in food. Indian J. Med. Res. 134, 22–25.

ILSI–India, 2012. Guidelines and Criteria for Evaluation of Efficacy, Safety and Health Claim of Probiotic in Food Products in India.

Kochan, P., Chmielarczyk, A., Szymaniak, L., Brykczynski, M., Galant, K., Zych, A., Pakosz, K., Giedrys-Kalemba, S., Lenouvel, E., Heczko, P.B., 2011. *Lactobacillus rhamnosus* administration causes sepsis in a cardiosurgical patient–is the time right to revise probiotic safety guidelines? Clin. Microbiol. Infect. 17, 1589–1592.

Kopeloff, N., 1926. *Lactobacillus acidophilus*. The Williams and Wilkins Company, Baltimore.

Lilly, D.M., Stillwell, R.H., 1965. Probiotics: growth promoting factors produced by microorganisms. Science 147, 747–748.

López-Velázquez, G., Díaz-García, L., Anzo, A., Parra-Ortiz, M., Llamosas-Gallardo, B., Ortiz-Hernández, A.A., Mancilla-Ramírez, J., Cruz-Rubio, J.M., Gutiérrez-Castrellón, P., 2013. Safety of a dual potential prebiotic system from Mexican agave "Metlin® and Metlos®", incorporated to an infant formula for term newborn babies: a randomized controlled trial. Rev. Invest. Clín. 65, 483–490.

Marcos, A., Wärnberg, J., Nova, E., Gómez, S., Alvarez, A., Alvarez, R., Mateos, J.A., Cobo, J.M., 2004. The effect of milk fermented by yogurt cultures plus *Lactobacillus casei* DN-114001 on the immune response of subjects under academic examination stress. Eur. J. Nutr. 43, 381–389.

Metchnikoff, E., 1907. Lactic acid as inhibiting intestinal putrefaction. In: Heinemann, W. (Ed.), London, the Prolongation of Life: Optimistic Studies, pp. 161–183.

Messaoudi, M., Lalonde, R., Violle, N., Javelot, H., Desor, D., Nejdi, A., Bisson, J.F., Rougeot, C., Pichelin, M., Cazaubiel, M., Cazaubiel, J.M., 2011a. Assessment of psychotropic-like properties of a probiotic formulation (*Lactobacillus helveticus* R0052 and *Bifidobacterium longum* R0175) in rats and human subjects. Brit. J. Nutr. 105, 755–764.

Messaoudi, M., Violle, N., Bisson, J.F., Desor, D., Javelot, H., Rougeot, C., 2011b. Beneficial psychological effects of a probiotic formulation (*Lactobacillus helveticus* R0052 and *Bifidobacterium longum* R0175) in healthy human volunteers. Gut Microbes 2, 256–261.

Mohammadi, A.A., Jazayeri, S., Khosravi-Darani, K., Solati, Z., Mohammadpour, N., Asemi, Z., Adab, Z., Djalali, M., Tehrani-Doost, M., Hosseini, M., Eghtesadi, S., 2015. The effects of probiotics on mental health and hypothalamic-pituitary-adrenal axis: a randomized, double-blind, placebo-controlled trial in petrochemical workers. Nutr. Neurosci. http://dx.doi.org/10.1179/1476830515Y.0000000023 [Published online 2015 April 16].

Morotomi, M., 1996. Properties of *Lactobacillus casei* Shirota strain as probiotics. Asia Pac. J. Clin. Nutr. 5, 29–30.

Möllenbrink, M., Bruckschen, E., 1994. Treatment of chronic constipation with physiologic *Escherichia coli* bacteria. Results of a clinical study of the effectiveness and tolerance of microbiological therapy with the *E. coli* Nissle 1917 strain (Mutaflor). Med. Klin. (Munich) 89, 587–593.

Van den Nieuwboer, M., Brummer, R.J., Guarner, F., Morelli, L., Cabana, M., Claassen, E., 2015a. Safety of probiotics and synbiotics in children under 18 years of age. Benef. Microbes 25, 1–16 [Published online 2015 March 25].

Van den Nieuwboer, M., Brummer, R.J., Guarner, F., Morelli, L., Cabana, M., Claassen, E., 2015b. The administration of probiotics and synbiotics in immune compromised adults: is it safe? Benef. Microbes 6, 3–17.

Van den Nieuwboer, M., Claassen, E., Morelli, L., Guarner, F., Brummer, R.J., 2014. Probiotic and synbiotic safety in infants under two years of age. Benef. Microbes 5, 45–60.

Narbona López, E., Uberos Fernández, J., Armadá Maresca, M.I., Couce Pico, M.L., Rodríguez Martínez, G., Saenz de Pipaon, M., 2014. Nutrition and Metabolism Group of the Spanish Neonatology Society: recommendations and evidence for dietary supplementation with probiotics in very low birth weight infants. An. Pediatr. (Barc.) 81, 397.e1–397.e8.

Ocaña, V.S., Pesce de Ruiz Holgado, A.A., Nader-Macías, M.E., 1999. Selection of vaginal H_2O_2-generating *Lactobacillus* species for probiotic use. Curr. Microbiol. 38, 279–284.

Ohr, L.M., 2010. Institute of Food Technologists. Health Benefits of Probiotics and Prebiotics. Available at: http://www.ift.org/food-technology/past-issues/2010/march/columns/nutraceuticals.aspx?page=viewall.

Parent, D., Bossens, M., Bayot, D., Kirkpatrick, C., Graf, F., Wilkinson, F.E., Kaiser, R.R., 1996. Therapy of bacterial vaginosis using exogenously-applied *Lactobacilli acidophili* and a low dose of estriol: a placebo-controlled multicentric clinical trial. Arzneimittelforschung 46, 68–73.

Publication of the superior health council no. 8651, 2012. Probiotics and Their Implications for Belgian Public Health. Available online at: http://health.belgium.be/internet2prd/groups/public/@public/@shc/documents/ie2divers/19097086.pdf.

Rao, A.V., Bested, A.C., Beaulne, T.M., Katzman, M.A., Iorio, C., Berardi, J.M., Logan, A.C., 2009. A randomized, double-blind, placebo-controlled pilot study of a probiotic in emotional symptoms of chronic fatigue syndrome. Gut Pathogens 19, 6.

Rettger, L.F., Levy, M.N., Weinstein, L., Weiss, J.E., 1935. *Lactobacillus acidophilus* and Its Therapeutic Application. Yale University Press, New Haven, Conn.

Reid, G., Sanders, M.E., Gaskins, H.R., Gibson, G.R., Mercenier, A., Rastall, R., Roberfroid, M., Rowland, I., Cherbut, C., Klaenhammer, T.R., 2003. New scientific paradigms for probiotics and prebiotics. J. Clin. Gastroenterol. 37, 105–118.

Roberfroid, M., 2007. Prebiotics: the concept revisited. J. Nutr. 137, 830S–837S.

Sanders, M.E., Klaenhammer, T.R., Ouwehand, A.C., Pot, B., Johansen, E., Heimbach, J.T., Marco, M.L., Tennilä, J., Ross, R.P., Franz, C., Pagé, N., Pridmore, R.D., Leyer, G., Salminen, S., Charbonneau, D., Call, E., Lenoir-Wijnkoop, I., 2014. Effects of genetic, processing, or product formulation changes on efficacy and safety of probiotics. Ann. N. Y. Acad. Sci. 1309, 1–18.

Schousboe, A., Waagepetersen, H.S., 2007. GABA: homeostatic and pharmacological aspects. In: Tepper, J.M., Abercrombie, E.D., Bolam, J.P. (Eds.), GABA and the Basal Ganglia: From Molecules to Systems. Elsevier Science Bv, Amsterdam, pp. 9–19.

Shanahan, F., 2012. A commentary on the safety of probiotics. Gastroenterol. Clin. North Am. 41, 869–876.

Steenbergen, L., Sellaro, R., van Hemert, S., Bosch, J.A., Colzato, L.S., 2015. A randomized controlled trial to test the effect of multispecies probiotics on cognitive reactivity to sad mood. Brain Behav. Immun. 48, 258–264. http://dx.doi.org/10.1016/j.bbi.2015.04.003 [Published online 2015 April 7].

Szajewska, H., Guarino, A., Hojsak, I., Indrio, F., Kolacek, S., Shamir, R., Vandenplas, Y., Weizman, Z., European Society for Pediatric Gastroenterology, Hepatology, and Nutrition, 2014. Use of probiotics for management of acute gastroenteritis: a position paper by the ESPGHAN Working Group for Probiotics and Prebiotics. J. Pediatr. Gastroenterol. Nutr. 58, 531–539.

Urben, L.M., Wiedmar, J., Boettcher, E., Cavallazzi, R., Martindale, R.G., McClave, S.A., 2014. Bugs or drugs: are probiotics safe for use in the critically ill? Curr. Gastroenterol. Rep. 16, 388.

US Pharmacopoeia, 2012. Microbial food cultures including probiotics, Appendix XV, first supplement. FCC 8, 1709.

Targeting the Microbiota: Considerations for Developing Probiotics as Functional Foods

Y. Sanz, K. Portune, E.M. Gómez Del Pulgar, A. Benítez-Páez

*Institute of Agrochemistry and Food Technology, National Research Council (IATA-CSIC),
Microbial Ecology, Nutrition & Health Research Group, Valencia, Spain*

THE PROBIOTIC CONCEPT AND EVOLUTION

The probiotic concept is based on the notion that the commensal microbiota contributes to human physiology; consequently, favorable modifications in its composition may help to maintain health and reduce disease risk (Neef and Sanz, 2013). The rationale behind the probiotic concept dates back to the times of Elie Metchnikoff (1907), who established associations between the consumption of fermented milk with lactic acid bacteria and longevity in rural populations of Bulgaria (Bibel, 1988). At around the same time (1900), bifidobacteria were isolated from healthy breast-fed infant feces by Henry Tissier, who suggested that they could prevent infections by displacing bacteria causing colitis in breast-fed infants (reviewed by Bertazzoni et al., 2013). The term *probiotic*, which originates from the Greek term *pro bios* ("for life"), was first used as such in 1965 by Lilly and Stillwell to describe substances produced by bacteria that, unlike antibiotics, stimulate the growth of other bacteria. Then in 1989 Roy Fuller finally suggested a description of probiotics similar to the currently accepted definition, indicating that they are "live microbial feed supplements which beneficially affect the host animal by improving its intestinal microbial balance." Since then, this term has been widely used on labels and in publicity to communicate a health benefit to consumers. The probiotic concept was finally defined by scientific consensus in 2001 in an attempt to categorize these functional food ingredients under harmonized criteria because of their increased commercialization. The currently accepted definition of a probiotic was developed in 2001 by an expert consultation group working under the umbrella of the Food and Agriculture Organization of the United Nations (FAO) and the World Health Organization (WHO) on the health benefits of probiotics in foods. Probiotics were then defined as "live microorganisms that, when administered in adequate amounts, confer a health benefit on the host" (FAO/WHO, 2001). In 2002 a joint FAO/WHO working group also published the first guidelines for the evaluation of probiotics in foods. This definition implies that probiotics must be alive and exert a measurable physiological benefit on the host at a defined dose. The criteria established for their evaluation also included basic recommendations such as the need to identify microorganisms at the species and strain level by appropriate molecular methods and to evaluate their efficacy in well-designed human trials. In October 2013, 13 years after the definition of probiotics and 12 years after the guidelines were published, an expert panel of the International Scientific Association for Probiotics and Prebiotics (ISAPP) reviewed the probiotic concept and related principles (Hill et al., 2014). The new recommendations of this expert panel are summarized in Table 2.1. In light of the findings of several recent human microbiome-related projects, a wider range of commensal bacteria is being

Table 2.1 Summary of Recommendations Related to the Probiotic Concept Update

Recommendations	Comment on the Update
Probiotics are defined as "live microorganisms that, when administered in adequate amounts, confer a health benefit on the host."	The generic definition is retained as in the FAO/WHO document (2001); it is only recommended to avoid inconsistencies in its use.
Microbial species shown in properly controlled studies to confer benefits to health are included in the framework for definition of probiotics.	The need to demonstrate their efficacy in controlled studies is emphasized, but this was already mentioned in the FAO/WHO document of 2002.
Any specific claim beyond "contains probiotics" must be further substantiated.	This lacks approval as a nutritional claim in the current EU legislation. It does not add to the previous definition or evaluation criteria.
Keep live cultures, traditionally associated with fermented foods and for which there is no evidence of a health benefit, outside of the probiotic framework.	This item emphasizes the need to prove a health benefit for a microbial culture to be called a probiotic.
Keep undefined, fecal microbiota transplants outside of the probiotic framework.	Exclude nonpurified and fully defined and characterized bacteria from the probiotic concept. This is according to the FAO/WHO document (2002) indicating the need to identify the bacteria at the species and strain level.
New commensals and consortia comprising defined strains from human samples, with adequate evidence of safety and efficacy, are "probiotics."	Extend the definition to new commensal bacteria of human origin that could be proven to confer health benefits in the future.

EU, European Union; FAO, Food and Agricultural Organization; WHO, World Health Organization.
Adapted from Hill, C., Guarner, F., Reid, G., Gibson, G.R., Merenstein, D.J., Pot, B., Morelli, L., Canani, R.B., Flint, H.J., Salminen, S., Calder, P.C., Sanders, M.E., 2014. Expert consensus document. The International Scientific Association for Probiotics and Prebiotics consensus statement on the scope and appropriate use of the term probiotic. Nat. Rev. Gastroenterol. Hepatol. 11, 506–514.

potentially considered as probiotic candidates. Accordingly, the ISAPP concluded that, with adequate evidence of safety and efficacy, these new commensal bacterial strains from human samples should be included in the probiotic concept, although the original definition was retained by the FAO/WHO (2001). This definition of probiotics represented an advance in harmonizing requirements for this category of food ingredient, but in practice it is too vague to identify different probiotic products or to inform consumers about the benefits of probiotic consumption because of the diverse range of potential biological effects. Moreover, all of the criteria proposed in the FAO/WHO (2002) guidelines for selection and evaluation of probiotics do not fully reflect what really matters for substantiating the benefits of probiotics. Furthermore, the requirements may largely vary depending on the target effects (eg, survival in the gastrointestinal tract, adhesion, etc.). For instance, survival through the gastrointestinal tract is unimportant for the effect of yogurt starter cultures on lactose maldigestion exerted by bacteria producing the enzyme β-galactosidase. In this regard we can foresee that our progress in understanding the mechanisms of action and molecules responsible for the so-called probiotic properties will facilitate the demonstration and communication of specific health benefits associated with these microorganisms, going far beyond the generic probiotic definition.

FUNCTIONAL FOOD VERSUS FOODS BEARING NUTRITIONAL OR HEALTH CLAIMS

In the last 2 decades an increasing number of foods have borne nutrition and health messages on their labels or other types of communications to the consumer (advertisement, etc.) implying a relationship between their consumption and health. These foods were categorized under the generic descriptor of "functional foods," including "probiotics." The use of health claims is currently regulated in most parts of the world, and manufacturers are now requested to provide scientific evidence to support these claims, although there are subtle differences in the legal requirements across countries. Therefore one must consider that functional foods currently comprise foods with approved health claims because no legal definition for functional foods exists.

In the European Union (EU), Regulation (EC) No. 1924/2006 of the European Parliament and the Council on Nutrition and Health Claims Made on Foods came into force on July 1, 2007. Accordingly, this regulation states that health claims should only be used in the EU in commercial communications after authorization by the European Commission and the European Parliament. This authorization is based on a scientific assessment of the evidence substantiating the claim, which is performed by the Panel on Dietetic Products, Nutrition, and Allergies (NDA) of the European Food Safety Authority (EFSA). This regulation aims to protect consumer rights and facilitate their choices by providing the accurate and necessary information to make choices in full knowledge of the facts and to avoid misleading messages. It also ensures fair competition between economic operators by establishing common rules for the use of health claims and protecting innovation. Fig. 2.1 outlines the type of nutritional and health claims permitted in the EU. The nutritional claims, based on the nutrients the food contains, imply that the nutrient in question has been proven to play a beneficial role in human physiology and health. Within this context, in December 2012, the Nutrition and Health Claims Regulation banned the use of the term *contains probiotic* from packaging in the EU because it was considered to constitute an unapproved health claim rather than a nutrition claim. Indeed, this is not considered factual nutritional information because the average consumer will associate this term with health connotations because of publicity in recent decades. However, this legal issue is under debate because, according to Article 1(4), generic descriptors, which have traditionally been used to indicate a particularity of a class of foods or beverages that could imply an effect on human health, are exempt from the application of this regulation. This seems to be the case for the term *probiotic* in Italy.

Regarding health claims, basically two types can be made (Fig. 2.1): (1) claims related to the role of a food on maintenance/improvement of normal physiological functions (Article 13.1 and Article 13.5) and (2) claims related to the role of a food in reducing a risk factor for disease (Article 14). In the regulatory text these two types of claims are divided into three different categories:

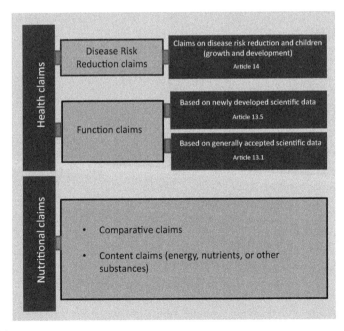

FIGURE 2.1

Types of nutritional and health claims according to the European Union Regulation (EC) No. 1924/2006.

1. Article 13.1 health claims, which relate to the role of a nutrient or food constituent (a) in growth, development, and bodily functions; (b) in psychological and/or behavioral functions; and (c) in slimming or weight control–related functions (eg, reducing hunger or increasing satiety). These claims must be based on generally accepted scientific principles.
2. Article 13.5 health claims, which also consider function claims based on newly established science.
3. Article 14 health claims, which include (a) reduction of disease risk claims and (b) claims related to children's development and health.

One of the major challenges of this regulatory framework is that claims should be intended for the general healthy population (or subgroups thereof) whereas many probiotic studies have been done on diseased populations. Indeed, to differentiate between foods and drugs, medicinal claims are not permitted (those referring to the ability of a substance to cure, treat, prevent, or diagnose a disease). Another important challenge is the paucity of generally accepted biomarkers associated with the risk of developing a disease, the modification of which should be assessed in disease risk–reduction claims. A few examples can be quoted, such as low-density lipoprotein cholesterol, blood pressure and cardiovascular disease, or pathogenic microorganisms and infections. The understanding of the mode of action could also help to demonstrate the biological plausibility of the effect and, therefore, to substantiate a claim. However, probiotics are in most cases expected to exert effects via multiple mechanisms, making it difficult to establish their mode of action.

Similarly, in the United States three categories of claims are defined by statute and/or the US Food and Drug Administration (FDA) regulation on food and dietary supplement labels: nutrient content claims, health claims (authorized or qualified), and structure/function claims (http://www.registrarcorp.com/fda-food/labeling). Health claims (authorized or qualified) describe a relationship between a food substance (a food, food component, dietary supplement, or ingredient) and reduced risk of a disease or health-related condition. The structure-function claims may describe (1) the role of a nutrient or dietary ingredient in the normal structure or function of the human body (eg, "calcium builds strong bones") or on maintaining such structure or function (eg, "fiber maintains bowel regularity"), (2) general well-being resulting from consumption of a nutrient or dietary ingredient, or (3) a benefit related to a nutrient deficiency disease (such as vitamin C and scurvy). In contrast to the EU regulations, qualified health claims are permitted in the United States when there is emerging evidence for a relationship between a food substance and reduced risk of a disease or health-related condition, but the evidence is not well enough established to meet the scientific standard required by the FDA to issue an authorizing regulation. Qualifying language is included in the claim to indicate that the evidence supporting the claim is limited to the consumers. In Canada five different claims categories can be distinguished: nutrient function claims, general health claims, disease risk-reduction claims, function claims, and therapeutic claims (http://www.hc-sc.gc.ca). In Japan Food for

Specified Health Uses (FOSHU) refers to foods bearing the following claims: (1) qualified FOSHU for food with a health function that is not substantiated by scientific evidence meeting FOSHU requirements, or food with certain effectiveness but without an established mechanism of the effective element responsible for its functionality; (2) standardized FOSHU for foods fulfilling the standards, specifications, and scientific evidence for FOSHU approval; and (3) reduction of disease risk FOSHU in the case of food for which reduction of disease risk is clinically and nutritionally established (http://www.mhlw.go.jp/english/).

CRITERIA FOR DEVELOPING PROBIOTICS AND CLAIMING THEIR BENEFITS ON FOODS IN EUROPE

Current regulations stipulate how the benefits of foods and food ingredients, including probiotics, should be substantiated. This regulatory system has also changed how benefits should be communicated to consumers. Therefore the evaluation criteria applied by authoritative bodies should necessarily be considered when developing probiotics or other types of food intended to bear a health claim on their labels. In the EU this evaluation is performed by the EFSA NDA Panel. In the evaluation process the NDA Panel considers whether or not (1) the food (constituent) is sufficiently characterized; (2) the claim effect is defined, measurable, and beneficial to human health; and (3) a cause-effect relationship has been established between the intake of the food (constituent) and the claimed effect in the target population group and under the proposed conditions of use.

CHARACTERIZATION OF THE FOOD (CONSTITUENT)

The requirements to consider that a food (constituent) or a food category is sufficiently characterized can differ depending on the type of food addressed and the claim. It should be sufficient to confirm the identity of the substance/object of the claim and to establish that the studies provided for substantiation of the health claim were performed with the food/constituent in question. For claims on microorganisms, data related to genus, species, and strain (genotyping) identification and characterization are required according to scientific consensus cited in the document of the FAO/WHO (2002). This is required because effects can be strain specific; therefore the effect of one strain cannot be extrapolated to another. An exception to this general principle can be found in the approved claim related to the role of yogurt starter cultures to improve lactose digestion. In this case the characterization of yogurt starter cultures down to the species level is considered sufficient in relation to the claimed effect because all strains within the species produce β-galactosidase (ie, the mechanism by which they improve lactose digestion). It is also strongly recommended that strains be deposited in an internationally recognized culture collection (with access number) for control purposes according to the FAO/WHO guidelines (2002).

DEFINITION OF THE HEALTH CLAIM AND RELEVANCE TO HUMAN HEALTH

For a health claim to be approved, the effect should be specific and measurable to make evaluation possible. In this context there are many examples of health claims presented in applications that have been considered as nondefined, including "gut health," "digestive health," "intestinal microbiota," or "immune system." For example, gut health is a broad concept that could include many different aspects of bowel function (eg, digestion, absorption, immune function). In contrast, maintenance of normal defecation is a specific health claim related to a well-defined aspect of bowel function that can be measured by generally accepted methods and therefore can be assessed.

To be acceptable the claim effect should also be considered as a beneficial physiological or health effect. For example, claims related to "maintaining a healthy/beneficial intestinal microbiota" or to "increasing the numbers of lactobacilli or bifidobacteria" have not been considered beneficial per se (EFSA, 2011a). In this regard the mere passage and survival of the microorganism administered (eg, lactobacilli) through the gastrointestinal tract and its detection in stools does not necessarily imply that it exerts any beneficial influence on host physiology. Moreover, current scientific knowledge is still insufficient to define the bacterial groups, and their relative abundances, that constitute a healthy microbiota. Many studies have tried to identify the specific bacteria that contribute to a normal microbiota by comparing its composition in healthy and diseased populations (eg, Miquel et al., 2013; Sanz et al., 2011, 2015). This has established associations between alterations in specific bacterial groups and certain conditions, but these alterations do not necessarily reflect causality of the underlying disease and the bacteria related to the disease may merely be bystanders. By contrast, claims such as "contribution to the (immune) defense against pathogens in the gastrointestinal tract" or "reduction (or beneficial alteration) of a risk factor for infections" have been considered beneficial. In 2011a the EFSA published guidelines on scientific requirements for health claims related to gut and immune function to facilitate study design for submissions. The aforementioned guide addressing the beneficial effects and outcome measures acceptable for substantiation of claims in these areas was updated in 2016 and recently published. Table 2.2 summarizes the health relationships considered defined and beneficial for claims related to the gastrointestinal tract, the immune system, and defense against pathogenic microorganisms (EFSA, 2016). Nevertheless, wording used in labeling may change because it does not depend completely on the scientific assessment and takes into consideration other issues, such as consumer understanding by risk managers. Other guidance documents have also been published in other scientific fields, some of which could also be of interest for probiotic claims. These include (1) bone, joints, and oral health; (2) appetite ratings, weight management, and blood glucose concentrations; (3) neurological and psychological functions; (4) antioxidants, oxidative damage, and cardiovascular health; and (5) physical performance (www.efsa.europa.eu/en/publications/efsajournal.htm). These guidance documents will also be

Table 2.2 Health Relationships Acceptable for Claims Related to the Gastrointestinal Tract, Immune System, and Defense Against Pathogenic Microorganisms

Type of Claim	Health Relationships
Function claims	Reduction of gastrointestinal discomfort in adults or infants
	Reduction of excessive intestinal gas accumulation
	Maintenance of normal defecation
	Improved digestion and/or absorption of nutrients
	Improved (immune) defense against pathogens in the gastrointestinal, respiratory, or urinary tract
	Beneficial change in response to allergens
Disease risk reduction claims	Claims on the reduction (or beneficial alteration) of a risk factor for infections (eg, the pathogen is an example of a risk factor)

Adapted from EFSA, 2011b. Scientific opinion in the maintenance of the list of QPS biological agents intentionally added to food and feed (2011 update). EFSA J. 9, 2497; EFSA, 2016. Guidance on the scientific requirements for health claims related to the immune system, the gastrointestinal tract and defence against pathogenic microorganisms. EFSA J. 14 (1), 4369.

updated regularly to help better define the beneficial effects and outcome measures to facilitate the chance of successful application in these areas.

SUBSTANTIATION OF THE HEALTH CLAIM

To determine the extent to which a cause-and-effect relationship is established between consumption of the food/constituent and claimed effect, the EFSA NDA Panel takes into consideration all of the evidence from pertinent studies. The overall strength, consistency, and biological plausibility of this evidence is assessed, as well as the quality of individual studies and their applicability to the target group and the conditions of use proposed.

Health claim substantiation is mainly based on human intervention studies conducted in the target population using the food and ingredient at the intended dose. This is especially important for claims based on new scientific knowledge (Article 13.5) intended for children's health or claims associated with reducing a risk factor for disease (Article 14). Double-blinded, randomized, placebo-controlled intervention studies are of primary importance to substantiate cause-and-effect relationships for other essential nutrients. In addition, other studies are considered in the evaluation process (eg, randomized noncontrolled studies, controlled nonrandomized studies, observational studies, etc.), but evidence derived from them is considered of second-order importance. In the EU regulatory framework, the population group for which the health claims on foods are intended is, in principle, the general (healthy) population or specific subgroups thereof (eg, elderly people, physically active subjects, or pregnant women). The NDA Panel considers, on a case-by-case basis, the extent to which it is established that extrapolation from other study groups to the target group is biologically justified (EFSA, 2011a, 2016). For example, data from irritable bowel syndrome patients have been accepted in the context of claims related to reduction of intestinal discomfort. However, data on patients with joint-osteoarthritis complaints were not considered acceptable to substantiate a claim on maintaining normal joints. The admissibility of applications for claims that specify target groups other than the general (healthy) population (disease) and/or under medication (eg, under antibiotic treatment) should first be checked by the EC and Member States (EFSA, 2016). Animal or in vitro studies may provide supportive evidence and mechanistic data, but they are not enough to substantiate a claim per se.

In the EU this scientific evaluation process constitutes the pillar for the authorization of claims on foods by risk managers of the EC and Member States. Thus a list of permitted claims and their specific conditions of use has been created and is available at the EU Register (http://ec.europa.eu/nuhclaims), which constitutes valuable examples for future applications.

SITUATION OF CLAIMS ON PROBIOTIC PRODUCTS IN DIFFERENT COUNTRIES

Many scientific articles on probiotics have been published (up to 13,420 in PubMed in November 2014), including a substantial number on human clinical trials (up to 1490). These studies have reported effects on several health-related outcomes, including incidence or duration of gastrointestinal infections, improving vitamin synthesis, normalizing intestinal transit, alleviating lactose intolerance, or reducing incidence of allergy. Nevertheless, in the EU only one health claim related to live yogurt cultures and their ability to improve lactose digestion has been approved under the current regulation of health claims made on foods. The high scientific standards applied during the evaluation of health claim applications, together with the legal constraints imposed by the European regulatory framework, have led the industry to seek alternative ways of advertising the proposed benefits of their products. Indeed, some food supplements are in the process of being registered as "medical devices," for which claims can be made without providing hard scientific evidence. The food industry is also using marketing strategies and combinations of probiotics with essential nutrients (eg, vitamins) to continue making claims (eg, those related to the immune system). Nevertheless, new scientific knowledge should be generated, taking into consideration the regulatory requirements to legally support the messages related to the benefits of probiotic microorganisms, to maintain consumer confidence in the long term.

In the United States the FDA has three ways to determine which health claims may be used on labels for conventional food or dietary supplements (The Nutrition Labeling and Education Act Authorized Health Claims; Health Claims Based on Authoritative Statements; Qualified Health Claims, FDA, 2015), but it has not approved any health claims related to reduced risk of disease or health-related conditions for probiotics to date. However, structure-function claims have been made for probiotics because these do not require FDA approval. In this case the manufacturer must have data proving that the claim is true and not misleading, and it must submit a notification with the text of the claim to the FDA and, for dietary supplements, the label including such a claim must also state that the FDA has not evaluated the said claim.

In Canada probiotic health claims can be made on foods and natural health products (NHPs) and they can be structure/function claims, risk-reduction claims, or treatment claims. Unlike the EU and FDA, in April 2009 Health Canada, which is the federal department dealing with Canadian health issues, accepted claims on what was called the Nature of Probiotic Microorganisms in Food (http://www.hc-sc.gc.ca). In this context the eligible claims on foods include "Probiotic that naturally forms part of the gut flora," "Provides live microorganisms that naturally form part of the gut flora contribute to healthy gut flora," or "Probiotic that contributes to healthy gut flora." The Canadian legislation has also developed a procedure to evaluate applications for specific claims on probiotics, the approval of which requires strain-specific human efficacy evidence and identification of the strains at the genus, species, and strain level in the labeling. An example of an NHP specific claim is that the strain *Lactobacillus johnsonii* La1 or *L. johnsonii* Lj1 can be used as "an adjunct to physician-supervised antibiotic therapy in patients with *Helicobacter pylori* infections" or that the strains *Lactobacillus rhamnosus* GG or *Saccharomyces boulardii* "help to reduce the risk of antibiotic-associated diarrhea."

In Japan specific probiotic claims can be made pursuant to FOSHU (Foods for Specified Health Uses, 2015, http://www.mhlw.go.jp/english/topics/foodsafety/fhc/02.html) regulations. These claims should be approved by its Consumer Affairs Agency, but the scientific standards differ from other regulatory frameworks. This country was pioneering in approving claims; by 1999 21 probiotic products had already received FOSHU approval in Japan. Current examples of eligible probiotic claims include that the yogurt (Meiji) containing *Lactobacillus delbrueckii* subsp. *bulgaricus* 2038 and *Streptococcus salivarius* subsp. *thermophilus* 113 helps regulate the balance of intestinal microflora to maintain a good gastrointestinal condition and the yogurt/lactic acid drink (Morinaga) containing *Bifidobacterium longum* BB536 and live bifidobacteria helps increase these bacteria in the intestines and maintains a healthy gastrointestinal environment.

Overall, differences in the criteria applied for approval and final use of health claims have generated marked differences in the probiotic industry across countries. There is a contradiction between the argument of the stakeholders that consumers should have the right to have information on all potential claims to facilitate their choices, even of those supported by weak scientific evidence, and the principles of the European legislation protecting consumer rights by approving only scientifically sound claims and avoiding misleading messages. Delineation of a limit between foods and drugs is also a particularly controversial issue that implies constraints on the scientific evidence required to substantiate a claim, the proposed wording, and the product category for which it can be used, particularly in the EU and United States. Overregulation regarding the evidence that should be provided to demonstrate the efficacy of probiotics in the health area is considered an important drawback for future scientific developments in this field. Despite this, there is general agreement on the need to develop a stronger scientific rationale behind probiotic selection and application and to improve the quality of human intervention studies to facilitate the approval of probiotic claims and regain consumer confidence, partly lost because of the limited numbers of claims approved in the EU and the absence of approved claims in the United States.

FUTURE PERSPECTIVES IN THE DEVELOPMENT OF PROBIOTICS

Our understanding of the complexity of the gut microbiota and its role in health and disease is growing rapidly because of high-throughput DNA sequencing and other omics technologies. Such studies aim to characterize microbial communities in different parts of the body, their variation within and across individuals, and their relationship with host factors (genetics, aging, diseases, etc.) or environmental challenges (diet, antibiotics, etc.). These studies are being conducted in progressively better controlled epidemiological and intervention studies within the context of different microbiome-related projects, which are providing more robust associations between the microbiota and health and disease (Hoffmann et al., 2013; Neef and Sanz, 2013). This vast amount of data is also helping to set a rationale for the selection of functionally distinct commensal bacteria, which could give rise to the next generation of probiotics and help design more efficient strategies to manipulate the microbiota to optimize its physiological functions. For example, many observational human studies report reductions in *Faecalibacterium prausnitzii* in the microbiota of patients with chronic inflammatory bowel diseases compared with controls. This species is also known to be a butyrate producer that could mediate anti-inflammatory effects (Miquel et al., 2013). In addition, strains of this species have been shown to be effective in treating inflammatory conditions in preclinical trials (Miquel et al., 2013); thus these may be potential new probiotic candidates. Likewise, associations between Bacteroidetes or *Bacteroides* spp. and a lean phenotype or weight loss and the clinical efficacy of species such as *Bacteroides uniformis* in preclinical trials in mouse obesity models would suggest its possible use as a new probiotic to prevent or treat obesity and its comorbidities in the future (Neef and Sanz, 2013).

The individual variability of the microbiota and its relationship with specific disease-prone genotypes will also lead to the future development of more personalized interventions with probiotics targeting specific population groups. For example, recent evidence suggests that the HLA-DQ2 genotype conferring a high risk of developing celiac disease is related to reduced numbers of *Bifidobacterium* spp. and *B. longum* and increased numbers of *Staphylococcus* spp. in the microbiota of infants, regardless of the type of milk-feeding (Olivares et al., 2014). Future confirmation that such shifts in the microbiota are causally related to disease onset could pave the way for intervening in the gut ecosystem with specific probiotics to restore the aberrant genotype-biased microbiota. This type of evidence on host-genotype microbe interactions could also help to explain an individual's microbiota-based resilience to change and differentiate between responders and nonresponders to specific probiotic interventions.

The discovery of new potential probiotic bacteria within our commensal microbiota is also raising new scientific, regulatory, and commercial questions. One example relates to whether these potential probiotics will be considered as foods or drugs because this will dictate the appropriate endpoints and study populations (disease or at-risk health populations) for the studies to be submitted for approval. The fact that these new potential probiotics have no history of use could also demand specific requirements for product characterization and safety assessments on a strain-by-strain basis. The risk could differ depending on the particular strain and its intended use. Within the EU regulatory framework, strains that were not consumed systematically as food before May 1997 are considered "Novel Foods," and their authorization is pursuant to the Novel Foods Regulation (EC 258/97). Currently, one strain (*Clostridium butyricum* CBM 588) has already been authorized under the Novel Foods Regulation in the EU. This strain was already approved as a microbial feed additive for chickens and piglets in the EU. However, the EFSA's BIOHAZ Panel in its 2011b update to the Qualified Presumption as Safe (QPS) list considered that the safety of *C. butyricum* is a strain-related property, that this species should not be recommended for the QPS list because a minority of strains contain a gene coding for botulinum neurotoxin type E, and there is limited knowledge of human and animal exposure to this species. It was also concluded that because QPS did not apply, this microorganism should undergo full novel food assessment. The safety assessment was based on verification of the absence of toxins and other virulence factors and confirmation that antibiotic resistance determinants detected in the strain were nonfunctional, as assessed by combining whole-genome sequencing and functional tests as well as toxicity studies (acute, semichronic, and chronic). This also constitutes an example of the procedure to gain authorization for new strains under the EU Novel Food Regulation, paving the way for the future commercialization of the so-called next generation of probiotics.

CONCLUSIONS

The approval and use of health claims for probiotics is regulated in most parts of the world, but the categorization and definition of products that can carry such claims (foods, dietary supplements, natural health products, etc.) and the different criteria applied for their authorization have created country-specific scenarios regarding their commercialization and communication of potential benefits. Advances in the identification of novel commensal bacteria and their influence on human health will soon create new opportunities for marketing those strains as foods, food supplements, or as products for specific nutritional or medicinal purposes. These developments are also raising new regulatory issues on these novel probiotics regarding their consideration as foods or drugs and safety requirements. A stronger consensus on the scientific criteria to evaluate the efficacy and safety of new probiotics for their intended use is necessary to facilitate legislators' and business operators' roles within a global market. The creation of foundational principles, applicable to health claims worldwide, would also boost investments in this research field and ultimately contribute to scientific advances that would benefit end consumers and society.

ACKNOWLEDGMENT

This work was supported by Grant No. 613979 (MyNewGut) under the Seventh Framework Program of the European Union.

REFERENCES

Bertazzoni, E., Donelli, G., Midtvedt, T., Nicoli, J., Sanz, Y., 2013. Probiotics and clinical effects: is the number what counts? J. Chemother. 25, 193–212.

Bibel, D., 1988. Elie Metchnikoff's bacillus of long life. ASM News 54, 661–665.

EFSA, 2011a. Guidance on the specific requirements for health claims related to gut and immune function. EFSA J. 9, 1984.

EFSA, 2011b. Scientific opinion in the maintenance of the list of QPS biological agents intentionally added to food and feed (2011 update). EFSA J. 9, 2497.

EFSA, 2016. Guidance on the scientific requirements for health claims related to the immune system, the gastrointestinal tract and defence against pathogenic microorganisms. EFSA J. 14 (1), 4369.

FAO/WHO, 2001. Report of a Joint FAO/WHO Expert Consultation on Evaluation of Health and Nutritional Properties of Probiotics in Food Including Powder Milk With Live Lactic Acid Bacteria. Food and Agriculture Organization of the United Nations & World Health Organization, Cordoba, Argentina.

FAO/WHO, 2002. Joint FAO/WHO Working Group – Guidelines for Evaluation of Probiotics in Food. Food and Agriculture Organization of the United Nations & World Health Organization, Ontario, Canada.

Hill, C., Guarner, F., Reid, G., Gibson, G.R., Merenstein, D.J., Pot, B., Morelli, L., Canani, R.B., Flint, H.J., Salminen, S., Calder, P.C., Sanders, M.E., 2014. Expert consensus document. The International Scientific Association for Probiotics and Prebiotics consensus statement on the scope and appropriate use of the term probiotic. Nat. Rev. Gastroenterol. Hepatol. 11, 506–514.

Hoffmann, D.E., Fraser, C.M., Palumbo, F.B., Ravel, J., Rothenberg, K., Rowthorn, V., Schwartz, J., 2013. Science and regulation. Probiotics: finding the right regulatory balance. Science 342, 314–315.

Miquel, S., Martin, R., Rossi, O., Bermudez-Humaran, L.G., Chatel, J.M., Sokol, H., Thomas, M., Wells, J.M., Langella, P., 2013. *Faecalibacterium prausnitzii* and human intestinal health. Curr. Opin. Microbiol. 16, 255–261.

Neef, A., Sanz, Y., 2013. Future for probiotic science in functional food and dietary supplement development. Curr. Opin. Clin. Nutr. Metab. Care 16, 679–687.

Olivares, M., Neef, A., Castillejo, G., Palma, G.D., Varea, V., Capilla, A., Palau, F., Nova, E., Marcos, A., Polanco, I., Ribes-Koninckx, C., Ortigosa, L., Izquierdo, L., Sanz, Y., 2014. The HLA-DQ2 genotype selects for early intestinal microbiota composition in infants at high risk of developing coeliac disease. Gut 64, 406–417.

Sanz, Y., De Pama, G., Laparra, M., 2011. Unraveling the ties between celiac disease and intestinal microbiota. Int. Rev. Immunol. 30, 207–218.

Sanz, Y., Olivares, M., Moya-Perez, A., Agostoni, C., 2015. Understanding the role of gut microbiome in metabolic disease risk. Pediatr. Res. 77, 236–244.

Perspectives on Microbiome Manipulation in People of Developing Countries

G. Reid

Lawson Health Research Institute, Canadian Center for Human Microbiome and Probiotic Research, London, ON, Canada; Western University, Department of Microbiology and Immunology, Division of Urology, Department of Surgery, London, ON, Canada

MICROBIOME NUANCES

An interest in the general bacterial population of the gut has been in the minority compared with studies pertaining to enteric pathogens. Nevertheless, as Dubos et al. (1967) profoundly stated, "the symbiotic species are of at least equal importance because…they are essential to the well-being of their host." It is difficult to comprehend that it has taken almost 50 years to fully appreciate this posit.

Some researchers have been fascinated by the differences in overall microbiota composition between people in developed and developing countries. On the basis of culture techniques, Williams (1973) noted higher bacterial ileal counts in Indian villagers and ten-fold higher *Bacteroides* in the feces of Ugandan subjects compared with British and American subjects. Although this predates the obesity epidemic that has presumably altered the microbiota of people living in the latter two nations, it illustrates that differences have existed for some time. However, largely because funding agencies have focused on diseases rather than health, the study of gut microbiota of people in the developing world has mostly been done to try and identify patterns that may be prerequisites for, or associated with, disease or aberrant conditions such as malnutrition. This is equally true for the vagina.

Investigations were performed to see if the composition of the vaginal microbiota differed in women infected with HIV only to discover the same organisms as in uninfected subjects (Hummelen et al., 2010, 2011). Even in Nairobi sex workers at risk of HIV but who remain recalcitrant to the virus, only elevated *Escherichia coli* levels in the vagina of some HIV-positive women were different from those free of the virus (Schellenberg et al., 2012). Again, the bacterial patterns did not differ between women in Africa and those in developed countries. Rather, higher diversity has been associated with concomitant bacterial vaginosis and HIV (Spear et al., 2008). However, differences may be much more subtle than can be found by simply identifying bacterial species by DNA, as

The Gut-Brain Axis. http://dx.doi.org/10.1016/B978-0-12-802304-4.00003-7

microbiota profiling does. For example, lactobacilli are able to inactivate viruses through their production of acid (Cadieux et al., 2002) and potentially also reduce viral infection by competitive binding through lectin molecules and promoting epithelial integrity (Petrova et al., 2013). Thus the type of lactobacilli present in the host could influence risk of infectivity, irrespective of where the woman lives.

In terms of the gut, researchers, and not only anthropologists, have been fascinated by human ancestry and their diet and ability to fight disease. This is understandable because in only very recent times have humans changed how they live and acquire their food. Very few, if any, humans inhabit the Earth without having had some sort of contact with modern humans and the by-products of their societies. Two groups with minimal exposure to urban dwellers and medications including vaccines have been studied: the Hadza wandering foragers of the East African Rift Valley ecosystem and Peruvian Amerindians. A study of the former reported extremely high taxonomic diversity and concluded that this indicates great ecosystem stability and flexibility (Schnorr, 2015). However, it may reflect more of an extremely seasonal and varied diet than stability per se. Although the theory that a hunter-gatherer's existence is more "natural" descending from human evolution, and that their microbiota have mutualistic functions that stabilize the body against foreign microorganisms, this is not easy to prove. Indeed, it is almost defeatist because it implies that modern society has produced more flaws than benefits in human–microbe interactions. Certainly, overuse of antibiotics has been responsible for many ecological aberrations (Levy and Marshall, 2004; Marshall and Levy, 2011; Cox and Blaser, 2015; Goneau et al., 2015), but these therapies and vaccines have saved millions of lives. Globalization and urbanization, and indeed any centralization process, can lessen diversity among the gene pool. However, the ability to provide fruit and vegetables all year round, to populations experiencing frigid winters for example, provides many attributes for health and surely cannot be blamed for lowering microbial diversity and consequently increasing the risk of obesity and allergy (Blaser, 2011). An Australian study of Aboriginals actually supports the concept that a developing world diet that alters the glycemic load, fatty acids, and macro- and micronutrient composition does modify the immune system and lead to allergic and other diseases (Walton and Williams, 2012). However, the indigenous Australians, similar to other hunter-gatherers, eat a lot of red meat, and for many years this has been blamed for cardiovascular disease and cancer (Micha et al., 2012; Kim et al., 2013).

So is it the exercise and high metabolism of the hunter-gatherers that is more important? Exercise does appear to help control the glycemic index in subjects with high fructose intake (Bidwell etal., 2014). Certainly, a stagnant lifestyle is detrimental to health, but tribes that have switched to Western diets appear to suffer from metabolic and allergic diseases, suggesting that diet has more effect than exercise on the microbiota (Danaei etal., 2013). In terms of the microbiota, which plays a huge role in the digestion of foods, it appears less modified by exercise than by diet, albeit it has been suggested that the microbiota can act similar to an endocrine organ, being sensitive to the homeostatic and physiological changes associated with exercise (Bermon etal., 2015). Interestingly, it is not the physical activity per se that equates with Hadza foragers being slimmer than Westerners, as reported by Pontzer et al. (2012), who showed that the average daily energy expenditure of traditional Hadza foragers was no different than that of Westerners after controlling for body size. This challenges the suggestion that obesity is due to a decreased energy expenditure component of the Western lifestyle.

The oral microbiome has been studied intensively, and a recent paper sheds light on the impact of dietary shifts due to the adoption of carbohydrate-rich Neolithic farming (beginning ~10,000 years ago) and the Industrial Revolution that introduced humans to processed flour and sugar (in ~1850; Alder et al., 2013). The authors showed that not only has bacterial diversity reduced with time, but the transition from hunter-gatherer to farming shifted the oral microbial community to a disease-associated profile, and cariogenic bacteria became dominant after the Industrial Revolution. It is not surprising that high sugar intake has altered the oral microbiota and fostered a massive dental hygiene industry. It is perhaps more surprising that humans have allowed this to happen!

The picture is further complicated by the story of *Helicobacter pylori*. Brought into the limelight by its discovery in the stomach and association with cancer (Marshall and Warren, 1984), it has recently been claimed that it may be a commensal that has evolved with humans; therefore its eradication will lead to other diseases, including allergy and asthma (Blaser, 2012). A problem with this theory is highlighted by a study of Baka Pygmies in Cameroon, a lineage of the oldest and most divergent San hunter-gatherers, who are one of the deepest branches of the human population tree. Following the logic that hunter-gatherers host a more beneficial and diverse microbiota, including "ancient" microbes now lost or depleted in urbanized humans (Blaser, 2012; von Hertzen et al., 2015), *H. pylori* would have evolved in these people and acted as commensals. However, a study showed that the Baka acquired their *H. pylori* via secondary contact with agriculturalist neighbors (Nell et al., 2013). Therefore is *H. pylori* an ancient microbe and one that humans should want to retain?

The search for humans who have not had contact with Westerners continues with the hope of uncovering microbiota nuances. A recent study of Amerindians from Venezuela purported to represent such a cohort (Clemente et al., 2015), but the fact that Westerners took samples from them and the tribe had outside health workers indicates the findings warrant caution. The Yanomami people were found to harbor a microbiome with the highest diversity of bacteria and genetic functions of any human group to date. The authors concluded that this provided proof that Westernization significantly affects human microbiome diversity. On the contrary, it shows that high diversity in the microbiome occurs in a small cohort of people who have inbred and have not associated with others in Venezuela or developed countries. In addition, the Yanomami use hallucinogenic drugs and various natural substances that could easily simulate exposure to antimicrobial and other pharmaceutical agents, and they consume the bones of deceased kinsmen, making them substantially different from Westerners or indeed most other humans.

Other microbial nuances have been reported in developing countries, such as in the stool samples obtained from children in a rural village in Burkina Faso. The significant enrichment in Bacteroidetes and depletion in Firmicutes along with a unique abundance of *Prevotella* and *Xylanibacter* was related to a high plant fiber diet

(De Filippo et al., 2010). The authors called for preservation of "this treasure of microbial diversity," but with an average lifespan of 55 years, even with obesity rates lower than 3%, more evidence is needed to verify that such diversity, and certain bacterial species within it, are absent in Westerners, and that this is actually beneficial to health and longevity. Isolation, propagation, and investigation of these rare species would be interesting, but even if they are shown to have significant attributes, developing them as probiotics would be challenging because they would have no safe history of use in foods and would likely be fastidious and difficult to scale up commercially. Under the Human Food Project, one researcher, Jeff Leach, who has been living with the Hadza in Tanzania, self-performed a fecal transplant from a hunter-gatherer; thus time will tell what imprint, if any, it has on his health.

FERMENTED FOODS AND PROBIOTICS FOR HEALTH

The origins of purposely administering live microbes to improve the health of humans is a relatively recent concept after the discovery of the microscope and culture techniques. The launch of the fermented Yakult drink in Japan in 1935 was likely the first such application. Of course, the purposeful fermentation in food and fluids has ancient roots (Selhub et al., 2014), but it was not with the knowledge of microbes being the catalysts, and it was mostly a means to improve food taste, texture, and to some extent fight off disease. The observation that yogurt might increase human longevity was notably made by a Russian scientist (Elie Metchnikoff) in a developing country setting (Bulgaria). This connectivity between science and society is an ideal illustration of the need for collective input into understanding how microbes influence life.

It is clear that fermented foods are an integral part of human evolution and health, and we dismiss them at our peril. However, they are ironically not a category on any food guide that recommends daily consumption of nutritious products. This seems ludicrous at worst and short-sighted at best. A case for inclusion of fermented foods has been made based upon the weight of evidence in conferring health benefits (Chilton et al., 2015). It is interesting that the list provided by Chilton and co-authors, of fermented foods and countries in which they are particularly popular with a long history of use, mostly comprises developing nations. This includes African countries where numerous fermented foods are part of the culinary history (Franz et al., 2014), but their use is no longer widespread or necessarily passed down to younger generations (Reid et al., 2014).

Fermented foods, including those containing probiotic organisms, confer a wide range of benefits as reviewed extensively by others (Ceapa et al., 2013; de Oliveira et al., 2013; Franz et al., 2014; Park et al., 2014; Vina et al., 2014; Chilton et al., 2015). They do this through the metabolic by-products of their fermentation before consumption and the compounds produced (eg, short-chain fatty acids, flavonoids, lactoferrin, and vitamins) as a result of their ingestion and metabolism in the intestine. This helps to reduce oxidative stress and inflammation, and recent studies suggest it may also have benefits to brain health (Selhub et al., 2014). The concept is that the amplification of certain nutrients and phytochemicals can influence the brain through the vagus nerve and indirect pathways. This is an exciting new element of microbiome research that will inevitably lead to fecal transplantation and probiotics being tested to try and influence various stages of illnesses such as Alzheimer's disease, autism spectrum disorders, Parkinson's disease, multiple sclerosis, anxiety, depression, and headache. Animal models show promise in some of these areas, and the ability of bacteria to produce neurochemicals and affect inflammation provides a rationale for further microbial endocrinology studies (Reid, 2011; Bhattacharjee and Lukiw, 2013; Lyte, 2014; Rosenfeld, 2015).

In the developing world, the ability to improve cognitive function, including learning and memory in children, would be a worthwhile target for microbiota manipulation (Gareau, 2014). Disease and malnutrition, as well as poor access to medical care and schooling, have caused severe deficits in the numbers of children educated sufficiently well to contribute to and advance developing countries. A study, albeit in rats, has shown that a probiotic comprising *Lactobacillus acidophilus* ATCC 4356, *Bifidobacterium lactis* DSM 10140, and *Lactobacillus fermentum* ATCC 9338 dissolved in drinking water efficiently reversed deteriorated brain functions in the levels of cognitive performances (Davari et al., 2013). If this proves feasible in humans, then it could transform some communities, for example through reducing mortality in the elderly (Paddick et al., 2015), helping to overcome stressful life events (Pilleron et al., 2015), and lowering later abuse of alcohol (Luczak et al., 2015). A key component will be to make effective, affordable probiotics available to economically challenged populations. There is a range of cognitive impairment and dementia in sub-Saharan Africa (Mavrodaris et al., 2013), and although it is unrealistic to suggest that this could be reduced through fermented food consumption, evidence is emerging that this could represent one factor in restoring cognitive function (Bangirana et al., 2006) as well as providing a good educational environment (Crowe et al., 2013). The provision of fermented food to schools would provide a means to contribute to both of these factors.

In the Tucuman and San Juan provinces of Argentina, approximately 180,000 children from humble social status receive Yogurito probiotic-supplemented fermented milk three times per week (Yogurito, 2015). This is made possible by the scientific studies of the Reference Center for Lactobacilli and cooperatives that produce the food under a government subsidized program. It not only provides the yogurt, but some schools also monitor anthropometric measurements to check that development is age-appropriate. The implementation of the social probiotic program has resulted in increased systemic immunity and reductions in respiratory and gastrointestinal infections (Villena et al., 2012). This incredible initiative is a model for the world to follow and shows clearly that social business can be effective and transformative.

Efforts to bring affordable probiotic fermented milk to Africa began in 2004 with the launch of a community kitchen in Mwanza, Tanzania, where a group of women (yogurt mamas) were taught how to produce yogurt supplemented with *Lactobacillus rhamnosus* GR-1 (Fiti). This Western Heads East program has blossomed over the past 11 years because of the commitment of local women in Tanzania and Kenya and the diligence and support of the National Institute for Medical Research, the Kivulini Women's Group, the Kenya Medical Research Institute, and the Jomo Kenyatta University for Agriculture and

Technology, as well as others. Despite multiple challenges of educating people about probiotics, ensuring hygienic and reproducible practices, providing training on small businesses and finance management, seasonality, and issues with milk provision and costing
(Whaling et al., 2011), the yogurt is consumed by approximately 5000 men, women,
and children each day. A project emanating from this one, but using a generic version of
L. rhamnosus GG, called Yoba, has been launched in Uganda with huge success, now
providing probiotic fermented milk to over 35,000 people each day (Kort et al., 2015). It
is important to note that these initiatives empower local women, provide them with nutritious food for their families as well as some income, and engage males through farming
and delivering the milk to the kitchens and yogurt to the community (Reid et al., 2013).

Many studies, albeit small, have been undertaken on the impact on health of the
yogurt with and without micronutrient supplementation. These have shown some
improvements in CD4 counts and energy levels of subjects infected with HIV (Irvine
et al., 2010; Reid, 2010; Hummelen et al., 2011; Hemsworth et al., 2012). In the most
recent study, daily Fiti consumption supplemented with micronutrient-rich Moringa was
found to be safe for pregnancy (Fig. 3.1). It did not alter the gut microbiota of pregnant
women, as determined by stool collection and analysis using 16S rRNA gene sequencing. However, the consumption did increase the relative abundance of *Bifidobacterium*
and decrease *Enterobacteriaceae* in the feces of newborns (Bisanz et al., 2015). This lack
of a major modification of the gut microbiota after probiotic consumption is in agreement with another study (McNulty et al., 2011). Nevertheless, metabolic changes do

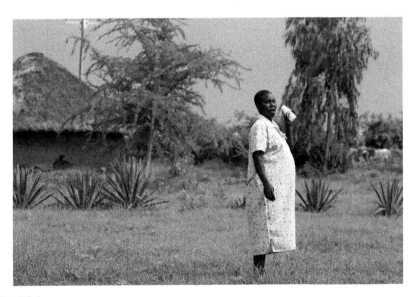

FIGURE 3.1

Photograph of pregnant Kenyan woman, Mary, drinking Fiti yogurt in Kadem, Migori
County, Kenya on May 12, 2015.

Photo taken by Kevin Gitau, assisted by Kathleen Walsh and copyright of Gregor Reid.

occur after intake of therapeutic food (Smith et al., 2013), indicating alterations in how the organisms function. This is important because many distant site effects of probiotics have been shown emanating from the gut, including to the brain, lungs, liver, vagina, bladder, skin, and heart (Reid et al., 2001; Beerepoot et al., 2012; Perez-Burgos et al., 2013; Al-Ghazzewi et al., 2014; Ettinger et al., 2014; King et al., 2014; Steenbergen et al., 2015). The finding that daily intake of Fiti yogurt in Mwanza, reduced heavy metal uptake in children and pregnant women illustrates that benefits can accrue without major gut microbiota changes (Bisanz et al., 2014). More insightful transcriptomic studies are needed to determine how the gut bacteria are altering their metabolism, as they clearly do in the vagina (Macklaim et al., 2013). In one human study, oral microbes that survived transit to the gut were found to express minimal transcriptional ability, although this does not rule out their effect on the host (Franzosa et al., 2014). The study, albeit of only eight subjects, also showed that many (41%) microbial transcripts were not differentially regulated relative to their genomic abundances, and overall there was subject-specific whole-community regulation. This approach is important to understand how bacteria react to food intake, hormonal fluctuations, circadian rhythm, and exposure to pharmaceutical agents and incoming microbes. Comparisons between subjects in the developing and developed world might then be more revealing.

CONCLUSIONS

Understanding the dynamics of the human microbiome is in its infancy. Still, although in vitro and animal studies will provide interesting insights, the focus should be on how the microbes affect human health and especially how their manipulation and/or their metabolic activity can restore it. Populations in the developing world are worthy of such studies, and should probiotic or prebiotic interventions be tested there, such products must be made available at affordable prices after completion of the studies for ethical and humanitarian reasons. Training personnel and providing research infrastructure will be critical for countries to develop their own expertise and control the way forward. This is occurring through many channels, but retention of highly qualified personnel in African countries remains a challenge.

The issues are not on a one-way street. Vaginal birthing and breastfeeding rates are significantly higher in the developing world, providing a lesson for Westerners whose economic independence and societal framework offers choices that are not always in the best interest of the health of the mother and infant. If the argument is that breastfeeding is avoided because of pollutants in the milk, then the greater societal problem is to reduce pollution or its damage to the newborn rather than to use formula or donor milk devoid of its microbes. There are many factors to consider when acquiring data from people in developing countries, especially if the studies are primarily coordinated by outsiders (Table 3.1). Full engagement and collaboration with local researchers is strongly encouraged where possible. As the research infrastructure grows and more highly qualified personnel take up leadership positions, we should expect to see many insightful microbiome projects reported in the years to come.

Table 3.1 Factors to Consider when Studying the Microbiome of populations in the Developing World

Diet	Dietary recalls are useful to provide information on what the subjects are eating. The potential for exposure to environmental pollutants should be considered.
Local medications	Efforts must be made to understand what substances are used to prevent and treat ailments. These could have similar properties to drugs used in developed countries, thereby countering the belief that the population has been "untouched" by modern medicine. This can certainly influence microbiota.
Interventions	These need to be suitable, practical, and affordable so that the study subjects can continue to gain access after completion.
Societal	One cannot assume to understand societal structure, practices, roles, habits, beliefs, and how people interact with "outsiders." All of these can influence participation, sampling, and the microbiome.
Behavior	Compliance must be carefully monitored. This can be challenging given location of homes. Behavior may differ significantly when people emigrate, urging caution when studying "Asian Americans" or "Caribbean Brits."
Analytical methods	In an ideal world, analysis of transcription by the organisms and host cells and metabolic readouts will be the most revealing. Sample collection and transportation issues cannot be underestimated in terms of logistics, power outages, and cost.
Outcomes	Although death and serious illness are valid outcomes, studies are needed on how to change practice—whether it is intake of contaminated water and food, seeking care for pregnancy, or changing food intake to a Western pattern. Identification of microbes to the species level is preferable by DNA sequencing, and efforts are needed to isolate more of these. Understanding and measuring cognitive outcomes related to the microbiome and probiotic/prebiotic interventions will be extremely useful. Safety of study personnel, subjects, and any products for testing is paramount.

ACKNOWLEDGMENTS

The author is funded by Grand Challenges Canada for his work in Africa.

REFERENCES

Adler, C.J., Dobney, K., Weyrich, L.S., Kaidonis, J., Walker, A.W., Haak, W., Bradshaw, C.J., Townsend, G., Sołtysiak, A., Alt, K.W., Parkhill, J., Cooper, A., 2013. Sequencing ancient calcified dental plaque shows changes in oral microbiota with dietary shifts of the Neolithic and Industrial revolutions. Nat. Genet. 45 (4), 450–455.

Al-Ghazzewi, F.H., Tester, R.F., 2014. Impact of prebiotics and probiotics on skin health. Benef. Microbes 5 (2), 99–107.

Bangirana, P., Idro, R., John, C.C., Boivin, M.J., 2006. Rehabilitation for cognitive impairments after cerebral malaria in African children: strategies and limitations. Trop. Med. Intl. Health 11 (9), 1341–1349.

Beerepoot, M.A., ter Riet, G., Nys, S., van der Wal, W.M., de Borgie, C.A., de Reijke, T.M., Prins, J.M., Koeijers, J., Verbon, A., Stobberingh, E., Geerlings, S.E., 2012. Lactobacilli vs antibiotics to prevent urinary tract infections: a randomized, double-blind, noninferiority trial in postmenopausal women. Arch. Intern. Med. 172 (9), 704–712.

Bermon, S., Petriz, B., Kajėnienė, A., Prestes, J., Castell, L., Franco, O.L., 2015. The microbiota: an exercise immunology perspective. Exerc. Immunol. Rev. 21, 70–79.

Bhattacharjee, S., Lukiw, W.J., 2013. Alzheimer's disease and the microbiome. Front. Cell. Neurosci. 7, 153.

Bidwell, A.J., Fairchild, T.J., Wang, L., Keslacy, S., Kanaley, J.A., 2014. Effect of increased physical activity on fructose-induced glycemic response in healthy individuals. Eur. J. Clin. Nutr. 68 (9), 1048–1054.

Bisanz, J.E., Enos, M.K., Mwanga, J.R., Changalucha, J., Burton, J.P., Gloor, G.B., Reid, G., 2014. Randomized open-label pilot study of the influence of probiotics and the gut microbiome on toxic metal levels in Tanzanian pregnant women and school children. mBio 5 (5), e01580–14.

Bisanz, J.E., Enos, M.K., PrayGod, G., Seney, S., Macklaim, J.M., Chilton, S., Willner, D., Knight, R., Fusch, C., Fusch, G., Gloor, G.B., Burton, J.P., Reid, G., 2015. Microbiota at multiple body sites during pregnancy in a rural Tanzanian population and effects of moringa-supplemented probiotic yogurt. Appl. Environ. Microbiol. 81 (15), 4965–4975.

Blaser, M., 2011. Antibiotic overuse: stop the killing of beneficial bacteria. Nature 476 (7361), 393–394.

Blaser, M.J., 2012. Equilibria of humans and our indigenous microbiota affecting asthma. Proc. Am. Thorac. Soc. 9 (2), 69–71.

Cadieux, P., Burton, J., Kang, C.Y., Gardiner, G., Braunstein, I., Bruce, A.W., Reid, G., 2002. *Lactobacillus* strains and vaginal ecology. JAMA 287, 1940–1941.

Ceapa, C., Wopereis, H., Rezaïki, L., Kleerebezem, M., Knol, J., Oozeer, R., 2013. Influence of fermented milk products, prebiotics and probiotics on microbiota composition and health. Best Pract. Res. Clin. Gastroenterol. 27 (1), 139–155.

Chilton, S.N., Burton, J.P., Reid, G., 2015. Inclusion of fermented foods in food guides around the world. Nutrients 7 (1), 390–404.

Clemente, J.C., Pehrsson, E.C., Blaser, M.J., Sandhu, K., Gao, Z., Wang, B., Magris, M., Hidalgo, G., Contreras, M., Noya-Alarcón, O., Lander, O., McDonald, J., Cox, M., Walter, J., Lyn Oh, P., Ruiz, J.F., Rodriguez, S., Shen, N., Song, S.J., Metcalf, J., Knight, R., Dantas, G., Dominguez-Bello, M.G., 2015. The microbiome of uncontacted Amerindians. Sci. Adv. 1 (3), e1500183.

Cox, L.M., Blaser, M.J., 2015. Antibiotics in early life and obesity. Nat. Rev. Endocrinol. 11 (3), 182–190.

Crowe, M., Clay, O.J., Martin, R.C., Howard, V.J., Wadley, V.G., Sawyer, P., Allman, R.M., 2013. Indicators of childhood quality of education in relation to cognitive function in older adulthood. J. Gerontol. A Biol. Sci. Med. Sci. 68 (2), 198–204.

Danaei, G., Singh, G.M., Paciorek, C.J., Lin, J.K., Cowan, M.J., Finucane, M.M., Farzadfar, F., Stevens, G.A., Riley, L.M., Lu, Y., Rao, M., Ezzati, M., Global Burden of Metabolic Risk Factors of Chronic Diseases Collaborating Group, 2013. The global cardiovascular risk transition: associations of four metabolic risk factors with national income, urbanization, and Western diet in 1980 and 2008. Circulation 127 (14), 1493–1502.

Davari, S., Talaei, S.A., Alaei, H., Salami, M., 2013. Probiotics treatment improves diabetes-induced impairment of synaptic activity and cognitive function: behavioral and electrophysiological proofs for microbiome-gut-brain axis. Neuroscience 240, 287–296.

De Filippo, C., Cavalieri, D., Di Paola, M., Ramazzotti, M., Poullet, J.B., Massart, S., Collini, S., Pieraccini, G., Lionetti, P., 2010. Impact of diet in shaping gut microbiota revealed by a comparative study in children from Europe and rural Africa. Proc. Natl. Acad. Sci. U.S.A. 107 (33), 14691–14696.

Dubos, R.J., Savage, D.C., Schaedler, R.W., 1967. The indigenous flora of the gastrointestinal tract. Dis. Colon Rectum 10, 23–34.

Ettinger, G., MacDonald, K., Burton, J.P., Reid, G., 2014. Cardiovascular health in relation to the human microbiome and probiotics. Gut Microbes 5 (6), 719–728.

Franz, C.M., Huch, M., Mathara, J.M., Abriouel, H., Benomar, N., Reid, G., Galvez, A., Holzapfel, W.H., 2014. African fermented foods and probiotics. Int. J. Food Microbiol. 190, 84–96.

Franzosa, E.A., Morgan, X.C., Segata, N., Waldron, L., Reyes, J., Earl, A.M., Giannoukos, G., Boylan, M.R., Ciulla, D., Gevers, D., Izard, J., Garrett, W.S., Chan, A.T., Huttenhower, C., 2014. Relating the metatranscriptome and metagenome of the human gut. Proc. Natl. Acad. Sci. U.S.A. 111 (22), E2329–E2338.

Gareau, M.G., 2014. Microbiota-gut-brain axis and cognitive function. Adv. Exp. Med. Biol. 817, 357–371.

Goneau, L.W., Hannan, T.J., MacPhee, R.A., Schwartz, D.J., Macklaim, J.M., Gloor, G.B., Razvi, H., Reid, G., Burton, J.P., Hultgren, S.J., 2015. Inadequate antibiotic therapy induces uropathogen virulence, persistence, and pathogenesis in a murine model of recurrent urinary tract infection. mBio 6 (2), e00356–15.

Hemsworth, J., Hekmat, S., Reid, G., 2012. Micronutrient- supplemented probiotic yogurt for HIV-infected adults taking HAART in London, Canada. Gut Microbes 3 (5), 1–6.

Hummelen, R., Macklaim, J.M., Bisanz, J.E., Hammond, J.-A., McMillan, A., Vongsa, B., Koenig, D., Gloor, G.B., Reid, G., 2011. Vaginal microbiome diversity and epithelial cell changes in post-menopausal women with dryness and atrophy. PLoS One 6 (11), e26602.

Hummelen, R., Macklaim, J., Fernandes, A., Dickson, R., Changalucha, J., Gloor, G.B., Reid, G., 2010. Deep sequencing of the vaginal microbiome in HIV patients. PLoS One 5 (8), e12078.

Irvine, S.L., Hummelen, R.B.S., Hekmat, S., Looman, C., Changalucha, J., Habbema, D.F., Reid, G., 2010. Probiotic yogurt consumption is associated with an increase of CD4 count among people living with HIV/AIDS. J. Clin. Gastroenterol. 44 (9), e201–e205.

King, S., Glanville, J., Sanders, M.E., Fitzgerald, A., Varley, D., 2014. Effectiveness of probiotics on the duration of illness in healthy children and adults who develop common acute respiratory infectious conditions: a systematic review and meta-analysis. Br. J. Nutr. 112 (1), 41–54.

Kim, E., Coelho, D., Blachier, F., 2013. Review of the association between meat consumption and risk of colorectal cancer. Nutr. Res. 33 (12), 983–994.

Kort, R., Westerik, N., Mariela Serrano, L., Douillard, F.P., Gottstein, W., Mukisa, I.M., Tuijn, C.J., Basten, L., Hafkamp, B., Meijer, W.C., Teusink, B., de Vos, W.M., Reid, G., Sybesma, W., 2015. A novel consortium of *Lactobacillus rhamnosus and Streptococcus thermophilus* for increased access to functional fermented foods. Microb. Cell Fact. 14 (1), 195.

Levy, S.B., Marshall, B., 2004. Antibacterial resistance worldwide: causes, challenges and responses. Nat. Med. 10 (12 Suppl), S122–S129.

Luczak, S.E., Yarnell, L.M., Prescott, C.A., Raine, A., Venables, P.H., Mednick, S.A., January 26, 2015. Childhood cognitive measures as predictors of alcohol use and problems by mid-adulthood in a non-Western cohort. Psychol. Addict. Behav. 29 (2), 365–370 [Epub ahead of print].

Lyte, M., 2014. Microbial endocrinology and the microbiota-gut-brain axis. Adv. Exp. Med. Biol. 817, 3–24.

Macklaim, J.M., Fernandes, A.D., Reid, G., Gloor, G.B., 2013. Comparative meta-RNA-seq of the vaginal microbiota and differential expression by *Lactobacillus iners* in health and dysbiosis. Microbiome 1, 12.

Marshall, B.M., Levy, S.B., 2011. Food animals and antimicrobials: impacts on human health. Clin. Microbiol. Rev. 24 (4), 718–733.

Marshall, B.J., Warren, J.R., 1984. Unidentified curved bacilli in the stomach of patients with gastritis and peptic ulceration. Lancet 1 (8390), 1311–1315.

Mavrodaris, A., Powell, J., Thorogood, M., 2013. Prevalences of dementia and cognitive impairment among older people in sub-Saharan Africa: a systematic review. Bull. WHO 91 (10), 773–783.

McNulty, N.P., Yatsunenko, T., Hsiao, A., Faith, J.J., Muegge, B.D., Goodman, A.L., Henrissat, B., Oozeer, R., Cools-Portier, S., Gobert, G., Chervaux, C., Knights, D., Lozupone, C.A., Knight, R., Duncan, A.E., Bain, J.R., Muehlbauer, M.J., Newgard, C.B., Heath, A.C., Gordon, J.I., 2011. The impact of a consortium of fermented milk strains on the gut microbiome of gnotobiotic mice and monozygotic twins. Sci. Transl. Med. 3 (106), 106ra106.

Micha, R., Michas, G., Mozaffarian, D., 2012. Unprocessed red and processed meats and risk of coronary artery disease and type 2 diabetes–an updated review of the evidence. Curr. Atheroscler. Rep. 14 (6), 515–524.

Nell, S., Eibach, D., Montano, V., Maady, A., Nkwescheu, A., Siri, J., Elamin, W.F., Falush, D., Linz, B., Achtman, M., Moodley, Y., Suerbaum, S., 2013. Recent acquisition of *Helicobacter pylori* by Baka pygmies. PLoS Genet. 9 (9), e1003775.

de Oliveira Leite, A.M., Miguel, M.A., Peixoto, R.S., Rosado, A.S., Silva, J.T., Paschoalin, V.M., 2013. Microbiological, technological and therapeutic properties of kefir: a natural probiotic beverage. Braz. J. Microbiol. 44 (2), 341–349.

Paddick, S.M., Kisoli, A., Dotchin, C.L., Gray, W.K., Chaote, P., Longdon, A., Walker, R.W., April 26, 2015. Mortality rates in community-dwelling Tanzanians with dementia and mild cognitive impairment: a 4-year follow-up study. Age Ageing 44 (4), 636–641. pii: afv048. [Epub ahead of print].

Park, K.Y., Jeong, J.K., Lee, Y.E., Daily 3rd, J.W., 2014. Health benefits of kimchi (Korean fermented vegetables) as a probiotic food. J. Med. Food 17 (1), 6–20.

Perez-Burgos, A., Wang, B., Mao, Y.K., Mistry, B., McVey Neufeld, K.A., Bienenstock, J., Kunze, W., 2013. Psychoactive bacteria *Lactobacillus rhamnosus* (JB-1) elicits rapid frequency facilitation in vagal afferents. Am. J. Physiol. Gastrointest. Liver Physiol. 304 (2), G211–G220.

Petrova, M.I., van den Broek, M., Balzarini, J., Vanderleyden, J., Lebeer, S., 2013. Vaginal microbiota and its role in HIV transmission and infection. FEMS Microbiol. Rev. 37 (5), 762–792.

Pilleron, S., Guerchet, M., Ndamba-Bandzouzi, B., Mbelesso, P., Dartigues, J.F., Preux, P.M., Clément, J.P., 2015. Association between stressful life events and cognitive disorders in Central Africa: results from the EPIDEMCA program. Neuroepidemiology 44 (2), 99–107.

Pontzer, H., Raichlen, D.A., Wood, B.M., Mabulla, A.Z., Racette, S.B., Marlowe, F.W., 2012. Hunter-gatherer energetics and human obesity. PLoS One 7 (7), e40503.

Reid, G., 2010. The potential role for probiotic yogurt for people living with HIV/AIDS. Gut Microbes 1 (6), 411–414.

Reid, G., 2011. Neuroactive probiotics. Bioessays 33 (8), 562.

Reid, G., Bruce, A.W., Fraser, N., Heinemann, C., Owen, J., Henning, B., 2001. Oral probiotics can resolve urogenital infections. FEMS Immunol. Med. Microbiol. 30, 49–52.

Reid, G., Nduti, N., Sybesma, W., Kort, R., Kollmann, T.R., Adam, R., Boga, H., Brown, E.M., Einerhand, A., El-Nezami, H., Gloor, G.B., Kavere, I.I., Lindahl, J., Manges, A., Mamo, W., Martin, R., McMillan, A., Obiero, J., Ochieng', P.A., Onyango, A., Rulisa, S., Salminen, E., Salminen, S., Sije, A., Swann, J.R., Van Treuren, W., Waweru, D., Kemp, S., 2014. Harnessing microbiome and probiotic research in sub-Saharan Africa: recommendations from an African workshop. Microbiome 2, 12.

Reid, M.K.E., Gough, R., Enos, M., Reid, G., 2013. Social businesses in Tanzania tackling health issues of the Millenium Development Goals, one community kitchen at a time. J. Soc. Bus. 3 (1), 24–38.

Rosenfeld, C.S., 2015. Microbiome disturbances and autism spectrum disorders. Drug Metab. Dispos. 43 (10), 1557–1571. April 7.

Schellenberg, J.J., Dumonceaux, T.J., Hill, J.E., Kimani, J., Jaoko, W., Wachihi, C., Mungai, J.N., Lane, M., Fowke, K.R., Ball, T.B., Plummer, F.A., 2012. Selection, phenotyping and identification of acid and hydrogen peroxide producing bacteria from vaginal samples of Canadian and East African women. PLoS One 7 (7), e41217.

Schnorr, S.L., 2015. The diverse microbiome of the hunter-gatherer. Nature 518 (7540), S14–S15.

Selhub, E.M., Logan, A.C., Bested, A.C., 2014. Fermented foods, microbiota, and mental health: ancient practice meets nutritional psychiatry. J. Physiol. Anthropol. 33, 2.

Spear, G.T., Sikaroodi, M., Zariffard, M.R., Landay, A.L., French, A.L., Gillevet, P.M., 2008. Comparison of the diversity of the vaginal microbiota in HIV-infected and HIV-uninfected women with or without bacterial vaginosis. J. Infect. Dis. 198 (8), 1131–1140.

Smith, M.I., Yatsunenko, T., Manary, M.J., Trehan, I., Mkakosya, R., Cheng, J., Kau, A.L., Rich, S.S., Concannon, P., Mychaleckyj, J.C., Liu, J., Houpt, E., Li, J.V., Holmes, E., Nicholson, J., Knights, D., Ursell, L.K., Knight, R., Gordon, J.I., 2013. Gut microbiomes of Malawian twin pairs discordant for kwashiorkor. Science 339 (6119), 548–554.

Steenbergen, L., Sellaro, R., van Hemert, S., Bosch, J.A., Colzato, L.S., 2015. A randomized controlled trial to test the effect of multispecies probiotics on cognitive reactivity to sad mood. Brain Behav. Immun. http://dx.doi.org/10.1016/j.bbi.2015.04.003. April 7.

Villena, J., Salva, S., Núñez, M., Corzo, J., Tolaba, R., Faedda, J., Font, G., Alvarez, S., 2012. Probiotics for everyone! The novel immunobiotic *Lactobacillus rhamnosus* CRL1505 and the beginning of social probiotic programs in Argentina. Intl. J. Biotechnol. Wellness Ind. 1, 189–198.

Vīna, I., Semjonovs, P., Linde, R., Deniņa, I., 2014. Current evidence on physiological activity and expected health effects of kombucha fermented beverage. J. Med. Food 17 (2), 179–188.

von Hertzen, L., Beutler, B., Bienenstock, J., Blaser, M., Cani, P.D., Eriksson, J., Färkkilä, M., Haahtela, T., Hanski, I., Jenmalm, M.C., Kere, J., Knip, M., Kontula, K., Koskenvuo, M., Ling, C., Mandrup-Poulsen, T., von Mutius, E., Mäkelä, M.J., Paunio, T., Pershagen, G., Renz, H., Rook, G., Saarela, M., Vaarala, O., Veldhoen, M., de Vos, W.M., 2015. Helsinki alert of biodiversity and health. Ann. Med. 1–8. http://dx.doi.org/10.3109/07853890.2015.1010226. April 23.

Walton, S.F., Weir, C., 2012. The interplay between diet and emerging allergy: what can we learn from Indigenous Australians? Int. Rev. Immunol. 31 (3), 184–201.

Whaling, M., Luginaah, I., Reid, G., Hekmat, S., Thind, A., Mwanga, J., Changalucha, J., 2011. Perceptions of probiotic yogurt for health and nutrition in the context of HIV/AIDS in Mwanza, Tanzania. J. Health Popul. Nutr. 30, 31–40.

Williams, R.E.O., 1973. Geographical differences in the bacterial flora of the gut. Pathol. Microbiol. 39, 249–250.

Yogurito, 2015. http://translate.google.ca/translate?hl=en&sl=es&u=http://www.tucumanalas7.com.ar/nota.php%3Fid%3D36650&prev=search.

Value of Microbial Genome Sequencing for Probiotic Strain Identification and Characterization: Promises and Pitfalls

C.M. Guinane
Teagasc Food Research Centre, Cork, Ireland

F. Crispie, P.D. Cotter
Teagasc Food Research Centre, Fermoy, Cork, Ireland; University College Cork, APC Microbiome Institute, Cork, Ireland

INTRODUCTION

Research into probiotics and associated health claims is at an all-time high, driven by (and driving) the emergence of more and more new products on the market. However, the long-term success of probiotics is dependent on several factors, including the further generation of reliable scientific and clinical research supporting health claims, rational probiotic strain selection, and subsequent accurate identification and detailed characterization of the strains in use. For many strains within the gastrointestinal tract (GIT) there is growing evidence of specific probiotic effects; however, the genetic determinants for many of these features are, as yet, not fully known. Crucially, the availability of the microbial genomes of probiotic strains will assist in deciphering these underlying molecular mechanisms. Indeed, in addition to understanding the health benefits of a strain, it is now becoming necessary to generate this information to investigate its safety profile. Fortunately, whole genome sequencing of bacterial organisms has now become routine and is certainly starting to play a role in probiotic strain selection. However, it is important to note that there are also obstacles and pitfalls with these technologies and in the functional interpretation of the data generated.

This chapter focuses on the role of next-generation sequencing (NGS) technologies and whole genome microbial sequencing in probiotic strain selection. We highlight the value of these technologies in probiotic research while also drawing attention to the difficulties that can occur in data analysis.

The Gut-Brain Axis. http://dx.doi.org/10.1016/B978-0-12-802304-4.00004-9

PROBIOTIC SELECTION AND IDENTIFICATION

There are no specific criteria in place to define probiotic traits, although characteristics such as adherence to intestinal mucosa and an ability to tolerate gastrointestinal stresses such as bile or acid have traditionally been regarded as desirable (Dunne et al., 1999; Salminen et al., 2005). Probiotic traits have generally been thought to be strain specific, which is likely to be true for certain attributes including production of a bioactive or for specific immunomodulatory or neurological effects. However, in addition to this, certain characteristics can now also be attributed at the species level, such as bile salt hydrolase activity or vitamin synthesis (reviewed by Hill et al., 2014). Even more generally, Health Canada, for example, accepts that several *Bifidobacterium* spp. and *Lactobacillus* spp. can confer a general health benefit (ie, by contributing to an overall gut microbial balance) if consumed in high enough numbers per serving (Health Canada, 2009).

As specific probiotic attributes can be linked to individual strains, strain identity and the preparation of a full dossier describing the culture's attributes is of great importance. Use of inappropriate methods to type a strain or species can lead to mislabeling, inevitably resulting in consumer distrust and an overall reduced confidence in probiotics. Genome sequencing of potential probiotic strains ensures accurate taxonomic assignment while also providing information with respect to potential metabolic activities, the presence/absence of probiotic traits, and the overall safety assessment of the strain (ie, the presence or absence of specific virulence genes or antibiotic resistance genes as outlined in the following sections).

TAXONOMIC IDENTIFICATION

As previously mentioned, it is extremely important that probiotic cultures have the correct taxonomic assignment. In Europe the European Food Safety Authority (EFSA) states that characterization at a genetic level by internationally recognized molecular methods is necessary, and they encourage that strains are deposited in an internationally recognized culture collection with an accession number for control purposes (EFSA, 2009). Identification to the species level is a key first step in the safety assessment of a strain because it immediately allows linkage to relevant species-specific information. Speciation traditionally relied on a combination of phenotypic and biochemical techniques including examination of cell morphology or carbohydrate fermentation patterns. However, many phenotypic identification approaches are inadequate for species-level designation. This is true also of several molecular-based methods, including pulsed-field gel electrophoresis or random amplified polymorphic DNA techniques, although these methods can be helpful for strain differentiation. As a consequence, 16S rDNA sequencing is most frequently used to ascertain the species of an isolate. 16S rDNA is generally seen as a reliable phylogenetic marker for assigning evolutionary markers among species (Schleifer and Ludwig, 1995) because of its presence in all bacteria and its resistance to evolutionary change. However, there are potential pitfalls associated with the use of the 16S gene because of the volume of uncurated deposits in public databases, which can lead to incorrect assignments. In addition, this gene does not always discriminate between closely related species, such as *Lactobacillus plantarum* and *Lactobacillus pentosus* (Collins et al., 1991; Quere et al., 1997). For the *Lactobacillus* genus, other housekeeping genes including *pheS* and *rpoA* have been found to be much more robust than the 16S rDNA gene in discriminating to the species level (Naser et al., 2007). Similarly, species within the genus *Bifidobacterium* display high similarity in 16S rDNA gene sequences; therefore to facilitate greater discrimination there are often a set of further housekeeping genes used for more accurate typing purposes. Some approaches have focused on one or two gene targets, including *hsp60* (polymerase chain reaction [PCR]-restriction fragment length polymorphism; Baffoni et al., 2013), *tuf*, and/or *recA* (Ventura and Zink, 2003). Another approach has been to utilize a multilocus approach for *Bifidobacterium* species discrimination (*tuf, recA, hsp60, atpD,* and *dnaK*; Ventura et al., 2006).

More recently, as a consequence of the emergence of NGS technologies and a large reduction in sequencing costs (section: Next-Generation Sequencing Tools), whole genome sequences are now being used for taxonomic designation of potential probiotic strains as an alternative to exhaustive molecular typing methods. The use of bacterial genome sequences has the major advantage of making all of the genetic information for a strain available for analysis, thereby facilitating the detection of antibiotic resistance genes, virulence genes, mobile genetic elements, and any loci that may be attributed to a particular probiotic trait (Fig. 4.1).

NEXT-GENERATION SEQUENCING TOOLS

There are several options that are available with respect to the sequencing of microbial genomes. Indeed, the technology has evolved considerably since 1995 when the first complete microbial genome, *Haemophilus influenza*, was sequenced by traditional (Sanger) DNA sequencing technology (Fleischmann et al., 1995). The subsequent revolution in genomics led to a demand for the development of new, cheaper, and faster sequencing methods and the advent of NGS. NGS platforms perform parallel sequencing on an enormous scale, during which millions of fragments of DNA can be sequenced in tandem. As a consequence, it is now possible to sequence many microbial genomes in a matter of days or hours (depending on the sequencing platform chosen) and at greatly reduced costs (Edwards and Holt, 2013; Liu et al., 2012). In 2005 the microbial genomics revolution began to gather considerably greater momentum when 454 Life Sciences (which subsequently became part of Roche Diagnostics) published a paper detailing the sequencing of the 580-kb bacterial genome of *Mycoplasma genitalium* in a single run (Margulies et al., 2005). There are some drawbacks to NGS, including that the relatively short read lengths produced by many of the NGS platforms can make sequence assembly difficult and the

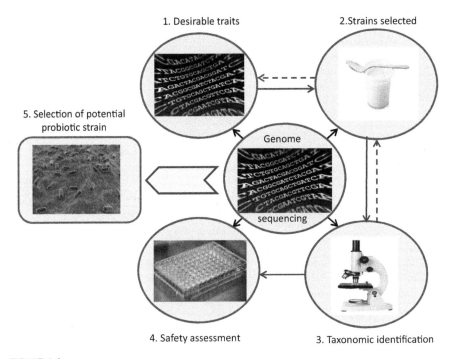

FIGURE 4.1

Utility of genome sequencing in the selection of probiotic strains. Genome sequencing contributes to the identification to desirable traits, taxonomic classification, safety assessment, and overall strain selection to take forward for further analysis.

sensitivity of the technology runs the risk of contaminating DNA being sequenced, particularly in samples with a low biomass (Salter et al., 2014). Library construction methods, GC content, and homopolymer stretches can also introduce significant bias that needs to be accounted for (Ross et al., 2013). Despite this, since 2005 NGS technologies have been implemented in many applications, including whole genome sequencing, de novo assembly sequencing, resequencing, compositional sequencing, and transcriptome sequencing at the DNA and RNA levels.

There are currently several companies that provide different NGS technologies. Although Roche is in the process of shutting down its 454 sequencing business, Illumina (www.illumina.com), Life Technologies (www.lifetechnologies.com), Pacific Biosystems (www.pacificbiosciences.com), and Oxford Nanopore (www.nanoporetech.com) are among those that are still active in the area.

ROCHE/454 LIFE SCIENCES

The Roche/454 platforms relied on a sequencing technology known as pyrosequencing. In pyrosequencing the incorporation of a nucleotide by DNA polymerase results in the release of pyrophosphate, which initiates several downstream reactions that ultimately produce light by the enzyme luciferase (Mardis, 2008). The resulting light signal captured is linear and reflects the number of nucleotides incorporated (reviewed in Buermans and den Dunnen, 2014; Liu et al., 2012; Mardis, 2008). In the original microbial genome paper, Margulies et al. reported achieving approximately 300,000 sequencing reads with read lengths of 80–120 bp when sequencing *M. genitalium* (Margulies et al., 2005). Since then, the technology has been used in various applications as well as serving as the major sequencing tool for the Human Microbiome Project (HMP; Human Microbiome Project, 2012). In 2008 the 454 GS FLX Titanium system was launched, and this was upgraded in 2011 to the FLX+ system, generating approximately 1 million reads with read lengths of more than 700 bp. In 2009 Roche developed the GS Junior, a bench-top sequencer that simplified library preparation and data processing with outputs of up to 70 Mb. However, the advent of newer sequencing technologies that could provide longer read lengths (Pacific Biosystems, Oxford Nanopore) or a greater number of reads (at a lower cost per read; Illumina, Life Technologies) led to a move away from this technology.

ILLUMINA

Illumina technology relies on an approach known as sequencing by synthesis (SBS; www.illumina.com). Illumina offers a range of sequencers catering for different sequencing requirements, including the MiSeqDX, the MiSeq, the NextSeq, the HiSeq 2500, and the HiSeq X 10. The MiSeqDX is the first and only in vitro diagnostic NGS system approved by the US Food and Drug Administration. Designed specifically for the clinical laboratory, it has an output of more than 1 Gb and read lengths of 2×150 bp (paired end [PE]). Illumina also has two other bench-top sequencers: the MiSeq, which can achieve up to 25 million reads with maximum read length 2×300 bp, and the NextSeq, which can achieve up to 400 million PE reads of 2×150 bp. Finally, they supply the HiSeq 2500 and the HiSeq X 10, the latter being a set of 10 ultrahigh throughput sequencers that have been designed to break the $1000 human genome barrier because collectively they can each achieve up to 600 Gb/day. Illumina claims that they can collectively sequence 18,000 human genomes in a year, at 30× coverage, for less than $1000 per human genome, including the library preparation, instrument depreciation, and estimated labor costs for a high-throughput laboratory (Buermans and den Dunnen, 2014; Pennisi, 2014). Given that the average bacterial genome is only a fraction of the size of a human genome, it has been extrapolated that sequencing a bacterial genome for $1 is not entirely unrealistic (Loman et al., 2012).

LIFE TECHNOLOGIES

The SOLiD (Sequencing by Oligo Ligation Detection) DNA sequencing system was originally released by Agencourt, who were purchased by Applied Biosystems, a subsidiary of Life Technologies, in 2006 (Di Bella et al., 2013; Liu et al., 2012). The technology was based on beads containing amplified DNA, which are deposited onto a flowcell glass slide while sequencing is performed by ligating fluorescently labeled di-base probes. The method was accepted as being highly accurate, with even the original system having an accuracy of 99.85% (Liu et al., 2012). Originally, the SOLiD system read length was 35 bp, with total output of 3 Gb data per run. The SOLiD 5500xl released in 2010 can reach read lengths of 75 bp and can reach outputs of 300 Gb (Buermans and den Dunnen, 2014). However, the short read lengths limit its potential applications; therefore Life Technologies have changed their focus to the Ion platforms.

Life technologies also provide two bench-top sequencers, the Ion Torrent Personal Genome Machine (PGM) and the Ion Torrent Proton. The PGM was released by Ion Torrent in 2010 and the Proton in 2012. The PGM and Proton systems use an SBS approach involving emulsion PCR. However, unlike other technologies they use semiconductor sequencing technology, in which they detect the change in pH that occurs when H^+ ions are released as nucleotides and are incorporated into DNA molecules. Ion technology has evolved very rapidly. The first chip for the Ion PGM had an output of only 10 Mb; however, improvements in the chip design, increasing the surface area and sensor well density alongside improvements in the chemistry now means that the PGM offers outputs of up to 2 Gb per chip (Di Bella et al., 2013; Buermans and den Dunnen, 2014). The read lengths for the PGM have also increased from 100 to 400 bp. The Proton generates larger quantities of data with a current output of approximately 10 Gb for the currently available Proton chip (PI chip). An improved chip design has been promised to be in the pipeline, these "PII" chips are forecast to have an output of approximately 32 Gb (Buermans and den Dunnen, 2014).

THIRD-GENERATION DNA SEQUENCERS

There have also been further developments leading to different types of sequencing technology. Commonly referred to as third-generation sequencers, the technologies involved are very different from those mentioned earlier. First of all PCR is not needed before sequencing, and the technology involves single molecule detection. Secondly, the signal is captured in real time. Three such third-generation sequencers are Helicos Biosciences Corporation's Heliscope, the Pacific Biosciences Single Molecule Real-Time (SMRT) system, and the Oxford Nanopore system.

The Pacific Biosciences SMRT technology uses a nanophotonic structure known as a zero-mode waveguide. Unlike other technologies, the nucleotides used in SMRT technology do not contain a terminator group, allowing continuous extension of the growing DNA strand (reviewed in Buermans and den Dunnen, 2014; Di Bella et al., 2013; Liu et al., 2012). This enables very long reads, with an average read length of 8–10 kb, whereas read lengths of up to 40 kb have been reported (Buermans and den Dunnen, 2014). Other advantages of the technology include the fast cycle time and the fact that sample preparation is short, simple, and cheap. The main disadvantage is a high error rate in the growing DNA strand (>10%). As a result, SMRT sequencing was originally only used in combination with other higher accuracy sequencing technologies (Koren and Phillippy, 2015). However, it should be noted that the long read lengths achievable using SMRT sequencing can overcome the shortfalls of other technologies that can be negatively impacted by the presence of repeats or elements such as prophages (Brown et al., 2014). In addition, SMRT sequencing also exhibits relatively little sequencing bias, and, in contrast to other sequencing technologies, the errors are randomly distributed and do not occur more frequently at the end of reads; thus with good coverage, a consensus accuracy of greater than 99.99% can be achieved (reviewed in Buermans and den Dunnen, 2014).

The basic principle of Oxford Nanopore DNA sequencing involves the passing of molecules through a pore that separates two compartments. The physical presence of the molecule passing through the pore causes a characteristic temporary change in the potential between the two compartments, which can allow for identification of the specific molecule because, for instance, the different sizes of each deoxyribonucleoside cause different changes (reviewed in Buermans and den Dunnen, 2014; Di Bella et al., 2013; Liu et al., 2012). In 2012 Oxford Nanopore Technologies announced that they had used a prototype of a hand-held portable device to decode the genome of a virus in a single pass of a complete strand of its DNA (Pennisi, 2014). More recently, they have released the GridION and the MinION (Di Bella et al., 2013). Early publications that arose from Oxford Nanopore's early release of the MinION criticized its accuracy, claiming that at most one-quarter of reads map to the reference (Mikheyev and Tin, 2014). However, Quick et al. (2014) have demonstrated the ability of the MinION to sequence the entire genome from *Escherichia coli* K12 substr. M91655 in one run and also noted that the newer chemistry (R7.3) improved the accuracy of the reads and suggested that as the technology evolves, the accuracy will further improve (Quick et al., 2014).

FROM SEQUENCE TO FUNCTION

Because of the advancements in the aforementioned NGS technologies, there has been an exponential increase in the number of whole bacterial genomes that are available. Indeed, the cost of sequencing has decreased 10-fold over the last 5 years and as a consequence high-throughput DNA sequencing has become more accessible for scientists. However, this revolution in DNA sequencing technologies has led to new challenges. The first of these relates to the storage of the vast volumes of sequence data generated. Developments in this area are focusing on the Cloud, where data can be stored in off-site centers that can then be accessed on demand (for review see Marx, 2013).

Further downstream, the challenge is to extract valuable information from the large volumes of raw sequence data generated. As sequencing technologies have evolved, the major bottleneck has moved from being associated with data generation to performing the subsequent analysis. Analysis of raw NGS sequence reads for whole microbial genome data is a complex process that includes multiple initial quality analysis steps and is dependent on several different software programs, up-to-date databases, and subsequently a high level of expertise to handle the data. Although several novel tools have been developed to analyze NGS outputs, choosing and using these is not always a trivial task, in particular for inexperienced users. As outlined in section "Next-Generation Sequencing Tools," there is now much choice in the types of sequencing technology that can be used and scientists need to keep in mind the read length, number, and quality provided by these technologies when deciding which path to take.

There are now a vast number of genomes from species of most bacterial genera available within public databases and, indeed, a multitude of genomes from species generally used as probiotics are available for analysis (section: Probiogenomics). Sequence data repositories include the Sequence Read Archive (www.ncbi.nlm.nih.gov/sra), Genbank (www.ncbi.nlm.nih.gov/genbank), and the European Bioinformatics Institute (www.ebi.ac.uk). In addition, MetaHIT (Metagenomics of the Human Intestinal Tract; www.metahit.eu) and the HMP (hmpdacc.org) are two major research consortia that generated large amounts of sequence data relating to human intestinal communities, including potentially probiotic strains. However, harnessing of all of these data is a challenge.

As the volume of bacterial genome sequences increases, the time spent on and quality of the annotation is certainly decreasing. Indeed, many of the genomes in public databases are deposited in a draft format and made available without annotation or, in some cases, automated annotation servers are used, which can often result in inaccurate annotation and require a lot of subsequent manual curation. For example, two-thirds of the more than 6500 genomes in the Genbank database in 2013 were in "draft" format (reviewed in Edwards and Holt, 2013), and most of the species for which completed sequences are available are not type strains (Chun and Rainey, 2014). Software such as the Rapid Annotation of microbial genomes using Subsystems Technology (RAST) and the SEED viewer (Overbeek et al., 2014) are often used, and although these are very valuable software, they can have their limitations when dealing with more complex genomes, such as those with a high GC content or where there are operons with small open reading frames that can get missed by gene prediction programs and thus require manual gene prediction. Many automated annotation pipelines rely on homology (Basic Local Alignment Search Tool [BLAST]) methods to transfer information from closely related reference genomes. This may cause errors because they rely on data that may be outdated. This can result in an inconsistency because orthologues can vary with respect to how they are annotated across different genomes; furthermore, misannotations can propagate in subsequent genome analyses (Richardson and Watson, 2013).

Despite the issues associated with automatic annotation, manual annotation and genome annotation can be an exhaustive process, and given the rate at which genomes are being sequenced, it is becoming less feasible for all probiotic genomes to be fully manually annotated. Furthermore, simply transferring annotation from a close homolog to a potential probiotic strain can be limiting because even close relatives can have many differences. In the absence of a functional homolog, the protein generally gets assigned as "hypothetical" without a predicted function. However, web-based servers are being generated to allow easier analysis and are designed to be more user friendly for the scientist that is not bioinformatically trained. In some cases specific domain and sequence analysis may uncover a putative function. Therefore it is more optimal to have dedicated databases for different functional groups (eg, antibiotic resistance and virulence genes) as described in section "Probiotic Safety Assessments Using Genomic Data."

PROBIOTIC SAFETY ASSESSMENTS USING GENOMIC DATA

Probiotics have an excellent safety record, and most strains are from the lactic acid bacteria genera that are considered to be part of the normal gut microbiota. Probiotics approved for commercial use undergo functional characterization and traditional safety assessments including several in vitro and in vivo tests (for review see Sanders et al., 2010). In addition to this, whole genome sequences can provide reassurance with respect to safety in relation to the presence of antibiotic resistance genes, virulence-related loci, or the likelihood of the strain producing an adverse bacterial metabolite. Information can also be given in relation to genome stability (ie, the presence of mobile elements, insertion sequences, and if horizontal gene transfer is likely to play a role in the evolution of the strain).

Specifically, EFSA guidelines stipulate the requirement for the absence of transferrable antimicrobial resistance genes and virulence factors within probiotic strains (EFSA, 2008). Antibiotic resistance in itself within these organisms does not have a safety concern; in fact, it could confer an advantage to the strain within the gut when exposed to an antibiotic treatment (Gueimonde et al., 2013). However, antibiotic resistance genes that occur on putative mobile or transferable elements within probiotic strains could pose a potential health threat because these strains may provide a reservoir for antibiotic resistance that could be transferred to pathogenic organisms within the gut. Antibiotic resistance can be assessed in vitro, but this does not give information as to whether the resistance genes are chromosomally encoded and therefore innate to the strain or if they have been acquired and can be further transmitted by gene transfer. Thus in such circumstances it is necessary to determine by whole genome sequencing whether the resistance determinant is stable or transmissible. There are several reports of antibiotic resistance among strains of *Lactobacillus* and *Bifidobacterium* (for review Gueimonde et al., 2013), several of which confer resistance to tetracycline, chloramphenicol, and erythromycin and are found on mobile elements (Jacobsen et al., 2007; Thumu and Halami, 2012a,b; van Hoek et al., 2008)

At present there are several antibiotic resistance databases that have been created for analyzing complete and draft genomes for the presence of antibiotic resistance genes. In general, the databases run on the principle of performing BLAST searches using known resistance genes against sequences of the complete or draft bacterial genomes. The Antibiotic Resistance Genes Online database was released in

2005 and focuses specifically on vancomycin and β-lactam resistance genes (Scaria et al., 2005). The Antibiotic Resistance Database (ARDB) was published in 2009 and comprises genes for 380 types of antimicrobial resistance, but it is currently not being updated or curated (Liu and Pop, 2009). Also of note are the Comprehensive Antibiotic Resistance Database, which was developed with an integrated antibiotic resistance ontology for the classification of antibiotic resistance gene data (McArthur et al., 2013), and the recently launched ResFinder tool, which is a web-based server that uses genomic data for identifying acquired resistance genes in bacteria (Zankari et al., 2012). ResFinder can detect 1862 different resistance genes that provide resistance to 12 classes of antimicrobials. The program focuses specifically on acquired resistance; therefore it is particularly suitable for the purposes of probiotic strain analysis. This database was built from data within the ARDB and other databases and from information provided in publications (Zankari et al., 2012). ARG-ANNOT (Antibiotic Resistance Gene Annotation) is another recently described tool that was created to detect existing and putative new antibiotic resistance genes in bacterial genomes. This software does not require a web platform because it is based on a locally installed BLAST program (Gupta et al., 2014).

In addition to antibiotic resistance genes, it is also necessary to analyze potential probiotic strains for the presence of any potential virulence genes or adverse metabolites. There are several dedicated databases that have centralized microbial virulence and toxin genes that can be used for this purpose. The Virulence Factor Database has served as a repository for bacterial virulence factors since 2004 and comprises data relating to toxins, enzymes, secreted effectors or cell wall–associated factors, host cell attachment, invasion, bacterial secretion systems, and iron-acquisition genes (Chen et al., 2005). An updated release of this database was created in 2008 and currently contains sequences of 2353 genes representing 408 virulence factors and 24 pathogenicity islands (Yang et al., 2008). The Center for Genomic Epidemiology (www.genomicepidemiology.org) has also created databases, including Pathogen Finder and Virulence Finder, which are relatively user friendly. In addition, the MvriDB developed in 2007 serves as a microbial database of proteins, toxins, virulence factors, and antibiotic resistance genes (Zhou et al., 2007).

Given the availability of such tools to assess genome sequences, it is not surprising that several isolates have undergone probiotic safety assessments using genomic analysis (Wei et al., 2012; Zhang et al., 2012). There are obviously drawbacks to an overreliance on these tools in the absence of sufficient, accurate, up-to-date curation and the use of correct parameters for BLAST searches.

PROBIOGENOMICS

Probiogenomics, a term coined by Ventura et al. (2012), is a growing area of interest that encompasses the genomics, genetics, and molecular biology of potential probiotic strains, with the emphasis to date primarily on *Bifidobacterium* and *Lactobacillus* isolates. Of course this can also include transcriptomics and proteomics in addition to whole genome sequencing of probiotic strains (Johnson and Klaenhammer, 2014). Genome sequencing is a first step in identifying genes of interest, which can then be studied to further decipher function. In the early days of genome sequencing, pathogenic organisms took priority as researchers sought to elucidate the genetic basis for their virulence. Although virulent strains are still widely sequenced, whole genome sequencing of probiotic strains is now a growing research area, especially as the molecular mechanisms underlying the health-promoting attributes of many such strains are still not fully clear. At the time of writing there are representative complete annotated genome sequences available for 13 species of *Bifidobacterium* and 23 species of *Lactobacillus* (www.ebi.ac.uk). It is interesting to note that the phylogeny of these two genera is different, having evolved from within distinct bacterial phyla and, at a molecular level, are very different. For several species, such as *Bifidobacterium longum*, *Bifidobacterium animalis*, *Lactobacillus johnsonii*, and *Lactobacillus rhamnosus*, there are multiple strain genomes available with many more in draft format (http://ebi.ac.uk; https://gold.jgi-psf.org). Among the strains sequenced are many that are used commercially and are regarded as having probiotic-associated traits. These include *L. rhamnosus* GG (Kankainen et al., 2009), *Lactobacillus acidophilus* NCFM (Altermann et al., 2005), and non-lactic acid bacteria (LAB)–associated commercial probiotic cultures such as *Pediococcus acidolactici* MA18/5M (Barreau et al., 2012).

There are many health claims associated with probiotic strains. However, in many instances the molecular mechanisms underlying these traits are not well elucidated. Probiogenomics can help to provide an insight into the genetic mechanisms of how probiotic strains sense their environment, cell adhesion mechanisms, microbial–host interactions, and how they adapt specifically to the GIT (Johnson and Klaenhammer, 2014; Ventura et al., 2012). For example, the genetic capacity to metabolize and transport carbohydrates was deciphered in the genome of *B. longum* NCC2705 (Schell et al., 2002). Further to this, genome mining of the *Bifidobacterium breve* UCC2003 strain revealed that it can produce fimbria-like structures that were found to be critical to effective colonization of the gut of a murine model (O'Connell Motherway et al., 2011). Bioinformatic analysis of intestinal lactobacilli has also suggested several traits that help explain how this bacterium has adapted to its niche. Genomic studies on *L. rhamnosus* GG identified sortase-independent pili that function in adhesion and colonization of the epithelial mucus layer within the GIT (Kankainen et al., 2009).

In terms of identifying putative probiotic traits, in silico analysis for specific gene clusters can be used to identify certain attributes such as potential bacteriocin production, exopolysaccharide production, cell surface proteins, stress tolerance genes, and others. For example, bacteriocin operons can be searched for, with relative ease, within sequenced genomes using the web-based program Bagel3 (van Heel et al., 2013). After the identification of gene clusters of interest, manual analysis is then required to narrow the selection to a lower number of potential producers that can then be assessed in vitro. This approach has recently been applied to identify novel bacteriocin producers from gut-derived isolates for potential probiotic use (Walsh et al., 2015).

In addition to beneficial traits, it is important to note that probiotics encounter several stresses in the GIT such as low pH, osmotic stress, or the detergent properties of bile that need to be overcome to remain viable. Furthermore, from a food processing perspective, the ability to withstand technological hurdles is extremely important to probiotic strain selection. Genome-wide and functional studies have been performed in *Lactobacillus* spp. to investigate gene loci involved in stress responses; the focus of such studies has varied, but some examples include analysis of the role of two-component system regulators, cell envelope-associated loci, and bile salt hydrolases (Altermann et al., 2004; Azcarate-Peril et al., 2004; Klaenhammer et al., 2005; Lambert et al., 2007). Genomics can potentially help identify stress response genes and provide insight into the overall industrial stability of the strain.

CONCLUSION

Probiotic microorganisms are attracting a growing research interest, and in addition to the plethora of in vitro testing that they undergo, more strains are now being sequenced for genetic analysis. Whole genome sequencing has the advantage of revealing the genetic blueprint of a strain from which beneficial attributes, potential virulence genes, or antibiotic resistance genes can be identified. Although there are many benefits to whole genome analysis in the field of probiogenomics, it is also evident that there are some challenges associated with some NGS technologies and difficulties in the downstream analysis. As discussed, although care needs to be taken in the interpretation of the data, genome sequencing certainly will have a pivotal role in the future of probiotic research (Fig. 4.1).

ACKNOWLEDGMENTS

Research in P.D.C lab is supported by Science Foundation of Ireland (SFI) funded Center for Science, Engineering and Technology, the APC Microbiome Institute and P.D.C. is also supported by an SFI PI award "Obesibiotics" (11/PI/1137).

REFERENCES

Altermann, E., Buck, L.B., Cano, R., Klaenhammer, T.R., 2004. Identification and phenotypic characterization of the cell-division protein CdpA. Gene 342, 189–197.

Altermann, E., Russell, W.M., Azcarate-Peril, M.A., Barrangou, R., Buck, B.L., McAuliffe, O., Souther, N., Dobson, A., Duong, T., Callanan, M., Lick, S., Hamrick, A., Cano, R., Klaenhammer, T.R., 2005. Complete genome sequence of the probiotic lactic acid bacterium *Lactobacillus acidophilus* NCFM. Proc. Natl. Acad. Sci. U.S.A. 102, 3906–3912.

Azcarate-Peril, M.A., Altermann, E., Hoover-Fitzula, R.L., Cano, R.J., Klaenhammer, T.R., 2004. Identification and inactivation of genetic loci involved with *Lactobacillus acidophilus* acid tolerance. Appl. Environ. Microbiol. 70, 5315–5322.

Baffoni, L., Stenico, V., Strahsburger, E., Gaggia, F., Di Gioia, D., Modesto, M., Mattarelli, P., Biavati, B., 2013. Identification of species belonging to the *Bifidobacterium* genus by PCR-RFLP analysis of a hsp60 gene fragment. BMC Microbiol. 13, 149.

Barreau, G., Tompkins, T.A., de Carvalho, V.G., 2012. Draft genome sequence of probiotic strain *Pediococcus acidilactici* MA18/5M. J. Bacteriol. 194, 901.

Brown, S.D., Nagaraju, S., Utturkar, S., De Tissera, S., Segovia, S., Mitchell, W., Land, M.L., Dassanayake, A., Kopke, M., 2014. Comparison of single-molecule sequencing and hybrid approaches for finishing the genome of *Clostridium autoethanogenum* and analysis of CRISPR systems in industrial relevant *Clostridia*. Biotechnol. Biofuels 7, 40.

Buermans, H.P., den Dunnen, J.T., 2014. Next generation sequencing technology: advances and applications. Biochim. Biophys. Acta 1842, 1932–1941.

Chen, L., Yang, J., Yu, J., Yao, Z., Sun, L., Shen, Y., Jin, Q., 2005. VFDB: a reference database for bacterial virulence factors. Nucleic Acids Res. 33, D325–D328.

Chun, J., Rainey, F.A., 2014. Integrating genomics into the taxonomy and systematics of the Bacteria and Archaea. Int. J. Syst. Evol. Microbiol. 64, 316–324.

Collins, M.D., Rodrigues, U., Ash, C., Aguirre, M., Farrow, J.A.E., Martinez-Murcia, A., Phillips, B.A., Williams, A.M., Wallbanks, S., 1991. Phylogenetic analysis of the genus *Lactobacillus* and related lactic acid bacteria as determined by reverse transcriptase sequencing of 16S rRNA. FEMS Microbiol. Lett. 77.

Di Bella, J.M., Bao, Y., Gloor, G.B., Burton, J.P., Reid, G., 2013. High throughput sequencing methods and analysis for microbiome research. J. Microbiol. Methods 95, 401–414.

Dunne, C., Murphy, L., Flynn, S., O'Mahony, L., O'Halloran, S., Feeney, M., Morrissey, D., Thornton, G., Fitzgerald, G., Daly, C., Kiely, B., Quigley, E.M., O'Sullivan, G.C., Shanahan, F., Collins, J.K., 1999. Probiotics: from myth to reality. Demonstration of functionality in animal models of disease and in human clinical trials. Antonie Van Leeuwenhoek 76, 279–292.

Edwards, D.J., Holt, K.E., 2013. Beginner's guide to comparative bacterial genome analysis using next-generation sequence data. Microb. Inform Exp. 3, 2.

EFSA, 2008. Update of the criteria used in the assessment of bacterial resistance to antibiotics of human or veterinary importance. EFSA J. 732, 1–15.

EFSA, 2009. In: Scientific Opinion on the Substantiation of Health Claims Related to Non-characterised Microorganisms Pursuant to Article 13(1) of Regulation (EC) No 1924/20061, p. 7.

Fleischmann, R.D., Adams, M.D., White, O., Clayton, R.A., Kirkness, E.F., Kerlavage, A.R., Bult, C.J., Tomb, J.F., Dougherty, B.A., Merrick, J.M., et al., 1995. Whole-genome random sequencing and assembly of *Haemophilus influenzae* Rd. Science 269, 496–512.

Gueimonde, M., Sanchez, B., G de Los Reyes-Gavilán, C., Margolles, A., 2013. Antibiotic resistance in probiotic bacteria. Front. Microbiol. 4, 202.

Gupta, S.K., Padmanabhan, B.R., Diene, S.M., Lopez-Rojas, R., Kempf, M., Landraud, L., Rolain, J.M., 2014. ARG-ANNOT, a new bioinformatic tool to discover antibiotic resistance genes in bacterial genomes. Antimicrob. Agents Chemother. 58, 212–220.

Health Canada, 2009. Accepted Claims About the Nature of Probitoic Microorganisms in Food. Health Canada (online). http://www.hc-sc.gc.ca/fn-an/label-etiquet/claims-reclam/probiotics_claims-allegations_probiotiques-eng.php%20.

Hill, C., Guarner, F., Reid, G., Gibson, G.R., Merenstein, D.J., Pot, B., Morelli, L., Canani, R.B., Flint, H.J., Salminen, S., Calder, P.C., Sanders, M.E., 2014. Expert consensus document. The International Scientific Association for Probiotics and Prebiotics consensus statement on the scope and appropriate use of the term probiotic. Nat. Rev. Gastroenterol. Hepatol. 11, 506–514.

Human Microbiome Project, C, 2012. A framework for human microbiome research. Nature 486, 215–221.

Jacobsen, L., Wilcks, A., Hammer, K., Huys, G., Gevers, D., Andersen, S.R., 2007. Horizontal transfer of tet(M) and erm(B) resistance plasmids from food strains of *Lactobacillus plantarum* to *Enterococcus faecalis* JH2-2 in the gastrointestinal tract of gnotobiotic rats. FEMS Microbiol. Ecol. 59, 158–166.

Johnson, B.R., Klaenhammer, T.R., 2014. Impact of genomics on the field of probiotic research: historical perspectives to modern paradigms. Antonie Van Leeuwenhoek 106, 141–156.

Kankainen, M., Paulin, L., Tynkkynen, S., von Ossowski, I., Reunanen, J., Partanen, P., Satokari, R., Vesterlund, S., Hendrickx, A.P., Lebeer, S., De Keersmaecker, S.C., Vanderleyden, J., Hamalainen, T., Laukkanen, S., Salovuori, N., Ritari, J., Alatalo, E., Korpela, R., Mattila-Sandholm, T., Lassig, A., Hatakka, K., Kinnunen, K.T., Karjalainen, H., Saxelin, M., Laakso, K., Surakka, A., Palva, A., Salusjarvi, T., Auvinen, P., de Vos, W.M., 2009. Comparative genomic analysis of *Lactobacillus rhamnosus* GG reveals pili containing a human- mucus binding protein. Proc. Natl. Acad. Sci. U.S.A. 106, 17193–17198.

Klaenhammer, T.R., Barrangou, R., Buck, B.L., Azcarate-Peril, M.A., Altermann, E., 2005. Genomic features of lactic acid bacteria effecting bioprocessing and health. FEMS Microbiol. Rev. 29, 393–409.

Koren, S., Phillippy, A.M., 2015. One chromosome, one contig: complete microbial genomes from long-read sequencing and assembly. Curr. Opin. Microbiol. 23C, 110–120.

Lambert, J.M., Bongers, R.S., Kleerebezem, M., 2007. Cre-lox-based system for multiple gene deletions and selectable-marker removal in *Lactobacillus plantarum*. Appl. Environ. Microbiol. 73, 1126–1135.

Liu, B., Pop, M., 2009. ARDB–Antibiotic resistance genes database. Nucleic Acids Res. 37, D443–D447.

Liu, L., Li, Y., Li, S., Hu, N., He, Y., Pong, R., Lin, D., Lu, L., Law, M., 2012. Comparison of next-generation sequencing systems. J. Biomed. Biotechnol. 2012, 251364.

Loman, N.J., Constantinidou, C., Chan, J.Z., Halachev, M., Sergeant, M., Penn, C.W., Robinson, E.R., Pallen, M.J., 2012. High-throughput bacterial genome sequencing: an embarrassment of choice, a world of opportunity. Nat. Rev. Microbiol. 10, 599–606.

Mardis, E.R., 2008. Next-generation DNA sequencing methods. Annu. Rev. Genomics Hum. Genet. 9, 387–402.

Margulies, M., Egholm, M., Altman, W.E., Attiya, S., Bader, J.S., Bemben, L.A., Berka, J., Braverman, M.S., Chen, Y.J., Chen, Z., Dewell, S.B., Du, L., Fierro, J.M., Gomes, X.V., Godwin, B.C., He, W., Helgesen, S., Ho, C.H., Irzyk, G.P., Jando, S.C., Alenquer, M.L., Jarvie, T.P., Jirage, K.B., Kim, J.B., Knight, J.R., Lanza, J.R., Leamon, J.H., Lefkowitz, S.M., Lei, M., Li, J., Lohman, K.L., Lu, H., Makhijani, V.B., McDade, K.E., McKenna, M.P., Myers, E.W., Nickerson, E., Nobile, J.R., Plant, R., Puc, B.P., Ronan, M.T., Roth, G.T., Sarkis, G.J., Simons, J.F., Simpson, J.W., Srinivasan, M., Tartaro, K.R., Tomasz, A., Vogt, K.A., Volkmer, G.A., Wang, S.H., Wang, Y., Weiner, M.P., Yu, P., Begley, R.F., Rothberg, J.M., 2005. Genome sequencing in microfabricated high-density picolitre reactors. Nature 437, 376–380.

Marx, V., 2013. Biology: the big challenges of big data. Nature 498, 255–260.

McArthur, A.G., Waglechner, N., Nizam, F., Yan, A., Azad, M.A., Baylay, A.J., Bhullar, K., Canova, M.J., De Pascale, G., Ejim, L., Kalan, L., King, A.M., Koteva, K., Morar, M., Mulvey, M.R., O'Brien, J.S., Pawlowski, A.C., Piddock, L.J., Spanogiannopoulos, P., Sutherland, A.D., Tang, I., Taylor, P.L., Thaker, M., Wang, W., Yan, M., Yu, T., Wright, G.D., 2013. The comprehensive antibiotic resistance database. Antimicrob. Agents Chemother. 57, 3348–3357.

Mikheyev, A.S., Tin, M.M., 2014. A first look at the Oxford Nanopore MinION sequencer. Mol. Ecol. Resour. 14, 1097–1102.

Naser, S.M., Dawyndt, P., Hoste, B., Gevers, D., Vandemeulebroecke, K., Cleenwerck, I., Vancanneyt, M., Swings, J., 2007. Identification of lactobacilli by pheS and rpoA gene sequence analyses. Int. J. Syst. Evol. Microbiol. 57, 2777–2789.

O'Connell Motherway, M., Zomer, A., Leahy, S.C., Reunanen, J., Bottacini, F., Claesson, M.J., O'Brien, F., Flynn, K., Casey, P.G., Munoz, J.A., Kearney, B., Houston, A.M., O'Mahony, C., Higgins, D.G., Shanahan, F., Palva, A., de Vos, W.M., Fitzgerald, G.F., Ventura, M., O'Toole, P.W., van Sinderen, D., 2011. Functional genome analysis of *Bifidobacterium breve* UCC2003 reveals type IVb tight adherence (Tad) pili as an essential and conserved host-colonization factor. Proc. Natl. Acad. Sci. U.S.A. 108, 11217–11222.

Overbeek, R., Olson, R., Pusch, G.D., Olsen, G.J., Davis, J.J., Disz, T., Edwards, R.A., Gerdes, S., Parrello, B., Shukla, M., Vonstein, V., Wattam, A.R., Xia, F., Stevens, R., 2014. The SEED and the Rapid Annotation of microbial genomes using Subsystems Technology (RAST). Nucleic Acids Res. 42, D206–D214.

Pennisi, E., 2014. Genomics. DNA sequencers still waiting for the nanopore revolution. Science 343, 829–830.

Quere, F., Deschamps, A., Urdaci, M.C., 1997. DNA probe and PCR-specific reaction for *Lactobacillus plantarum*. J. Appl. Microbiol. 82, 783–790.

Quick, J., Quinlan, A.R., Loman, N.J., 2014. A reference bacterial genome dataset generated on the MinION portable single-molecule nanopore sequencer. Gigascience 3, 22.

Richardson, E.J., Watson, M., 2013. The automatic annotation of bacterial genomes. Brief Bioinform. 14, 1–12.

Ross, M.G., Russ, C., Costello, M., Hollinger, A., Lennon, N.J., Hegarty, R., Nusbaum, C., Jaffe, D.B., 2013. Characterizing and measuring bias in sequence data. Genome Biol. 14, R51.

Salminen, S., Nurmi, J., Gueimonde, M., 2005. The genomics of probiotic intestinal microorganisms. Genome Biol. 6, 225.

Salter, S.J., Cox, M.J., Turek, E.M., Calus, S.T., Cookson, W.O., Moffatt, M.F., Turner, P., Parkhill, J., Loman, N.J., Walker, A.W., 2014. Reagent and laboratory contamination can critically impact sequence-based microbiome analyses. BMC Biol. 12, 87.

Sanders, M.E., Akkermans, L.M., Haller, D., Hammerman, C., Heimbach, J., Hormannsperger, G., Huys, G., Levy, D.D., Lutgendorff, F., Mack, D., Phothirath, P., Solano-Aguilar, G., Vaughan, E., 2010. Safety assessment of probiotics for human use. Gut Microbes 1, 164–185.

Scaria, J., Chandramouli, U., Verma, S.K., 2005. Antibiotic Resistance Genes Online (ARGO): a Database on vancomycin and beta-lactam resistance genes. Bioinformation 1, 5–7.

Schell, M.A., Karmirantzou, M., Snel, B., Vilanova, D., Berger, B., Pessi, G., Zwahlen, M.C., Desiere, F., Bork, P., Delley, M., Pridmore, R.D., Arigoni, F., 2002. The genome sequence of *Bifidobacterium longum* reflects its adaptation to the human gastrointestinal tract. Proc. Natl. Acad. Sci. U.S.A. 99, 14422–14427.

Schleifer, K.H., Ludwig, W., 1995. Phylogeny of the genus *Lactobacillus* and related genera. Syst. Appl. Microbiol. 18, 461–467.

Thumu, S.C., Halami, P.M., 2012a. Acquired resistance to macrolide-lincosamide-streptogramin antibiotics in lactic acid bacteria of food origin. Indian J. Microbiol. 52, 530–537.

Thumu, S.C., Halami, P.M., 2012b. Presence of erythromycin and tetracycline resistance genes in lactic acid bacteria from fermented foods of Indian origin. Antonie Van Leeuwenhoek 102, 541–551.

van Heel, A.J., de Jong, A., Montalban-Lopez, M., Kok, J., Kuipers, O.P., 2013. BAGEL3: automated identification of genes encoding bacteriocins and (non-)bactericidal posttranslationally modified peptides. Nucleic Acids Res. 41, W448–W453.

van Hoek, A.H.A.M., Mayrhofer, S., Domig, K.J., Flóres, A.B., Ammor, M.S., Mayo, B., Aarts, H.J.M., 2008. Mosaic tetracycline resistance genes and their flanking regions in *Bifidobacterium thermophilum* and *Lactobacillus johnsonii*. Antimicrob. Agents Chemother. 52.

Ventura, M., Canchaya, C., Del Casale, A., Dellaglio, F., Neviani, E., Fitzgerald, G.F., van Sinderen, D., 2006. Analysis of bifidobacterial evolution using a multilocus approach. Int. J. Syst. Evol. Microbiol. 56, 2783–2792.

Ventura, M., Turroni, F., van Sinderen, D., 2012. Probiogenomics as a tool to obtain genetic insights into adaptation of probiotic bacteria to the human gut. Bioeng. Bugs 3, 73–79.

Ventura, M., Zink, R., 2003. Comparative sequence analysis of the tuf and recA genes and restriction fragment length polymorphism of the internal transcribed spacer region sequences supply additional tools for discriminating *Bifidobacterium lactis* from *Bifidobacterium animalis*. Appl. Environ. Microbiol. 69, 7517–7522.

Walsh, C.J., Guinane, C.M., Hill, C., Ross, R.P., O'Toole, P.W., Cotter, P.D., 2015. In silico identification of bacteriocin gene clusters in the gastrointestinal tract, based on the Human Microbiome Project's reference genome database. BMC Microbiol. 15, 183.

Wei, Y.X., Zhang, Z.Y., Liu, C., Malakar, P.K., Guo, X.K., 2012. Safety assessment of *Bifidobacterium longum* JDM301 based on complete genome sequences. World J. Gastroenterol. 18, 479–488.

Yang, J., Chen, L., Sun, L., Yu, J., Jin, Q., 2008. VFDB 2008 release: an enhanced web-based resource for comparative pathogenomics. Nucleic Acids Res. 36, D539–D542.

Zankari, E., Hasman, H., Cosentino, S., Vestergaard, M., Rasmussen, S., Lund, O., Aarestrup, F.M., Larsen, M.V., 2012. Identification of acquired antimicrobial resistance genes. J. Antimicrob. Chemother. 67, 2640–2644.

Zhang, Z.Y., Liu, C., Zhu, Y.Z., Wei, Y.X., Tian, F., Zhao, G.P., Guo, X.K., 2012. Safety assessment of *Lactobacillus plantarum* JDM1 based on the complete genome. Int. J. Food Microbiol. 153, 166–170.

Zhou, C.E., Smith, J., Lam, M., Zemla, A., Dyer, M.D., Slezak, T., 2007. MvirDB–a microbial database of protein toxins, virulence factors and antibiotic resistance genes for bio-defence applications. Nucleic Acids Res. 35, D391–D394.

Probiotics as Curators of a Healthy Gut Microbiota: Delivering the Solution

5

A.B. Murphy

University College Cork, APC Microbiome Institute, Cork, Ireland; Teagasc Food Research Centre, Fermoy, Cork, Ireland; University College Cork, School of Microbiology, Cork, Ireland

T.G. Dinan

University College Cork, APC Microbiome Institute, Cork, Ireland; University College Cork, Department of Psychiatry and Neurobehavioural Science, Cork, Ireland

J.F. Cryan

University College Cork, APC Microbiome Institute, Cork, Ireland; University College Cork, Department of Anatomy and Neuroscience, Cork, Ireland

C. Stanton

Teagasc Food Research Centre, Fermoy, Cork, Ireland; University College Cork, APC Microbiome Institute, Cork, Ireland

R.P. Ross

University College Cork, APC Microbiome Institute, Cork, Ireland; University College Cork, College of Science, Engineering and Food Science, Cork, Ireland

INTRODUCTION

The gut microbiota plays a vital role in human health and is essential for key processes such as nutrition, metabolism, and pathogen resistance (Lozupone et al., 2012). Recent advances in sequencing technologies have increased our understanding and appreciation of the complexity of the gut microbiota and the importance of a healthy gut ecosystem. Large-scale projects (Human Microbiome Project Consortium, 2012) have made significant progress in the characterization of microbial communities in the gut that are crucial to human health. Defining the features of a healthy gut microbiota is essential to identify and examine the key alterations that can lead to disease.

The dominant influence of the gut microbiota in host physiology is becoming evident; thus disruptions in the normal gut microbiota composition and function can have significant consequences for affected individuals. Microbiota disturbances are associated with an increased risk of disease development in infants and adults (Lozupone et al., 2012). Moreover, a role for the gut microbiota in the regulation

The Gut-Brain Axis. http://dx.doi.org/10.1016/B978-0-12-802304-4.00005-0

of several processes relating to brain function and mental health has emerged. Gut-brain interaction has recently become an area of considerable investigation, with a multitude of preclinical studies suggesting that alterations in the gut-brain axis are involved in the development of several gastrointestinal(GI) and psychiatric disorders such as irritable bowel syndrome (IBS), anxiety, and depression (Mayer et al., 2015).

Given the prominent role of the gut microbiota in several functions that are essential to the maintenance of human health, modulation of the gut microbiota using functional food-based approaches is a rapidly growing area of research. Evidence from epidemiological and animal studies suggest a role for probiotics in the restoration of normal gut microbiota function (Derrien and van Hylckama Vlieg, 2015). Moreover, probiotics have been used as potential therapies for psychiatric disorders with some promising initial results.

In this review we describe the development of a healthy gut microbiota from infancy to adulthood, followed by the range of factors known to disrupt its composition in infants and adults, including mode of delivery, antibiotic treatment, diet, stress, and infection. We then examine the use of probiotics as a possible therapeutic strategy for the reversal of gut microbiota alterations and, subsequently, the beneficial effects of probiotics on human health. Finally, strategies for effective delivery of probiotics are discussed, with examples of food- and nonfood-based probiotic carriers.

GUT MICROBIOTA COMPOSITION IN INFANTS AND ADULTS

It has recently emerged that the infant gut is not sterile, as was previously assumed. Several reports have shown that low levels of bacteria are present in amniotic fluid, placenta, and the meconium of healthy newborns (Jiménez et al., 2005; Martín et al., 2004). Preclinical studies indicate that bacteria found in meconium are transported from the mother to the fetus, via the bloodstream and through the placenta, where amniotic fluid is swallowed by the fetus (Jiménez et al., 2005, 2008). The diversity of bacteria inhabiting the fetus is still largely unknown. It has been proposed that fetal microbes may prepare the infant for the rapid colonization that takes place at birth (Rodríguez et al., 2015). The concept of a "placental microbiome" has also recently emerged with studies reporting that the placenta contains nonpathogenic commensal bacteria with a similar profile to that of an oral microbiome (Aagaard et al., 2014). It has been suggested that there are associations between the prevalence of certain bacteria such as *Pernibacillus* and *Burkholdaria* in the placenta and preterm birth (Aagaard et al., 2014); however, further investigations are necessary to provide a deeper understanding of the implications of fetal microbial interaction on the infant and the mother. At birth, the infant gut is rapidly colonized by either maternal fecal and vaginal bacteria or microbes from the hospital environment depending on the mode of delivery (Adlerberth and Wold, 2009). Initial colonizers of standard vaginally delivered (SVD) infants such as Enterobacteriaceae, *Staphylococcus*, and *Streptococcus* consume oxygen in the gut that prepares the environment for the establishment of strict anaerobes such as *Bifidobacterium* and *Bacteroides*

(Adlerberth and Wold, 2009; Penders et al., 2006). During the first months of life, the infant gut is unstable and can undergo many compositional changes until approximately 2 years of age when the microbial community is similar to that of an adult (Mändar and Mikelsaar, 1996; Sekirov et al., 2010).

Defining a healthy adult gut microbiota is vital to illustrate the compositional differences associated with disease (Lozupone et al., 2012). In recent years, because of substantial improvements in sequencing technologies, it has become clear that four main phyla (Firmicutes, Bacteroidetes, Actinobacteria, and Proteobacteria) dominate the healthy adult gut microbiota with members from the Firmicutes and Bacteroidetes phyla being most abundant (Eckburg et al., 2005; Qin et al., 2010; Turnbaugh et al., 2009). Although these four phyla make up a healthy phylogenetic core in adults, there is considerable interindividual diversity at lower taxonomic levels with some studies suggesting that at the species or strain level, the gut microbiota profile is highly unique and person specific (Eckburg et al., 2005; Turnbaugh et al., 2010). It has been suggested that three enterotypes or core bacterial clusters exist based on the dominance of a particular genus—*Bacteroides*, *Prevotella*, or *Ruminococcus* (Arumugam et al., 2011). However, this concept has been debated recently, with suggestions that this approach may be an oversimplification of the gut microbiota composition (Jeffery et al., 2012). This is supported by a recent study in which Knights and colleagues reported that over the course of a year a healthy individual's microbiota profile can fluctuate between clusters and is not restricted to a single enterotype (Knights et al., 2014). Alternatively, it has been proposed that rather than discrete groups or clusters, the gut microbiota composition is dynamic and should be viewed as a continuous gradient (Jeffery et al., 2012). It has recently been shown that some bacterial groups are bimodally distributed; either being highly prevalent or nearly absent (Lahti et al., 2014). It was reported that these contrasting states are stable whereas intermediate abundance appears to be unstable. These stable states are associated with human health and can be influenced by many host and environmental factors. In addition, it has been reported that a combination of diversity and functionality are necessary to maintain a stable microbiota. Given that the microbiome—the gene pool of the microbiota—is highly conserved among individuals (Qin et al., 2010; Turnbaugh et al., 2009), the concept of functional redundancy has been suggested, whereby essential processes may be performed by several taxa (Jalanka-Tuovinen et al., 2011). Furthermore, it has been proposed that there are key species that may contribute considerably to the functional profile and play a vital role in maintaining gut microbiota stability (Flint et al., 2012).

FACTORS DISRUPTING THE GUT MICROBIOTA

It is well established that colonization of the infant gut at birth influences normal development (Mueller et al., 2015). Although caesarean section (CS) delivery rates have increased rapidly over the last decade (Roberts et al., 2012), it has become apparent that CS delivery can greatly affect the infant gut colonization pattern and can result in negative consequences for the infant. When compared with SVD newborns, infants born by CS are colonized with less beneficial microbes, including lower numbers of *Bifidobacterium* and *Bacteroides* and higher numbers of potentially detrimental bacterial species such as *Clostridium difficile* (Biasucci et al., 2010; Penders et al., 2006). This disruption of maternal bacterial transmission in CS delivered infants was illustrated in a recent study that showed that in SVD infants, 72% of the initial bacterial species colonizing the gut match species from the mother whereas only 41% of the maternal bacterial species are found in CS infants (Bäckhed et al., 2015). It has been suggested that these initial microbial alterations can persist for months (Bäckhed et al., 2015) or years after delivery (Jakobsson et al., 2014). In addition, these colonization disturbances at birth are associated with an increased risk of developing several disorders later in life such as inflammatory bowel disease, asthma, obesity, and type I diabetes (Hyde and Modi, 2012). Epidemiological studies have also suggested that CS delivery may negatively affect normal CNS development (Juárez et al., 2008). It has been proposed that this influence is dependent on alterations in gut-brain signaling during critical neurodevelopmental time windows (Borre et al., 2014). Given that microbiota disruption due to CS delivery can influence development and lead to an increased risk of developing mental and immune-related disorders, it is of relevance to investigate the use of early microbiota-targeted interventions to reduce later risk.

Antibiotic use is widespread, with almost 50% of adults and 70% of children receiving antibiotics each year (Morgun et al., 2015). Antibiotic use in infancy can considerably disrupt the gut microbiota colonization pattern and has been linked to childhood asthma and obesity (Murphy et al., 2014; Penders et al., 2011). Furthermore, short-term treatment with antibiotics after birth has been shown to reduce bacterial diversity and has been associated with a significant reduction in *Bifidobacterium* spp. (Hussey et al., 2010; Savino et al., 2011) accompanied by increased levels of Proteobacteria (Fouhy et al., 2012). These initial disruptions can result in prolonged consequences and the altered microbiota composition can persist for at least 1 year after perinatal antibiotic exposure (Persaud et al., 2014). The adult gut microbiota is also susceptible to the effects of antibiotic use with some reports suggesting that the postantibiotic compositional shift may take years to return to pretreatment state and in some cases may never fully recover (Dethlefsen and Relman, 2011; Jakobsson et al., 2010; Jernberg et al., 2007). It has also been reported that intestinal disturbances due to antimicrobials can influence behavior and brain chemistry (Bercik et al., 2011; Desbonnet et al., 2015; O'Mahony et al., 2014). Indeed, antibiotics have been used positively to treat schizophrenia and depression. For example, Ghanizadeh et al. (2014) reported that using minocycline, which acts on gram-positive and gram-negative bacteria, as an adjuvant treatment with risperidone yielded positive results when administered to schizophrenia patients compared with placebo.

Diet is a key factor affecting the colonization and diversity of the human gut microbiota. From birth, the effects of diet can be seen between infants who are exclusively breastfed and infants who are formula fed. Human breast milk contains various lipids, proteins, and an abundance of human milk oligosaccharides (Subramanian et al., 2015), which promote the growth of *Bifidobacterium* spp. and have been associated with many beneficial effects on health, including enhanced intestinal barrier function (Weng et al., 2014) and improved response to vaccinations (Huda et al., 2014). Bacterial diversity and stability was found to differ between breast-fed and formula-fed infants, with breast-fed infants having a lower overall bacterial diversity (Azad et al., 2013) but a more stable and uniform bacterial community (Bezirtzoglou et al., 2011). It has been reported that once breastfeeding concludes and solid food is introduced, the microbial community dominated by *Lactobacillus*, *Bifidobacterium*, and Enterobacericeae becomes colonized by *Clostridium* spp. and *Bacteroides* spp. (Bergström et al., 2014; Fallani et al., 2011). Several studies have shown strong links between adult diet and microbial diversity in the gut (Doré and Blottière, 2015). A diet rich in animal protein and fat is associated with high levels of *Bacteroides* whereas individuals consuming a diet high in fiber, fruit, and vegetables and low in meat and dairy are dominated by *Prevotella* (Wu et al., 2011).

Stress can have a substantial effect on gut microbiota composition (Cryan and Dinan, 2012). This is particularly evident in studies investigating the effects of prenatal stress and early life stress. Maternal stress during pregnancy has been shown to disrupt the gut microbiota in offspring and is also associated with a higher prevalence of neurodevelopmental disorders (Jašarević et al., 2015; Golubeva et al., 2015). Early maternal separation can also result in various behavioral and physiological alterations accompanied by gut microbiota disturbances (O'Mahony et al., 2009). In addition, chronic stress in adulthood has been associated with altered microbiota composition characterized by a decrease in *Bacteroides* spp. accompanied by an increase in *Clostridium* spp. (Cryan and Dinan, 2012).

Accumulating evidence has indicated that maternal infection during pregnancy is associated with brain and behavioral impairments in the offspring (Atladóttir et al., 2010; Brown and Derkits, 2010). Preclinical investigations have reported that offspring of mice infected with influenza show significant alterations in the expression of genes associated with neurodevelopmental disorders accompanied by brain atrophy in several regions and altered levels of neurochemicals including serotonin and taurine (Fatemi et al., 2008). It was recently shown that offspring of a maternal immune activation mouse model show GI abnormalities accompanied by alterations in gut microbiota composition (Hsiao et al., 2013), indicating that in addition to influencing behavior, maternal infection can also impact the gut microbiota.

It is evident that various factors can influence the gut microbiota of the infant and adult and may contribute to alterations in brain function and behavior. Therefore it is of great importance to investigate new therapies that may have the potential to reverse the gut microbiota disturbances and prophylactic therapies, which may help to prevent microbial alterations in the gut that can lead to disease.

PREBIOTICS AND PROBIOTICS
POTENTIAL BENEFITS OF PREBIOTICS AND PROBIOTICS

It has become apparent that many neurological and GI conditions are linked with gut bacterial disruptions (Clemente et al., 2012). Dietary habits can have a large influence on the gut microbiota composition. Consequently, modulation of the gut microbiota through functional foods containing such ingredients as prebiotics and probiotics may be a promising intervention strategy to alleviate symptoms associated with GI and mental conditions.

Prebiotics are nondigestible short-chain carbohydrates that act as substrates for probiotic bacteria in the gut such as *Lactobacillus* and *Bifidobacterium* (Langlands et al., 2004). The most well-known prebiotics include galactooligosaccharides, fructooligosaccharides, and inulin (Al-Sheraji et al., 2013) and can be found naturally in various foods, including asparagus, garlic, tomato, and banana (Sangeetha et al., 2005). They can also be found in human breast milk as a substrate for *Bifidobacterium* (Kunz and Rudloff, 1993). Prebiotics exert many positive effects on human health through the stimulation of beneficial microbes including improving host immunity, gut barrier function, while reducing potentially pathogenic bacteria. Fermentation of dietary fibers also increases short chain fatty acid (SCFA) production which can reduce the pH in the lumen and in stool, further preventing the growth of pathogens (Slavin, 2013). Prebiotics have been shown to stimulate the bifidogenic effects of human breast milk and reduce the incidence of allergies and infection in infants for up to 2 years (Arslanoglu et al., 2008; Boehm and Moro, 2008). In addition, prebiotic treatment in mice has been shown to alter the cecal microbiota composition with differences seen in over 100 taxa when compared with controls (Everard et al., 2011). Prebiotics can also be used in combination with probiotics (synbiotic) to enhance the effects of a probiotic. This has been shown to be more effective at altering the gut microbiota composition than using a probiotic alone (Saulnier et al., 2008).

The most commonly used probiotics are *Lactobacillus* spp. and *Bifidobacterium* spp. (Cammarota et al., 2014). Probiotics exert beneficial effects through several mechanisms, including the inhibition of pathogenic species through the production of antimicrobial compounds or direct competition for adhesive sites. Furthermore, they enhance epithelial barrier function and modulate immune responses (Power et al., 2014). Probiotics have been reported to have various beneficial effects on humans. For example, *Lactobacillus plantarum* 299v and *Lactobacillus rhamnosus* GG increase the production of intestinal mucins that prevent adherence to epithelial cells by pathogenic microbes (Mack et al., 1999). *Lactobacillus* GG, *Bifidobacterium lactis* Bb-12, and *Saccharomyces boulardii* have also been reported to enhance immunoglobulin A (IgA) production and secretion (Rautava et al., 2006; Rodrigues et al., 2000). Because IgA maintains homeostasis in the mucosal barrier, increased secretion can protect the epithelium and defend against pathogens (Mantis et al., 2011). Other studies have shown the protective effects of probiotics against pathogenic strains, including the production of bacteriocins (Rea et al., 2011) and the ability to increase production of human β-defensins (Kabeerdoss et al., 2011). Probiotics should have "Generally Recognized As Safe" (GRAS) status (Nagpal et al., 2012b), be stable during processing and drying, and be capable of withstanding conditions encountered in the GI tract (Iannitti and Palmieri, 2010).

DELIVERY OF VIABLE AND FUNCTIONAL PROBIOTICS

For a probiotic to exert beneficial effects, it must remain viable and reach the GI tract in adequate numbers (at least 10^6–10^7 CFU/g; Bosnea et al., 2009). Thus, there are many challenges in the successful delivery of probiotics because the fate of ingested probiotics needs to be considered. Probiotic strains ingested orally pass through the GI tract, where they are subjected to low pH levels in the stomach and high enzyme levels in the duodenum. After this, cells are exposed to bile, pancreatin, and lipase in the small intestine (Derrien and van Hylckama Vlieg, 2015). Survival in these harsh physiochemical conditions appears to be strain specific with strains of *Bifidobacterium animalis*, *Lactobacillus casei*, *L. rhamnosus*, and *L. plantarum* proving to be most resilient (Derrien and van Hylckama Vlieg, 2015).

An attractive solution to increase viability of probiotic cells in the GI tract is encapsulation. Microencapsulation must protect the probiotic cells from chemical degradation and must produce capsules large enough to allow for a sufficient bacterial load to be delivered (McClements et al., 2009). Moreover, the microencapsulation method needs to allow for controlled release of the probiotic into the GI tract (Cook et al., 2012). Microencapsulation of probiotics is performed using three main methods: extrusion, emulsion, and spray drying (Kailasapathy, 2002). A range of materials are used for microencapsulation, including alginate, gellan gum, chitosan, starch, and milk proteins (Burgain et al., 2011). The process involves the production of microcapsules through the formation of water-in-oil emulsions, stabilized by surfactants. Microencapsulation using extrusion is a physical technique that projects a solution containing the probiotic cells through a nozzle at high pressure whereas spray drying involves dissolving the probiotic and polymer matrix and subsequently atomizing in heated air (de Vos et al., 2010). In addition, spray freeze drying is used in combination with cryoprotectants, which produces microcapsules by drying a frozen sample under vacuum (Cook et al., 2012). Encapsulation is also used to protect cells from heat and moisture, which is frequent during processing of food products for probiotic delivery (D'Orazio et al., 2015).

The benefits of microencapsulation were highlighted in a recent study investigating the effects of this technique on the viability of several strains in conditions mimicking the GI tract, storage, and production (D'Orazio et al., 2015). It was found that the nonencapsulated strains were destroyed on exposure to GI conditions as well as exposure to heat and osmotic stress. Chitosan-coated alginate microcapsules were found to significantly enhance protection and probiotic viability. The benefits of microbial encapsulation were demonstrated in a study that investigated the survival of commercial probiotics (Millette et al., 2013). Twenty-nine commercially available probiotics in various different forms (fermented milk, powder, capsules, and yogurt) were assessed for bacterial viability in simulated gastric and intestinal fluids. It was found that probiotic in capsules covered with an enteric coating had a higher rate of survival than uncoated forms. Only one fermented milk product and one probiotic powder showed high probiotic survival rates. It is evident that further research is needed on viability of commercial probiotic products because the majority of those examined were unable to survive conditions consistent with the GI tract; thus they may not exert beneficial effects on the consumer. In addition to survival in the gut, probiotic strains must reach the area in the GI tract where they can benefit the host. The addition of specific excipients can allow probiotics to be released in a controlled manner. The use of chitosan has been shown to retain bacterial strains in vitro for more than 2 h in simulated gastric and intestinal juices before release (Cook et al., 2011). However, given the timing of passage through the GI tract, these capsules would only allow for probiotic release into the small intestine whereas the target area for various conditions is the large intestine (Cook et al., 2012). However, a study by Lin and colleagues described the use of alginate microcapsules coated with chitosan followed by a second coat of alginate and reported that these capsules were stable and remained intact in the GI tract of rats for 6 h (Lin et al., 2008). A study evaluating various encapsulation materials showed that microcapsules composed of alginate, xanthan gum, and carrageenan are very effective at enhancing probiotic survival (Ding and Shah, 2009).

NONFOOD-BASED PROBIOTIC DELIVERY

Probiotic products are currently available in various nonfood-based forms, including chewing gum, lozenges, sachets, and capsules (Klayraung et al., 2009). Tablet-based delivery systems have several benefits, including accurate dosage administration and targeted delivery to the site of action (e Silva et al., 2013). In addition, they are very stable during storage and easy to administer (Dash et al., 1999). However, a disadvantage of tablets is the level of heat produced during compression with temperatures reaching up to 60°C, which can be detrimental to the survival of many bacterial strains (Roueche et al., 2006). Several attempts have been made to prevent this damage through the use of various tablet excipients. Tablets have been shown to act as good carriers for probiotics. Several functional polymer compositions have been investigated for probiotic viability in simulated GI conditions. For example, a hydrophilic tablet was proposed containing carboxy-methyl high amylose starch and chitosan for the delivery of *L. rhamnosus* (Calinescu and Mateescu, 2008). It was found that alterations in the molecular weight and percentage of chitosan used affected the timing of bacterial release in simulated GI conditions and improved the percentage of bacteria delivered, suggesting that this formulation may have potential as a carrier for probiotics intended for colonic release. Klayraung and colleagues investigated the use of tablets as delivery systems for freeze-dried *Lactobacillus fermentum* 2311 (Klayraung et al., 2009). It was found that tablets containing hydroxypropyl methylcellulose phthalate were successful for enhancing survival of the probiotic bacterial strain (80% viability). Incorporation of sodium alginate further increased viability in simulated GI conditions (>90%), and the tablets were found to have a slow disintegration time (~5 h). A novel tablet excipient was proposed by Poulin and colleagues (Poulin et al., 2011). These tablets containing *Bifidobacterium longum* HA-135 were assessed in simulated gastric conditions, and it was found that increased compression during tablet formation decreased bacterial viability whereas compression at 67 MPa resulted in tablets containing 10^9 viable cells. Viability decreased rapidly for noncompressed freeze-dried cells during gastric incubation. This was also true for tablets composed of β-lactoglobulin, which dissolved after 30 min in gastric fluid. However, tablets were also prepared using succinylated β-lactoglobulin at 50% and 100%, resulting in survival of 10^7 CFU/tablet 2 h after exposure to gastric conditions. It was also noted that the tablets were stable for 3 months at 4°C. Therefore, 67 MPa appears to be a stable pressure at which to manufacture tablets to allow for tablet formation but also to reduce probiotic viability loss.

Several other formulations have been examined as tablet-based probiotic carriers and have shown some promising results, including sodium alginate; hydroxypropylcellulose (Chan and Zhang, 2005); hydroxypropylmethylcellulose acetate succinate (Stadler and Viernstein, 2003); cellulose acetate phthalate in combination with sodium croscarmellose (e Silva et al., 2013); and a bilayered mini-tablet-in-tablet system containing ovalbumin, lactose, and eudragit S100 (Govender et al., 2015). In addition to tablet carriers, there are various well-known commercial probiotics available, including Probio-Tec® probiotic strains available in various dosage forms, BioGaia probiotic straws, chewable tablets and drops, Align (Proctor & Gamble), Florastor (Biocodex), Idoform/Bifiform (Ferrosan), Probiotica (McNeil Consumer Healthcare), and many others (Sreeja and Prajapati, 2013).

FOOD-BASED PROBIOTIC DELIVERY

The demand for "functional foods" that provide a health benefit to the consumer has gained popularity in recent years (Tripathi and Giri, 2014), and in this respect various food products have been evaluated as delivery systems for probiotics (see Table 5.1). The dairy industry in particular has developed several probiotic carriers, including fermented milks, yogurt, powdered infant milk, butter, cheese, mayonnaise, and ice cream (Cruz et al., 2009). Many factors need to be considered when developing functional food products harboring viable probiotics given that several aspects of food processing and storage can negatively affect the viability of probiotic strains, including pH; the presence of salt, sugar, and artificial flavorings; heat treatment; and oxygen levels (Tripathi and Giri, 2014). In addition to the stability of the probiotic strain, the sensory aspects of the food product also need to be considered. As such, a high number of probiotic cells are necessary to exert a beneficial effect, and this can result in some unpleasant flavors in the food product, such as the undesirable flavors associated with acetic or lactic acids produced by *Bifidobacterium*. This may require the addition of extra ingredients to mask undesirable flavors (Granato et al., 2010a). Some common food products and their effectiveness as probiotic carriers are discussed in the following subsections.

Table 5.1 Food Products Investigated as Potential Probiotic Carriers

Carrier	Products	Probiotic	References
Dairy based	Yogurt	*L. casei,* *L. acidophilus, L. casei,* *B. bifidum*	Aryana and McGrew (2007) Sendra et al. (2008)
	Ice cream	*L. casei, B. lactis* *L. johnsonii*	Homayouni et al. (2008) Alamprese et al. (2002)
	Chocolate	*L. helveticus, L. acidophilus*	Possemiers et al. (2010)
	Whey protein drink	*B. breve, B. infantis, B. lactis,* *L. plantarum, L. casei,* *Streptococcus thermophilus*	Dalev et al. (2006)
	Cheddar cheese	*B. longum, B. lactis,* *L. casei, L. acidophilus*	Ong and Shah (2009)
	Feta cheese	*L. acidophilus, B. lactis*	Kailasapathy and Mason-dole (2005)
Soy based	Soy milk	*L. acidophilus, L. gasseri* *L. plantarum*	Ewe et al. (2010) Bao et al. (2012)
	Soy cream cheese	*L. acidophilus*	Liong et al. (2009)
Fruit and vegetable based	Carrot juice	*B. lactis* Bb12, *B. bifidum* B7.1, B3.2	Kun et al. (2008)
	Tomato, orange, and grape juice	*L. plantarum, L. acidophilus* *L. casei* A4, *L. delbrueckii* D7	Nagpal et al. (2012a) Yoon et al. (2004)
	Cabbage juice	*L. plantarum, L. acidophilus*	Yoon et al. (2006)
	Banana puree	*L. acidophilus*	Tsen et al. (2009)
	Blackcurrant juice	*L. plantarum* 299v	Luckow and Delahunty (2004)
Oat based	Oat-based drink	*L. plantarum* B28	Angelov et al. (2006)
	Malt-based drink	*L. reuteri*	Kedia et al. (2007)
	Oat bran pudding	*Lactobacillus* and *Bifidobacteria*	Blandino et al. (2003)

Yogurt

Fermented milks and yogurts have been used for the delivery of several probiotic strains (Lourens-Hattingh and Viljoen, 2001). Because yogurts are natural carriers of bacteria and have a high consumer acceptance, they can be considered a good food-based probiotic carrier (Sanders and Marco, 2010). Several studies have examined the sensory impact of the addition of probiotics to yogurt. Yogurt containing *L. rhamnosus* and *Lactobacillus reuteri* was found to have the same appearance, flavor, texture, and overall quality as nonprobiotic yogurt (Hekmat and Reid, 2006). Likewise, probiotic Greek yogurt containing *Lactobacillus paracasei* had a rich, smooth, and traditional taste and good acceptance among consumers (Maragkoudakis et al., 2006). However, it has been noted that there is a texture change in yogurt that has been modified with encapsulated probiotics (Kailasapathy, 2006). Different types of yogurt have shown changes in probiotic viability levels; skimmed-set yogurt retains higher levels of viable probiotics than whole-set yogurt (Birollo et al., 2000). In addition, it has also been noted that plain yogurt sustains probiotic viability during storage better than fruit yogurts (Kailasapathy et al., 2008). This appears to be due to reductions in pH that occur after addition of fruit pulp (Ranadheera et al., 2010). The addition of prebiotics such as inulin and fructooligosaccharides to yogurt products to create a synbiotic has also proven effective for probiotic viability enhancement (Capela et al., 2006). A recent study reported that probiotic yogurt containing *L. rhamnosus* GG, *B. lactis* Bb-12, and *Lactobacillus acidophilus* La-5 was effective for the reduction of antibiotic-associated diarrhea in children (Fox et al., 2015).

Although yogurt appears to be an effective probiotic carrier, there are many challenges during processing that need to be taken into consideration. These include the fact that dairy products such as yogurt have a low pH and it has been suggested that previous strain exposure to lower pH values is useful to allow for acid tolerance during processing (Granato et al., 2010a; Sanz, 2007). In addition, care should be taken to prevent the introduction of oxygen during processing because several anaerobic strains may lose viability upon exposure (Ahn et al., 2001). It is also necessary to consider the compatibility between starter cultures and probiotic strains (Vinderola et al., 2002b).

Ice Cream and Desserts

Ice cream as a potential probiotic carrier has been demonstrated to provide greater protection than milk and yogurt (Ranadheera et al., 2012). It is also highly consumer friendly and is attractive to children and adults (Cruz et al., 2009). Ice cream has several properties that make it an effective probiotic carrier, including the presence of milk proteins, fat, and lactose in addition to relatively high pH (5.5–6.5; Cruz et al., 2009). Several studies have demonstrated the potential of ice cream as a delivery vector for probiotics. Two different ice cream formulations containing *L. acidophilus*, *Lactobacillus agilis*, and *L. rhamnosus* and either sucrose and aspartame were stable for 6 months stored at −20°C (Başyiğit et al., 2006). It was also found that the probiotic strains were resistant to various conditions, including bile salts and antibiotics. Ice creams containing *Lactobacillus johnsonii* La1 with different fat and sugar amounts were found to retain high probiotic viability after 8 months of storage at −16°C and −28°C (Alamprese et al., 2005). *L. acidophilus* La-5 and *B. animalis* Bb-12 showed increased probiotic survival in ice cream containing inulin and fructooligosaccharides (Akalın and Erişir, 2008). It was also noted that the prebiotic containing ice cream was firmer and had less variation in melting properties compared with control product.

Several studies have examined the sensory properties of probiotic ice cream and desserts. Ice cream containing *L. acidophilus* and *B. lactis* was shown to have good overall sensory qualities, and no "probiotic flavors" were detected (Akın et al., 2007). Strawberry ice cream supplemented with *L. acidophilus* was found to be acceptable with the addition of fruit improving the taste, suggesting that acidic fruit may be a useful additive to ensure masking of any unpleasant "probiotic flavors" (Belgec

Varder and Öksüz, 2007). A symbiotic chocolate mousse containing *L. paracasei* and/or inulin was evaluated for sensory characteristics (Aragon-Alegro et al., 2007), and no significant differences were found among the probiotic, symbiotic, and control mousse. However, upon sensory evaluation of each chocolate mousse, the probiotic mousse was preferred, followed by the symbiotic product. Sensory evaluation was performed on a probiotic coconut flan containing *B. lactis* and *L. paracasei* (Corrêa et al., 2008). Although several sensory parameters, such as flavor and texture, were found to be similar at 7, 14, and 21 days of storage, there was a tendency for preference of the probiotic flan over the control product.

Because of the high acceptance among testers and the probiotic viability noted during storage, ice cream shows potential as a probiotic carrier. However, as with yogurt, many manufacturing and processing concerns need to be addressed. Most notable is the fact that oxygen incorporation is a key step in the manufacture of ice cream and is vital for texture properties of the final product; thus it cannot be avoided (Sofjan and Hartel, 2004). Therefore it may be necessary to select oxygen-tolerant probiotic strains or use encapsulated probiotics during manufacture. It has been reported that microencapsulation of *L. casei* and *B. lactis* in ice cream increased the probiotic survival by 30% (Homayouni et al., 2008). However, the effect of microencapsulation on the sensory and texture properties of the ice cream should be considered.

Cheese

Several cheese varieties have been successfully used as probiotic delivery systems, including cheddar cheese, goat cheese, Crescenza cheese, cottage cheese, and fresh cheese (Ross et al., 2002). Cheese has a relatively high pH when compared with other food carriers and has a high fat content, which can help to protect the probiotics during transit through the GI tract (Stanton et al., 1998). These properties provide a stable medium for the bacteria and may support long-term viability (Vinderola et al., 2002a). Various studies have examined the potential of cheese as a probiotic carrier. For example, survival of *L. rhamnosus* and *L. acidophilus* was shown to be enhanced in simulated GI conditions (using GI tract and colon simulator) when present in Gouda cheese (Mäkeläinen et al., 2009). Furthermore, the cheese appeared to increase the levels of *Lactobacillus* in the simulation and increased the concentrations of fatty acids produced. Cheddar cheese containing *L. acidophilus*, *L. casei*, *L. paracasei*, and *Bifidobacterium* spp. was produced, and strains showed high viability during manufacturing (Ong et al., 2006). This was also seen in a recent study containing the same probiotic species in cheddar cheese (Ganesan et al., 2014). Two *Lactobacillus salivarius* strains were shown to remain viable in fresh cheese for up to 21 days, and their presence did not modify cheese texture (Cárdenas et al., 2014). Addition of *L. paracasei*, *Bifidobacterium bifidum*, and *L. acidophilus* did not negatively impact sensory properties after storage for 15 days at 5°C (Vinderola et al., 2009). This was noted in probiotic cheese supplemented with *L. fermentum* and *L. plantarum* with reports of similar flavor, texture, and appearance in probiotic and control cheeses (Kılıç et al., 2009). Health benefits associated with the consumption of probiotic cheese include improvements in blood pressure, increased phagocytic activity, and reduction of salivary yeast counts based on clinical and animal studies (Lollo et al., 2015; Ouwehand et al., 2010).

Beverages and Other Probiotic Foods

Several nondairy and vegetarian foods have been used to deliver probiotics (Heenan et al., 2004), including fruits (Lavermicocca et al., 2005), vegetables (Yoon et al., 2006), and cereal products (Helland et al., 2004) as well as probiotic beverages, such as fruit and vegetable juices. It has been shown that several probiotic strains can tolerate the low pH environment of orange, pineapple, and cranberry juices, surviving above 10^6 CFU/mL for at least 12 weeks (Sheehan et al., 2007). Carrot juice has been shown to promote the viability of *B. bifidum* and *B. lactis* for up to 24 h (Kun et al., 2008). In addition, probiotics have been shown to remain viable in tomato juice for up to 4 weeks at 4°C (Yoon et al., 2004). Although these juices may be potentially effective probiotic carriers, the sensory properties need to be examined because strong or unpleasant flavors can result in a negative perception of probiotic juices (Granato et al., 2010b). This was evident in a study by Luckow and Delahunty, who reported that consumers were able to distinguish between orange juice containing probiotics and conventional orange juice and described the flavors as "medicinal," "dairy," and "dirty" (Luckow and Delahunty, 2004). Sensory properties of whey beverages were enhanced after incorporation of probiotic *B. longum* and *L. acidophilus* (Zoellner et al., 2009), whereas fermented goat milk containing probiotic *L. acidophilus* and *B. bifidum* were also found to be highly acceptable (Martın-Diana et al., 2003; Vinderola et al., 2000).

Several other foods have been examined as probiotic carriers, including soy cheese, soy milk, and table olives (Peres et al., 2012). The use of table olives is an interesting choice because a serving of 10–15 olives can carry 10^9–10^{10} *Lactobacillus* spp., which suggests that olives may be an effective probiotic delivery vector (Lavermicocca, 2006). The colonization of the surface of olives was investigated using *L. paracasei* (De Bellis et al., 2010), and it was found that the probiotic successfully colonized the surface of the olives. The addition of probiotics to vegetables provides an attractive option for consumers who are lactose intolerant or prefer nondairy products. In addition, several other fruits have been investigated as probiotic delivery vectors, including strawberry and apple (Peres et al., 2012).

It is evident that chemical composition and physical structure of the proposed food carrier are important parameters for probiotic viability. Moreover, it is clear that slight changes in the fat and sugar composition can greatly impact bacterial survival (Ranadheera et al., 2010). In many of these food products, stability has been enhanced through the use of microencapsulation methods mentioned previously, with encapsulation proving to significantly enhance probiotic viability in comparison to free cells, during exposure to simulated gastric conditions and during storage (Capela et al., 2006; McMaster et al., 2005). However, further investigation is necessary to examine the sensory properties associated with encapsulated bacterial cells so as to enhance food products as optimal delivery systems for probiotic bacteria.

GUT MICROBIOTA MODULATION USING PROBIOTICS AND PREBIOTICS

INFANT MICROBIOTA MODULATION

The use of probiotics during the perinatal period is an important area of investigation because of the role of initial colonization of the infant gut in health and disease prevention (Mueller et al., 2015). Disruption in the colonization pattern of the infant gut microbiota during critical developmental windows can have long-lasting heath consequences (Cox et al., 2014). Because the gut microbiota in infancy is relatively simple and unstable, the use of probiotics could potentially have large and long-lasting impact on the composition. The administration of probiotics during pregnancy is still a somewhat new concept, with relatively few clinical trials conducted to date. Many studies have focused on pregnancy outcomes and associated conditions, including preterm delivery, gestational diabetes, gestational weight gain, and preeclampsia (Arango et al., 2015). In addition, probiotic supplementation to pregnant women and their newly born infants has resulted in health benefits. For example, administration of *L. acidophilus* LA-5, *B. lactis* Bb12, and *L. rhamnosus* reduced the risk of atopic eczema in infants at 6 months (Bertelsen et al., 2014) while *L. rhamnosus* GG administration alone was also shown to reduce the risk of atopic eczema in children up to 7 years old (Kalliomäki et al., 2007). Beneficial effects of probiotics have also been noted for the treatment/prevention of allergies, diarrhea, and necrotizing enterocolitis in preterm infants (Di Gioia et al., 2014). In a recent clinical trial, *Bifidobacterium breve* M-16V and *B. longum* BB536 were given to pregnant mothers 1 month before delivery and to their infants for the first 6 months of life to assess the effects of a probiotic formulation on the prevention of allergic diseases (Enomoto et al., 2014). It was found that infants who showed symptoms of eczema/atopic dermatitis (AD) at 4 months had lower proportions of Actinobacteria and higher proportions of Proteobacteria than those without symptoms. It was also noted that mothers given probiotics had a significantly lower abundance of Proteobacteria whereas infants in the probiotic group had higher levels of Bacteroidetes at 4 months of age. No differences in gut microbiota composition were seen between infants in the probiotic and placebo groups at 10 months of age. It is interesting to note that the occurrence of AD tended to be lower in the infants given probiotics at 4 months of age and was significantly reduced in this group at 10 and 18 months. Several studies have indicated that children affected with allergic diseases have more *Clostridium* spp. accompanied by decreases in *Bifidobacterium* and Enterobacteriacae (Enomoto et al., 2014). Moreover, it is of interest to note that in this study, differences in microbial composition between AD symptomatic infants and healthy infants were apparent at 4 months but not at 10 months, suggesting that the early microbiota plays an important role in AD and related conditions. The gut microbiota modifications reported here suggest a role for *B. breve* M-16V and *B. longum* BB536 during the perinatal period as a possible prophylactic treatment to reduce the risk of AD development. However, further analyses of the composition of the infant gut at lower taxonomic levels are necessary to examine the use of this probiotic formula as a possible intervention strategy. Other studies have shown that the use of *L. rhamnosus* GG in infants and pregnant mothers can result in higher levels of *Bifidobacterium*, specifically *B. longum* and *B. breve* (Gueimonde et al., 2006; Lahtinen et al., 2009). Because breast milk is the gold standard for early infant nutrition (Hassiotou et al., 2013), because of the range of health benefits provided for the developing infant, interventions with strains targeted to the increase of beneficial microbes is a desirable outcome of probiotic treatment. Moreover, it has recently been proposed that strains isolated from human breast milk for use in infant formula may be more beneficial than probiotics isolated from infant microbiota or fermented foods (Chassard et al., 2014). This may prove to be a promising avenue of investigation; however, further clinical studies are necessary.

ADULT MICROBIOTA MODULATION

Several clinical trials have examined the use of probiotics in adult cohorts to promote health or alleviate disease. A recent study by Zhang and colleagues investigated the use of the potential probiotic *L. casei* Zhang, which was isolated from fermented mare's milk (Zhang et al., 2014). The probiotic was administered to adults in the form of chewable tablets over a 28-day period. Significant differences in the gut microbiota composition were observed during and after treatment with the probiotic. It was found that consumption of *L. casei* Zhang was associated with increases in *Prevotella*, *Lactobacillus*, *Faecalibacterium*, *Propionibacterium*, and *Bifidobacterium* whereas *Clostridium*, *Phascolarctobacterium*, *Serratia*, *Enterococcus*, *Shigella*, and *Shewanella* either decreased in abundance or were eliminated during the treatment period. Similar clinical studies have also indicated that *B. lactis* and *L. casei* Shirota can result in increases of *Bifidobacterium* (Matsumoto et al., 2006). Administration of probiotic biscuits containing *Lactobacillus helveticus* Barl3 and *B. longum* Bar33 to elderly subjects reversed age-related increases of opportunistic intestinal pathogens, such as *Clostridium* cluster XI, *C. difficile*, *Clostridium perfringens*, *Enterococcus faecium*, and *Campylobacter* (Rampelli et al., 2013). By reversing the increase of pathobionts in the gut associated with inflammaging (Biagi et al., 2012), the probiotic may help to maintain healthy gut function in elderly adults. The beneficial effect of probiotics on adults has been demonstrated in additional studies with reports concluding that four main probiotic treatments are effective for primary prevention of *C. difficle* infection: *S. boulardii*, *L. casei* DN1140011, a mixture of *L. acidophilus* and *B. bifidum*, and a mixture of *L. acidophilus*, *L. casei*, and *L. rhamnosus* (McFarland, 2015). *L. rhamnosus* LC705, *L. rhamnosus* GG, *Propionibacterium freundenreichii* ssp. *shermanii* JS and *B. animalis* ssp. *lactis* Bb12 have also proven to be effective for IBS with reductions in distension and abdominal pain reported, accompanied by stabilization of the gut microbiota (Kajander et al., 2008).

It is important to note that although the clinical trials discussed here are examples of positive effects on the gut microbiota, there are a substantial number of studies in which similar probiotic strains have had little or no effect (Derrien and van Hylckama Vlieg, 2015). There are many factors to consider when drawing conclusions about the effects of particular probiotics used in clinical studies. Considerable variability exists with respect to the potential probiotic used and the dosage. Likewise, the delivery of probiotics varies among studies, with several examples of food-based delivery and more conventional delivery such as tablets or capsules (Govender et al., 2014). The duration of administration also needs to be taken into consideration, in addition to the health status of subjects in the study. In healthy individuals probiotic-induced gut microbiota modulation has been reported in some studies whereas in others no effects were apparent. This has been noted in studies in which the treatment conditions and strain did not differ among participants, which suggests that in some cases the effect of probiotics may depend on a person's own intestinal ecosystem before the intervention (Ferrario et al., 2014).

CONCLUSION

Consumer interest in probiotic-containing functional foods and supplements has increased in recent years. This review examined the latest literature with regard to what defines a healthy gut microbiota from infancy to adulthood, the factors that disrupt it, and the effectiveness of probiotic interventions in prophylaxis alongside strategies to improve probiotic delivery. A stable microbiota appears to be the prerequisite for host health, although there is still much debate on what constitutes this stability in terms of bacterial composition. It is accepted that diversity and functionality are key elements to a healthy microbiota, which is now accepted as being person specific at the species, or indeed, strain level. Disruptions in normal colonization patterns increase the risk of disease development in infancy and adulthood, and these effects are as far reaching as brain function. From womb to tomb, several factors can disrupt the microbiota, beginning at the very earliest stages of life from maternal infection during pregnancy to mode of delivery, antibiotic usage, diet, and stress. Indeed, colonization disturbances at birth or indeed as a result of antibiotic usage throughout life can persist for months or years and have been linked to disorders including IBD, asthma, obesity, diabetes, and allergies and negatively affect CNS development and function. Restoration of the gut microbiota using prebiotics and probiotics has emerged as an attractive intervention strategy. Indeed, in terms of probiotics, several clinical studies have yielded positive results ranging from reduction in diarrhea, necrotizing enterocolitis, and the development of allergies in preterm infants and children in receipt of antibiotics to an increase in beneficial gut microbiota profiles in adults with a concomitant reduction in intestinal pathogens and a proven ability to reduce the symptoms of IBS. However, not all studies have yielded such outcomes, with many failing to demonstrate the ability of probiotic interventions to positively impact human health. Several factors have to be considered when selecting a potential probiotic, which span the spectrum from strain selection to the individual's own ecosystem. For example, strains from human breast milk may be more beneficial for use in infant formula than strains isolated from the infant intestine (Chassard et al., 2014). The timing of delivery is also essential, with recent studies touting the benefits of probiotic administration during pregnancy. Another major hurdle is the mode of probiotic delivery because viable bacteria must reach the target site in sufficient numbers to exert an effect. Food-based delivery systems are already in use and available in the marketplace. Probiotic cheese and yogurts have the advantage of appealing to the "ready-to-go" consumer market. It is interesting to note that ice cream has proven to be an effective matrix to protect bacterial viability. However, ice cream itself is not considered a healthy option because of its high fat and sugar contents. In this respect, one has to consider the conflicting message of such a product and ensure delivery of effective probiotic numbers in a healthy-size portion. In addition to dairy products, other food-based options have emerged, including soy-based products, fruits, and cereal, important alternatives for nondairy consumers. Nonfood-based probiotic delivery systems have also gained acceptance with various tablets, powders, straws, and chewing gums on the market. Such carriers have the advantage of eliminating many of the technological challenges associated with food vectors, including interactions with starter cultures, detrimental pH levels, and negative effects on sensory aspects. However, this method does not benefit from the advantages of a food-based carrier, which include growth promotion, increased probiotic viability, and enhanced protection in the GI tract after consumption. In addition to carrier choice, methods for enhancing probiotic survival are necessary to ensure that a sufficient number of bacterial cells are ingested and delivered to the target site, generally the large intestine. These include microencapsulation, protective agents, packaging materials that protect against oxygen, and optimal storage conditions.

In conclusion, research continues to illustrate the benefits of a healthy gut microbiota on host health, linking gut microbiota perturbations to increased risk of disease. Probiotic intervention is a promising avenue with regard to restoring a stable microbiota and hence positively influencing health. However, the variability of effectiveness reported in clinical studies continues to be a cause for concern. Various factors can influence outcomes, ranging from the choice of probiotic strain to the processing procedures used for probiotic delivery. Carefully designed clinical trials are essential, in which selected probiotic strains, along with their carrier systems, are tested in the appropriate population.

ACKNOWLEDGMENTS

The authors received funding from Science Foundation Ireland Alimentary Pharmabiotic Centre (APC) Microbiome Institute; the European Community's Seventh Framework Program Grant MyNewGut under Grant Agreement No. FP7/2007–2013; and the Department of Agriculture, Food, and the Marine, Ireland.

REFERENCES

Aagaard, K., Ma, J., Antony, K.M., Ganu, R., Petrosino, J., Versalovic, J., 2014. The placenta harbors a unique microbiome. Sci. Transl. Med. 6 (237), 237ra65.

Adlerberth, I., Wold, A.E., 2009. Establishment of the gut microbiota in Western infants. Acta Paediatr. 98, 229–238.

Ahn, J.B., Hwang, H.-J., Park, J.-H., 2001. Physiological responses of oxygen-tolerant anaerobic *Bifidobacterium longum* under oxygen. J. Microbiol. Biotechnol. 11, 443–451.

Akalın, A., Erişir, D., 2008. Effects of inulin and oligofructose on the rheological characteristics and probiotic culture survival in low-fat probiotic ice cream. J. Food Sci. 73, M184–M188.

Akın, M., Akın, M., Kırmacı, Z., 2007. Effects of inulin and sugar levels on the viability of yogurt and probiotic bacteria and the physical and sensory characteristics in probiotic ice-cream. Food Chem. 104, 93–99.

Al-Sheraji, S.H., Ismail, A., Manap, M.Y., Mustafa, S., Yusof, R.M., Hassan, F.A., 2013. Prebiotics as functional foods: a review. J. Funct. Foods 5, 1542–1553.

Alamprese, C., Foschino, R., Rossi, M., Pompei, C., Corti, S., 2005. Effects of *Lactobacillus rhamnosus* GG addition in ice cream. Int. J. Dairy Technol. 58, 200–206.

Alamprese, C., Foschino, R., Rossi, M., Pompei, C., Savani, L., 2002. Survival of *Lactobacillus johnsonii* La1 and influence of its addition in retail-manufactured ice cream produced with different sugar and fat concentrations. Int. Dairy J. 12, 201–208.

Angelov, A., Gotcheva, V., Kuncheva, R., Hristozova, T., 2006. Development of a new oat-based probiotic drink. Int. J. Food Microbiol. 112, 75–80.

Aragon-Alegro, L.C., Alegro, J.H.A., Cardarelli, H.R., Chiu, M.C., Saad, S.M.I., 2007. Potentially probiotic and synbiotic chocolate mousse. LWT Food Sci. Technol. 40, 669–675.

Arango, L.F.G., Barrett, H.L., Callaway, L.K., Nitert, M.D., 2015. Probiotics and pregnancy. Curr. Diab. Rep. 15, 1–9.

Arslanoglu, S., Moro, G.E., Schmitt, J., Tandoi, L., Rizzardi, S., Boehm, G., 2008. Early dietary intervention with a mixture of prebiotic oligosaccharides reduces the incidence of allergic manifestations and infections during the first two years of life. J. Nutr. 138, 1091–1095.

Arumugam, M., Raes, J., Pelletier, E., Le Paslier, D., Yamada, T., Mende, D.R., Fernandes, G.R., Tap, J., Bruls, T., Batto, J.-M., 2011. Enterotypes of the human gut microbiome. Nature 473, 174–180.

Aryana, K.J., McGrew, P., 2007. Quality attributes of yogurt with *Lactobacillus casei* and various prebiotics. LWT Food Sci. Technol. 40, 1808–1814.

Atladóttir, H.O., Thorsen, P., Østergaard, L., Schendel, D.E., Lemcke, S., Abdallah, M., Parner, E.T., 2010. Maternal infection requiring hospitalization during pregnancy and autism spectrum disorders. J. Autism Dev. Disord. 40, 1423–1430.

Azad, M.B., Konya, T., Maughan, H., Guttman, D.S., Field, C.J., Chari, R.S., Sears, M.R., Becker, A.B., Scott, J.A., Kozyrskyj, A.L., 2013. Gut microbiota of healthy Canadian infants: profiles by mode of delivery and infant diet at 4 months. CMAJ 185, 385–394.

Bäckhed, F., Roswall, J., Peng, Y., Feng, Q., Jia, H., Kovatcheva-Datchary, P., Li, Y., Xia, Y., Xie, H., Zhong, H., 2015. Dynamics and stabilization of the human gut microbiome during the first year of life. Cell Host Microbe 17, 690–703.

Bao, Y., Zhang, Y., Li, H., Liu, Y., Wang, S., Dong, X., Su, F., Yao, G., Sun, T., Zhang, H., 2012. In vitro screen of *Lactobacillus plantarum* as probiotic bacteria and their fermented characteristics in soymilk. Ann. Microbiol. 62, 1311–1320.

Başyiğit, G., Kuleaşan, H., Karahan, A.G., 2006. Viability of human-derived probiotic lactobacilli in ice cream produced with sucrose and aspartame. J. Ind. Microbiol. Biotechnol. 33, 796–800.

Belgec Varder, N., Öksüz, Ö., 2007. Artisan strawberry ice cream made with supplementation of *Lactococci* or *Lactobacillus acidophilus*. Italian J. Food Sci. 19, 403–412.

Bercik, P., Denou, E., Collins, J., Jackson, W., Lu, J., Jury, J., Deng, Y., Blennerhassett, P., Macri, J., McCoy, K.D., 2011. The intestinal microbiota affect central levels of brain-derived neurotropic factor and behavior in mice. Gastroenterology 141, 599–609. e3.

Bergström, A., Skov, T.H., Bahl, M.I., Roager, H.M., Christensen, L.B., Ejlerskov, K.T., Mølgaard, C., Michaelsen, K.F., Licht, T.R., 2014. Establishment of intestinal microbiota during early life: a longitudinal, explorative study of a large cohort of Danish infants. Appl. Environ. Microbiol. 80, 2889–2900.

Bertelsen, R.J., Brantsæter, A.L., Magnus, M.C., Haugen, M., Myhre, R., Jacobsson, B., Longnecker, M.P., Meltzer, H.M., London, S.J., 2014. Probiotic milk consumption in pregnancy and infancy and subsequent childhood allergic diseases. J. Allergy Clin. Immunol. 133, 165–171. e8.

Bezirtzoglou, E., Tsiotsias, A., Welling, G.W., 2011. Microbiota profile in feces of breast- and formula-fed newborns by using fluorescence in situ hybridization (FISH). Anaerobe 17, 478–482.

Biagi, E., Candela, M., Fairweather-Tait, S., Franceschi, C., Brigidi, P., 2012. Ageing of the human metaorganism: the microbial counterpart. Age 34, 247–267.

Biasucci, G., Rubini, M., Riboni, S., Morelli, L., Bessi, E., Retetangos, C., 2010. Mode of delivery affects the bacterial community in the newborn gut. Early Human Dev. 86, 13–15.

Birollo, G., Reinheimer, J., Vinderola, C., 2000. Viability of lactic acid microflora in different types of yoghurt. Food Res. Int. 33, 799–805.

Blandino, A., Al-Aseeri, M., Pandiella, S., Cantero, D., Webb, C., 2003. Cereal-based fermented foods and beverages. Food Res. Int. 36, 527–543.

Boehm, G., Moro, G., 2008. Structural and functional aspects of prebiotics used in infant nutrition. J. Nutr. 138, 1818S–1828S.

Borre, Y.E., O'Keeffe, G.W., Clarke, G., Stanton, C., Dinan, T.G., Cryan, J.F., 2014. Microbiota and neurodevelopmental windows: implications for brain disorders. Trends Mol. Med. 20, 509–518.

Bosnea, L.A., Kourkoutas, Y., Albantaki, N., Tzia, C., Koutinas, A.A., Kanellaki, M., 2009. Functionality of freeze-dried *L. casei* cells immobilized on wheat grains. LWT Food Sci. Technol. 42, 1696–1702.

Brown, A.S., Derkits, E.J., 2010. Prenatal infection and schizophrenia: a review of epidemiologic and translational studies. Am. J. Psychiatry. 167, 261–280.

Burgain, J., Gaiani, C., Linder, M., Scher, J., 2011. Encapsulation of probiotic living cells: from laboratory scale to industrial applications. J. Food Eng. 104, 467–483.

Calinescu, C., Mateescu, M.A., 2008. Carboxymethyl high amylose starch: chitosan self-stabilized matrix for probiotic colon delivery. Eur. J. Pharm. Biopharm. 70, 582–589.

Cammarota, G., Ianiro, G., Bibbò, S., Gasbarrini, A., 2014. Gut microbiota modulation: probiotics, antibiotics or fecal microbiota transplantation? Intern. Emerg. Med. 9, 365–373.

Capela, P., Hay, T., Shah, N., 2006. Effect of cryoprotectants, prebiotics and microencapsulation on survival of probiotic organisms in yoghurt and freeze-dried yoghurt. Food Res. Int. 39, 203–211.

Cárdenas, N., Calzada, J., Peirotén, Á., Jiménez, E., Escudero, R., Rodríguez, J.M., Medina, M., Fernández, L., 2014. Development of a potential probiotic fresh cheese using two *Lactobacillus salivarius* strains isolated from human milk. BioMed. Res. Int. 2014.

Chan, E.S., Zhang, Z., 2005. Bioencapsulation by compression coating of probiotic bacteria for their protection in an acidic medium. Process Biochem. 40, 3346–3351.

Chassard, C., de Wouters, T., Lacroix, C., 2014. Probiotics tailored to the infant: a window of opportunity. Curr. Opin. Biotechnol. 26, 141–147.

Clemente, J.C., Ursell, L.K., Parfrey, L.W., Knight, R., 2012. The impact of the gut microbiota on human health: an integrative view. Cell 148, 1258–1270.

Cook, M.T., Tzortzis, G., Charalampopoulos, D., Khutoryanskiy, V.V., 2011. Production and evaluation of dry alginate-chitosan microcapsules as an enteric delivery vehicle for probiotic bacteria. Biomacromolecules 12, 2834–2840.

Cook, M.T., Tzortzis, G., Charalampopoulos, D., Khutoryanskiy, V.V., 2012. Microencapsulation of probiotics for gastrointestinal delivery. J. Control. Release 162, 56–67.

Corrêa, S., Castro, I.A., Saad, S.M., 2008. Probiotic potential and sensory properties of coconut flan supplemented with *Lactobacillus paracasei* and *Bifidobacterium lactis*. Int. J. Food Sci. Technol. 43, 1560–1568.

Cox, L.M., Yamanishi, S., Sohn, J., Alekseyenko, A.V., Leung, J.M., Cho, I., Kim, S.G., Li, H., Gao, Z., Mahana, D., 2014. Altering the intestinal microbiota during a critical developmental window has lasting metabolic consequences. Cell 158, 705–721.

Cruz, A.G., Antunes, A.E., Sousa, A.L.O., Faria, J.A., Saad, S.M., 2009. Ice-cream as a probiotic food carrier. Food Res. Int. 42, 1233–1239.

Cryan, J.F., Dinan, T.G., 2012. Mind-altering microorganisms: the impact of the gut microbiota on brain and behaviour. Nat. Rev. Neurosci. 13, 701–712.

D'Orazio, G., Di Gennaro, P., Boccarusso, M., Presti, I., Bizzaro, G., Giardina, S., Michelotti, A., Labra, M., La Ferla, B., 2015. Microencapsulation of new probiotic formulations for gastrointestinal delivery: in vitro study to assess viability and biological properties. Appl. Microbiol. Biotechnol. 1–11.

Dalev, D., Bielecka, M., Troszynska, A., Ziajka, S., Lamparski, G., 2006. Sensory quality of new probiotic beverages based on cheese whey and soy preparation. Polish J. Food Nutr. Sci. 15/56.

Dash, S., Spreen, A.N., Ley, B.M., 1999. Health Benefits of Probiotics. Bl Publications.

De Bellis, P., Valerio, F., Sisto, A., Lonigro, S.L., Lavermicocca, P., 2010. Probiotic table olives: microbial populations adhering on olive surface in fermentation sets inoculated with the probiotic strain *Lactobacillus paracasei* IMPC2. 1 in an industrial plant. Int. J. Food Microbiol. 140, 6–13.

Derrien, M., van Hylckama Vlieg, J.E., 2015. Fate, activity, and impact of ingested bacteria within the human gut microbiota. Trends Microbiol. 23, 354–366.

Desbonnet, L., Clarke, G., Traplin, A., O'Sullivan, O., Crispie, F., Moloney, R.D., Cotter, P.D., Dinan, T.G., Cryan, J.F., 2015. Gut microbiota depletion from early adolescence in mice: implications for brain and behaviour. Brain Behav. Immun. 48, 165–173.

Dethlefsen, L., Relman, D.A., 2011. Incomplete recovery and individualized responses of the human distal gut microbiota to repeated antibiotic perturbation. Proc. Natl. Acad. Sci. 108, 4554–4561.

Di Gioia, D., Aloisio, I., Mazzola, G., Biavati, B., 2014. Bifidobacteria: their impact on gut microbiota composition and their applications as probiotics in infants. Appl. Microbiol. Biotechnol. 98, 563–577.

Ding, W., Shah, N.P., 2009. Effect of various encapsulating materials on the stability of probiotic bacteria. J. Food Sci. 74, M100–M107.

Doré, J., Blottièrc, H., 2015. The influence of diet on the gut microbiota and its consequences for health. Curr. Opin. Biotechnol. 32, 195–199.

Eckburg, P.B., Bik, E.M., Bernstein, C.N., Purdom, E., Dethlefsen, L., Sargent, M., Gill, S.R., Nelson, K.E., Relman, D.A., 2005. Diversity of the human intestinal microbial flora. Science 308, 1635–1638.

Enomoto, T., Sowa, M., Nishimori, K., Shimazu, S., Yoshida, A., Yamada, K., Furukawa, F., Nakagawa, T., Yanagisawa, N., Iwabuchi, N., 2014. Effects of bifidobacterial supplementation to pregnant women and infants in the prevention of allergy development in infants and on fecal microbiota. Allergol. Int. 63, 575–585.

Everard, A., Lazarevic, V., Derrien, M., Girard, M., Muccioli, G.G., Neyrinck, A.M., Possemiers, S., Van Holle, A., François, P., de Vos, W.M., 2011. Responses of gut microbiota and glucose and lipid metabolism to prebiotics in genetic obese and diet-induced leptin-resistant mice. Diabetes 60, 2775–2786.

Ewe, J.-A., Wan-Abdullah, W.-N., Liong, M.-T., 2010. Viability and growth characteristics of Lactobacillus in soymilk supplemented with B-vitamins. Int. J. Food Sci. Nutr. 61, 87–107.

Fallani, M., Amarri, S., Uusijarvi, A., Adam, R., Khanna, S., Aguilera, M., Gil, A., Vieites, J.M., Norin, E., Young, D., 2011. Determinants of the human infant intestinal microbiota after the introduction of first complementary foods in infant samples from five European centres. Microbiology 157, 1385–1392.

Fatemi, S.H., Reutiman, T.J., Folsom, T.D., Huang, H., Oishi, K., Mori, S., Smee, D.F., Pearce, D.A., Winter, C., Sohr, R., 2008. Maternal infection leads to abnormal gene regulation and brain atrophy in mouse offspring: implications for genesis of neurodevelopmental disorders. Schizophr. Res. 99, 56–70.

Ferrario, C., Taverniti, V., Milani, C., Fiore, W., Laureati, M., De Noni, I., Stuknyte, M., Chouaia, B., Riso, P., Guglielmetti, S., 2014. Modulation of fecal clostridiales bacteria and butyrate by probiotic intervention with Lactobacillus paracasei DG varies among healthy adults. J. Nutr. 144, 1787–1796.

Flint, H.J., Scott, K.P., Louis, P., Duncan, S.H., 2012. The role of the gut microbiota in nutrition and health. Nat. Rev. Gastroenterol. Hepatol. 9, 577–589.

Fouhy, F., Guinane, C.M., Hussey, S., Wall, R., Ryan, C.A., Dempsey, E.M., Murphy, B., Ross, R.P., Fitzgerald, G.F., Stanton, C., 2012. High-throughput sequencing reveals the incomplete, short-term recovery of infant gut microbiota following parenteral antibiotic treatment with ampicillin and gentamicin. Antimicrob. Agents Chemother. 56, 5811–5820.

Fox, M.J., Ahuja, K.D.K., Robertson, I.K., Ball, M.J., Eri, R.D., 2015. Can probiotic yogurt prevent diarrhoea in children on antibiotics? A double-blind, randomised, placebo-controlled study. BMJ Open 5.

Ganesan, B., Weimer, B., Pinzon, J., Dao Kong, N., Rompato, G., Brothersen, C., McMahon, D., 2014. Probiotic bacteria survive in cheddar cheese and modify populations of other lactic acid bacteria. J. Appl. Microbiol. 116, 1642–1656.

Ghanizadeh, A., Dehbozorgi, S., OmraniSigaroodi, M., Rezaei, Z., 2014. Minocycline as add-on treatment decreases the negative symptoms of schizophrenia; a randomized placebo-controlled clinical trial. Recent Pat. Inflam. Allergy Drug Discov. 8, 211–215.

Golubeva, A.V., Crampton, S., Desbonnet, L., Edge, D., O'Sullivan, O., Lomasney, K.W., Zhdanov, A.V., Crispie, F., Moloney, R.D., Borre, Y.E., 2015. Prenatal stress-induced alterations in major physiological systems correlate with gut microbiota composition in adulthood. Psychoneuroendocrinology 60, 58–74.

Govender, M., Choonara, Y.E., Kumar, P., du Toit, L.C., van Vuuren, S., Pillay, V., 2014. A review of the advancements in probiotic delivery: conventional versus non-conventional formulations for intestinal flora supplementation. AAPS PharmSciTech 15, 29–43.

Govender, M., Choonara, Y.E., Vuuren, S., Kumar, P., Toit, L.C., Pillay, V., 2015. A gastro-resistant ovalbumin bi-layered mini-tablet-in-tablet system for the delivery of *Lactobacillus acidophilus* probiotic to simulated human intestinal and colon conditions. J. Pharm. Pharmacol. 67 (7), 939–950.

Granato, D., Branco, G.F., Cruz, A.G., Faria, J.D.A.F., Shah, N.P., 2010a. Probiotic dairy products as functional foods. Compr. Rev. Food Sci. Food Saf. 9, 455–470.

Granato, D., Branco, G.F., Nazzaro, F., Cruz, A.G., Faria, J.A., 2010b. Functional foods and nondairy probiotic food development: trends, concepts, and products. Compr. Rev. Food Sci. Food Saf. 9, 292–302.

Gueimonde, M., Sakata, S., Kalliomäki, M., Isolauri, E., Benno, Y., Salminen, S., 2006. Effect of maternal consumption of lactobacillus GG on transfer and establishment of fecal bifidobacterial microbiota in neonates. J. Pediatr. Gastroenterol. Nutr. 42, 166–170.

Hassiotou, F., Geddes, D.T., Hartmann, P.E., 2013. Cells in human milk state of the science. J. Hum. Lact. 29 (2), 171–182, 0890334413477242.

Heenan, C., Adams, M., Hosken, R., Fleet, G., 2004. Survival and sensory acceptability of probiotic microorganisms in a nonfermented frozen vegetarian dessert. LWT Food Sci. Technol. 37, 461–466.

Hekmat, S., Reid, G., 2006. Sensory properties of probiotic yogurt is comparable to standard yogurt. Nutr. Res. 26, 163–166.

Helland, M.H., Wicklund, T., Narvhus, J.A., 2004. Growth and metabolism of selected strains of probiotic bacteria in milk-and water-based cereal puddings. Int. Dairy J. 14, 957–965.

Homayouni, A., Azizi, A., Ehsani, M., Yarmand, M., Razavi, S., 2008. Effect of microencapsulation and resistant starch on the probiotic survival and sensory properties of synbiotic ice cream. Food Chem. 111, 50–55.

Hsiao, E.Y., McBride, S.W., Hsien, S., Sharon, G., Hyde, E.R., McCue, T., Codelli, J.A., Chow, J., Reisman, S.E., Petrosino, J.F., 2013. Microbiota modulate behavioral and physiological abnormalities associated with neurodevelopmental disorders. Cell 155, 1451–1463.

Huda, M.N., Lewis, Z., Kalanetra, K.M., Rashid, M., Ahmad, S.M., Raqib, R., Qadri, F., Underwood, M.A., Mills, D.A., Stephensen, C.B., 2014. Stool microbiota and vaccine responses of infants. Pediatrics 134, e362–e372.

Human Microbiome Project Consortium, 2012. Structure, function and diversity of the healthy human microbiome. Nature 486, 207–214.

Hussey, S., Wall, R., Gruffman, E., O'Sullivan, L., Ryan, C.A., Murphy, B., Fitzgerald, G., Stanton, C., Ross, R.P., 2010. Parenteral antibiotics reduce bifidobacteria colonization and diversity in neonates. Int. J. Microbiol. 2011.

Hyde, M.J., Modi, N., 2012. The long-term effects of birth by caesarean section: the case for a randomised controlled trial. Early Hum. Dev. 88, 943–949.

Iannitti, T., Palmieri, B., 2010. Therapeutical use of probiotic formulations in clinical practice. Clin. Nutr. 29, 701–725.

Jakobsson, H.E., Abrahamsson, T.R., Jenmalm, M.C., Harris, K., Quince, C., Jernberg, C., Björkstén, B., Engstrand, L., Andersson, A.F., 2014. Decreased gut microbiota diversity, delayed Bacteroidetes colonisation and reduced Th1 responses in infants delivered by caesarean section. Gut 63, 559–566.

Jakobsson, H.E., Jernberg, C., Andersson, A.F., Sjölund-Karlsson, M., Jansson, J.K., Engstrand, L., 2010. Short-term antibiotic treatment has differing long-term impacts on the human throat and gut microbiome. PLoS One 5, e9836.

Jalanka-Tuovinen, J., Salonen, A., Nikkilä, J., Immonen, O., Kekkonen, R., Lahti, L., Palva, A., de Vos, W.M., 2011. Intestinal microbiota in healthy adults: temporal analysis reveals individual and common core and relation to intestinal symptoms. PloS One 6, e23035.

Jašarević, E., Rodgers, A.B., Bale, T.L., 2015. A novel role for maternal stress and microbial transmission in early life programming and neurodevelopment. Neurobiol. Stress 1, 81–88.

Jeffery, I.B., Claesson, M.J., O'Toole, P.W., Shanahan, F., 2012. Categorization of the gut microbiota: enterotypes or gradients? Nat. Rev. Microbiol. 10, 591–592.

Jernberg, C., Löfmark, S., Edlund, C., Jansson, J.K., 2007. Long-term ecological impacts of antibiotic administration on the human intestinal microbiota. ISME J. 1, 56–66.

Jiménez, E., Fernández, L., Marín, M.L., Martín, R., Odriozola, J.M., Nueno-Palop, C., Narbad, A., Olivares, M., Xaus, J., Rodríguez, J.M., 2005. Isolation of commensal bacteria from umbilical cord blood of healthy neonates born by cesarean section. Curr. Microbiol. 51, 270–274.

Jiménez, E., Marín, M.L., Martín, R., Odriozola, J.M., Olivares, M., Xaus, J., Fernández, L., Rodríguez, J.M., 2008. Is meconium from healthy newborns actually sterile? Res. Microbiol. 159, 187–193.

Juárez, I., Gratton, A., Flores, G., 2008. Ontogeny of altered dendritic morphology in the rat prefrontal cortex, hippocampus, and nucleus accumbens following cesarean delivery and birth anoxia. J. Comp. Neurol. 507, 1734–1747.

Kabeerdoss, J., Devi, R.S., Mary, R.R., Prabhavathi, D., Vidya, R., Mechenro, J., Mahendri, N., Pugazhendhi, S., Ramakrishna, B.S., 2011. Effect of yoghurt containing *Bifidobacterium lactis* Bb12® on faecal excretion of secretory immunoglobulin A and human beta-defensin 2 in healthy adult volunteers. Nutr. J. 10, 138.

Kailasapathy, K., 2002. Microencapsulation of probiotic bacteria: technology and potential applications. Curr. Issues Intest. Microbiol. 3, 39–48.

Kailasapathy, K., 2006. Survival of free and encapsulated probiotic bacteria and their effect on the sensory properties of yoghurt. LWT Food Sci. Technol. 39, 1221–1227.

Kailasapathy, K., Harmstorf, I., Phillips, M., 2008. Survival of *Lactobacillus acidophilus* and *Bifidobacterium animalis* ssp. lactis in stirred fruit yogurts. LWT Food Sci. Technol. 41, 1317–1322.

Kailasapathy, K., Masondole, L., 2005. Survival of free and microencapsulated *Lactobacillus acidophilus* and *Bifidobacterium lactis* and their effect on texture of feta cheese. Aust. J. Dairy Technol. 60, 252.

Kajander, K., Myllyluoma, E., Rajilić-Stojanović, M., Kyrönpalo, S., Rasmussen, M., Järvenpää, S., Zoetendal, E., De Vos, W., Vapaatalo, H., Korpela, R., 2008. Clinical trial: multispecies probiotic supplementation alleviates the symptoms of irritable bowel syndrome and stabilizes intestinal microbiota. Aliment. Pharmacol. Ther. 27, 48–57.

Kalliomäki, M., Salminen, S., Poussa, T., Isolauri, E., 2007. Probiotics during the first 7 years of life: a cumulative risk reduction of eczema in a randomized, placebo-controlled trial. J. Allergy Clin. Immunol. 119, 1019–1021.

Kedia, G., Wang, R., Patel, H., Pandiella, S.S., 2007. Use of mixed cultures for the fermentation of cereal-based substrates with potential probiotic properties. Process Biochem. 42, 65–70.

Kılıç, G.B., Kuleaşan, H., Eralp, İ., Karahan, A.G., 2009. Manufacture of Turkish Beyaz cheese added with probiotic strains. LWT Food Sci. Technol. 42, 1003–1008.

Klayraung, S., Viernstein, H., Okonogi, S., 2009. Development of tablets containing probiotics: effects of formulation and processing parameters on bacterial viability. Int. J. Pharm. 370, 54–60.

Knights, D., Ward, T.L., McKinlay, C.E., Miller, H., Gonzalez, A., McDonald, D., Knight, R., 2014. Rethinking "enterotypes". Cell Host Microbe 16, 433–437.

Kun, S., Rezessy-Szabó, J.M., Nguyen, Q.D., Hoschke, Á., 2008. Changes of microbial population and some components in carrot juice during fermentation with selected *Bifidobacterium* strains. Process Biochem. 43, 816–821.

Kunz, C., Rudloff, S., 1993. Biological functions of oligosaccharides in human milk. Acta Paediatr. 82, 903–912.

Lahti, L., Salojärvi, J., Salonen, A., Scheffer, M., de Vos, W.M., 2014. Tipping elements in the human intestinal ecosystem. Nat. Commun. 5.

Lahtinen, S.J., Boyle, R.J., Kivivuori, S., Oppedisano, F., Smith, K.R., Robins-Browne, R., Salminen, S.J., Tang, M.L., 2009. Prenatal probiotic administration can influence *Bifidobacterium microbiota* development in infants at high risk of allergy. J. Allergy Clin. Immunol. 123, 499–501. e8.

Langlands, S., Hopkins, M., Coleman, N., Cummings, J., 2004. Prebiotic carbohydrates modify the mucosa associated microflora of the human large bowel. Gut 53, 1610–1616.

Lavermicocca, P., 2006. Highlights on new food research. Dig. Liver Dis. 38, S295–S299.

Lavermicocca, P., Valerio, F., Lonigro, S.L., De Angelis, M., Morelli, L., Callegari, M.L., Rizzello, C.G., Visconti, A., 2005. Study of adhesion and survival of lactobacilli and bifidobacteria on table olives with the aim of formulating a new probiotic food. Appl. Environ. Microbiol. 71, 4233–4240.

Lin, J., Yu, W., Liu, X., Xie, H., Wang, W., Ma, X., 2008. In vitro and in vivo characterization of alginate-chitosan-alginate artificial microcapsules for therapeutic oral delivery of live bacterial cells. J. Biosci. Bioeng. 105, 660–665.

Liong, M.T., Easa, A.M., Lim, P.T., Kang, J.Y., 2009. Survival, growth characteristics and bioactive potential of *Lactobacillus acidophilus* in a soy-based cream cheese. J. Sci. Food Agric. 89, 1382–1391.

Lollo, P.C., Morato, P.N., Moura, C.S., Almada, C.N., Felicio, T.L., Esmerino, E.A., Barros, M.E., Amaya-Farfan, J., Sant'Ana, A.S., Raices, R.R., 2015. Hypertension parameters are attenuated by the continuous consumption of probiotic Minas cheese. Food Res. Int. 76, 611–617.

Lourens-Hattingh, A., Viljoen, B.C., 2001. Yogurt as probiotic carrier food. Int. Dairy J. 11, 1–17.

Lozupone, C.A., Stombaugh, J.I., Gordon, J.I., Jansson, J.K., Knight, R., 2012. Diversity, stability and resilience of the human gut microbiota. Nature 489, 220–230.

Luckow, T., Delahunty, C., 2004. Which juice is 'healthier'? A consumer study of probiotic non-dairy juice drinks. Food Qual. Preference 15, 751–759.

Mack, D.R., Michail, S., Wei, S., McDougall, L., Hollingsworth, M.A., 1999. Probiotics inhibit enteropathogenic *E. coli* adherence in vitro by inducing intestinal mucin gene expression. Am. J. Physiol. Gastrointest. Liver Physiol. 276, G941–G950.

Mäkeläinen, H., Forssten, S., Olli, K., Granlund, L., Rautonen, N., Ouwehand, A., 2009. Probiotic lactobacilli in a semi-soft cheese survive in the simulated human gastrointestinal tract. Int. Dairy J. 19, 675–683.

Mändar, R., Mikelsaar, M., 1996. Transmission of mother's microflora to the newborn at birth. Neonatology 69, 30–35.

Mantis, N.J., Rol, N., Corthésy, B., 2011. Secretory IgA's complex roles in immunity and mucosal homeostasis in the gut. Mucosal Immunol. 4, 603–611.

Maragkoudakis, P.A., Miaris, C., Rojez, P., Manalis, N., Magkanari, F., Kalantzopoulos, G., Tsakalidou, E., 2006. Production of traditional Greek yoghurt using lactobacillus strains with probiotic potential as starter adjuncts. Int. Dairy J. 16, 52–60.

Martın-Diana, A., Janer, C., Peláez, C., Requena, T., 2003. Development of a fermented goat's milk containing probiotic bacteria. Int. Dairy J. 13, 827–833.

Martín, R.O., Langa, S., Reviriego, C., Jiménez, E., Marín, M.A.L., Olivares, M., Boza, J., Jiménez, J., Fernández, L., Xaus, J., Rodríguez, J.M., 2004. The commensal microflora of human milk: new perspectives for food bacteriotherapy and probiotics. Trends Food Sci. Technol. 15, 121–127.

Matsumoto, K., Takada, T., Shimizu, K., Kado, Y., Kawakami, K., Makino, I., Yamaoka, Y., Hirano, K., Nishimura, A., Kajimoto, O., 2006. The effects of a probiotic milk product containing *Lactobacillus casei* strain Shirota on the defecation frequency and the intestinal microflora of sub-optimal health state volunteers: a randomized placebo-controlled cross-over study. Biosci. Microflora 25, 39–48.

Mayer, E.A., Tillisch, K., Gupta, A., 2015. Gut/brain axis and the microbiota. J. Clin. Invest. 125, 926–938.

McClements, D.J., Decker, E.A., Park, Y., Weiss, J., 2009. Structural design principles for delivery of bioactive components in nutraceuticals and functional foods. Critical Rev. Food Sci. Nutr. 49, 577–606.

McFarland, L.V., 2015. Probiotics for the primary and secondary prevention of *C. difficile* infections: a meta-analysis and systematic review. Antibiotics 4, 160–178.

McMaster, L., Kokott, S., Reid, S., Abratt, V., 2005. Use of traditional African fermented beverages as delivery vehicles for *Bifidobacterium lactis* DSM 10140. Int. J. Food Microbiol. 102, 231–237.

Millette, M., Nguyen, A., Amine, K.M., Lacroix, M., 2013. Gastrointestinal survival of bacteria in commercial probiotic products. Int. J. Probiotics Prebiotics 8, 149.

Morgun, A., Dzutsev, A., Dong, X., Greer, R.L., Sexton, D.J., Ravel, J., Schuster, M., Hsiao, W., Matzinger, P., Shulzhenko, N., 2015. Uncovering effects of antibiotics on the host and microbiota using transkingdom gene networks. Gut 64 (11), 1732–1743, gutjnl-2014-308820.

Mueller, N.T., Bakacs, E., Combellick, J., Grigoryan, Z., Dominguez-Bello, M.G., 2015. The infant microbiome development: mom matters. Trends Mol. Med. 21, 109–117.

Murphy, R., Stewart, A., Braithwaite, I., Beasley, R., Hancox, R., Mitchell, E., 2014. Antibiotic treatment during infancy and increased body mass index in boys: an international cross-sectional study. Int. J. Obes. 38, 1115–1119.

Nagpal, R., Kumar, A., Kumar, M., 2012a. Fortification and fermentation of fruit juices with probiotic lactobacilli. Ann. Microbiol. 62, 1573–1578.

Nagpal, R., Kumar, A., Kumar, M., Behare, P.V., Jain, S., Yadav, H., 2012b. Probiotics, their health benefits and applications for developing healthier foods: a review. FEMS Microbiol. Lett. 334, 1–15.

O'Mahony, S., Felice, V., Nally, K., Savignac, H., Claesson, M., Scully, P., Woznicki, J., Hyland, N., Shanahan, F., Quigley, E., 2014. Disturbance of the gut microbiota in early-life selectively affects visceral pain in adulthood without impacting cognitive or anxiety-related behaviors in male rats. Neuroscience 277, 885–901.

O'Mahony, S.M., Marchesi, J.R., Scully, P., Codling, C., Ceolho, A.-M., Quigley, E.M., Cryan, J.F., Dinan, T.G., 2009. Early life stress alters behavior, immunity, and microbiota in rats: implications for irritable bowel syndrome and psychiatric illnesses. Biol. Psychiatry 65, 263–267.

Ong, L., Henriksson, A., Shah, N., 2006. Development of probiotic cheddar cheese containing *Lactobacillus acidophilus*, *Lb. casei*, *Lb. paracasei* and *Bifidobacterium* spp. and the influence of these bacteria on proteolytic patterns and production of organic acid. Int. Dairy J. 16, 446–456.

Ong, L., Shah, N.P., 2009. Probiotic cheddar cheese: influence of ripening temperatures on survival of probiotic microorganisms, cheese composition and organic acid profiles. LWT Food Sci. Technol. 42, 1260–1268.

Ouwehand, A.C., Ibrahim, F., Forssten, S.D., 2010. Cheese as a carrier for probiotics: in vitro and human studies. Aust. J. Dairy Technol. 65, 165.

Penders, J., Kummeling, I., Thijs, C., 2011. Infant antibiotic use and wheeze and asthma risk: a systematic review and meta-analysis. Eur. Respir. J. 38, 295–302.

Penders, J., Thijs, C., Vink, C., Stelma, F.F., Snijders, B., Kummeling, I., van den Brandt, P.A., Stobberingh, E.E., 2006. Factors influencing the composition of the intestinal microbiota in early infancy. Pediatrics 118, 511–521.

Peres, C.M., Peres, C., Hernández-Mendoza, A., Malcata, F.X., 2012. Review on fermented plant materials as carriers and sources of potentially probiotic lactic acid bacteria–with an emphasis on table olives. Trends Food Sci Technol 26, 31–42.

Persaud, R., Azad, M.B., Konya, T., Guttman, D.S., Chari, R.S., Sears, M.R., Becker, A.B., Scott, J.A., Kozyrskyj, A.L., Investigators, C.S., 2014. Impact of perinatal antibiotic exposure on the infant gut microbiota at one year of age. Allergy Asthma Clin. Immunol. 10, A31.

Possemiers, S., Marzorati, M., Verstraete, W., Van de Wiele, T., 2010. Bacteria and chocolate: a successful combination for probiotic delivery. Int. J. Food Microbiol. 141, 97–103.

Poulin, J.-F., Caillard, R., Subirade, M., 2011. β-Lactoglobulin tablets as a suitable vehicle for protection and intestinal delivery of probiotic bacteria. Int. J. Pharm. 405, 47–54.

Power, S.E., O'Toole, P.W., Stanton, C., Ross, R.P., Fitzgerald, G.F., 2014. Intestinal microbiota, diet and health. Br. J. Nutr. 111, 387–402.

Qin, J., Li, R., Raes, J., Arumugam, M., Burgdorf, K.S., Manichanh, C., Nielsen, T., Pons, N., Levenez, F., Yamada, T., 2010. A human gut microbial gene catalogue established by metagenomic sequencing. Nature 464, 59–65.

Rampelli, S., Candela, M., Severgnini, M., Biagi, E., Turroni, S., Roselli, M., Carnevali, P., Donini, L., Brigidi, P., 2013. A probiotics-containing biscuit modulates the intestinal microbiota in the elderly. J. Nutr. Health Aging 17, 166–172.

Ranadheera, C.S., Evans, C., Adams, M., Baines, S., 2012. In vitro analysis of gastrointestinal tolerance and intestinal cell adhesion of probiotics in goat's milk ice cream and yogurt. Food Res. Int. 49, 619–625.

Ranadheera, R., Baines, S., Adams, M., 2010. Importance of food in probiotic efficacy. Food Res. Int. 43, 1–7.

Rautava, S., Arvilommi, H., Isolauri, E., 2006. Specific probiotics in enhancing maturation of IgA responses in formula-fed infants. Pediatr. Res. 60, 221–224.

Rea, M.C., Dobson, A., O'Sullivan, O., Crispie, F., Fouhy, F., Cotter, P.D., Shanahan, F., Kiely, B., Hill, C., Ross, R.P., 2011. Effect of broad- and narrow-spectrum antimicrobials on *Clostridium difficile* and microbial diversity in a model of the distal colon. Proc. Natl. Acad. Sci. 108, 4639–4644.

Roberts, C.L., Algert, C.S., Ford, J.B., Todd, A.L., Morris, J.M., 2012. Pathways to a rising caesarean section rate: a population-based cohort study. BMJ Open 2, e001725.

Rodrigues, A., Cara, D., Fretez, S., Cunha, F., Vieira, E., Nicoli, J., Vieira, L., 2000. *Saccharomyces boulardii* stimulates sIgA production and the phagocytic system of gnotobiotic mice. J. Appl. Microbiol. 89, 404–414.

Rodríguez, J.M., Murphy, K., Stanton, C., Ross, R.P., Kober, O.I., Juge, N., Avershina, E., Rudi, K., Narbad, A., Jenmalm, M.C., 2015. The composition of the gut microbiota throughout life, with an emphasis on early life. Microb. Ecol. Health Dis. 26.

Ross, R., Fitzgerald, G., Collins, K., Stanton, C., 2002. Cheese delivering biocultures–probiotic cheese. Aust. J. Dairy Technol. 57, 71.

Roueche, E., Serris, E., Thomas, G., Périer-Camby, L., 2006. Influence of temperature on the compaction of an organic powder and the mechanical strength of tablets. Powder Technol. 162, 138–144.

e Silva, J.S., Sousa, S.C., Costa, P., Cerdeira, E., Amaral, M.H., Lobo, J.S., Gomes, A.M., Pintado, M.M., Rodrigues, D., Rocha-Santos, T., 2013. Development of probiotic tablets using microparticles: viability studies and stability studies. AAPS PharmSciTech 14, 121–127.

Sanders, M.E., Marco, M.L., 2010. Food formats for effective delivery of probiotics. Food Sci. Technol. 1.

Sangeetha, P., Ramesh, M., Prapulla, S., 2005. Recent trends in the microbial production, analysis and application of fructooligosaccharides. Trends Food Sci. Technol. 16, 442–457.

Sanz, Y., 2007. Ecological and functional implications of the acid-adaptation ability of *Bifidobacterium*: a way of selecting improved probiotic strains. Int. Dairy J. 17, 1284–1289.

Saulnier, D.M., Gibson, G.R., Kolida, S., 2008. In vitro effects of selected synbiotics on the human faecal microbiota composition. FEMS Microbiol. Ecol. 66, 516–527.

Savino, F., Roana, J., Mandras, N., Tarasco, V., Locatelli, E., Tullio, V., 2011. Faecal microbiota in breast-fed infants after antibiotic therapy. Acta Paediatr. 100, 75–78.

Sekirov, I., Russell, S.L., Antunes, L.C.M., Finlay, B.B., 2010. Gut microbiota in health and disease. Physiol. Rev. 90, 859–904.

Sendra, E., Fayos, P., Lario, Y., Fernandez-Lopez, J., Sayas-Barbera, E., Perez-Alvarez, J.A., 2008. Incorporation of citrus fibers in fermented milk containing probiotic bacteria. Food Microbiol. 25, 13–21.

Sheehan, V.M., Ross, P., Fitzgerald, G.F., 2007. Assessing the acid tolerance and the technological robustness of probiotic cultures for fortification in fruit juices. Innovative Food Sci. Emerging Technol. 8, 279–284.

Slavin, J., 2013. Fiber and prebiotics: mechanisms and health benefits. Nutrients 5, 1417–1435.

Sofjan, R.P., Hartel, R.W., 2004. Effects of overrun on structural and physical characteristics of ice cream. Int. Dairy J. 14, 255–262.

Sreeja, V., Prajapati, J.B., 2013. Probiotic formulations: application and status as pharmaceuticals—a review. Probiotics Antimicrob. Proteins 5, 81–91.

Stadler, M., Viernstein, H., 2003. Optimization of a formulation containing viable lactic acid bacteria. Int. J. Pharm. 256, 117–122.

Stanton, C., Gardiner, G., Lynch, P., Collins, J., Fitzgerald, G., Ross, R., 1998. Probiotic cheese. Int. Dairy J. 8, 491–496.

Subramanian, S., Blanton, L.V., Frese, S.A., Charbonneau, M., Mills, D.A., Gordon, J.I., 2015. Cultivating healthy growth and nutrition through the gut microbiota. Cell 161, 36–48.

Tripathi, M., Giri, S., 2014. Probiotic functional foods: survival of probiotics during processing and storage. J. Funct. Foods 9, 225–241.

Tsen, J.H., Lin, Y.P., King, V., 2009. Response surface methodology optimisation of immobilised *Lactobacillus acidophilus* banana puree fermentation. Int. J. Food Sci. Technol. 44, 120–127.

Turnbaugh, P.J., Hamady, M., Yatsunenko, T., Cantarel, B.L., Duncan, A., Ley, R.E., Sogin, M.L., Jones, W.J., Roe, B.A., Affourtit, J.P., Egholm, M., Henrissat, B., Heath, A.C., Knight, R., Gordon, J.I., 2009. A core gut microbiome in obese and lean twins. Nature 457, 480–484.

Turnbaugh, P.J., Quince, C., Faith, J.J., McHardy, A.C., Yatsunenko, T., Niazi, F., Affourtit, J., Egholm, M., Henrissat, B., Knight, R., 2010. Organismal, genetic, and transcriptional variation in the deeply sequenced gut microbiomes of identical twins. Proc. Natl. Acad. Sci. 107, 7503–7508.

de Vos, P., Faas, M.M., Spasojevic, M., Sikkema, J., 2010. Encapsulation for preservation of functionality and targeted delivery of bioactive food components. Int. Dairy J. 20, 292–302.

Vinderola, C., Costa, G., Regenhardt, S., Reinheimer, J., 2002a. Influence of compounds associated with fermented dairy products on the growth of lactic acid starter and probiotic bacteria. Int. Dairy J. 12, 579–589.

Vinderola, C., Gueimonde, M., Delgado, T., Reinheimer, J., De Los Reyes-Gavilan, C., 2000. Characteristics of carbonated fermented milk and survival of probiotic bacteria. Int. Dairy J. 10, 213–220.

Vinderola, C., Mocchiutti, P., Reinheimer, J., 2002b. Interactions among lactic acid starter and probiotic bacteria used for fermented dairy products. J. Dairy Sci. 85, 721–729.

Vinderola, G., Prosello, W., Molinari, F., Ghiberto, D., Reinheimer, J., 2009. Growth of *Lactobacillus paracasei* A13 in Argentinian probiotic cheese and its impact on the characteristics of the product. Int. J. Food Microbiol. 135, 171–174.

Weng, M., Ganguli, K., Zhu, W., Shi, H.N., Walker, W.A., 2014. Conditioned medium from *Bifidobacteria infantis* protects against *Cronobacter sakazakii*-induced intestinal inflammation in newborn mice. Am. J. Physiol. Gastrointest. Liver Physiol. 306, G779–G787.

Wu, G.D., Chen, J., Hoffmann, C., Bittinger, K., Chen, Y.-Y., Keilbaugh, S.A., Bewtra, M., Knights, D., Walters, W.A., Knight, R., 2011. Linking long-term dietary patterns with gut microbial enterotypes. Science 334, 105–108.

Yoon, K.Y., Woodams, E.E., Hang, Y.D., 2004. Probiotication of tomato juice by lactic acid bacteria. J. Microbiol. (Seoul, Korea) 42, 315–318.

Yoon, K.Y., Woodams, E.E., Hang, Y.D., 2006. Production of probiotic cabbage juice by lactic acid bacteria. Biores. Technol. 97, 1427–1430.

Zhang, J., Wang, L., Guo, Z., Sun, Z., Gesudu, Q., Kwok, L., Zhang, H., 2014. 454 pyrosequencing reveals changes in the faecal microbiota of adults consuming *Lactobacillus casei* Zhang. FEMS Microbiol. Ecol. 88, 612–622.

Zoellner, S., Cruz, A., Faria, J., Bolini, H., Moura, M., Carvalho, L., Sant'ana, A., 2009. Whey beverage with acai pulp as a food carrier of probiotic bacteria. Aust. J. Dairy Technol. 64, 177.

Microbial Endocrinology: Context and Considerations for Probiotic Selection

M. Lyte

*Iowa State University, Department of Veterinary Microbiology and Preventive Medicine,
Ames, IA, United States*

HISTORICAL CONTEXT

It is often surprising to learn that what one considers to be a relatively new field, the term *microbial endocrinology*, first appearing in the literature in 1993 (Lyte, 1993), has in fact been around for a very long time. The consideration of past historical references, some of which date back to the early days of microbiology, should be viewed more than just a pure academic exercise; they not only provide important confirmatory data for what is presently being described but can also inform changes in current experimental design that may yield more translatable results. The first demonstration of a bacterium, and ostensibly what we now use today as a probiotic, to produce a neurochemical was shown in the early part of the 20th century. In 1937 a report describing the production of acetylcholine in "*Bact. acetylcholini*" was published (Habs, 1937–1938). It is interesting to note that the report described the isolation of bacteria capable of producing acetylcholine from the colon of white rats as well as from human feces (Habs, 1937–1938). It would be another 10 years until the detailed biochemical analysis of acetylcholine in a microorganism, *Lactobacillus plantarum*, would be described (Stephenson and Rowatt, 1947). These reports are not unique. The scientific literature contains numerous examples, as discussed in the following section, detailing the ability of a wide range of microorganisms to produce what otherwise would be thought of exclusively as mammalian in origin (Lyte, 2010). What is perhaps most surprising is that the use of neurochemical-secreting probiotics in influencing behavior through the microbiota-gut-brain axis was not envisioned until recently (Dinan et al., 2013; Lyte, 2011, 2014; Wall et al., 2014).

Note regarding definitions: Attempting to reconcile certain aspects of two seemingly distinct entities of study (ie, neurobiology and microbiology) requires clarifying the meaning and origin of mutually used terms. The use of the terms *neurotransmitter*, *neuromodulator*, and *neurohormone* are designations that are associated with neurobiology and not microbiology. These terms are deeply rooted in the language of neurobiology and do not have any counterparts in microbiology. A neurotransmitter, as defined in neurobiology, is a form of chemical communication between neurons in close proximity to one another. The extracellular space that physically separates one neuron from another is called a synaptic cleft. To allow communication between these two neurons, neurotransmitters are released by one neuron into this cleft to act upon the receptors of the recipient neuron. In this way neurotransmitters are chemical messengers that allow for the communication and potential propagation of signals between neurons. A neuromodulator is similar to a neurotransmitter, but it does not need to be released at a synaptic site and can act across longer distances and possibly through second messenger pathways. The term *neurohormone* specifically refers to neuroendocrine cell-produced signaling molecules that are secreted into the systemic circulation to effect an action at distant sites. Adding to the complexity of resolving a distinct terminology, any chemical may simultaneously be correctly described with more than one role; for example, a neurochemical (eg, norepinephrine) can both be a neurotransmitter and a neurohormone. Given that microorganisms can form communities, a case can be made that the local release by microbial cells within one community adjacent to another fulfills the requirement of a neurotransmitter. Likewise, release by one community in the cecum can have downstream effects on another microbial community in the colon, thus fulfilling a neurohormone-style definition.

Consensus does not currently exist across the disciplines of neurobiology and microbiology as to how these neurobiology-based terms should be applied within microbiology. As such, for the purpose of clarity and precision of meaning (and not incidentally simplicity), any chemical produced by a microorganism that is also recognized within neurobiology as a neurotransmitter, neuromodulator, or neurohormone in a mammalian system will be referred to in this chapter as simply a neurochemical. For a deeper understanding of the spectrum of biological activities in animals encompassing the role of neurochemicals in homeostasis and various disease pathologies, the reader is referred to any standard neuroendocrinology reference book, such as Fink et al. (2012).

MICROBIAL ENDOCRINOLOGY: RELEVANCE TO PROBIOTICS
CONCEPTUAL BASIS

Microbial endocrinology is defined as the study of the ability of microorganisms to produce and recognize neurochemicals that originate from either production by the microorganisms themselves or from within the host that they inhabit. As shown in Fig. 6.1, microbial endocrinology represents the intersection of the fields of microbiology and neurobiology.

Neurochemicals produced by probiotic microorganisms can potentially exert their effects on host immunological competence through neuroimmunological-mediated mechanisms or on host behavior through neurobehavioral mechanisms (Fig. 6.2). Although not shown in Fig. 6.2, neurochemicals secreted by probiotics can influence neighboring microbial communities that then can influence host physiology.

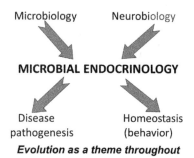

FIGURE 6.1 The conceptual basis of microbial endocrinology represents the intersection of microbiology and neurobiology and is based on the commonly shared neurochemicals that form the evolutionary basis of cell-to-cell communication in vertebrates.

(see text for in-depth discussion and references).

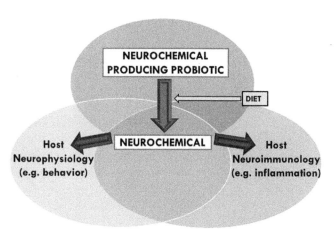

FIGURE 6.2 Microbial endocrinology-based mechanism by which neurochemical-producing probiotic can influence host.

As shown in figure, diet plays an important role in providing the necessary substrate(s) and cofactor(s) needed by the probiotic for the in vivo production of the neurochemical of interest (see text for more in-depth discussion).

In addition, although not specifically a point of discussion in this probiotics-focused chapter, host-produced neurochemicals that are secreted into the intestinal lumen can affect probiotic microorganisms; for example, the biogenic amine norepinephrine has been shown to increase the growth of certain probiotics such as *Lactobacillus acidophilus* ASF360 and *Streptococcus thermophilus* NCIMB 41,856 (Bailey et al., 2011). Because other biogenic amines, such as serotonin and dopamine, are also produced by the host and are present in the lumen of the intestinal tract (Eisenhofer et al., 1995, 1997; Eldrup and Richter, 2000), this observation further raises the issue of the ability of the host to influence the growth and presumably function of probiotics or commensal organisms.

It should also be noted that although the concept of microbial endocrinology, from a microbial species perspective, has been largely applied to bacteria, it also applies to other microorganisms, most notably yeasts. Given that yeasts constitute a significant fraction of the probiotics in use, their consideration from a microbial endocrinology-based perspective will be explored further here (for a more comprehensive review on yeasts and endocrinology see Clemons et al., 2010). Furthermore, the term *psychobiotics* has recently been coined to describe those probiotics that may have the capacity to produce a health benefit in patients suffering from psychiatric illness, potentially as a consequence of their production of neuroactive substances such as gamma-aminobutyric acid (GABA) and serotonin (Dinan et al., 2013). As such, psychobiotics operate via a microbial endocrinology-based mechanism.

That a microorganism, such as a probiotic bacterium or yeast, should be able to produce a neurochemical that is exactly the same as that found in mammalian systems may seem surprising; however, what are commonly considered to be exclusively vertebrate neurochemicals, and their cognate receptors, are, in fact, widely dispersed throughout nature from bacteria to plants and insects. There is a large body of literature documenting the presence of what otherwise would be considered exclusively mammalian neurochemicals in normal plant physiology extending from pollen germination to the stimulation of flowering (Kang et al., 2009; Roshchina, 2001). For example, stress responses in plants, such as tomatoes and potatoes, involves the production of the same catecholamines that are involved in the mammalian response to stress (Kulma and Szopa, 2007; Swiedrych et al., 2004; Von Roepenack-Lahaye et al., 2003). In addition to being identified in plants (Kulma and Szopa, 2007), neurochemicals such as norepinephrine have also been shown in insects (Pitman, 1971) and fish (Guerrero et al., 1990).

This wide prevalence in nature from plants to insects to vertebrates also includes microorganisms, both prokaryotic and eukaryotic. Both the range of neurochemicals and the variety of microorganisms in which they have been identified is very large (Lenard, 1992). Neurochemicals isolated from microorganisms, which have been demonstrated to show biological activity in mammalian cells, include serotonin (Sridharan et al., 2014); histamine (Landete et al., 2007b; Leuschner et al., 1998; Maijala, 1993; Masson et al., 1996; Thomas et al., 2012); catecholamines, such as norepinephrine and dopamine (Asano et al., 2012; Malikina et al., 2010; Ozogul, 2011; Shishov et al., 2009; Tsavkelova et al., 2000); agmatine (Arena and Manca de Nadra, 2001; Griswold et al., 2004; Raasch et al., 1995); corticotrophin (Janakidevi et al., 1966); somatostatin (LeRoith et al., 1985); progesterone (Schar et al., 1986); and GABA (Barrett et al., 2012; Hiraga et al., 2008; Ko et al., 2013; Komatsuzaki et al., 2005, 2008; Rizzello et al., 2008; Siragusa et al., 2007). A listing of some of the probiotic-specific genera and their associated neurochemical production is shown in Table 6.1. Numerous other neurochemicals identified by radioimmunoassay and chromatographic behavior, as well as the presence of their corresponding putative receptor(s), have also been demonstrated in various microorganisms (for reviews

Table 6.1 Diversity of Neurochemicals Isolated From Various Microbial Species

Genus	Neurochemical	References
Lactobacillus, Bifidobacterium	GABA	Barrett et al. (2012), Hiraga et al. (2008), Ko et al. (2013), Komatsuzaki et al. (2005, 2008), Rizzello et al. (2008), and Siragusa et al. (2007)
Escherichia, Bacillus, Saccharomyces, Serratia	Catecholamines: norepinephrine, dopamine	Asano et al. (2012), Malikina et al. (2010), Ozogul (2011), Shishov et al. (2009), and Tsavkelova et al. (2000)
Candida, Streptococcus, Escherichia, Enterococcus	Serotonin	Hurley et al. (1971), Ozogul (2011), and Shishov et al. (2009)
Escherichia, Streptococcus, Lactobacillus	Agmatine	Arena and Manca de Nadra (2001), Griswold et al. (2004), and Raasch et al. (1995)
Lactobacillus, Lactococcus, Streptococcus, Enterococcus	Histamine	Landete et al. (2007a,b), Leuschner et al. (1998), Maijala (1993), Masson et al. (1996), and Thomas et al. (2012)
Lactobacillus, Bacillus	Acetylcholine	Girvin and Stevenson (1954), Habs (1937–1938), Horiuchi et al. (2003), Kawashima et al. (2007), and Stephenson and Rowatt (1947)

As can be seen in the table, members of an individual genus are capable of producing more than one neurochemical. Additional references for specific neurochemicals can be found in text.

see Lenard, 1992; Roth et al., 1982). Investigators have debated the significance of such neurochemicals in microorganisms for decades. The most widely accepted theory concerns the use of such substances as a form of intercellular communication (Dohler, 1986; LeRoith et al., 1986). Indeed, studies have shown that the growth of colonies of *Escherichia coli* involves a high degree of specialization of function by individual bacteria (Budrene and Berg, 1995; Shapiro and Hsu, 1989) and presumably the need for some form of intercellular communication to accomplish this goal.

In light of this, the consideration of probiotics from a microbial endocrinology-based perspective led to the concept that they could function as therapeutic "drug delivery vehicles" with potential for the treatment or management of behavioral and other pathophysiological conditions (Lyte, 2011). Many psychoactive drugs, as well as others used to treat nonbehavioral issues, represent parent neurochemicals themselves or are a related analog of the same. Therefore it should not be considered inappropriate that live microorganisms that produce such chemicals are classified as neurochemical drug delivery vehicles not dissimilar to their pill-based counterparts (Lyte, 2011). Although the definition of a probiotic is that of a live microorganism, it may be argued that probiotic microorganisms that become nonviable, either after manufacture or ingestion, can still act as drug delivery vehicles because they can contain neurochemicals within their cell structure that may be released after their destruction by other microbes or by the host's digestive system. It is well accepted that live and nonviable microorganisms can be equally efficacious (Iannitti and Palmieri, 2010). Even the need to administer the probiotic itself to achieve a desired effect has been questioned because it has been demonstrated that simple administration of bacterial culture medium, in which the probiotic has been grown, is sufficient to achieve the same changes in colonic motility as the probiotic itself (Bar et al., 2009). As such, the amount of a neurochemical found within, or produced by, a probiotic microorganism is most likely sufficient to influence the localized immune and neurophysiological processes in the gut because immune and neuronal cells have been well documented to respond to nanomolar concentrations of mediators such as GABA (Barrett et al., 2012; Hiraga et al., 2008; Ko et al., 2013; Komatsuzaki et al., 2005, 2008; Rizzello et al., 2008; Siragusa et al., 2007). Therefore the delivery of neurochemicals by probiotics may represent the amount of neurochemical contained within the bacterium at the time of ingestion or of that which is actively produced once inside of the gastrointestinal tract. Thus, in delivering a neurochemical to a specific anatomical site in which various cellular processes are influenced, the utilization of neurochemical-containing or -producing probiotic bacteria can be viewed essentially as delivery vehicles for neuroactive compounds.

When considering the conceptual basis for the design of probiotics based on microbial endocrinology, the question of the degree of intestinal colonization after ingestion of the probiotic has important implications with respect to the physiological consequences on the host just as it does for the use of probiotics in general. Given the relatively poor ability of probiotic bacteria to successfully colonize large segments of the intestine, it is not surprising that increasing the daily frequency of probiotic ingestion increases the purported beneficial effects on physiological measures such as inflammation as well as for psychological measures such as anxiety-like behavior. This is wholly consistent with the microbial endocrinology-based theory of probiotics acting as delivery vehicles for neurochemicals because continued administration of a neurochemical that suppresses cytokine production (ie, GABA) would be expected to be more efficacious if administered multiple times over a defined time period rather than at a single time point. As such, the selection of probiotic strains that combine successful colonization with robust production of the desired neurochemical should be viewed as dual essential criteria in the design of any microbial delivery vehicle developed for in vivo applications. The possibility of establishing, within the intestinal environment, a neurochemical-secreting probiotic may offer substantial therapeutic benefit over more conventional drug dosing regimens because actively growing probiotic organisms would provide a continual supply of the neurochemical that would presumably avoid the peaks and troughs associated with per oral administered pharmacotherapy.

PROBIOTIC MICROORGANISMS KNOWN TO PRODUCE NEUROCHEMICALS

As discussed at the start of this chapter, the ability of probiotics to produce neurochemicals has been known for nearly a century. The genera range of probiotics is fairly extensive as shown in Table 6.1. This section provides a description of selective genera of probiotics and is meant to be illustrative of the capacity of probiotics to produce neurochemicals. For a more exhaustive discussion of the neurochemical-producing capacity of probiotics, the reader is also directed to recent excellent reviews on the subject of neurochemical production by microorganisms in general (Roshchina, 2010; Wall et al., 2014). In addition, there is an extensive food-based literature that has documented the ability of several genera, both bacterial and yeast, to produce neurochemicals in a food-based environment. Many of these studies concern the production of biogenic amines, such as histamine, that result from the use of microorganisms as starter cultures as part of the fermentative process involved in the production of foods and beverages (Karmas, 1981; Landete et al., 2007a; Moret et al., 1992; Silla Santos, 1996; Tarjan and Janossy, 1978). Because levels of certain biogenic amines, such as histamine, can reach toxic levels during the food manufacturing process, their presence must be monitored according to approved national standards to avoid cases of toxic food poisoning (Ienistea, 1971).

ESCHERICHIA

The most well-known probiotic belonging to this genus is *E. coli* Nissle 1917 (Bernstein, 2014; Trebichavsky et al., 2010). Originally isolated during World War I, *E. coli* Nissle 1917 has been used in numerous studies over the past decades with varying degrees of efficacy reported in the treatment of a wide range of gastrointestinal conditions (Bernstein, 2014). *E. coli* Nissle 1917 has also been demonstrated to enhance immune responsiveness in newborn infants (Cukrowska et al., 2002). Members belonging to the genus *Escherichia* have also been shown to possess the capacity for the production of the biogenic amines dopamine, norepinephrine, and epinephrine (Tsavkelova et al., 2000). This finding was also one of the reasons that the acquisition of neurochemical signaling pathways between cells has been proposed to have originated from late gene horizontal transfer (Iyer et al., 2004). As shown in Table 6.1, production of other neurochemicals such as serotonin (Shishov et al., 2009) has also been observed in various *Escherichia* spp. Dover and Halpern (1972) were among the first to describe the ability of *E. coli* K-12 to utilize GABA as their sole source of nitrogen. Although this obviously does not indicate production, but instead utilization, it nonetheless points out that bacteria can use substances more commonly associated with the mammalian nervous system for their own benefit. It also suggests that if a bacterium can utilize a specific substance, it may also have the capacity to produce it. Although the ability of *E. coli* Nissle 1917 to produce neurochemicals has not yet been reported, preliminary data obtained in our laboratory have shown that it is capable of producing several neurochemicals ranging from GABA to agmatine (Lyte, M., unpublished observations). It is interesting to note that the commercial production of GABA has been achieved through the use of a recombinant bacterium that expresses a glutamate decarboxylase gene obtained from *E. coli* (Takahashi et al., 2012). Furthermore, a putative role for utilization of GABA by pathogenic strains of *E. coli*, also shown in *Lactobacilli*, is to confer acid resistance in regions of the gastrointestinal tract with low pH (Richard and Foster, 2003).

Likewise, it is well recognized that agmatine can be utilized by several lactic acid bacteria, especially with regards to acid resistance (Arena et al., 2008; Lucas et al., 2007). The possible provision of agmatine by other bacterial genera has not been extensively examined, especially within the neuroscience community, although its bacterial origin is well known (Haenisch et al., 2008; Raasch et al., 1995).

LACTOBACILLI

As mentioned earlier, *Lactobacillus* spp. were among the first probiotics to be shown to produce large amounts of neurochemicals, specifically acetylcholine (Stephenson and Rowatt, 1947). Lactic acid bacteria are also well recognized histamine producers (Bover-Cid and Holzapfel, 1999; Coton et al., 1998). Recent work by Thomas et al. (2012) demonstrated that histamine production by *Lactobacillus reuteri* was sufficient to suppress inflammatory cytokine production in a Toll-like receptor-2–activated human monocytoid line. However, the most highly investigated neurochemical produced by *Lactobacilli* is unquestionably GABA. A recent report by Barrett et al. (2012) demonstrated the prodigious ability of various strains isolated from the human intestine, such as *Lactobacillus brevis*, to produce GABA from the added precursor substrate monosodium glutamate. What was very notable in this study was that this particular isolate of *L. brevis* was able to convert 100% of monosodium glutamate to GABA in a simple anaerobic fermentation.

The ability of Lactobacilli to produce large quantities of GABA has been utilized by food researchers as a means to create functional foods. Recently, a functional food study used the GABA-producing *L. brevis* FPA 3709 strain as a means to enrich black soybean milk with GABA, which was then fed to rats subjected to a forced swim test to assess depressive-like behavior (Ko et al., 2013). This study demonstrated that GABA-enriched soybean milk significantly reduced the immobility time before rats began to swim and was as effective as the antidepressant fluoxetine (Ko et al., 2013). This study provides suggestive evidence that the provision of a GABA-secreting probiotic could exert similar effects to those observed with the use of functional foods enriched with probiotic-derived neurochemicals. In another study, the ability of per oral fed *Lactobacillus rhamnosus* to reduce anxiety- and depressive-like behaviors in mice was associated with changes in central GABA receptor expression in the brain (Bravo et al., 2011). In particular, levels of $GABA_{A\alpha2}$ mRNA were altered in those brain regions associated with specific behaviors (Bravo et al., 2011). Furthermore, animals in which the vagus nerve (the longest of the cranial nerves that innervates the gut as well as other visceral organs) had been severed did not show any behavioral or brain GABA mRNA-related changes. This suggested that it was nerve signaling from the gut to the brain that was responsible for the observation of altered behavior in the animals fed *L. rhamnosus*. Although they did not quantify the amount of GABA produced by the administered *L. rhamnosus* strain, the demonstration of a mechanism, such as that mediated via alterations in central GABA receptor expression, provides evidence that probiotics may have the ability to influence behavior, potentially through a microbial endocrinology-based route.

SACCHAROMYCES

Although it may appear from a cursory examination of the literature that prokaryotic microorganisms, namely bacteria, constitute the overwhelming majority of publications dealing with the capacity of a microorganism to produce neurochemicals, this would be an incorrect impression. Eukaryotic microorganisms, chiefly yeasts, have been recognized for decades to possess the biochemical machinery to produce neurochemicals, including ones that are often surprising to learn about. For example, the production of melatonin by *Saccharomyces cerevisiae* during winemaking has been described (Rodriguez-Naranjo et al., 2013). Moreover, Malikina et al. (2010) demonstrated the ability of dopamine and serotonin to increase growth of *S. cerevisiae*.

OTHER BACTERIAL GENERA

As shown in Table 6.1, other bacterial genera have been reported to produce neurochemicals. These include *Bifidobacterium* spp., which has been shown to produce GABA (Barrett et al., 2012). Production of the catecholamine dopamine by *Bacillus* spp. and *Streptococcus* spp. has also been shown (Ozogul, 2011). As interest in the potential of probiotics to serve as a neurochemical delivery vehicle grows, the description of neurochemical production by other probiotics species will undoubtedly result in more comprehensive examination of neurochemical-producing capacity. Critical to these investigations will be consideration of the experimental issues that are discussed in the following section.

EXPERIMENTAL ISSUES ASSOCIATED WITH EVALUATION OF PROBIOTICS FOR NEUROCHEMICAL PRODUCTION
IN VITRO TESTING ISSUES

It should be appreciated that any investigation of the neurochemical-producing capacity of a probiotic microorganism cannot simply be determined by its evaluation in an off-the-shelf microbiological medium. One of the principal reasons for this is that different types of rich microbiological media will contain highly variable amounts of substrates and cofactors that can be used by the probiotic in the production of a wide array of neurochemicals. It is often surprising to learn that although the formulations of standardized media (eg, MRS and BHI) do not differ among companies, the actual composition can. This is because a number of the source ingredients, such as those of animal origin, have different suppliers and are often sourced from animals raised on different feeds in different countries. Side-by-side comparison of even simple medium, such as buffered peptone water, from different companies often reveals a wide variation in color. This implies that the concentration of neurochemical precursors and cofactors that are needed as part of the biochemical synthesis pathway for a particular neurochemical will vary greatly between companies and even between different batches from the same company, leading to incorrect conclusions concerning the ability of a probiotic to produce a particular neurochemical. Thus there is an excellent case to be made for the inclusion of defined media in the evaluation of probiotics and their ability to produce a particular neurochemical.

EXPERIMENTAL RUBRIC TO ADDRESS IN VITRO TO IN VIVO DESIGN ISSUES

An experimental rubric has been proposed by which the ability of a candidate probiotic to affect brain and behavior by a microbial endocrinology-based mechanism can be developed (Lyte, 2011). Unequivocal demonstration of such a neurochemical-based pathway is unquestionably the most important, and at the same time most difficult, of the experimental issues. To date there has been little, if any, scientific evidence to show that neurochemicals secreted by probiotics, or any other microorganism, can directly influence behavior. That is mainly because of the issue of correlation versus causation. The literature contains many well-designed probiotic studies that have demonstrated the ability of probiotic species to effect behavioral change in laboratory animal and human studies (Desbonnet et al., 2008; Mayer et al., 2015; Messaoudi et al., 2011; Petschow et al., 2013). Only a subset of these studies specifically examined the mechanisms by which probiotics could effect a change in behavior, and, of these, few, if any, specifically looked at a microbial endocrinology-based mechanism. This is not surprising given the exceedingly slow pace at which the recognition that such neurochemical-based production by probiotics has entered the scientific and medical spheres (discussed here and Lyte, 2010). Regardless, most probiotic-based studies on behavior have been largely, but certainly not exclusively, correlative in nature.

To conclusively demonstrate that a microbial endocrinology-based mechanism is operative, several experimental steps must be followed to conclusively demonstrate causation. To illustrate the steps shown in Table 6.2, GABA has been chosen as the prototypical example because it satisfies several of the fundamental requirements, including the ability of several probiotic species to produce large amounts under varying conditions such as by *Lactobacillus* and *Bifidobacterium* (Barrett et al., 2012; Hiraga et al., 2008; Ko et al., 2013; Komatsuzaki et al., 2005, 2008; Rizzello et al., 2008; Siragusa et al., 2007). The concentration of GABA produced, which is in the micro- to millimolar range, would undoubtedly effect activation of neuronal elements within the intestine and extraintestinally based on the GABA-related neurophysiology-based literature (Krantis, 2000). For example, in the production of fermented foodstuffs, such as Japanese funa-sushi and Chinese traditional *pao-cai*, which use lactobacilli as part of the manufacturing processing, GABA levels in the millimolar range have been demonstrated in the final products (Higuchi et al., 1997; Komatsuzaki et al., 2005; Li et al., 2008). Secondly, as the predominant inhibitory neurotransmitter in the nervous system, GABA also serves a receptor-mediated role in several immunological (Bjurstom et al., 2008) and intestinal neurophysiological (Krantis, 2000; Page et al., 2006) processes. Because dysregulation of such

Table 6.2 Microbial Endocrinology-Based Rubric to Evaluate Ability of Neurochemical-Producing Probiotics to Influence Behavior and/or Disease Pathobiology

Step	Purpose	Comments
1	Determine neurochemical of interest to be produced by probiotic based on desired physiological and/or behavioral effect in host.	Physiological and/or behavioral measures should be readily quantifiable. Measures that are receptor-based with known antagonists are preferred because they can subsequently be used at in vivo steps involving animal models. Do not rely solely on published metabolic pathways for candidate probiotics because these are often incomplete and have not been performed in more than one media (see text and below).
2	Screen candidate probiotic in vitro for neurochemical production using robust assay to determine if neurochemical of interest as well as other neurochemicals are produced.	More than one microbiological growth medium should be used. Targeted and quantifiable (not relative units because does not allow comparison over time) metabolomics assay preferred. If metabolomics is not an option (because of cost/availability), then enzyme-linked immunoabsorbent-based assay for single neurochemical may instead be used. However, it may miss production of other relevant neurochemicals. Preferred use of a medium that reflects the regional gut environment where probiotic may influence behavior (ie, adjacent to enteric nervous system–vagal route) and or disease pathology.
3	Define kinetics (ie, time-dependent achievable intra- and extracellular concentrations) of neurochemical production.	Identify in vitro growth conditions that result in sustained levels of neurochemical production throughout growth period. Utilize food-based substrates that can then be incorporated into diet to enable probiotic to have substrate(s) and cofactor(s) necessary for optimal in vivo production.
4	Obtain non-neurochemical producer mutant (either through in vitro screening or site-directed mutagenesis procedure).	A mutant that does not produce the neurochemical will provide critical control for in vivo experiments. Repeat all neurochemical production assays with mutant to ensure that not only neurochemical of interest is not produced but also any other neurochemical that may influence biological endpoints is also not produced.
5	Conduct time and dose-dependent per oral administration of neurochemical-producing probiotic using normal animals to determine ability of probiotic to produce neurochemical in vivo. Use vehicle-only animals as control.	Supplement diet with substrate(s) and cofactor(s) needed by probiotic to produce neurochemical of interest before and after probiotic administration to maximize potential for production of neurochemicals in vivo. Measure levels of neurochemical of interest in intestinal luminal fluid and plasma. Utilize both molecular and culture-based techniques to determine presence of probiotic in gastrointestinal tract to determine proximity of probiotic to area of interest that may mediate desired biological response. Perform gross pathology and immunohistopathology of relevant tissue and compare to control (vehicle-only) animals.

Continued

Table 6.2 Microbial Endocrinology-Based Rubric to Evaluate Ability of Neurochemical-Producing Probiotics to Influence Behavior and/or Disease Pathobiology—cont'd

Step	Purpose	Comments
6	Perform per oral administration of probiotic in an animal model that involves a neurochemical-responsive element.	Animal models of specific disease pathology or behavior are suitable candidates. Select dosage of neurochemical-secreting probiotic from prior step that is found to result in high and sustainable levels of neurochemical within the gut. If known receptor antagonists are available, then give antagonist to block neurochemical-responsive element of disease or behavioral process.
7	Perform control experiments utilizing per oral administration of mutant (non-neurochemical–secreting) probiotic.	Quantifiable changes in animal model that are obtained by administration of neurochemical-secreting probiotic in previous step should not be present (or at lower levels) with mutant strain.

Modified from Lyte, M., 2011. Probiotics function mechanistically as delivery vehicles for neuro-active compounds: microbial endocrinology in the design and use of probiotics. Bioessays 33, 574–581.

GABA-sensitive elements in the gut has often been implicated in the pathophysiology of intestinal diseases, such as inflammatory bowel disease (IBD), the potential use of a GABA-secreting probiotic to ameliorate a specific pathophysiological condition such as IBD makes for an ideal system in which to test the validity of the hypothesis.

In the Table 6.2 rubric, the guiding element is the initial selection of the neurochemical itself, such as GABA, and the desired physiological/behavioral endpoint, not the probiotic species. This is admittedly a clinically based approach that is more akin to the strategy used in drug development in which selection of the appropriate drug is based on what condition it is meant to treat. The choice of whether one formulation or another in which the drug can be obtained is secondary to first identifying the drug. This similarly applies to the choice of the probiotic meant to deliver the desired neurochemical to achieve the intended physiological/behavioral clinical outcome. This comment is not meant to be facetious but is only intended to acknowledge that the rationale behind the selection of one probiotic over another in any one study is often not clearly apparent.

Once the neurochemical of choice is identified, screening of candidate probiotics should begin utilizing appropriate in vivo and ex vivo model systems (steps 2 and 3, Table 6.2). Although static in vitro models are by far the easiest to perform, the use of more in vivo reflective systems, such as multistage fermenters (Mills et al., 2015), offers the possibility to study the candidate probiotic's ability to produce neurochemicals in a dynamic environment where multiple factors can be altered. These model gut systems (also referred to as batch culture fermentation) offer significant advantages over the more limited traditional system of single experimental vessels in which there is limited ability to add fresh substrate or real-time monitoring of growth. For example, in the batch culture system fresh substrate can be continually introduced and spent medium removed. This can simulate, in part, the intestinal environment following the digestion of food over time.

One of the most important aspects of evaluating probiotics for putative neurochemical production is to not screen for the neurochemical of interest but other neurochemicals as well. It should not be assumed that a case of "one probiotic-one neurochemical" exists. For example, probiotics belonging to *Lactobacilli* and *Bifidobacterium* have been shown to produce more neurochemicals than just GABA alone (Table 6.1). Metabolic maps only identify known pathways. Utilizing a targeted panel encompassing an array of neurochemicals can help identify the co-production of other neurochemicals by a probiotic. Such a targeted metabolomics panel that provides for quantitative determination of a range of neurochemicals has been utilized by our laboratory to demonstrate the ability of *L. reuteri* to produce a range of neurochemicals in defined and rich media (data not shown). The identification of a range of neurochemicals by a single probiotic microorganism presents a new set of issues because more than one neurophysiological target may be involved in the host response to the probiotic when administered in vivo. This would further complicate the demonstration of a unique, single mechanism being restricted to only one target.

Identifying a mutant of the candidate probiotic that does not produce the neurochemical of interest also represents an important part of the design rubric (step 4, Table 6.2). Such a non-neurochemical–producing mutant will serve as an in vivo control as part of the approach demonstrating that the observed neurophysiological/behavioral effect is indeed due to a microbial endocrinology-based mechanism. The in vitro identification of sets of high and non-GABA–producing probiotics could be performed using standard growth methodology combined with analysis of GABA production in place of the more involved generation of mutants by site-directed mutagenesis. The feasibility of finding high and non-GABA–producing isolates has already been reported in the case for *L. brevis* strains isolated from Chinese traditional *paocai* (Li et al., 2008). If the same behavioral endpoint is observed with the mutant as with the neurochemical-producing microbe, then a microbial endocrinology-based mechanism is likely not responsible for the observed effect.

In vivo testing (steps 5–7, Table 6.2) is designed to provide the quality of experimental results that will unequivocally demonstrate that neurochemical production by the probiotic is needed to obtain the desired behavioral or neurophysiological endpoint. These include measurement of the concentration of the neurochemical of interest in the intestinal luminal fluid and in the plasma before and after the administration of the probiotic (step 5, Table 6.2).

Use of animal models with specific disease pathology (step 6, Table 6.2), and with elements known to be responsive to modulation by a particular neurochemical, will allow for kinetic-based experiments testing dosage and timing of administration. For example, a gut inflammation model would provide for an ideal test of the microbial endocrinology-based mechanisms of action for probiotics. Once identified in step 1

(Table 6.2), candidate probiotic strains would then be administered to normal and preclinical disease-representative animal models (ie, dextran sulfate-induced colitis; Johansson et al., 2010). Changes in pathophysiology (eg, indices of gut inflammation in the context of IBD) could be coupled with assessment of neurochemical levels in the intestinal tract (Wikoff et al., 2009) and enumeration of numbers of probiotic bacteria in the lumen mucosa to establish a cause-and-effect relationship. An additional control shown in step 7 (Table 6.2) should be used to demonstrate that any observed endpoint is actually due to the production of the putative ascribed neurochemical by the probiotic. For example, a specific GABA receptor antagonist could be used before the introduction of the GABA-secreting probiotic to examine if the prior observed change in gut inflammation that occurred when the probiotic was given alone still occurred or not. Finally, if administration of the non-neurochemical–producing mutant in the animal model did not produce the same endpoint as that observed with the neurochemical-producing probiotic, it could then be concluded that a microbial endocrinology-based mechanism was responsible for the observed host effect.

DIETARY ISSUES

In an analogous manner to that previously described for the selection of media with which to identify candidate probiotic strains for the production of neurochemicals, a similar set of experimental issues are involved when the issue of diet is raised. From a biochemical synthesis standpoint, the in vivo production of neurochemicals by probiotics will be entirely dependent on the dietary intake of appropriate and adequate amounts of substrates and cofactors. One way to achieve this is through the design of the diet itself (ie, specific foods or food groups) or through supplementation of the diet with specific substrates/cofactors. Selection of the food and/or supplements that contain substrates and cofactors is a relatively easy process because the biochemical synthetic pathways for neurochemicals in mammals have been known for decades as well as the foods that contain the required substrates and cofactors. In this fashion the inclusion of these dietary elements should be considered as a "prebiotic" because they may result in "...specific changes, both in the composition and/or activity in the gastrointestinal microflora that confers benefits upon host well-being and health" (Roberfroid, 2007). However, the preceding quote only refers to prebiotics as those substances that originate from "...selectively fermented ingredients..." (Gibson et al., 2010). A recent editorial has called for a reconsideration of the definition of what constitutes a prebiotic that is not tied to terms such as *selective and specific* but should recognize more general attributes that take into consideration the growing body of knowledge concerning diet-microbiome-host interactions (Bindels et al., 2015).

Regardless, the recognition that diet itself is a powerful modulator of the microbiome is widely accepted (for review, see Scott et al., 2013). However, understanding how diet affects interactions among different bacterial species is still in its infancy. Although we may understand how one specific diet changes the microbiome, we do not yet understand how diet may drive members of one specific phylum to change the growth/activity of another. A recent example of this can be found in work by Strandwitz et al. (2014), who showed that production of GABA by one gut bacterial species is required for the growth of another. As described in this preliminary work, growth and subsequent isolation of the gut microbe *Flavonifractor* spp. from fecal matter were dependent on a neighboring GABA-producing bacterium, such as *Bacteroides fragilis*. This preliminary report suggests that production of any neurochemical by a probiotic may also affect neighboring microbial communities as well as the intended target in the host. Whether the consequences of a neurochemical-producing probiotic are beneficial or harmful for neighboring microbial communities in the gastrointestinal tract has yet to be investigated for any known probiotic. Much will depend on several factors, such as where in the gut the probiotic is primarily located (ie, luminal- or mucosal-associated). Neurochemical production associated with attachment to the gut mucosal surface will most likely ensure that the main beneficiary of such production by the probiotic will be the host. On the other hand, luminal production of a neurochemical will undoubtedly influence other microbial populations.

CONCLUDING THOUGHTS

The consideration of probiotics from the perspective of microbial endocrinology to influence the microbiota-gut-brain axis as first proposed in 2011 (Lyte, 2011) offers considerable opportunities to effect host physiological and behavioral changes that may influence host health and pathophysiology of certain disease states. However, given the lack of extensive in vivo studies that specifically select probiotics based on their neurochemical-producing capacity as well as considering the dietary provision of substrates and cofactors necessary for the probiotic, it is not surprising that the full clinical potential is not yet understood or fully realized. Considering the growing publications addressing the neurochemical capacity of microorganisms in general, and probiotics in particular, for impacting the microbiota-gut-brain axis (for review see Lyte and Cryan, 2014), this hopefully will change in the foreseeable future.

REFERENCES

Arena, M.E., Landete, J.M., Manca de Nadra, M.C., Pardo, I., Ferrer, S., 2008. Factors affecting the production of putrescine from agmatine by *Lactobacillus hilgardii* XB isolated from wine. J. Appl. Microbiol. 105, 158–165.

Arena, M.E., Manca de Nadra, M.C., 2001. Biogenic amine production by *Lactobacillus*. J. Appl. Microbiol. 90, 158–162.

Asano, Y., Hiramoto, T., Nishino, R., Aiba, Y., Kimura, T., Yoshihara, K., Koga, Y., Sudo, N., 2012. Critical role of gut microbiota in the production of biologically active, free catecholamines in the gut lumen of mice. Am. J. Physiol. Gastrointest. Liver Physiol. 303, G1288–G1295.

Bailey, J.R., Probert, C.S., Cogan, T.A., 2011. Identification and characterisation of an iron-responsive candidate probiotic. PLoS One 6, e26507.

Bar, F., Von Koschitzky, H., Roblick, U., Bruch, H.P., Schulze, L., Sonnenborn, U., Bottner, M., Wedel, T., 2009. Cell-free supernatants of *Escherichia coli* Nissle 1917 modulate human colonic motility: evidence from an in vitro organ bath study. Neurogastroenterol. Motil. 21, 559–566, e516–e557.

Barrett, E., Ross, R.P., O'Toole, P.W., Fitzgerald, G.F., Stanton, C., 2012. gamma-Aminobutyric acid production by culturable bacteria from the human intestine. J. Appl. Microbiol. 113, 411–417.

Bernstein, C.N., 2014. Antibiotics, probiotics and prebiotics in IBD. Nestle Nutr. Inst. Workshop Ser. 79, 83–100.

Bindels, L.B., Delzenne, N.M., Cani, P.D., Walter, J., 2015. Towards a more comprehensive concept for prebiotics. Nat. Rev. Gastroenterol. Hepatol. 12 (5), 303–310.

Bjurstom, H., Wang, J., Ericsson, I., Bengtsson, M., Liu, Y., Kumar-Mendu, S., Issazadeh-Navikas, S., Birnir, B., 2008. GABA, a natural immunomodulator of T lymphocytes. J. Neuroimmunol. 205, 44–50.

Bover-Cid, S., Holzapfel, W.H., 1999. Improved screening procedure for biogenic amine production by lactic acid bacteria. Int. J. Food Microbiol. 53, 33–41.

Bravo, J.A., Forsythe, P., Chew, M.V., Escaravage, E., Savignac, H.M., Dinan, T.G., Bienenstock, J., Cryan, J.F., 2011. Ingestion of *Lactobacillus* strain regulates emotional behavior and central GABA receptor expression in a mouse via the vagus nerve. Proc. Natl. Acad. Sci. U.S.A. 108, 16050–16055.

Budrene, E.O., Berg, H.C., 1995. Dynamics of formation of symmetrical patterns by chemotactic bacteria. Nature 376, 49–53.

Clemons, K.V., Shankar, J., Stevens, D.A., 2010. Mycologic endocrinology. In: Lyte, M., Freestone, P.P.E. (Eds.), Microbial Endocrinology. Interkingdom Signaling in Infectious Disease and Health. Springer, New York, pp. 269–290.

Coton, E., Rollan, G., Bertrand, A., Lonvaud-Funel, A., 1998. Histamine producing lactic acid bacteria: early detection, frequency and distribution. Am. J. Enol. Vitic. 49, 199–204.

Cukrowska, B., LodInova-ZadnIkova, R., Enders, C., Sonnenborn, U., Schulze, J., Tlaskalova-Hogenova, H., 2002. Specific proliferative and antibody responses of premature infants to intestinal colonization with nonpathogenic probiotic *E. coli* strain Nissle 1917. Scand. J. Immunol. 55, 204–209.

Desbonnet, L., Garrett, L., Clarke, G., Bienenstock, J., Dinan, T.G., 2008. The probiotic *Bifidobacteria infantis*: an assessment of potential antidepressant properties in the rat. J. Psychiatr. Res. 43, 164–174.

Dinan, T.G., Stanton, C., Cryan, J.F., 2013. Psychobiotics: a novel class of psychotropic. Biol. Psychiatry 74 (10), 720–726.

Dohler, K.D., 1986. Development of hormone receptors: conclusion. Experientia 42, 788–794.

Dover, S., Halpern, Y.S., 1972. Control of the pathway of γ-aminobutyrate breakdown in *Escherichia coli* K-12. J. Bacteriol. 110, 165–170.

Eisenhofer, G., Aneman, A., Friberg, P., Hooper, D., Fandriks, L., Lonroth, H., Hunyady, B., Mezey, E., 1997. Substantial production of dopamine in the human gastrointestinal tract. J. Clin. Endocrinol. Metab. 82, 3864–3871.

Eisenhofer, G., Aneman, A., Hooper, D., Holmes, C., Goldstein, D.S., Friberg, P., 1995. Production and metabolism of dopamine and norepinephrine in mesenteric organs and liver of swine. Am. J. Physiol. 268, G641–G649.

Eldrup, E., Richter, E.A., 2000. DOPA, dopamine, and DOPAC concentrations in the rat gastrointestinal tract decrease during fasting. Am. J. Physiol. Endocrinol. Metab. 279, E815–E822.

Fink, G., Pfaff, D.W., Levine, J.E., 2012. Handbook of Neuroendocrinology, first ed. Academic Press/Elsevier, Amsterdam; Boston.

Gibson, G.R., Scott, K.P., Rastall, R.A., Tuohy, K.M., Hotchkiss, A., Dubert-Ferrandon, A., Gareau, M., Murphy, E.F., Saulnier, D., Loh, G., Macfarlane, S., Delzenne, N., Ringel, Y., Kozianowski, G., Dickman, R., Lenoir-Wijnkoop, I., Walker, C., Buddington, R., 2010. Dietary prebiotics: current status and new definition. Food Sci. Technol. Bull. Funct. Foods 7, 1–19.

Girvin, G.T., Stevenson, J.W., 1954. Cell free choline acetylase from *Lactobacillus plantarum*. Can. J. Biochem. Physiol. 32, 131–146.

Griswold, A.R., Chen, Y.Y., Burne, R.A., 2004. Analysis of an agmatine deiminase gene cluster in *Streptococcus mutans* UA159. J. Bacteriol. 186, 1902–1904.

Guerrero, H.Y., Caceres, G., Paiva, C.L., Marcano, D., 1990. Hypothalamic and telencephalic catecholamine content in the brain of the teleost fish, *Pygocentrus notatus*, during the annual reproductive cycle. Gen. Comp. Endocrinol. 80, 257–263.

Habs, H., 1937–1938. Untersuchungen uber das *Bact. acetylcholini*. II. Die Stellung des *Bact. acetylcholini* im System der Bakterien. Zbl. Bact. 97, 194–200.

Haenisch, B., von Kugelgen, I., Bonisch, H., Gothert, M., Sauerbruch, T., Schepke, M., Marklein, G., Hofling, K., Schroder, D., Molderings, G.J., 2008. Regulatory mechanisms underlying agmatine homeostasis in humans. Am. J. Physiol. Gastrointest. Liver Physiol. 295, G1104–G1110.

Higuchi, T., Hayashi, H., Abe, K., 1997. Exchange of glutamate and gamma-aminobutyrate in a *Lactobacillus* strain. J. Bacteriol. 179, 3362–3364.

Hiraga, K., Ueno, Y., Oda, K., 2008. Glutamate decarboxylase from *Lactobacillus brevis*: activation by ammonium sulfate. Biosci. Biotechnol. Biochem. 72, 1299–1306.

Horiuchi, Y., Kimura, R., Kato, N., Fujii, T., Seki, M., Endo, T., Kato, T., Kawashima, K., 2003. Evolutional study on acetylcholine expression. Life Sci. 72, 1745–1756.

Hurley, R., Leask, B.G., Ruthven, C.R., Sandler, M., Southgate, J., 1971. Investigation of 5-hydroxytryptamine production by *Candida albicans in vitro* and *in vivo*. Microbios 4, 133–143.

Iannitti, T., Palmieri, B., 2010. Therapeutical use of probiotic formulations in clinical practice. Clin. Nutr. 29, 701–725.

Ienistea, C., 1971. Bacterial production and destruction of histamine in foods, and food poisoning caused by histamine. Nahrung 15, 109–113.

Iyer, L.M., Aravind, L., Coon, S.L., Klein, D.C., Koonin, E.V., 2004. Evolution of cell-cell signaling in animals: did late horizontal gene transfer from bacteria have a role? Trends Genet. 20, 292–299.

Janakidevi, K., Dewey, V.C., Kidder, G.W., 1966. The biosynthesis of catecholamines in two genera of protozoa. J. Biol. Chem. 241, 2576–2578.

Johansson, M.E., Gustafsson, J.K., Sjoberg, K.E., Petersson, J., Holm, L., Sjovall, H., Hansson, G.C., 2010. Bacteria penetrate the inner mucus layer before inflammation in the dextran sulfate colitis model. PLoS One 5, e12238.

Kang, K., Park, S., Kim, Y.S., Lee, S., Back, K., 2009. Biosynthesis and biotechnological production of serotonin derivatives. Appl. Microbiol. Biotechnol. 83, 27–34.

Karmas, E., 1981. Biogenic amines as indicators of seafood freshness. Food Sci. Technol. 5, 108–109.

Kawashima, K., Misawa, H., Moriwaki, Y., Fujii, Y.X., Fujii, T., Horiuchi, Y., Yamada, T., Imanaka, T., Kamekura, M., 2007. Ubiquitous expression of acetylcholine and its biological functions in life forms without nervous systems. Life Sci. 80, 2206–2209.

Ko, C.Y., Lin, H.-T.V., Tsai, G.J., 2013. Gamma-aminobutyric acid production in black soybean milk by *Lactobacillus brevis* FPA 3709 and the antidepressant effect of the fermented product on a forced swimming rat model. Process Biochem. 48, 559–568.

Komatsuzaki, N., Nakamura, T., Kimura, T., Shima, J., 2008. Characterization of glutamate decarboxylase from a high gamma-aminobutyric acid (GABA)-producer, *Lactobacillus paracasei*. Biosci. Biotechnol. Biochem. 72, 278–285.

Komatsuzaki, N., Shima, J., Kawamoto, S., Momose, H., Kimura,. T., 2005. Production of gamma-aminobutyric acid (GABA) by *Lactobacillus paracasei* isolated from traditional fermented foods. Food Microbiol. 22, 497–504.

Krantis, A., 2000. GABA in the mammalian enteric nervous system. News Physiol. Sci. 15, 284–290.

Kulma, A., Szopa, J., 2007. Catecholamines are active compounds in plants. Plant Sci. 172, 433–440.

Landete, J.M., de Las Rivas, B., Marcobal, A., Munoz, R., 2007a. Molecular methods for the detection of biogenic amine-producing bacteria on foods. Int. J. Food Microbiol. 117, 258–269.

Landete, J.M., Ferrer, S., Pardo, I., 2007b. Biogenic amine production by lactic acid bacteria, acetic bacteria and yeast isolated from wine. Food Control 18, 1569–1574.

Lenard, J., 1992. Mammalian hormones in microbial cells. Trends Biochem. Sci. 17, 147–150.

LeRoith, D., Pickens, W., Vinik, A.I., Shiloach, J., 1985. *Bacillus subtilis* contains multiple forms of somatostatin-like material. Biochem. Biophys. Res. Commun. 127, 713–719.

LeRoith, D., Roberts, C.J., Lesniak, M.A., Roth, J., 1986. Receptors for intercellular messenger molecules in microbes: similarities to vertebrate receptors and possible implications for diseases in man. Experientia 42, 782–788.

Leuschner, R.G., Heidel, M., Hammes, W.P., 1998. Histamine and tyramine degradation by food fermenting microorganisms. Int. J. Food Microbiol. 39, 1–10.

Li, H.X., Gao, D.D., Cao, Y.S., Xu, H.Y., 2008. A high gamma-aminobutyric acid-producing *Lactobacillus brevis* isolated from Chinese traditional paocai. Ann. Microbiol. 58, 649–653.

Lucas, P.M., Blancato, V.S., Claisse, O., Magni, C., Lolkema, J.S., Lonvaud-Funel, A., 2007. Agmatine deiminase pathway genes in *Lactobacillus brevis* are linked to the tyrosine decarboxylation operon in a putative acid resistance locus. Microbiology 153, 2221–2230.

Lyte, M., 1993. The role of microbial endocrinology in infectious disease. J. Endocrinol. 137, 343–345.

Lyte, M., 2010. Microbial endocrinology: a personal journey. In: Lyte, M., Freestone, P.P.E. (Eds.), Microbial Endocrinology: Interkingdom Signaling in Infectious Disease and Health. Springer, New York, pp. 1–16.

Lyte, M., 2011. Probiotics function mechanistically as delivery vehicles for neuroactive compounds: microbial endocrinology in the design and use of probiotics. Bioessays 33, 574–581.

Lyte, M., 2014. Microbial endocrinology and the microbiota-gut-brain axis. Adv. Exp. Med. Biol. 817, 3–24.

Lyte, M., Cryan, J.F., 2014. Microbial Endocrinology: The Microbiota-gut-brain axis in Health and Disease. Springer, New York.

Maijala, R.L., 1993. Formation of histamine and tyramine by some lactic acid bacteria in MRS-broth and modified decarboxylation agar. Lett. Appl. Microbiol. 17, 40–43.

Malikina, K.D., Shishov, V.A., Chuvelev, D.I., Kudrin, V.S., Oleskin, A.V., 2010. [Regulatory role of monoamine neurotransmitters in *Saccharomyces cerevisiae* cells]. Prikl. Biokhim. Mikrobiol. 46, 672–677.

Masson, F., Talon, R., Montel, M.C., 1996. Histamine and tyramine production by bacteria from meat products. Int. J. Food Microbiol. 32, 199–207.

Mayer, E.A., Tillisch, K., Gupta, A., 2015. Gut/brain axis and the microbiota. J. Clin. Investig. 125, 926–938.

Messaoudi, M., Lalonde, R., Violle, N., Javelot, H., Desor, D., Nejdi, A., Bisson, J.F., Rougeot, C., Pichelin, M., Cazaubiel, M., Cazaubiel, J.M., 2011. Assessment of psychotropic-like properties of a probiotic formulation (*Lactobacillus helveticus* R0052 and *Bifidobacterium longum* R0175) in rats and human subjects. Br. J. Nutr. 105, 755–764.

Mills, C.E., Tzounis, X., Oruna-Concha, M.J., Mottram, D.S., Gibson, G.R., Spencer, J.P., 2015. In vitro colonic metabolism of coffee and chlorogenic acid results in selective changes in human faecal microbiota growth. Br. J. Nutr. 1–8.

Moret, S., Bortolomeazzi, R., Lercker, G., 1992. Improvement of extraction procedure for biogenic amines in foods and their high-performance liquid chromatographic determination. J. Chromatogr. 591, 175–180.

Ozogul, F., 2011. Effects of specific lactic acid bacteria species on biogenic amine production by foodborne pathogens. Int. J. Food Sci. Technol. 46, 478–484.

Page, A.J., O'Donnell, T.A., Blackshaw, L.A., 2006. Inhibition of mechanosensitivity in visceral primary afferents by GABAB receptors involves calcium and potassium channels. Neuroscience 137, 627–636.

Petschow, B., Dore, J., Hibberd, P., Dinan, T., Reid, G., Blaser, M., Cani, P.D., Degnan, F.H., Foster, J., Gibson, G., Hutton, J., Klaenhammer, T.R., Ley, R., Nieuwdorp, M., Pot, B., Relman, D., Serazin, A., Sanders, M.E., 2013. Probiotics, prebiotics, and the host microbiome: the science of translation. Ann. N.Y. Acad. Sci. 1306, 1–17.

Pitman, R.M., 1971. Transmitter substances in insects: a review. Comp. Gen. Pharmacol. 2, 347–371.

Raasch, W., Regunathan, S., Li, G., Reis, D.J., 1995. Agmatine, the bacterial amine, is widely distributed in mammalian tissues. Life Sci. 56, 2319–2330.

Richard, H.T., Foster, J.W., 2003. Acid resistance in *Escherichia coli*. Adv. Appl. Microbiol. 52, 167–186.

Rizzello, C.G., Cassone, A., Di Cagno, R., Gobbetti, M., 2008. Synthesis of angiotensin I-converting enzyme (ACE)-inhibitory peptides and gamma-aminobutyric acid (GABA) during sourdough fermentation by selected lactic acid bacteria. J. Agric. Food Chem. 56, 6936–6943.

Roberfroid, M., 2007. Prebiotics: the concept revisited. J. Nutr. 137, 830S–837S.

Rodriguez-Naranjo, M.I., Ordonez, J.L., Callejon, R.M., Cantos-Villar, E., Garcia-Parrilla, M.C., 2013. Melatonin is formed during winemaking at safe levels of biogenic amines. Food Chem. Toxicol. 57, 140–146.

Roshchina, V.V., 2001. Neurotransmitters in Plant Life. Science Publishers, Enfield, (NH).

Roshchina, V.V., 2010. Evolutionary considerations of neurotransmitters in microbial, plant and animal cells. In: Lyte, M., Freestone, P.P. (Eds.), Microbial Endocrinology: Interkingdom Signaling in Infectious Disease and Health. Springer, New York, pp. 17–52.

Roth, J., LeRoith, D., Shiloach, J., Rosenzweig, J.L., Lesniak, M.A., Havrankova, J., 1982. The evolutionary origins of hormones, neurotransmitters, and other extracellular chemical messengers: implications for mammalian biology. N. Engl. J. Med. 306, 523–527.

Schar, G., Stover, E.P., Clemons, K.V., Feldman, D., Stevens, D.A., 1986. Progesterone binding and inhibition of growth in *Trichophyton mentagrophytes*. Infect. Immun. 52, 763–767.

Scott, K.P., Gratz, S.W., Sheridan, P.O., Flint, H.J., Duncan, S.H., 2013. The influence of diet on the gut microbiota. Pharmacol. Res. 69, 52–60.

Shapiro, J.A., Hsu, C., 1989. *Escherichia coli* K-12 cell–cell interactions seen by time-lapse video. J. Bacteriol. 171, 5963–5974.

Shishov, V.A., Kirovskaia, T.A., Kudrin, V.S., Oleskin, A.V., 2009. [Amine neuromediators, their precursors, and oxidation products in the culture of *Escherichia coli* K-12]. Prikl. Biokhim. Mikrobiol. 45, 550–554.

Silla Santos, M.H., 1996. Biogenic amines: their importance in foods. Int. J. Food Microbiol. 29, 213–231.

Siragusa, S., De Angelis, M., Di Cagno, R., Rizzello, C.G., Coda, R., Gobbetti, M., 2007. Synthesis of gamma-aminobutyric acid by lactic acid bacteria isolated from a variety of Italian cheeses. Appl. Environ. Microbiol. 73, 7283–7290.

Sridharan, G.V., Choi, K., Klemashevich, C., Wu, C., Prabakaran, D., Pan, L.B., Steinmeyer, S., Mueller, C., Yousofshahi, M., Alaniz, R.C., Lee, K., Jayaraman, A., 2014. Prediction and quantification of bioactive microbiota metabolites in the mouse gut. Nat. Commun. 5, 5492.

Stephenson, M., Rowatt, E., 1947. The production of acetylcholine by a strain of *Lactobacillus plantarum*. J. Gen. Microbiol. 1, 279–298.

Strandwitz, P., Kim, K.-H., Stewart, E., Clardy, J., Lewis, K., 2014. GABA Modulating Bacteria in the Human Gut Microbiome, RISE:2014. Abstract ID#: 417. Northeastern University.

Swiedrych, A., Lorenc-Kukula, K., Skirycz, A., Szopa, J., 2004. The catecholamine biosynthesis route in potato is affected by stress. Plant Physiol. Biochem. 42, 593–600.

Takahashi, C., Shirakawa, J., Tsuchidate, T., Okai, N., Hatada, K., Nakayama, H., Tateno, T., Ogino, C., Kondo, A., 2012. Robust production of gamma-amino butyric acid using recombinant *Corynebacterium glutamicum* expressing glutamate decarboxylase from *Escherichia coli*. Enzyme Microb. Technol. 51, 171–176.

Tarjan, V., Janossy, G., 1978. The role of biogenic amines in foods. Nahrung 22, 285–289.

Thomas, C.M., Hong, T., van Pijkeren, J.P., Hemarajata, P., Trinh, D.V., Hu, W., Britton, R.A., Kalkum, M., Versalovic, J., 2012. Histamine derived from probiotic *Lactobacillus reuteri* suppresses TNF via modulation of PKA and ERK signaling. PLoS One 7, e31951.

Trebichavsky, I., Splichal, I., Rada, V., Splichalova, A., 2010. Modulation of natural immunity in the gut by *Escherichia coli* strain Nissle 1917. Nutr. Rev. 68, 459–464.

Tsavkelova, E.A., Botvinko, I.V., Kudrin, V.S., Oleskin, A.V., 2000. Detection of neurotransmitter amines in microorganisms with the use of high-performance liquid chromatography. Dokl. Biochem. 372, 115–117.

Von Roepenack-Lahaye, E., Newman, M.A., Schornack, S., Hammond-Kosack, K.E., Lahaye, T., Jones, J.D., Daniels, M.J., Dow, J.M., 2003. p-Coumaroylnoradrenaline, a novel plant metabolite implicated in tomato defense against pathogens. J. Biol. Chem. 278, 43373–43383.

Wall, R., Cryan, J.F., Ross, R.P., Fitzgerald, G.F., Dinan, T.G., Stanton, C., 2014. Bacterial neuroactive compounds produced by psychobiotics. Adv. Exp. Med. Biol. 817, 221–239.

Wikoff, W., Anfora, A., Liu, J., Schultz, P., Lesley, S., Peters, E., Siuzdak, G., 2009. Metabolomics analysis reveals large effects of gut microflora on mammalian blood metabolites. Proc. Natl. Acad. Sci. U.S.A. 106, 3698–3703.

Germ-Free Animals: A Key Tool in Unraveling How the Microbiota Affects the Brain and Behavior

P. Luczynski, K.A. McVey Neufeld
University College Cork, APC Microbiome Institute, Cork, Ireland

G. Clarke, T.G. Dinan
*University College Cork, APC Microbiome Institute, Cork, Ireland; University College Cork,
Department of Psychiatry and Neurobehavioural Science, Cork, Ireland*

J.F. Cryan
*University College Cork, APC Microbiome Institute, Cork, Ireland; University College Cork,
Department of Anatomy and Neuroscience, Cork, Ireland*

INTRODUCTION

Humans coexist in a mutualistic relationship with trillions of microorganisms, collectively known as the microbiota. These microorganisms can be found on all body surfaces, including the gastrointestinal (GI) tract, skin, oral cavity, nasal passages, and urogenital tract (Costello et al., 2009). The microbiota is not limited to bacteria. It also includes protozoa, fungi, nematodes, and viruses. Research examining the relationship between these microorganisms and their host has largely focused on those living within the intestinal tract and encompass more than 1000 bacterial species totaling approximately 100 trillion organisms (Frank and Pace, 2008). The gut microbiome, all genes present in the microorganisms colonizing the GI tract, encodes more than 3.3 million nonredundant genes; 150 times more genes than the human host genome (Qin et al., 2010). The gut microbiota is well known to be critical for processes such as digestion (Hooper and Gordon, 2001), immune responses (Bäckhed et al., 2005; Hooper and Macpherson, 2010), the absorption of nutrients (Hooper and Gordon, 2001), and growth (Nicholson et al., 2012). There is now a rapidly growing body of evidence supporting the view that these commensal microorganisms also affect the development of the CNS (Collins et al., 2012; Cryan and Dinan, 2012; Dinan and Cryan, 2012; Foster and Neufeld, 2013; Rhee et al., 2009; Sampson and Mazmanian, 2015).

The Gut-Brain Axis. http://dx.doi.org/10.1016/B978-0-12-802304-4.00007-4

COMMUNICATION ALONG THE MICROBIOTA-GUT-BRAIN AXIS

Although the bidirectional communication of the microbiota-gut-brain axis has been well established preclinically and clinically (Mayer, 2000; Rhee et al., 2009; Bercik, 2011; Cryan and OMahony, 2011), the exact mechanisms by which this communication occurs are largely unknown but are slowly being elucidated. Several systems are simultaneously likely to be involved in the transmission of information between microbiota and brain, with research focusing on autonomic and enteric nervous systems (ENS), immune, and endocrine pathways (Cryan and Dinan, 2012; El Aidy et al., 2015; Foster and Neufeld, 2013; Mayer et al., 2015). All of these systems have been shown to be directly affected by intestinal microbial status, and each in turn exhibit alterations in models of microbiota-gut-brain dysfunction. The human gut is innervated by approximately 50,000 extrinsic sensory neurons and 100 million intrinsic afferent neurons (Blackshaw et al., 2007; Furness, 2006). Given this level of innervation, it is perhaps not surprising that neural pathways are one of the major routes of communication between the gut and the brain. Preclinical work examining the importance of the vagal nerve for microbiota and gut-to-brain communication seems to be largely dependent on the specific bacterial species under investigation. However, in addition to this vagal pathway (Bercik et al., 2011b; Bravo et al., 2011; Lyte et al., 2006), vagal-independent communication also occurs (Bercik et al., 2010, 2011a). The neurons of the ENS are also responsive to bacteria, with studies demonstrating changes to the sensory neurons found in the myenteric plexus after addition of probiotic bacteria (Kunze et al., 2009) as well as changes in excitability in the absence of bacteria (Mcvey Neufeld et al., 2013). The immune system has similarly been shown to be important for microbiota-gut-brain communication under certain conditions. For example, infection studies examining subclinical doses of pathogenic bacteria demonstrate central changes in behavior and neurochemistry despite an absence of increased peripheral cytokine production (Lyte et al., 2006). Mice lacking bacteria show undeveloped adaptive and innate immune systems (Bengmark, 2013; Grenham et al., 2011; Macpherson and Harris, 2004; Shanahan, 2002), which likely contributes to the CNS dysfunction observed. Hypothalamic-pituitary-adrenal (HPA) axis reactivity is also sensitive to changes in the intestinal microbiota, with many studies showing altered endocrine signaling in response to microbial manipulation, both of which are known to induce CNS changes (Bravo et al., 2011; Clarke et al., 2013; Gareau et al., 2011; Neufeld et al., 2011; Sudo et al., 2004).

THE MICROBIOTA-BRAIN-GUT AXIS IN HEALTH AND DISEASE

Several lines of clinical evidence exist that support the idea that a stable gut microbial community is important for optimal health. Indeed, unstable microbial profiles have been documented in patients with irritable bowel syndrome (IBS) (Jeffery et al., 2012; Salonen et al., 2010; Tana et al., 2010; Wu, 2012), obesity (Ley et al., 2006; Tremaroli and Backhed, 2012; Turnbaugh et al., 2009a), type 2 diabetes (Karlsson et al., 2013; Qin et al., 2012; Vrieze et al., 2012), and cardiovascular disease (Hansen et al., 2015; Howitt and Garrett, 2012; Karlsson et al., 2012; Koren et al., 2011; Tuohy et al., 2014).

As yet, there is a paucity of studies describing a clear link between the microbiota and clinical disease manifestation with respect to disorders of the brain; however, a burgeoning preclinical literature exists. Several strategies have been used to investigate communication along the microbiota-brain-gut axis. These include exploring the effects of pathogenic bacteria on the brain and behavior. As mentioned earlier, administration of subclinical doses of pathogenic bacterial strains, such as *Campylobacter jejuni* or *Citrobacter rodentium*, to mice results in states of increased anxiety, and the latter strain also induces deficits in learning and memory (Gareau et al., 2011; Goehler et al., 2008; Lyte et al., 1998, 2006). Another commonly used method to induce intestinal dysbiosis in animal models is the administration of antibiotics. Antibiotic-treated mice display fewer anxiety-like and more exploratory behaviors, which are reversed after a 2-week washout period (Bercik et al., 2011a). Moreover, early-life exposure to antibiotics alters the composition of gut microbiota in adulthood (Nobel et al., 2015). Exposure to stressors early in life also affects the adult brain-gut axis: maternally separated pups show increased HPA axis activity, immune system reactivity, visceral sensitivity, and altered fecal microbial composition in adulthood (O'Mahony et al., 2009). Probiotics, live organisms that exert health benefits on the host when ingested in adequate quantities, have been used to study the effect of beneficial microorganisms on brain function, behavior, and brain-gut communication. The *Bifidobacteria* and *Lactobacillus* genera have been shown to reduce anxiety in humans and mice (Bravo et al., 2011; Messaoudi et al., 2011). Indeed, a growing body of literature demonstrates that probiotics of the *Lactobacillus* strain can normalize HPA axis responsivity, reverse stress-induced colonic alterations, and improve cognitive function (Savignac et al., 2015). We have coined the term *psychobiotic* to refer to bacteria with positive mental health effects (Dinan et al., 2013). Several studies have now demonstrated that probiotics can reverse the maladaptive stress-responsivity and cognitive function induced by chemical colitis and bacterial and parasitic infections (Bercik et al., 2010, 2011b; Gareau et al., 2007).

Perhaps the most compelling evidence for a role of the microbiota in gut-brain signaling has come from studies utilizing germ-free (GF) mice (mice raised without any exposure to microorganisms). Such analyses have generated exciting data that aim to directly answer the question, "Can the gut microbiota affect brain and behavior?". This chapter will summarize lessons learned from GF mice and the importance of commensal intestinal microbiota in nervous system development and function, particularly in the context of neuropsychiatric disorders. Tables 7.1 and 7.2 recapitulate what we now know about how growing up GF affects behavior and brain function, respectively.

Table 7.1 Behavioral Phenotypes of Germ-Free Mice

Parameter	Phenotype	Strain and Sex	Test	Reversible?	References
Anxiety	Reduced basal anxiety	Swiss Webster (m)	LDB	Yes	Clarke et al. (2013)
Anxiety	No change in basal anxiety	Swiss Webster (f)	LDB		Gareau et al. (2011)
Anxiety	Reduced basal anxiety	NMRI (m)	OF, LDB, EPM	Yes: EPM No: LDB, OF	Heijtz et al. (2011)
Anxiety	Reduced basal anxiety	Swiss Webster (f)	EPM		Neufeld et al. (2011)
Learning and memory	Normal olfactory memory	Swiss Webster (m)	STFP		Desbonnet et al. (2014)
Learning and memory	Impaired (short-term) recognition and working memory	Swiss Webster (f)	NOR, TM		Gareau et al. (2011)
Locomotion	Hyperlocomotion and increased rearing	NMRI (m)	OF	Yes	Heijtz et al. (2011)
Self-groom-ing	Increased time spent self-grooming	Swiss Webster (m)	–		Desbonnet et al. (2014)
Social cognition	No preference for novel conspecific	Swiss Webster (m > f)	TCS	Yes	Desbonnet et al. (2014)
Social preference	Avoidance of conspecifics	Swiss Webster (m > f)	TCS	No	Desbonnet et al. (2014)

Numerous behavioral parameters are altered in germ-free mice. Experiments demonstrating reversibility or irreversibility with bacterial colonization are labeled Yes *or* No, *respectively. EPM,* Elevated plus maze; f, female; LDB, *light–dark box;* m, male; m>f, *phenotype expressed more strongly in males than females;* NOR, *novel object recognition test;* OF, *open-field test;* STFP, *social transmission of food preference test;* TM, *T-maze;* TCS, *three-chambered sociability test.*

THE GERM-FREE MOUSE

In the biological sciences, a common way to study the impact of a part of a system is to entirely abrogate it. For example, to determine the effect of a gene on an organism, scientists often compare knock-out animals, animals lacking the gene in question, to their wild-type counterparts. Therefore it was a logical step for scientists studying the effect of bacteria on health and disease to ask how the absence of microbiota would affect host physiology. GF animals were generated to help answer this question. Here we focus on the GF mouse; however, GF rats and pigs have also been studied (Crumeyrolle-Arias et al., 2014; Gordon and Pesti, 1971; Gordon and Wostmann, 1960; Wang and Donovan, 2015). GF mice are an invaluable research tool, allowing scientists to explicitly study how microbiota

Table 7.2 Biochemical, Molecular, and Cellular Alterations in Germ-Free Mice

Parameter	Phenotype	Strain and Sex	Tissue/Brain Region	Reversible?	References
Adrenocorticotropin hormone	Increased ACTH after 1 h restraint stress	BALB/c (m)	Blood: plasma	Yes	Sudo et al. (2004)
Brain-derived neurotrophic factor	Decreased *Bdnf* expression	Swiss Webster (m)	HC		Clarke et al. (2013)
Brain-derived neurotrophic factor	Decreased BDNF expression	Swiss Webster (f)	CA1		Gareau et al. (2011)
Brain-derived neurotrophic factor	Decreased *Bdnf* expression	NMRI (m)	Basolateral AMY, CA1, cingulate CTX		Heijtz et al. (2011)
Brain-derived neurotrophic factor	Increased *Bdnf* expression	Swiss Webster (f)	DG		Neufeld et al. (2011)
Brain-derived neurotrophic factor	Decreased BDNF expression	BALB/c (m)	CTX, HC		Sudo et al. (2004)
Blood–brain barrier	Increased BBB permeability	NMRI (m)	–		
cFos	Decreased cFos expression after 1 h water avoidance stress	Swiss Webster (f)	CA1		Gareau et al. (2011)
Corticosterone	Increased CORT after 30-min novel environment stress	Swiss Webster (m, f)	Blood: plasma		Clarke et al. (2013)
Corticosterone	Increased basal CORT	Swiss Webster (f)	Blood: plasma		Neufeld et al. (2011)
Corticosterone	Increased CORT after 1 h restraint stress	BALB/c (m)	Blood: plasma	Yes	Sudo et al. (2004)
Dopamine receptor	Increased *Drd1a* expression	NMRI (m)	HC		Heijtz et al. (2011)
Glucocorticoid receptor	Decreased GR mRNA expression	BALB/c (m)	CTX		Sudo et al. (2004)
Glutamate receptor	Decreased *Nr1* expression	BALB/c (m)	CTX		Sudo et al. (2004)

Continued

Table 7.2 Biochemical, Molecular, and Cellular Alterations in Germ-Free Mice—cont'd

Parameter	Phenotype	Strain and Sex	Tissue/Brain Region	Reversible?	References
Glutamate receptor	Decreased *Nr2* expression	BALB/c (m)	CTX, HC		Sudo et al. (2004)
Glutamate receptor	Decreased *Nr2* expression	Swiss Webster (f)	Central AMY		Neufeld et al. (2011)
Kynurenine:tryptophan ratio	Decreased kynurenine:tryptophan ratio	Swiss Webster (m, f)	Blood: plasma	Yes	Clarke et al. (2013)
Microglia	Altered cellular properties and immature morphology	C57BL/6 (m, f)	CTX, corpus callosum, HC, olfactory bulb, CB	Yes	Erny et al. (2015)
Monoamine turnover	Increased NA, DA, and 5-HT turnover	NMRI (m)	STR		Heijtz et al. (2011)
Neurogenesis	Increased cell and neuron survival	Swiss Webster	SGZ	No	Ogbonnaya et al. (2015)
NGFI-A	Decreased *Ngfi-a* expression	NMRI (m)	AMY, HC, PFC, STR		Heijtz et al. (2011)
Serotonin	Increased 5-HT levels	Swiss Webster (m)	HC	No	Clarke et al. (2013)
Serotonin receptor	Reduced *Htr1a* expression	Swiss Webster (f)	DG		Neufeld et al. (2011)
Synapse-related genes	Reduced synaptophysin and PSD-95 expression	NMRI (m)	STR		Heijtz et al. (2011)
Transcriptome	Differential expression	NMRI (m)	CB > HC > STR > CTX		Heijtz et al. (2011)
Tryptophan	Increased tryptophan concentration	Swiss Webster (m)	Blood: plasma	Yes	Clarke et al. (2013)

Numerous biochemical and molecular parameters are altered in germ-free mice. Experiments demonstrating reversibility or irreversibility with bacterial colonization are labeled Yes or No, respectively.
5-HT, serotonin; ACTH, adrenocorticotropic hormone; AMY, amygdala; BBB, blood–brain barrier; BDNF, brain-derived neurotrophic factor; CA1, region CA1 of the hippocampus; CB, cerebellum; CORT, corticosterone; CTX, cortex; DA, dopamine; DG, dentate gyrus; GR, glucocorticoid receptor; HC, hippocampus; NA, noradrenaline; NGFI-A, nerve growth factor-inducible clone; PSD-95, postsynaptic density protein 95; PFC, prefrontal cortex; SGZ, subgranular zone of the hippocampus; STR, striatum.

affects brain development and function. These animals also offer the opportunity for monocolonization studies in which researchers can introduce identified strains of bacteria (eg, a probiotic) and study their effects without interference from other commensal microorganisms. Moreover, studies using GF mice allow researchers to study the "humanization" of the gut microbiota (ie, the transplantation of fecal microbiota from humans or animal models of a given disease; Aroniadis and Brandt, 2013; Bercik et al., 2011a; Borody and Khoruts, 2012; Cryan and Dinan, 2012; Turnbaugh et al., 2009b).

Historically, the concept of gnotobiotic animals, organisms that contain a known composition of microorganisms, can be traced back to Louis Pasteur in 1885 (Gordon and Pesti, 1971; Pasteur, 1885). Pasteur outlined potential gnotobiotic experiments and speculated that animals would not be able to survive when all microbiota is eliminated, as in the case of GF animals (Gordon and Pesti, 1971). He assumed that because of close and synergistic evolution, microbes are indispensable to their animal hosts. The first GF animals were produced at the end of the 19th century by Nuttal and Thierfelder: GF guinea pigs were delivered by aseptic caesarean section and maintained for 2 weeks (Nuttall and Thierfelder, 1897). In the 1940s, James Reyniers and his group at the Lobund Institute, University of Notre Dame, were the first to rear successive generations of GF rodents in sterile conditions (Reyniers, 1959; Reyniers et al., 1946), definitively proving that seemingly normal life is possible in animals lacking microbes. These advances made studying gnotobiotic and GF possible for the first time, and, almost one century later, this area of research is still growing.

The generation of GF animals has not changed significantly since it was first pioneered by Reyniers in the mid-20th century. To initially generate a GF colony of animals, offspring must be carefully delivered by caesarean section to avoid exposure to the microorganisms on the mother's skin and vagina (Bibiloni, 2012; Faith et al., 2010; Macpherson and Harris, 2004; Reyniers, 1959; Smith et al., 2007; Stilling et al., 2014b). Newly born animals are then hand reared aseptically in isolators and fed sterile milk. Mice are raised free from microbial colonization by only being exposed to sterile food, water, and bedding (Bibiloni, 2012; Macpherson and Harris, 2004; Reyniers, 1959). Another method to initially generate GF rodents involves the transfer of an embryo at the two-cell stage to a pseudopregnant recipient (Bibiloni, 2012; Faith et al., 2010; Smith et al., 2007). Further generations can then be derived in a much less labor-intensive process: GF mice are interbred and mothers can give birth naturally without exposing their offspring to microbes (Faith et al., 2010; Macpherson and Harris, 2004; Reyniers, 1959; Smith et al., 2007). These colonies are maintained in isolators in a GF unit ventilated with sterile, filtered air under positive pressure (Bibiloni, 2012; Macpherson and Harris, 2004). On an approximately weekly basis, a technician swabs the cages and analyzes fecal samples to make certain that the GF unit has not been contaminated by any microbes (Bibiloni, 2012; Williams, 2014). Through these methods it is ensured that GF mice are never exposed to bacteria, not only in their gut but also on any other body surfaces.

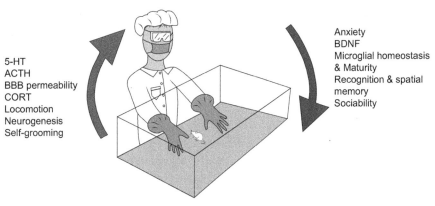

5-HT
ACTH
BBB permeability
CORT
Locomotion
Neurogenesis
Self-grooming

Anxiety
BDNF
Microglial homeostasis
& Maturity
Recognition & spatial
memory
Sociability

FIGURE 7.1

Schematic summarizing the physiological and behavioral changes observed in GF mice. GF mice are housed in an isolator under aseptic conditions. *GF*, Germ-free; *5-HT*, serotonin; *ACTH*, adrenocorticotropin hormone; *BBB*, blood–brain barrier; *CORT*, corticosterone ; *BDNF*, brain-derived neurotrophic factor.

However, it is important to note that increasing evidence suggests that caesarean-derived newborns are not sterile, as previously thought (Funkhouser and Bordenstein, 2013). Contamination in the GF unit is monitored through culture methods, which may not adequately detect bacteria, fungi, protozoans, and viruses that are not easily cultured (Stilling et al., 2014b). Stilling et al. (2014b) suggest that the only way to definitively determine the microbial status of GF animals is to use deep gene sequencing. This is because targeted amplification of 16S ribosomal DNA, a section of DNA found in all bacteria, by polymerase chain reaction would only be useful to determine which bacteria are present but would not give any information as to which fungi or viruses the host animal harbors (see Fig. 7.1).

THE GERM-FREE MOUSE AND HEALTH

To what extent was Pasteur correct in his claims of the importance of the microbiota for an organism's health? We now know that GF animals are functionally immature in many systems. Studies of GF mice have shown that the microbiota is required for normal aging and immunological, metabolic, protective, GI, and enteric neural functions (Grenham et al., 2011).

AGING

The gut microbiota plays a central role in aging and age-related diseases. GF mice live significantly longer than conventionally colonized (CC) animals (Gordon et al., 1966; Tazume et al., 1991). This increased longevity is likely due to a reduction in pathological infections. In humans, microbial diversity and stability decline with aging and are accompanied by reduced brain function and cognitive ability (Borre et al., 2014; O'Toole and Claesson, 2010). These findings have prompted the notion of modulating the microbiota in the elderly to restore microbial diversity, thereby improving general and mental health.

IMMUNE STATUS

GF studies have revealed that the microbiota is required for the normal development of the mucosal immune system. To differentiate potentially pathogenic bacteria from other harmless commensal microbiota, the innate mucosal immune system uses toll-like receptors (TLRs), which recognize pathogen-associated molecular patterns (Akira and Hemmi, 2003). When TLRs recognize these molecules, a downstream signaling pathway triggers the activation of T cells, the production of cytokines, and the activation of the HPA axis (Ulevitch, 1999). In GF animals the expression of certain TLRs is decreased or absent, suggesting that exposure to normal commensal bacteria is essential to mount adequate immune responses (Grenham et al., 2011; Shanahan, 2002). Indeed, in GF animals IgA secretion is decreased and Peyer's patches, lymphoid follicles in the intestine, are fewer and smaller (Abrams et al., 1962; Wostmann et al., 1970). GF mice have a blunted immune response: both males and females produce reduced levels of the cytokine tumor necrosis factor-α after splenocyte stimulation with lipopolysaccharide (Clarke et al., 2013). It is important to note that recolonization of GF animals with intestinal bacteria is sufficient to restore the function of the mucosal immune system (Umesaki et al., 1995).

METABOLISM AND DIGESTION

The microbiota is critical for normal digestion and metabolism. GF mice consume more food compared with control mice to maintain the same body weight (Wostmann et al., 1983). Moreover, GF mice are protected against diet-induced obesity even when fed a Western-style, high-fat, sugar-rich diet (Bäckhed et al., 2004, 2007). This lean phenotype is associated with elevated levels of fatty acid oxidization enzymes, suggesting that the microbiota modulates host metabolism and energy storage (Bäckhed et al., 2007).

GF mice are also prone to nutritional deficiencies (Gustafsson, 1959; Sumi et al., 1977). The microbiota maximizes nutrient availability through the release of calories from otherwise unavailable oligosaccharides and by modulating absorption (Grenham et al., 2011; Sekirov et al., 2010). The gut microbiota is required to synthesize vital nutrients (Sekirov et al., 2010). When GF rats are fed a diet containing radiolabeled thiamine, large quantities are found in the feces but little to none in the tissue (Wostmann et al., 1962). GF rats fed a diet lacking vitamin K rapidly develop a hemorrhagic condition whereas controls do not (Gustafsson, 1959). GF mice are also unable survive without vitamin B in their diet, indicating that bacteria are required for its production (Sumi et al., 1977). To prevent these nutritional deficiencies, GF mice are fed a diet supplemented with increased vitamin K and B (Grenham et al., 2011).

GASTROINTESTINAL HEALTH

The microbiota is necessary for normal structural development and function of the GI system, as evidenced by the alterations to gut morphology in GF mice. Greatly enlarged cecums, reduced intestinal surface areas, smaller Peyer's patches, and thinner villi are all characteristics of the gut of GF mice (Abrams et al., 1962; Gordon and Bruckner-Kardoss, 1961; Shanahan, 2002; Wostmann and Bruckner-Kardoss, 1959). In addition, enterochromaffin cells, cells in the GI tract that synthesize serotonin, are larger in GF animals (Shanahan, 2002). The protective consequences of growing up GF are evidenced by the reduction in epithelial cell turnover observed in GF mice (Abrams et al., 1962). The recognition of gut microbes by TLRs is required to induce the proliferation of epithelial cells in the intestine (Rakoff-Nahoum et al., 2004). GF mice likely have reduced protection after GI insults because epithelial cell turnover accelerates healing after an injury (Grenham et al., 2011). Paneth cells, secretory cells in the intestine, secrete antimicrobial factors in response to TLR activation by enteric microbes (Vaishnava et al., 2008). The reduction of TLR activation under GF conditions renders the intestinal barrier more susceptible to pathogenic bacteria.

ENTERIC NERVOUS SYSTEM FUNCTION

The observed alterations in the GI tract of GF mice extend to the ENS. The first neural point of contact for the bacteria housed in the intestinal lumen are the sensory neurons of the ENS, the ganglia of which are embedded within the gut wall (Forsythe and Kunze, 2013). Work examining the electrophysiological properties of these myenteric sensory neurons, the so-called afterhyperpolarization (AH) neurons named for their pronounced refractory slow afterhyperpolarizing period after an action potential, has shown that these neurons are less excitable in adult GF mice as compared with controls (Mcvey Neufeld et al., 2013, 2015). Intracellular recordings from these cells demonstrate a longer than normal refractory period after an action potential in GF mice as compared with controls. It is interesting to note that colonizing GF mice with commensal bacteria in adulthood normalizes this neuronal dysfunction (Mcvey Neufeld et al., 2013). Previous work has shown that these same sensory neurons are altered after 9 days of feeding *Lactobacillus rhamnosus* (JB-1) to healthy rats (Kunze et al., 2009). After feeding of this probiotic bacteria, AH cells demonstrate an attenuated inhibitory slow afterhyperpolarizing period and thus an increase in intrinsic excitability. These sensory neurons synapse on enteric motor neurons, which control gut motility; thus they may in part provide a mechanistic explanation for findings of altered motility in GF rats (Husebye et al., 1994, 2001).

It is intriguing that these AH neurons also form anatomical and functional synapses with vagal nerve endings in the gut (Perez-Burgos et al., 2014; Powley et al., 2008), thus highlighting one of the potential mechanisms by which the intestinal luminal bacterial status could be transmitted to the brain. In fact, extracellular recordings of the mixed vagal and spinal mesenteric afferent nerve again show altered function in GF mice when compared with controls and conventionalized adult GF mice (McVey Neufeld et al., 2015).

The intestinal microbiota has been demonstrated to be crucial to the normal postnatal development of the enteric sensory and motor neurons. At postnatal day 3, enteric neurons in the jejunum and ileum of GF mice are structurally, functionally, and neurochemically different from controls (Collins et al., 2014). Specifically, GF mice show a decrease in overall nerve density in the small intestine, with fewer neuronal cell bodies in myenteric ganglia and fewer connective nerve fibers between ganglia (Collins et al., 2014). Consistent with previous reports (Abrams and Bishop, 1967; Husebye et al., 1994, 2001), these authors found altered motility in the absence of colonizing microbiota—GI function that is in part controlled by myenteric motor neuron output.

It is interesting to note that to date there has been little published regarding neurochemical expression in the enteric neurons of GF mice, but what has been reported shows alterations here too as compared with controls. Adult GF mice show decreased expression of calcium-binding protein calbindin in myenteric sensory neurons compared with control mice and GF animals conventionalized with commensal microbiota in adulthood (McVey Neufeld et al., 2015). This may indicate alterations in calcium signaling in the absence of microbiota, which may explain some of the observed differences in neuronal function. In addition, early postnatal GF mice show a significant increase in numbers of small intestine myenteric neurons positive for neuronal nitric oxide synthase (nNOS), a neurotransmitter expressed in inhibitory motor neurons (Collins et al., 2014), whereas another report found significant increases in colonic nNOS neurons at 4 weeks of age (Anitha et al., 2012). Although it remains unclear how these neurochemical differences contribute to the altered intestinal function we observe in the absence of colonizing microbiota, what remains obvious is that just as in the brain, the input from commensal bacteria is required for normal neurodevelopment and function.

GNOTOBIOTICS, HUMANIZATION, AND FECAL MICROBIAL THERAPY

The colonization of GF mice with identified compositions of microbiota (gnotobiotics) has provided important insights into the role of gut bacteria in metabolic disorders. The microbiome from obese animals has an increased capacity to harvest energy from the diet compared with lean mice (Turnbaugh et al., 2006). When microbiota from obese mice is transplanted into GF mice, animals gain significantly more weight than those transplanted with lean microbiota (Turnbaugh et al., 2006). Transplantation of fecal microbiota from obese humans to GF mice also induces more weight gain than the transplantation of lean human microbiota (Ridaura et al., 2013). Furthermore, the monoassociation of GF mice with the *Enterobacter* strain of bacteria from an obese human patient induces weight gain (Fei and Zhao, 2013). Metabolic activity is coordinated with the circadian rhythms of the host. It is interesting to note that the gut microbiota also displays a diurnal variation in composition and function (Leone et al., 2015). Time-shifted or "jet-lagged" mice display altered microbial compositions and enhanced weight gain when they are fed a high-fat diet (Leone et al., 2015). When fecal microbiota from jet-lagged mice is transferred into GF mice, these recipients exhibit increased body fat and glucose intolerance (Thaiss et al., 2014). This is also true for time shifts in humans: colonization of GF mice with fecal microbiota from jet-lagged humans induces weight gain (Thaiss et al., 2014). A recent study found that mice fed calorie-free artificial sweeteners developed glucose intolerance through functional alterations to the gut microbiota (Suez et al., 2014). It is interesting to note that glucose intolerance is fully transmissible to GF mice through fecal transplantation of microbiota from sweetener-consuming mice (Suez et al., 2014). Taken together, findings from bacterial colonization studies suggest that there are transmissible interactions between diet and microbiota that can influence the host metabolism.

Fecal microbial transplantation (FMT) is the process of transferring stool from a healthy donor to a recipient. This process has been used to treat *Clostridium difficile* infection for over 50 years, but new research has raised the possibility that FMT could treat other illnesses with microbial dysfunction, including neuropsychiatric disorders. Currently, only single-case reports or anecdotal evidence exists supporting FMT as a treatment for diseases of the CNS such as multiple sclerosis, Parkinson's disease, and autism (Borody and Campbell, 2012; Borody and Khoruts, 2012; Collins et al., 2013). Therefore further clinical investigation of FMT as a potential treatment of neuropsychiatric disorders in which the microbiota is implicated is warranted.

ANXIETY AND STRESS RESPONSIVITY

There is now a significant body of evidence indicating that microorganisms in the gut influence the development and later function of the stress system (Collins et al., 2012; Dinan and Cryan, 2012; Foster and Neufeld, 2013; Grenham et al., 2011; Rhee et al., 2009; Sampson and Mazmanian, 2015). Signals from the gut have been demonstrated to drive HPA axis activation: both enteric pathogens and vagal stimulation can elicit increases in corticosterone levels (Hosoi et al., 2000; Zimomra et al., 2011). The contribution of signaling along the microbiota-brain-gut axis is particularly significant for GI disorders such as IBS (Kennedy et al., 2014a). Patients with IBS have altered microbial compositions and display HPA axis hyperactivity (Jeffery et al., 2012; Kennedy et al., 2014b). However, the clinical evidence linking abnormal gut function to the development of maladaptive stress responsivity is limited as of yet. Most of what is presently known about how gut microbes can affect the stress system has been gleaned from preclinical models.

ALTERATIONS IN HPA FUNCTION

The use of GF animals has provided significant insights into the role of the microbiota in regulating the development of the HPA axis. The landmark study by Sudo et al. (2004)

was the first to show alterations in stress responsivity in GF mice. However, there is conflicting evidence as to whether basal corticosterone levels are altered in GF mice; both normal (Clarke et al., 2013; Sudo et al., 2004) and increased (Neufeld et al., 2011) levels have been reported in the literature. These inconsistent findings could be due to differences in methodology, acclimatization period, mode of euthanasia, strain, and sex.

ALTERATIONS IN STRESS CIRCUITRY

Accumulating evidence indicates that the microbiota alters stress responsivity; however, little is known about the underlying neural circuitry. Sudo et al. (2004) sought to determine if the visceral communication involved in the normalization of the HPA axis after bacterial recolonization occurred through a neural or immunological route. In this study, GF mice were recolonized with *Bifidobacterium infantis* at 5 weeks of age. Plasma cytokines, interleukin (IL)-6 and IL-1β, and c-Fos expression in the paraventricular nucleus (PVN) of the brain were then subsequently analyzed. The PVN is a neuronal nucleus of the hypothalamus and contains neurons that release corticotrophin-releasing hormone. c-Fos, a marker for neuronal activation, is elevated in the PVN 6 h after inoculation and is accompanied by a concomitant increase in corticosterone. Although *B. infantis* treatment also causes IL-6 levels to increase, this effect seems to be independent of HPA axis activity; pretreatment with anti-IL-6 antibody fails to affect the elevated levels of c-Fos and corticosterone in the PVN and plasma, respectively. These findings strongly suggest that stress-relevant visceral information resulting from bacterial colonization is transmitted to the brain via a neuronal, humoral, cytokine-independent route.

ALTERATIONS IN ANXIETY BEHAVIOR

The logical question that emerged from the finding that GF mice display HPA axis hyperresponsivity was whether the microbiota could also influence stress-related behavior. Neufeld et al. (2011) were among the first to show that basal anxiety is reduced in female GF mice. This phenotype has since been reproduced in female and male GF animals (Clarke et al., 2013; Heijtz et al., 2011). Decreased anxiety-like behaviour in GF animals has been measured using the open-field, light–dark box, and elevated plus maze behavioral tests (Clarke et al., 2013; Heijtz et al., 2011; Neufeld et al., 2011). It is interesting to note that in some situations no change in anxiety-like behaviour in GF mice has been shown (Bercik et al., 2011a; Gareau et al., 2011). The recolonization of male GF mice postweaning normalizes the anxiolytic-like behavioral profile (Clarke et al., 2013). This anxiolytic-like behavioral profile appears to be amenable to microbial intervention: recolonization of male GF mice normalizes anxiety-like behavior (Clarke et al., 2013). It is interesting to note that reduced anxiety-like behaviour induced by the absence of microbiota seems to be a species-specific effect: GF rats exhibit an anxiogenic-like phenotype (Crumeyrolle-Arias et al., 2014). Although it may seem contradictory that GF animals display reduced basal anxiety-like behaviour and HPA axis overactivity, stress hormone signaling does not necessarily correlate to behavioral output (Rodgers et al., 1999). Regardless of this apparent disparity, these findings clearly demonstrate that the microbiota is required for the normal development of stress responsivity.

One of the main advantages of the GF model is that it provides the option to reintroduce bacteria and observe the effects that this transplantation has on host physiology and behavior. Bercik et al. (2011a) demonstrated that the introduction of bacteria from one mouse strain can alter the behavior of a different strain. When microbiota from Balb/C mice, a strain that consistently exhibits a high anxiety-like phenotype (Belzung and Griebel, 2001; O'Mahony et al., 2010), is transplanted to low anxiety-like GF NIH Swiss mice, an anxiogenic-like phenotype emerges. In contrast, the reverse microbiota transplantation, from NIH Swiss donors into Balb/C mice, attenuates the high anxiety-like phenotype. These findings raise the possibility that intestinal dysbiosis contributes to the physiological and behavioral aspects of GI diseases. For example, patients with IBS show psychiatric co-morbidity (most frequently the mood disorders), alterations to the gut microbiota, and HPA axis hyperactivity (Fond et al., 2014; Kennedy et al., 2014a,b). Therefore microbiota could be a suitable target for probiotics; altering the gut microbiota may infer positive health benefits for the GI and psychiatric symptoms of IBS and related disorders (Clarke et al., 2012). Moreover, that the microbiota can alter behavior also emphasizes the potential benefits of fecal transplantation as a therapy for disorders of the microbiota-brain-gut axis (Aroniadis and Brandt, 2013; Borody and Khoruts, 2012).

SOCIAL, REPETITIVE, AND LOCOMOTOR BEHAVIORS

Group living affords numerous evolutionary advantages including mutual protection, sharing of food, and increased access to mating partners (Hamilton, 1964; Stilling et al., 2014a). Therefore it is not surprising that the brain has evolved to accommodate social behavior. Unlike genes, microbes are contagious: they can be actively and passively transmitted to new habitats and hosts. This has led evolutionary biologists to speculate that natural selection has favored those microbes that can increase their own transmission, including through social interactions (Ezenwa et al., 2012; Lombardo, 2008; Montiel-Castro et al., 2013; Troyer, 1984; Tung et al., 2015). On the other hand, the exchange of microorganisms through contact with conspecifics could also impart evolutionary advantages to the host: bacterial symbionts aid in digestion and increase the resistance to other infectious agents (Lombardo, 2008; Stilling et al., 2014b; Troyer, 1984). As such, it can be hypothesized that sociability and microbial composition have both had significant and converging influences on the evolution of brain and behavior.

SOCIAL BEHAVIOR IN GERM-FREE MICE

One way to explore the interaction between the microbiota and social behaviors is to investigate how alterations to the microbiota affect the development of social capabilities. Recent data from our group have uncovered social deficits in GF mice, some of which are reversed by bacterial colonization (Desbonnet et al., 2014). Mice are social animals that are naturally predisposed to seek out stable and novel social situations. GF mice, particularly males, display social deficits in the three-chambered sociability test. These animals spend abnormally more time exploring an empty chamber compared with a chamber containing a mouse (social preference). Moreover, GF mice do not exhibit the normal preference for a novel over a familiar mouse (social cognition). Colonization of GF mice with gut bacteria postweaning reverses the social avoidance phenotype but has no effect on social cognition impairments; colonized mice prefer the social chamber but have no preference for a novel versus a familiar mouse. It is important to note that the ability to process information during social interaction is not affected in GF mice because they display normal partiality for the novel food in the social transmission of food preference test (Desbonnet et al., 2014). These findings indicate that the microbiota is crucial for the programming of normal social behaviors but not information processing. Moreover, this development of social cognition is permanently established during the preweaning period. However, it is important to note that the critical window during which social preference is amenable to microbial intervention is likely longer.

REPETITIVE AND LOCOMOTOR BEHAVIOR IN GERM-FREE MICE

In addition to social deficits, Desbonnet et al. (2014) noted that GF mice display alterations in stereotyped and repetitive behaviors. During the social transmission of food preference test, male GF mice spend a substantially greater proportion of time engaging in repetitive self-grooming behaviors, which is normalized with colonization postweaning (Desbonnet et al., 2014). GF mice also display increased hyper-locomotion and increased rearing during the open-field test whereas the colonized offspring of GF mice exhibit no such alterations in motor behavior (Heijtz et al., 2011). However, it is worth noting that Neufeld et al. (2011) report no difference in locomotor behavior in female GF mice. Together these results indicate that the microbiota is required for the normal development of the neural networks governing repetitive and motor behaviors.

PARALLELS TO AUTISM SPECTRUM DISORDERS

Investigations focusing on the influence of the microbiota on social, locomotor, and repetitive behaviors are particularly relevant to autism spectrum disorder (ASD). Patients with ASD have deficits in social interaction and communication and display repetitive and stereotyped behaviors. It is interesting to note that GI complications such as constipation, increased intestinal permeability, and an altered microbial composition are common in patients with ASD (Howard et al., 2000; Kang et al., 2013; Mayer et al., 2014; Mulle et al., 2013; Rosenfeld, 2015; Sampson and Mazmanian, 2015). Moreover, ASD individuals have a higher prevalence of inflammatory bowel disease and GI disorders compared with controls

(Kohane et al., 2012). These findings suggest that the microbiota could play a role in the development or pathophysiology of this disorder. Indeed, rodent models of microbial dysfunction and ASD exhibit autism-like behavioral profiles similar to those observed in GF mice. Mice exposed to maternal immune activation display deficits in social communicative behavior, increased anxiety, decreased sociability, and high levels of stereotyped behavior (Hsiao et al., 2013). Moreover, these animals also have defective intestinal integrity, dysbiosis of the gut microbiota, and alterations in serum metabolite levels (Hsiao et al., 2013). It is intriguing that treatment with the *Bacteroides fragilis* strain of bacteria ameliorates many of the behavioral and GI symptoms observed in mice exposed to maternal immune activation. This autism-like profile is also mirrored in another mouse model of ASD: mice exposed to valproate in utero also display deficits in social behavior and an altered gut microbiome (De Theije et al., 2014). The observations that GF mice and other murine models of ASD show both behavioral and microbial changes suggest that neurodevelopmental disorders, including autism, may have microbial etiologies. If correct, then targeting the gut microbiota with interventions such as diet, probiotics, and prebiotics could represent safe and effective treatments for neurodevelopmental disorders including ASD (Gilbert et al., 2013; Mayer et al., 2014; Sampson and Mazmanian, 2015).

LEARNING AND MEMORY

Given its widespread effects on social-, anxiety-, and stress-related behavior and physiology, it is not too surprising that the microbiota can influence cognition. Indeed, administration of potential probiotics of the *Lactobacillus* strain improves memory (Savignac et al., 2015). Probiotics could enhance memory by altering hippocampal long-term potentiation (LTP; Distrutti et al., 2014). Administration of a probiotic mixture prevented age-related LTP deficits in the rat hippocampus (Distrutti et al., 2014). In contrast, stressed mice infected with the enteric pathogen *C. rodentium* display learning and memory deficits (Gareau et al., 2011). Given these findings, it is possible that learning and memory are also altered in GF mice. To answer this question, Gareau et al., (2011) subjected GF mice to the novel object test and the T-maze and discovered that these animals indeed have significant deficits in learning and memory. GF mice explore novel objects and environments significantly less than controls. It is interesting to note that a one hour period of psychological stress (the water avoidance test) has no effect on these learning and memory deficits. However, it is important to note that GF mice display normal olfactory memory as measured in the social transmission of food preference test (Desbonnet et al., 2014). The authors speculate that the memory deficits in GF mice could be due to altered hippocampal activity. Indeed, after memory testing the number of c-Fos-positive CA1 hippocampal cells is reduced in GF animals. Together these results demonstrate that the absence of microbiota induces deficits in object and spatial but not olfactory memory, likely through a hippocampal-mediated mechanism.

NEUROCHEMICAL AND MOLECULAR ALTERATIONS

GF mice display abnormalities in cognition, stress responsivity, and sociability compared with their CC counterparts. However, the neurochemical and molecular underpinnings of such changes largely remain unknown. There is evidence now that the microbiota regulates neurotransmission and the expression of neurotrophic factors and synapse-related genes.

SEROTONERGIC SYSTEM

The neurotransmitter serotonin (5-hydroxytryptamine) is primarily known for its role in the brain although approximately 95% of the body's serotonin is located within the GI tract. Peripherally, serotonin is involved in the regulation of gut secretion, motility, and pain perception (Ridaura and Belkaid, 2015; Yano et al., 2015). In the brain, it plays an important role in mood, appetite, sleep, and cognition (Wrase et al., 2006). Serotonin modulates the development and plasticity of neural circuits involved in mood disorders (Albert et al., 2012; Young and Leyton, 2002). Given that GI and affective disorders are highly co-morbid, it is not surprising that drugs that affect serotonergic neurotransmission are effective in treating mood disorders and IBS (O'Mahony et al., 2015). Serotonin synthesis in the brain requires the availability of tryptophan, an essential amino acid. Reduction in tryptophan levels because of enzymatic degradation to kynurenine can induce depressive symptoms because of insufficient serotonin production (Myint et al., 2007).

Gut bacteria are required for normal digestion and absorption of nutrients; therefore tryptophan availability and serotonin signaling could be altered in mice lacking microbiota. Indeed, GF mice have increased plasma tryptophan levels and a decreased kynurenine:tryptophan ratio compared with controls (Clarke et al., 2013). Male, but not female, GF mice also have elevated hippocampal levels of serotonin and its metabolite 5-hydroxyindoleacetic acid (Clarke et al., 2013). It is interesting to note that bacterial colonization postweaning restores tryptophan availability and metabolism but not hippocampal serotonin (Clarke et al., 2013). These findings clearly indicate that serotonergic signaling is altered in GF mice given that levels of serotonin and its precursor differ compared with controls. Moreover, tryptophan availability could be a route by which the gut microbiota can influence serotonergic signaling in the brain.

SYNAPSE-RELATED TRANSCRIPTOMIC ALTERATIONS

Studies investigating the molecular correlates of the altered behavioral and physiological profile of GF mice are still ongoing. In addition to the altered serotonergic signaling, evidence demonstrating that the microbiota acts on a synaptic level is derived from observed differences in mRNA and protein expression between GF and control mice. Neurotransmitter receptor expression differs in GF mice. For example, dopamine receptor subunit *Drd1a* mRNA is increased in the hippocampus

(Heijtz et al., 2011). GF mice display reduced glutamate receptor *NR1* mRNA in the cortex and *NR2a* in the cortex, hippocampus, and central nucleus of the amygdala (Neufeld et al., 2011; Sudo et al., 2004). Protein levels of the synaptic markers synaptophysin and postsynaptic density protein-95 are also increased in the striatum of GF mice (Heijtz et al., 2011). A recent analysis of the amygdala transcriptome revealed the upregulation of immediate early genes (Stilling et al., 2015). Moreover, there is differential expression of genes involved in neurotransmission, neuronal plasticity, and morphology, which suggests that there is altered baseline activity in the amygdala of GF animals. Taken together, these results indicate that the microbiota induces changes on a synapse level in structures critical for stress responsivity, sociability, and cognition, all of which are altered in GF mice. It is clear that further experiments are required to improve our understanding of how the microbiota affects synaptic communication and structure.

BRAIN-DERIVED NEUROTROPHIC FACTOR

Brain-derived neurotrophic factor (BDNF) is a secretory growth factor that supports the survival of existing neurons and promotes synaptogenesis and differentiation of new neurons (Park and Poo, 2013). BDNF dysfunction is a hallmark of anxiety and depressive disorders (Autry and Monteggia, 2012), and stress exposure alters *Bdnf* levels in the CNS (Lakshminarasimhan and Chattarji, 2012). Several independent groups have now demonstrated BDNF dysfunction in the CNS of GF animals. *Bdnf* expression is decreased in the cortex and amygdala of GF mice (Heijtz et al., 2011). Contradicting evidence exists describing the changes in *Bdnf* expression in the hippocampus: studies report reduced (Clarke et al., 2013; Gareau et al., 2011; Heijtz et al., 2011; Sudo et al., 2004) and increased (Neufeld et al., 2011) expression. These contrasting findings are likely due to differences in mRNA quantification methodology, the hippocampal subregion studied, and the strain and sex of animals studied. What is clear from these findings is that the microbiota regulates central BDNF expression. Future studies should investigate how these microbiota-induced changes in neurotrophin factor signaling affect the activity and structure of neuronal networks underlying cognition and stress responses.

NEUROGENESIS

Neurogenesis, the birth of new neurons, is thought to play a key role in learning and memory, stress responsivity, and the efficacy of antidepressant drugs (Marín-Burgin and Schinder, 2012; Miller and Hen, 2015; Snyder et al., 2011). Several studies have suggested that brain functions and substrates mediated by hippocampal neurogenesis are altered in GF mice. These include learning and memory, anxiety-like behavior, corticosterone levels, serotonin signaling, BDNF expression, and proinflammatory cytokine levels (Clarke et al., 2013; Neufeld et al., 2011; Sudo et al., 2004). Ogbonnaya et al. (2015) investigated whether adult neurogenesis in the subgranular zone (SGZ) of the hippocampus is regulated by the gut microbiota. In GF animals, there is no change in cell proliferation across the total SGZ. In contrast, cell survival is increased in GF mice, and postweaning colonization does not prevent this effect. Likewise, GF mice exhibit increased survival of newly born neurons, which is maintained after postweaning colonization. Postweaning colonization does not prevent any microbiota-induced changes in cell and neuronal survival; therefore there is clearly a critical window in early life during which microbial colonization can affect adult hippocampal neurogenesis. These alterations in hippocampal neurogenesis could underlie the deficits in learning and memory observed in GF animals: increased neuronal survival occurs preferentially in the dorsal hippocampus, a region critical for spatial learning and memory (Moser et al., 1995; O'Leary and Cryan, 2014). It is important to note that increased neurogenesis is typically associated with improved learning and memory (Deng et al., 2010). Taken together, these findings indicate that neurogenesis may contribute to the behavioral and cognitive profile of GF mice.

BLOOD–BRAIN BARRIER

The blood–brain barrier (BBB) is a highly selective barrier that restricts the paracellular diffusion of water-soluble substances from the blood to the brain. The BBB begins to develop early in fetal life and consists of capillary endothelial cells sealed with tight junctions, astrocytes, and pericytes (Abbott et al., 2010; Ballabh et al., 2004; Hawkins and Davis, 2005). An intact BBB is necessary to protect the neonate against colonizing bacteria during this critical period of brain development (Hensch, 2004; Knudsen, 2004). Disruption of the BBB can compromise the CNS and cause illness (Abbott et al., 2010; Ballabh et al., 2004; Hawkins and Davis, 2005). Therefore it is important to understand how the BBB is affected by various factors, including the microbiota, early in life to determine how to treat and prevent various neurological illnesses.

Braniste et al. (2014) were the first to assess the role of the intestinal microbiota in the development and maintenance of BBB integrity in the mouse. First, the role of the maternal gut microbiota in prenatal BBB development was investigated. In control fetal mice from specific-pathogen-free (SPF) dams, the BBB prevents labeled immunoglobulin penetration by embryological day (E)15.5 to E17.5. In contrast, the brains of fetal mice from GF dams at E16.5 show diffuse immunoglobulin dispersal. The tight junction protein occludin is lower in the fetal GF brains, which could explain the increased BBB permeability in these animals. The BBB of adult GF mice is also more permeable than that of SPF controls, but this is not due to differences in vascular density or pericyte coverage. One possible mechanism explaining increased BBB permeability in adult GF mice is altered endothelial tight junction expression; indeed, expression of the tight junction proteins occludin and claudin-5 are reduced in the frontal cortex, striatum, and hippocampus. Moreover, tight junctions in the brains of GF animals are diffuse and less organized compared with controls. These results have important implications for neurodevelopment because increased BBB permeability might allow molecules in the blood such as glucocorticoids, which are known to be elevated in GF animals (Clarke et al., 2013; Neufeld et al., 2011; Sudo et al., 2004), to enter the growing brain and subsequently affect neurogenesis and synaptic connectivity.

In the second part of the study, Braniste et al. (2014) examined the effect of intestinal microbial interventions on BBB permeability in the adult mouse. Colonization of GF mice with bacteria from SPF mice reduces the permeability of the BBB and increases the expression of occludin and claudin-5 in the brain. This microbiota-induced change in permeability is likely due to short-chain fatty acids (SCFAs) or metabolites produced by intestinal bacteria. Monocolonization with *Clostridium tyrobutyricum*, a butyrate-producing bacterial strain, or *Bacteroides thetaiotaomicron*, an acetate-producing strain, decreases BBB permeability and increases tight junction protein expression. Moreover, administration of sodium butyrate alone has the same effect. Taken together, these findings clearly demonstrate that the microbiota is required for normal BBB development but that barrier function is malleable to some extent later in life. Future studies should explore whether microbiota-related interventions, such as probiotics or dietary changes, could be used to treat or prevent diseases with BBB pathologies.

MICROGLIA

Microglia are the macrophages of the brain and spinal cord, and they function as the main form of immune defense in the CNS. These cells maintain tissue homeostasis by scavenging pathogens, dying cells, and other potentially harmful molecules through microbial-associated molecular pattern (MAMP) receptor dependent and independent mechanisms (Kettenmann et al., 2011; Prinz and Priller, 2014; Ransohoff and Perry, 2009). Microglia are also important for normal brain development and sculpting synaptic circuits in the developing nervous system (Schafer and Stevens, 2013). Given their importance in protecting the CNS, it is not surprising that studies have now associated microglia-related genes with neurological and psychiatric diseases such as Alzheimer's disease and dementia (Prinz and Priller, 2014). These diseases are now being termed *microgliopathies* and continue to garner increasing research interest.

The role of the gut microbiota in the modulation of innate and adaptive immune responses has been well established; however, little was known until recently about how the host microbiota regulated the CNS immune system (Cryan and Dinan, 2015). Erny et al. (2015) examined the contribution of bacteria to microglia homeostasis and maturation. Initial experiments measuring the genome-wide mRNA expression profiles revealed marked differences of microglial genes between SPF and GF mouse brains, suggesting that the absence of microglia induces microglia dysregulation. A histopathological analysis of the brains of GF mice confirmed differences in microglia, demonstrating more

Iba-1-positive microglia throughout the brain located in gray and white matter. Microglia from GF mice are elongated and more complex and frequently overlap with adjacent microglia, indicating that they do not respect neighboring cell territories. It is important to note that these microbiota-induced microglial defects are not a result of altered levels of survival or growth factors. In response to bacterial and viral challenge, GF mice display a strongly attenuated induction of proinflammatory genes and a failure to exhibit activated microglial morphology. These results collectively indicate that in the absence of gut microbiota, the microglial immune response and the resistance to bacterial and viral infections are diminished.

Because GF mice are microbiota deficient from birth, the development of microglia may be affected by the complete absence of colonizing bacteria. To determine whether microglia require continuous inputs from the host microbiota, SPF mice were treated with antibiotics to deplete intestinal bacteria. Antibiotic-treated mice also display an immature microglial phenotype, similar to the GF condition. However, in contrast to GF mice, the number of microglia is unchanged in antibiotic-treated mice. Moreover, the full repertoire of microbes is required for normal microglial homeostasis. GF mice colonized with only three strains of bacteria from the Schaedler flora community exhibit an immature morphological phenotype. It is important to note that when Schaedler mice were colonized with a complex bacterial composition, microglia function and morphology are largely normalized. Erny et al. (2015) then sought to determine the signaling pathways by which gut bacteria promote microglial maturation and homeostasis. Treatment of GF mice with SCFAs, bacterial fermentation products, largely normalized microglia density, cell morphology, and maturity. Moreover, SCFA receptor free fatty acid receptor-2, but not MAMP receptors, are required for SCFA-mediated microglial normalization to occur. These findings suggest that microglia require constant input from a complex host microbiota for normal structure and function. Furthermore, the host microbiota could regulate microglial homeostasis via SCFA signaling.

THE GERM-FREE MOUSE: STRENGTHS, LIMITATIONS, AND ALTERNATIVES

Criticisms of the GF model tend to focus on the apparent lack of direct clinical relevance. Humans are never in a truly GF state. There is now evidence to suggest that even during the prenatal period, which was previously considered to be entirely aseptic, we are exposed to some form of colonizing bacteria (Funkhouser and Bordenstein, 2013). It is clear that the use of GF animals in preclinical work is not to exactly mimic any potential human health experience. Instead, the strength of the GF animal model is that it allows us to ascertain what role bacterial exposure of any kind plays on the development and function of a given system. It is a controlled state in which we can examine the dysfunction that arises because of the absence of any microbial input on anatomy and physiology. In addition, we can introduce either single strains of bacteria, such as in monocolonized animals, or a cocktail of commensal microbiota, thus conventionalizing the previously GF animals to a specific pathogen-free (or similar) status. In this way we can determine what role specific bacteria may play in any number of health-related issues. The timing of introduction of bacteria can also be varied, allowing us to examine the role of bacterial exposure and input on the development of systems. In fact, GF mice have already been used to begin to elucidate the role of intestinal microbiota on the development of the HPA stress axis and the existence of critical windows during which the stress circuitry in the brain is plastic enough to alter development in response to bacterial signals (Sudo et al., 2004).

GF animals are not exposed to microbiota from birth, and this can have permanent consequences for brain development. Although this is useful for studying the effect of the microbiota on neurodevelopment, some experimental questions require the microbiota to be altered in adulthood. Colonization of GF animals with bacteria are not sufficient for these types of experiments because critical developmental windows may have already closed and permanent alterations to brain and behavior may be present. Therefore the GF model is limited in that microbiota-free status cannot be induced at any time point; animals can only be born GF. Furthermore, because GF animals will be colonized with bacteria shortly after their removal from the GF unit, behavioral paradigms lasting more than a day are not possible without the confound of colonization. For these reasons we must find alternatives for GF rodents that allow the gut microbiota to be altered in adulthood and that can be exposed to the external environment for extended periods of time. Possible rodent models exist and include antibiotic treatment, probiotics, bacterial colonization, and humanization among others. Future studies should determine if the changes along the microbiota-brain-gut axis observed in GF animals can also be induced in these alternative rodent models.

CONCLUSIONS

In recent years there has been significant progress made in recognizing the importance of the commensal intestinal microbiota to brain function and development. GF mice have been an invaluable tool in gleaning much of this knowledge. Key findings demonstrate that the microbiota is required for normal stress responsivity, sociability, and cognition (Clarke et al., 2013; Desbonnet et al., 2014; Gareau et al., 2011; Heijtz et al., 2011; Neufeld et al., 2011; Sudo et al., 2004). Moreover, the microbiota is critical for innate immune system and BBB homeostasis (Braniste et al., 2014; Erny et al., 2015). Gut bacteria also affect neurotransmission, plasticity-related, and neurotrophic signaling systems (Clarke et al., 2013; Heijtz et al., 2011; Neufeld et al., 2011; Sudo et al., 2004). Going forward, there is still a significant amount of information we can learn from the GF mouse; this model is a blank slate that allows us to reintroduce various combinations of bacteria at different developmental periods. However, growing up GF can have profound neurodevelopmental effects that may deem them unsuitable for certain studies. In these cases it may be possible to supplant the GF model with antibiotic-treated rodents. An increasing understanding of the impact of the microbiota on brain and behavior will ultimately inform novel treatments for multiple neuropsychiatric and GI disorders.

REFERENCES

Abbott, N.J., Patabendige, A.A.K., Dolman, D.E.M., Yusof, S.R., Begley, D.J., 2010. Structure and function of the blood–brain barrier. Neurobiol. Dis. 37, 13–25.

Abrams, G.D., Bauer, H., Sprinz, H., 1962. Influence of the Normal Flora on Mucosal Morphology and Cellular Renewal in the Ileum. A Comparison of Germ-Free and Conventional Mice. (DTIC Document).

Abrams, G.D., Bishop, J.E., 1967. Effect of the normal microbial flora on gastrointestinal motility. Exp. Biol. Med. 126, 301–304.

Akira, S., Hemmi, H., 2003. Recognition of pathogen-associated molecular patterns by TLR family. Immunol. Lett. 85, 85–95.

Albert, P.R., Benkelfat, C., Descarries, L., 2012. The neurobiology of depression—revisiting the serotonin hypothesis. I. Cellular and molecular mechanisms. Philos. Trans. R. Soc. B Biol. Sci. 367, 2378–2381.

Anitha, M., Vijay–Kumar, M., Sitaraman, S.V., Gewirtz, A.T., Srinivasan, S., 2012. Gut microbial products regulate murine gastrointestinal motility via toll-like receptor 4 signaling. Gastroenterology 143, 1006–1016.

Aroniadis, O.C., Brandt, L.J., 2013. Fecal microbiota transplantation: past, present and future. Curr. Opin. Gastroenterol. 29, 79–84.

Autry, A.E., Monteggia, L.M., 2012. Brain-derived neurotrophic factor and neuropsychiatric disorders. Pharmacol. Rev. 64, 238–258.

Bäckhed, F., Ding, H., Wang, T., Hooper, L.V., Koh, G.Y., Nagy, A., Semenkovich, C.F., Gordon, J.I., 2004. The gut microbiota as an environmental factor that regulates fat storage. Proc. Natl. Acad. Sci. U.S.A. 101, 15718–15723. http://dx.doi.org/10.1073/pnas.0407076101.

Bäckhed, F., Ley, R.E., Sonnenburg, J.L., Peterson, D.A, Gordon, J.I., 2005. Host-bacterial mutualism in the human intestine. Science 307, 1915–1920. http://dx.doi.org/10.1126/science.1104816.

Bäckhed, F., Manchester, J.K., Semenkovich, C.F., Gordon, J.I., 2007. Mechanisms underlying the resistance to diet-induced obesity in germ-free mice. Proc. Natl. Acad. Sci. 104, 979–984. http://dx.doi.org/10.1073/pnas.0605374104.

Ballabh, P., Braun, A., Nedergaard, M., 2004. The blood–brain barrier: an overview: structure, regulation, and clinical implications. Neurobiol. Dis. 16, 1–13.

Belzung, C., Griebel, G., 2001. Measuring normal and pathological anxiety-like behaviour in mice: a review. Behav. Brain Res. 125, 141–149. http://dx.doi.org/10.1016/S0166-4328(01)00291-1.

Bengmark, S., 2013. Gut microbiota, immune development and function. Pharmacol. Res. 69, 87–113.

Bercik, P., Denou, E., Collins, J., Jackson, W., Lu, J., Jury, J., Deng, Y., Blennerhassett, P., Macri, J., McCoy, K.D., Verdu, E.F., Collins, S.M., 2011a. The intestinal microbiota affect central levels of brain-derived neurotropic factor and behavior in mice. Gastroenterology 141, 599–609. http://dx.doi.org/10.1053/j.gastro.2011.04.052. e3.

Bercik, P., Park, A.J., Sinclair, D., Khoshdel, A., Lu, J., Huang, X., Deng, Y., Blennerhassett, P.A., Fahnestock, M., Moine, D., Berger, B., Huizinga, J.D., Kunze, W., McLean, P.G., Bergonzelli, G.E., Collins, S.M., Verdu, E.F., 2011b. The anxiolytic effect of *Bifidobacterium longum* NCC3001 involves vagal pathways for gut–brain communication. Neurogastroenterol. Motil. 23, 1132–1139. http://dx.doi.org/10.1111/j.1365-2982.2011.01796.x.

Bercik, P., Verdu, E.F., Foster, J.A., Macri, J., Potter, M., Huang, X., Malinowski, P., Jackson, W., Blennerhassett, P., Neufeld, K.A., 2010. Chronic gastrointestinal inflammation induces anxiety-like behavior and alters central nervous system biochemistry in mice. Gastroenterology 139, 2102–2112.

Bibiloni, R., 2012. Rodent models to study the relationships between mammals and their bacterial inhabitants. Gut Microbe. 3, 536–543. http://dx.doi.org/10.4161/gmic.21905.

Blackshaw, L.A., Brookes, S.J.H., Grundy, D., Schemann, M., 2007. Sensory transmission in the gastrointestinal tract. Neurogastroenterol. Motil. 19, 1–19.

Borody, T.J., Campbell, J., 2012. Fecal microbiota transplantation: techniques, applications, and issues. Gastroenterol. Clin. North Am. 41, 781–803.

Borody, T.J., Khoruts, A., 2012. Fecal microbiota transplantation and emerging applications. Nat. Rev. Gastroenterol. Hepatol. 9, 88–96.

Borre, Y.E., O'Keeffe, G.W., Clarke, G., Stanton, C., Dinan, T.G., Cryan, J.F., 2014. Microbiota and neurodevelopmental windows: implications for brain disorders. Trends Mol. Med. 20, 509–518. http://dx.doi.org/10.1016/j.molmed.2014.05.002.

Braniste, V., Al-Asmakh, M., Kowal, C., Anuar, F., Abbaspour, A., Tóth, M., Korecka, A., Bakocevic, N., Ng, L.G., Kundu, P., Gulyás, B., Halldin, C., Hultenby, K., Nilsson, H., Hebert, H., Volpe, B.T., Diamond, B., Pettersson, S., 2014. The gut microbiota influences blood–brain barrier permeability in mice. Sci. Transl. Med. 6, 263ra158. http://dx.doi.org/10.1126/scitranslmed.3009759.

Bravo, J.A., Forsythe, P., Chew, M.V., Escaravage, E., Savignac, H.M., Dinan, T.G., Bienenstock, J., Cryan, J.F., 2011. Ingestion of lactobacillus strain regulates emotional behavior and central GABA receptor expression in a mouse via the vagus nerve. Proc. Natl. Acad. Sci. 108, 16050–16055.

Clarke, G., Cryan, J.F., Dinan, T.G., Quigley, E.M., 2012. Review article: probiotics for the treatment of irritable bowel syndrome–focus on lactic acid bacteria. Aliment. Pharmacol. Ther. 35, 403–413.

Clarke, G., Grenham, S., Scully, P., Fitzgerald, P., Moloney, R.D., Shanahan, F., Dinan, T.G., Cryan, J.F., 2013. The microbiome-gut-brain axis during early life regulates the hippocampal serotonergic system in a sex-dependent manner. Mol. Psychiatry 18, 666–673. http://dx.doi.org/10.1038/mp.2012.77.

Collins, J., Borojevic, R., Verdu, E.F., Huizinga, J.D., Ratcliffe, E.M., 2014. Intestinal microbiota influence the early postnatal development of the enteric nervous system. Neurogastroenterol. Motil. 26, 98–107. http://dx.doi.org/10.1111/nmo.12236.

Collins, S.M., Kassam, Z., Bercik, P., 2013. The adoptive transfer of behavioral phenotype via the intestinal microbiota: experimental evidence and clinical implications. Curr. Opin. Microbiol. 16, 240–245. http://dx.doi.org/10.1016/j.mib.2013.06.004.

Collins, S.M., Surette, M., Bercik, P., 2012. The interplay between the intestinal microbiota and the brain. Nat. Rev. Micro 10, 735–742.

Costello, E.K., Lauber, C.L., Hamady, M., Fierer, N., Gordon, J.I., Knight, R., 2009. Bacterial community variation in human body habitats across space and time. Science 326, 1694–1697. http://dx.doi.org/10.1126/science.1177486.

Crumeyrolle-Arias, M., Jaglin, M., Bruneau, A., Vancassel, S., Cardona, A., Daugé, V., Naudon, L., Rabot, S., 2014. Absence of the gut microbiota enhances anxiety-like behavior and neuroendocrine response to acute stress in rats. Psychoneuroendocrinology 42, 207–217.

Cryan, J.F., Dinan, T.G., 2015. Gut microbiota: microbiota and neuroimmune signalling—Metchnikoff to microglia. Nat. Rev. Gastroenterol. Hepatol. 12, 494–496. http://dx.doi.org/10.1038/nrgastro.2015.127.

Cryan, J.F., Dinan, T.G., 2012. Mind-altering microorganisms: the impact of the gut microbiota on brain and behaviour. Nat. Rev. Neurosci. 13, 701–712. http://dx.doi.org/10.1038/nrn3346.

Cryan, J.F., O'Mahony, S.M., 2011. The microbiome-gut-brain axis: from bowel to behavior. Neurogastroenterol. Motil. 23, 187–192. http://dx.doi.org/10.1111/j.1365-2982.2010.01664.x.

De Theije, C.G.M., Wopereis, H., Ramadan, M., van Eijndthoven, T., Lambert, J., Knol, J., Garssen, J., Kraneveld, A.D., Oozeer, R., 2014. Altered gut microbiota and activity in a murine model of autism spectrum disorders. Brain Behav. Immun. 37, 197–206.

Deng, W., Aimone, J.B., Gage, F.H., 2010. New neurons and new memories: how does adult hippocampal neurogenesis affect learning and memory? Nat. Rev. Neurosci. 11, 339–350.

Desbonnet, L., Clarke, G., Shanahan, F., Dinan, T.G., Cryan, J.F., 2014. Microbiota is essential for social development in the mouse. Mol. Psychiatry 19, 146–148. http://dx.doi.org/10.1038/mp.2013.65.

Dinan, T.G., Cryan, J.F., 2012. Regulation of the stress response by the gut microbiota: implications for psychoneuroendocrinology. Psychoneuroendocrinology 37, 1369–1378. http://dx.doi.org/10.1016/j.psyneuen.2012.03.007.

Dinan, T.G., Stanton, C., Cryan, J.F., 2013. Psychobiotics: a novel class of psychotropic. Biol. Psychiatry 74, 720–726.

Distrutti, E., O'Reilly, J.-A., McDonald, C., Cipriani, S., Renga, B., Lynch, M.A., Fiorucci, S., 2014. Modulation of intestinal microbiota by the probiotic VSL#3 resets brain gene expression and ameliorates the age-related deficit in LTP. PLoS One 9, e106503. http://dx.doi.org/10.1371/journal.pone.0106503.

El Aidy, S., Dinan, T.G., Cryan, J.F., 2015. Gut microbiota: the conductor in the orchestra of immune–neuroendocrine communication. Clin. Ther. 37, 954–967.

Erny, D., Hrabe de Angelis, A.L., Jaitin, D., Wieghofer, P., Staszewski, O., David, E., Keren-Shaul, H., Mahlakoiv, T., Jakobshagen, K., Buch, T., Schwierzeck, V., Utermohlen, O., Chun, E., Garrett, W.S., McCoy, K.D., Diefenbach, A., Staeheli, P., Stecher, B., Amit, I., Prinz, M., 2015. Host microbiota constantly control maturation and function of microglia in the CNS. Nat. Neurosci. 18 (7), 965–977.

Ezenwa, V.O., Gerardo, N.M., Inouye, D.W., Medina, M., Xavier, J.B., 2012. Animal behavior and the microbiome. Science 338, 198–199. http://dx.doi.org/10.1126/science.1227412.

Faith, J.J., Rey, F.E., O'Donnell, D., Karlsson, M., McNulty, N.P., Kallstrom, G., Goodman, A.L., Gordon, J.I., 2010. Creating and characterizing communities of human gut microbes in gnotobiotic mice. ISME J. 4, 1094.

Fei, N., Zhao, L., 2013. An opportunistic pathogen isolated from the gut of an obese human causes obesity in germfree mice. ISME J. 7, 880–884.

Fond, G., Loundou, A., Hamdani, N., Boukouaci, W., Dargel, A., Oliveira, J., Roger, M., Tamouza, R., Leboyer, M., Boyer, L., 2014. Anxiety and depression comorbidities in irritable bowel syndrome (IBS): a systematic review and meta-analysis. Eur. Arch. Psychiatry Clin. Neurosci. 264, 651–660. http://dx.doi.org/10.1007/s00406-014-0502-z.

Forsythe, P., Kunze, W.A., 2013. Voices from within: gut microbes and the CNS. Cell. Mol. life Sci. 70, 55–69.

Foster, J.A., Neufeld, K.-A.M., 2013. Gut–brain axis: how the microbiome influences anxiety and depression. Trends Neurosci. 36, 305–312.

Frank, D.N., Pace, N.R., 2008. Gastrointestinal microbiology enters the metagenomics era. Curr. Opin. Gastroenterol. 24, 4–10.

Funkhouser, L.J., Bordenstein, S.R., 2013. Mom knows best: the universality of maternal microbial transmission. PLoS Biol. 11, e1001631.

Furness, J.B., 2006. The organisation of the autonomic nervous system: peripheral connections. Auton. Neurosci. 130, 1–5.

Gareau, M.G., Jury, J., MacQueen, G., Sherman, P.M., Perdue, M.H., 2007. Probiotic treatment of rat pups normalises corticosterone release and ameliorates colonic dysfunction induced by maternal separation. Gut 56, 1522–1528.

Gareau, M.G., Wine, E., Rodrigues, D.M., Cho, J.H., Whary, M.T., Philpott, D.J., Macqueen, G., Sherman, P.M., 2011. Bacterial infection causes stress-induced memory dysfunction in mice. Gut 60, 307–317. http://dx.doi.org/10.1136/gut.2009.202515.

Gilbert, J.A., Krajmalnik-Brown, R., Porazinska, D.L., Weiss, S.J., Knight, R., 2013. Toward effective probiotics for autism and other neurodevelopmental disorders. Cell 155, 1446–1448.

Goehler, L.E., Park, S.M., Opitz, N., Lyte, M., Gaykema, R.P.A., 2008. *Campylobacter jejuni* infection increases anxiety-like behavior in the holeboard: possible anatomical substrates for viscerosensory modulation of exploratory behavior. Brain Behav. Immun. 22, 354–366.

Gordon, H.A., Bruckner-Kardoss, E., 1961. Effect of normal microbial flora on intestinal surface area. Am. J. Physiol. Content 201, 175–178.

Gordon, H.A., Bruckner-kardoss, E., Wostmann, B.S., 1966. Aging in germ-free mice: life tables and lesions observed at natural death. J. Gerontol. 21, 380–387.

Gordon, H.A., Pesti, L., 1971. The gnotobiotic animal as a tool in the study of host microbial relationships. Bact. Rev. 35, 390–429. http://dx.doi.org/10.1126/science.173.3992.171.

Gordon, H.A., Wostmann, B.S., 1960. Morphological studies on the germfree albino rat. Anat. Rec. 137, 65–70. http://dx.doi.org/10.1002/ar.1091370108.

Grenham, S., Clarke, G., Cryan, J., Dinan, T., 2011. Brain–gut–microbe communication in health and disease. Front. Physiol. 2, 94. http://dx.doi.org/10.3389/fphys.2011.00094.

Gustafsson, B.E., 1959. Vitamin K deficiency in germfree rats. Ann. N. Y. Acad. Sci. 78, 166–174.

Hamilton, W., 1964. The genetical evolution of social behaviour. J. Theortical Biol. 7, 1–52. http://dx.doi.org/10.1016/0022-5193(64)90038-4.

Hansen, T., Gobel, R., Hansen, T., Pedersen, O., 2015. The gut microbiome in cardio-metabolic health. Genome Med. 7, 33.

Hawkins, B.T., Davis, T.P., 2005. The blood–brain barrier/neurovascular unit in health and disease. Pharmacol. Rev. 57, 173–185. http://dx.doi.org/10.1124/pr.57.2.4.

Heijtz, R.D., Wang, S., Anuar, F., Qian, Y., Björkholm, B., Samuelsson, A., Hibberd, M.L., Forssberg, H., Pettersson, S., 2011. Normal gut microbiota modulates brain development and behavior. Proc. Natl. Acad. Sci. 108, 3047–3052.

Hensch, T.K., 2004. Critical period regulation. Annu. Rev. Neurosci. 27, 549–579.

Hooper, L.V., Gordon, J.I., 2001. Commensal host-bacterial relationships in the gut. Science 292, 1115–1118. http://dx.doi.org/10.1126/science.1058709.

Hooper, L.V., Macpherson, A.J., 2010. Immune adaptations that maintain homeostasis with the intestinal microbiota. Nat. Rev. Immunol. 10, 159–169.

Hosoi, T., Okuma, Y., Nomura, Y., 2000. Electrical stimulation of afferent vagus nerve induces IL-1β expression in the brain and activates HPA axis. Am. J. Physiol. Integr. Comp. Physiol. 279, R141–R147.

Howard, M.A, Cowell, P.E., Boucher, J., Broks, P., Mayes, A, Farrant, A, Roberts, N., 2000. Convergent neuroanatomical and behavioural evidence of an amygdala hypothesis of autism. Neuroreport 11, 2931–2935. http://dx.doi.org/10.1097/00001756-200009110-00020.

Howitt, M.R., Garrett, W.S., 2012. A complex microworld in the gut: gut microbiota and cardiovascular disease connectivity. Nat. Med. 18, 1188–1189.

Hsiao, E.Y., McBride, S.W., Hsien, S., Sharon, G., Hyde, E.R., McCue, T., Codelli, J.A., Chow, J., Reisman, S.E., Petrosino, J.F., Patterson, P.H., Mazmanian, S.K., 2013. Microbiota modulate behavioral and physiological abnormalities associated with neurodevelopmental disorders. Cell 155, 1451–1463. http://dx.doi.org/10.1016/j.cell.2013.11.024.

Husebye, E., Hellström, P.M., Midtvedt, T., 1994. Intestinal microflora stimulates myoelectric activity of rat small intestine by promoting cyclic initiation and aboral propagation of migrating myoelectric complex. Dig. Dis. Sci. 39, 946–956.

Husebye, E., Hellström, P.M., Sundler, F., Chen, J., Midtvedt, T., 2001. Influence of microbial species on small intestinal myoelectric activity and transit in germ-free rats. Am. J. Physiol. Liver Physiol. 280, G368–G380.

Jeffery, I.B., O'Toole, P.W., Ohman, L., Claesson, M.J., Deane, J., Quigley, E.M.M., Simren, M., 2012. An irritable bowel syndrome subtype defined by species-specific alterations in faecal microbiota. Gut 61, 997–1006. http://dx.doi.org/10.1136/gutjnl-2011-301501.

Kang, D.-W., Park, J.G., Ilhan, Z.E., Wallstrom, G., LaBaer, J., Adams, J.B., Krajmalnik-Brown, R., 2013. Reduced incidence of prevotella and other fermenters in intestinal microflora of autistic children. PLoS One 8, e68322.

Karlsson, F.H., Fåk, F., Nookaew, I., Tremaroli, V., Fagerberg, B., Petranovic, D., Bäckhed, F., Nielsen, J., 2012. Symptomatic atherosclerosis is associated with an altered gut metagenome. Nat. Commun. 3, 1245.

Karlsson, F.H., Tremaroli, V., Nookaew, I., Bergström, G., Behre, C.J., Fagerberg, B., Nielsen, J., Bäckhed, F., 2013. Gut metagenome in European women with normal, impaired and diabetic glucose control. Nature 498, 99–103.

Kennedy, P.J., Cryan, J.F., Dinan, T.G., Clarke, G., 2014a. Irritable bowel syndrome: a microbiome-gut-brain axis disorder? World J. Gastroenterol. 20, 14105.

Kennedy, P.J., Cryan, J.F., Quigley, E.M.M., Dinan, T.G., Clarke, G., 2014b. A sustained hypothalamic–pituitary–adrenal axis response to acute psychosocial stress in irritable bowel syndrome. Psychol. Med. 44, 3123–3134.

Kettenmann, H., Hanisch, U.-K., Noda, M., Verkhratsky, A., 2011. Physiology of microglia. Physiol. Rev. 91, 461–553.

Knudsen, E., 2004. Sensitive periods in the development of the brain and behavior. Cogn. Neurosci. J. 16, 1412–1425.

Kohane, I.S., McMurry, A., Weber, G., MacFadden, D., Rappaport, L., Kunkel, L., Bickel, J., Wattanasin, N., Spence, S., Murphy, S., 2012. The co-morbidity burden of children and young adults with autism spectrum disorders. PLoS One 7, e33224.

Koren, O., Spor, A., Felin, J., Fåk, F., Stombaugh, J., Tremaroli, V., Behre, C.J., Knight, R., Fagerberg, B., Ley, R.E., Bäckhed, F., 2011. Human oral, gut, and plaque microbiota in patients with atherosclerosis. Proc. Natl. Acad. Sci. 108, 4592–4598. http://dx.doi.org/10.1073/pnas.1011383107.

Kunze, W.A., Mao, Y., Wang, B., Huizinga, J.D., Ma, X., Forsythe, P., Bienenstock, J., 2009. *Lactobacillus reuteri* enhances excitability of colonic AH neurons by inhibiting calcium-dependent potassium channel opening. J. Cell. Mol. Med. 13, 2261–2270.

Lakshminarasimhan, H., Chattarji, S., 2012. Stress leads to contrasting effects on the levels of brain derived neurotrophic factor in the hippocampus and amygdala. PLoS One 7, e30481.

Leone, V., Gibbons, S.M., Martinez, K., Hutchison, A.L., Huang, E.Y., Cham, C.M., Pierre, J.F., Heneghan, A.F., Nadimpalli, A., Hubert, N., Zale, E., Wang, Y., Huang, Y., Theriault, B., Dinner, A.R., Musch, M.W., Kudsk, K.A., Prendergast, B.J., Gilbert, J.A., Chang, E.B., 2015. Effects of diurnal variation of gut microbes and high-fat feeding on host circadian clock function and metabolism. Cell Host Microbe 17, 681–689. http://dx.doi.org/10.1016/j.chom.2015.03.006.

Ley, R.E., Turnbaugh, P.J., Klein, S., Gordon, J.I., 2006. Microbial ecology: human gut microbes associated with obesity. Nature 444, 1022–1023.

Lombardo, M.P., 2008. Access to mutualistic endosymbiotic microbes: an underappreciated benefit of group living. Behav. Ecol. Sociobiol 62, 479–497.

Lyte, M., Li, W., Opitz, N., Gaykema, R.P.A., Goehler, L.E., 2006. Induction of anxiety-like behavior in mice during the initial stages of infection with the agent of murine colonic hyperplasia *Citrobacter rodentium*. Physiol. Behav. 89, 350–357.

Lyte, M., Varcoe, J.J., Bailey, M.T., 1998. Anxiogenic effect of subclinical bacterial infection in mice in the absence of overt immune activation. Physiol. Behav. 65, 63–68.

Macpherson, A.J., Harris, N.L., 2004. Interactions between commensal intestinal bacteria and the immune system. Nat. Rev. Immunol. 4, 478–485.

Marín-Burgin, A., Schinde r, A.F., 2012. Requirement of adult-born neurons for hippocampus-dependent learning. Behav. Brain Res. 227, 391–399.

Mayer, E.A., 2000. The neurobiology of stress and gastrointestinal disease. Gut 47, 861–869.

Mayer, E.A., Padua, D., Tillisch, K., 2014. Altered brain-gut axis in autism: comorbidity or causative mechanisms? BioEssays 36, 933–939.

Mayer, E.A., Tillisch, K., Gupta, A., 2015. Gut/brain axis and the microbiota. J. Clin. Invest. 125, 0.

Mcvey Neufeld, K.A., Mao, Y.K., Bienenstock, J., Foster, J.A., Kunze, W.A, 2013. The microbiome is essential for normal gut intrinsic primary afferent neuron excitability in the mouse. Neurogastroenterol. Motil. 25, 183. http://dx.doi.org/10.1111/nmo.12049. e88.

McVey Neufeld, K.A., Perez-Burgos, A., Mao, Y.K., Bienenstock, J., Kunze, W.A., 2015. The gut microbiome restores intrinsic and extrinsic nerve function in germ-free mice accompanied by changes in calbindin. Neurogastroenterol. Motil. 27, 627–636.

Messaoudi, M., Lalonde, R., Violle, N., Javelot, H., Desor, D., Nejdi, A., Bisson, J.-F., Rougeot, C., Pichelin, M., Cazaubiel, M., 2011. Assessment of psychotropic-like properties of a probiotic formulation (*Lactobacillus helveticus* R0052 and *Bifidobacterium longum* R0175) in rats and human subjects. Br. J. Nutr. 105, 755–764.

Miller, B.R., Hen, R., 2015. The current state of the neurogenic theory of depression and anxiety. Curr. Opin. Neurobiol. 30, 51–58.

Montiel-Castro, A.J., González-Cervantes, R.M., Bravo-Ruiseco, G., Pacheco-López, G., 2013. The microbiota-gut-brain axis: neurobehavioral correlates, health and sociality. Front. Integr. Neurosci. 7.

Moser, M.-B., Moser, E.I., Forrest, E., Andersen, P., Morris, R.G., 1995. Spatial learning with a minislab in the dorsal hippocampus. Proc. Natl. Acad. Sci. 92, 9697–9701.

Mulle, J.G., Sharp, W.G., Cubells, J.F., 2013. The gut microbiome: a new frontier in autism research. Curr. Psychiatry Rep. 15, 1–9.

Myint, A.-M., Kim, Y.K., Verkerk, R., Scharpé, S., Steinbusch, H., Leonard, B., 2007. Kynurenine pathway in major depression: evidence of impaired neuroprotection. J. Affect. Disord. 98, 143–151.

Neufeld, K.M., Kang, N., Bienenstock, J., Foster, J.A., 2011. Reduced anxiety-like behavior and central neurochemical change in germ-free mice. Neurogastroenterol. Motil. 23, 255–265. http://dx.doi.org/10.1111/j.1365-2982.2010.01620.x.

Nicholson, J., Holmes, E., Kinross, J., Burcelin, R., Gibson, G., Jia, W., Petttersen, S., 2012. Host-gut microbiota metabolic interactions. Science 336, 1262–1267. http://dx.doi.org/10.1126/science.1223813.

Nobel, Y.R., Cox, L.M., Kirigin, F.F., Bokulich, N.A., Yamanishi, S., Teitler, I., Chung, J., Sohn, J., Barber, C.M., Goldfarb, D.S., Raju, K., Abubucker, S., Zhou, Y., Ruiz, V.E., Li, H., Mitreva, M., Alekseyenko, A.V., Weinstock, G.M., Sodergren, E., Blaser, M.J., 2015. Metabolic and metagenomic outcomes from early-life pulsed antibiotic treatment. Nat. Commun. 6.

Nuttall, G.H.F., Thierfelder, H., 1897. Thierisches Leben ohne Bakterien im Verdauungskanal. (II. Mittheilung). Hoppe. Seylers. Z. Physiol. Chem. 22, 62–73.

O'Leary, O.F., Cryan, J.F., 2014. A ventral view on antidepressant action: roles for adult hippocampal neurogenesis along the dorsoventral axis. Trends Pharmacol. Sci. 35, 675–687.

O'Mahony, C.M., Sweeney, F.F., Daly, E., Dinan, T.G., Cryan, J.F., 2010. Restraint stress-induced brain activation patterns in two strains of mice differing in their anxiety behaviour. Behav. Brain Res. 213, 148–154.

O'Mahony, S.M., Clarke, G., Borre, Y.E., Dinan, T.G., Cryan, J.F., 2015. Serotonin, tryptophan metabolism and the brain-gut-microbiome axis. Behav. Brain Res. 277, 32–48.

O'Mahony, S.M., Marchesi, J.R., Scully, P., Codling, C., Ceolho, A.-M., Quigley, E.M.M., Cryan, J.F., Dinan, T.G., 2009. Early life stress alters behavior, immunity, and microbiota in rats: implications for irritable bowel syndrome and psychiatric illnesses. Biol. Psychiatry 65, 263–267.

O'Toole, P.W., Claesson, M.J., 2010. Gut microbiota: changes throughout the lifespan from infancy to elderly. Int. Dairy J. 20, 281–291.

Ogbonnaya, E.S., Clarke, G., Shanahan, F., Dinan, T.G., Cryan, J.F., O'Leary, O.F., 2015. Adult hippocampal neurogenesis is regulated by the microbiome. Biol. Psychiatry. http://dx.doi.org/10.1016/j.biopsych.2014.12.023.

Park, H., Poo, M., 2013. Neurotrophin regulation of neural circuit development and function. Nat. Rev. Neurosci. 14, 7–23.

Pasteur, L., 1885. Observations relatives à la note précédente de M. Duclaux. CR Acad. Sci. 100, 68.

Perez-Burgos, A., Mao, Y.-K., Bienenstock, J., Kunze, W.A., 2014. The gut-brain axis rewired: adding a functional vagal nicotinic "sensory synapse". FASEB J. 28, 3064–3074.

Powley, T.L., Wang, X.Y., Fox, E.A., Phillips, R.J., Liu, L.W.C., Huizinga, J.D., 2008. Ultrastructural evidence for communication between intramuscular vagal mechanoreceptors and interstitial cells of cajal in the rat fundus. Neurogastroenterol. Motil. 20, 69–79.

Prinz, M., Priller, J., 2014. Microglia and brain macrophages in the molecular age: from origin to neuropsychiatric disease. Nat. Rev. Neurosci. 15, 300–312.

Qin, J., Li, R., Raes, J., Arumugam, M., Burgdorf, K.S., Manichanh, C., Nielsen, T., Pons, N., Levenez, F., Yamada, T., 2010. A human gut microbial gene catalogue established by metagenomic sequencing. Nature 464, 59–65.

Qin, J., Li, Y., Cai, Z., Li, S., Zhu, J., Zhang, F., Liang, S., Zhang, W., Guan, Y., Shen, D., 2012. A metagenome-wide association study of gut microbiota in type 2 diabetes. Nature 490, 55–60.

Rakoff-Nahoum, S., Paglino, J., Eslami-Varzaneh, F., Edberg, S., Medzhitov, R., 2004. Recognition of commensal microflora by toll-like receptors is required for intestinal homeostasis. Cell 118, 229–241.

Ransohoff, R.M., Perry, V.H., 2009. Microglial physiology: unique stimuli, specialized responses. Annu. Rev. Immunol. 27, 119–145.

Reyniers, J.A., 1959. The pure culture concept and gnotobiotics. Ann. N. Y. Acad. Sci. 78, 3–16.

Reyniers, J.A., Trexler, P.C., Ervin, R.F., 1946. Rearing germ-free albino rats. Lobund Rep. 1.

Rhee, S.H., Pothoulakis, C., Mayer, E.A., 2009. Principles and clinical implications of the brain-gut-enteric microbiota axis. Nat. Rev. Gastroenterol. Hepatol. 6, 306–314.

Ridaura, V., Belkaid, Y., 2015. Gut microbiota: the link to your second brain. Cell 161, 193–194. http://dx.doi.org/10.1016/j.cell.2015.03.033.

Ridaura, V.K., Faith, J.J., Rey, F.E., Cheng, J., Duncan, A.E., Kau, A.L., Griffin, N.W., Lombard, V., Henrissat, B., Bain, J.R., 2013. Gut microbiota from twins discordant for obesity modulate metabolism in mice. Science 341, 1241214.

Rodgers, R., Haller, J., Holmes, A., Halasz, J., Walton, T., Brain, P., 1999. Corticosterone response to the plus-maze: high correlation with risk assessment in rats and mice. Physiol. Behav. 68, 47–53. http://dx.doi.org/10.1016/S0031-9384(99)00140-7.

Rosenfeld, C.S., 2015. Microbiome disturbances and autism spectrum disorders. Drug Metab. Dispos. 43 (10), 1557–1571.

Salonen, A., de Vos, W.M., Palva, A., 2010. Gastrointestinal microbiota in irritable bowel syndrome: present state and perspectives. Microbiology 156, 3205–3215.

Sampson, T.R., Mazmanian, S.K., 2015. Control of brain development, function, and behavior by the microbiome. Cell Host Microbe 17, 565–576. http://dx.doi.org/10.1016/j.chom.2015.04.011.

Savignac, H.M., Tramullas, M., Kiely, B., Dinan, T.G., Cryan, J.F., 2015. Bifidobacteria modulate cognitive processes in an anxious mouse strain. Behav. Brain Res. 287, 59–72. http://dx.doi.org/10.1016/j.bbr.2015.02.044.

Schafer, D.P., Stevens, B., 2013. Phagocytic glial cells: sculpting synaptic circuits in the developing nervous system. Curr. Opin. Neurobiol. 23, 1034–1040.

Sekirov, I., Russell, S.L., Antunes, L.C.M., Finlay, B.B., 2010. Gut microbiota in health and disease. Physiol. Rev. 90, 859–904.

Shanahan, F., 2002. The host–microbe interface within the gut. Best Pract. Res. Clin. Gastroenterol. 16, 915–931.

Smith, K., McCoy, K.D., Macpherson, A.J., 2007. Use of axenic animals in studying the adaptation of mammals to their commensal intestinal microbiota. In: Seminars in Immunology. Elsevier, pp. 59–69.

Snyder, J.S., Soumier, A., Brewer, M., Pickel, J., Cameron, H.A., 2011. Adult hippocampal neurogenesis buffers stress responses and depressive behaviour. Nature 476, 458–461.

Stilling, R.M., Bordenstein, S.R., Dinan, T.G., Cryan, J.F., 2014a. Friends with social benefits: host-microbe interactions as a driver of brain evolution and development? Front. Cell. Infect. Microbiol. 4.

Stilling, R.M., Dinan, T.G., Cryan, J.F., 2014b. Microbial genes, brain & behaviour–epigenetic regulation of the gut–brain axis. Genes, Brain Behav. 13, 69–86.

Stilling, R.M., Ryan, F.J., Hoban, A.E., Shanahan, F., Clarke, G., Claesson, M.J., Dinan, T.G., Cryan, J.F., 2015. Microbes & neurodevelopment - absence of microbiota during early life increases activity-related transcriptional pathways in the amygdala. Brain Behav. Immun. http://dx.doi.org/10.1016/j.bbi.2015.07.009.

Sudo, N., Chida, Y., Aiba, Y., Sonoda, J., Oyama, N., Yu, X.-N., Kubo, C., Koga, Y., 2004. Postnatal microbial colonization programs the hypothalamic-pituitary-adrenal system for stress response in mice. J. Physiol. 558, 263–275. http://dx.doi.org/10.1113/jphysiol.2004.063388.

Suez, J., Korem, T., Zeevi, D., Zilberman-schapira, G., Thaiss, C.a, Maza, O., Israeli, D., Zmora, N., Gilad, S., Weinberger, A., Kuperman, Y., Harmelin, A., Kolodkin-gal, I., Shapiro, H., 2014. Artificial sweeteners induce glucose intolerance by altering the gut microbiota. Nature 514, 181–186. http://dx.doi.org/10.1038/nature13793.

Sumi, Y., Miyakawa, M., Kanzaki, M., Kotake, Y., 1977. Vitamin B-6 deficiency in germfree rats. J. Nutr. 107, 1707–1714.

Tana, C., Umesaki, Y., Imaoka, A., Handa, T., Kanazawa, M., Fukudo, S., 2010. Altered profiles of intestinal microbiota and organic acids may be the origin of symptoms in irritable bowel syndrome. Neurogastroenterol. Motil. 22, 512. e115.

Tazume, S., Umehara, K., Matsuzawa, H., Aikawa, H., Hashimoto, K., Sasaki, S., 1991. Effects of germfree status and food restriction on longevity and growth of mice. Jikken Dobutsu 40, 517–522.

Thaiss, C.A., Zeevi, D., Levy, M., Zilberman-schapira, G., Suez, J., Tengeler, A.C., Abramson, L., Katz, M.N., Korem, T., Zmora, N., Kuperman, Y., Biton, I., Gilad, S., Harmelin, A., Shapiro, H., Halpern, Z., Segal, E., Elinav, E., 2014. Article transkingdom control of microbiota diurnal oscillations promotes metabolic homeostasis. Cell 159, 514–529. http://dx.doi.org/10.1016/j.cell.2014.09.048.

Tremaroli, V., Backhed, F., 2012. Functional interactions between the gut microbiota and host metabolism. Nature 489, 242–249.

Troyer, K., 1984. Microbes, herbivory and the evolution of social behavior. J. Theor. Biol. 106, 157–169.

Tung, J., Barreiro, L.B., Burns, M.B., Grenier, J.-C., Lynch, J., Grieneisen, L.E., Altmann, J., Alberts, S.C., Blekhman, R., Archie, E.A, 2015. Social networks predict gut microbiome composition in wild baboons. eLife 4, 1–18. http://dx.doi.org/10.7554/eLife.05224.

Tuohy, K.M., Fava, F., Viola, R., 2014. "The way to a man's heart is through his gut microbiota" – dietary pro- and prebiotics for the management of cardiovascular risk. Proc. Nutr. Soc. 73, 172–185.

Turnbaugh, P.J., Hamady, M., Yatsunenko, T., Cantarel, B.L., Duncan, A., Ley, R.E., Sogin, M.L., Jones, W.J., Roe, B.A., Affourtit, J.P., 2009a. A core gut microbiome in obese and lean twins. Nature 457, 480–484.

Turnbaugh, P.J., Ley, R.E., Mahowald, M.a, Magrini, V., Mardis, E.R., Gordon, J.I., 2006. An obesity-associated gut microbiome with increased capacity for energy harvest. Nature 444, 1027–1031. http://dx.doi.org/10.1038/nature05414.

Turnbaugh, P.J., Ridaura, V.K., Faith, J.J., Rey, F.E., Knight, R., Gordon, J.I., 2009b. The effect of diet on the human gut microbiome: a metagenomic analysis in humanized gnotobiotic mice. Sci. Transl. Med. 1, 6ra14.

Ulevitch, R.J., 1999. Endotoxin opens the toll gates to innate immunity. Nat. Med. 5, 144–145.

Umesaki, Y., Okada, Y., Matsumoto, S., Imaoka, A., Setoyama, H., 1995. Segmented filamentous bacteria are indigenous intestinal bacteria that activate intraepithelial lymphocytes and induce MHC class II molecules and fucosyl asialo GM1 glycolipids on the small intestinal epithelial cells in the ex-germ-free mouse. Microbiol. Immunol. 39, 555–562.

Vaishnava, S., Behrendt, C.L., Ismail, A.S., Eckmann, L., Hooper, L.V., 2008. Paneth cells directly sense gut commensals and maintain homeostasis at the intestinal host-microbial interface. Proc. Natl. Acad. Sci. 105, 20858–20863.

Vrieze, A., Van Nood, E., Holleman, F., Salojärvi, J., Kootte, R.S., Bartelsman, J.F.W.M., Dallinga–Thie, G.M., Ackermans, M.T., Serlie, M.J., Oozeer, R., Derrien, M., Druesne, A., Van Hylckama Vlieg, J.E.T., Bloks, V.W., Groen, A.K., Heilig, H.G.H.J., Zoetendal, E.G., Stroes, E.S., de Vos, W.M., Hoekstra, J.B.L., Nieuwdorp, M., 2012. Transfer of intestinal microbiota from lean donors increases insulin sensitivity in individuals with metabolic syndrome. Gastroenterology 143, 913–916. http://dx.doi.org/10.1053/j.gastro.2012.06.031. e7.

Wang, M., Donovan, S.M., 2015. Human microbiota-associated swine: current progress and future opportunities. ILAR J. 56, 63–73. http://dx.doi.org/10.1093/ilar/ilv006.

Williams, S.C.P., 2014. Gnotobiotics. Proc. Natl. Acad. Sci. 111, 1661.

Wostmann, B., Bruckner-Kardoss, E., 1959. Development of cecal distention in germ-free baby rats. Am. J. Physiol. Content 197, 1345–1346.

Wostmann, B.S., Knight, P.L., Keeley, L.L., Kan, D.F., 1962. Metabolism and function of thiamine and naphthoquinones in germfree and conventional rats. In: Federation Proceedings, pp. 120–124.

Wostmann, B.S., Larkin, C., Moriarty, A., Bruckner-Kardoss, E., 1983. Dietary intake, energy metabolism, and excretory losses of adult male germfree wistar rats. Lab. Anim. Sci. 33, 46–50.

Wostmann, B.S., Pleasants, J.R., Bealmear, P., Kincade, P.W., 1970. Serum proteins and lymphoid tissues in germ-free mice fed a chemically defined, water soluble, low molecular weight diet. Immunology 19, 443.

Wrase, J., Reimold, M., Puls, I., Kienast, T., Heinz, A., 2006. Serotonergic dysfunction: brain imaging and behavioral correlates. Cogn. Affect. Behav. Neurosci. 6, 53–61.

Wu, J.C.Y., 2012. Psychological co-morbidity in functional gastrointestinal disorders: epidemiology, mechanisms and management. J. Neurogastroenterol. Motil. 18, 13–18.

Yano, J.M., Yu, K., Donaldson, G.P., Shastri, G.G., Ann, P., Ma, L., Nagler, C.R., Ismagilov, R.F., Mazmanian, S.K., Hsiao, E.Y., 2015. Indigenous bacteria from the gut microbiota regulate host serotonin biosynthesis. Cell 161, 264–276. http://dx.doi.org/10.1016/j.cell.2015.02.047.

Young, S.N., Leyton, M., 2002. The role of serotonin in human mood and social interaction: insight from altered tryptophan levels. Pharmacol. Biochem. Behav. 71, 857–865.

Zimomra, Z.R., Porterfield, V.M., Camp, R.M., Johnson, J.D., 2011. Time-dependent mediators of HPA axis activation following live *Escherichia coli*. Am. J. Physiol. Integr. Comp. Physiol. 301, R1648–R1657.

Global and Epidemiological Perspectives on Diet and Mood

F.N. Jacka

Deakin University, Geelong, VIC, Australia

Noncommunicable diseases (NCDs) globally account for the largest burden of early mortality and are predicted to cost more than US$30 trillion over the next 20 years (Bloom et al., 2011). However, when the global burden of disease is viewed in terms of disability rather than mortality, mental and substance use disorders account for the leading cause of health-related disability worldwide, with unipolar depression alone accounting for the second highest number of years lost to disability (Murray et al., 2013). Although methodological challenges complicate attempts to assess possible increases in the prevalence of mental disorders, there are data to support such increases from the United States (Twenge et al., 2010), Britain (Collishaw et al., 2004), Taiwan (Fu et al., 2013), and Australia (O'Donnell et al., 2013), although upward trends in young people may be plateauing (Maughan et al., 2008).

Although three of the "Big Four" NCDs—cardiovascular disease (CVD), type 2 diabetes mellitus, and cancer—are well known to be directly influenced by unhealthy diet (WHO, 2011; Swinburn et al., 2011), there is now highly consistent evidence across age groups, cultures, and countries to suggest that unhealthy diet is also a key risk factor for common mental disorders, particularly depression. The following presents a discussion of the change to global eating patterns and the recent literature highlighting the relationships between diet and mental health.

CHANGES TO THE FOOD SUPPLY AND GLOBAL IMPACT ON HEALTH

Substantial changes in efficiencies of production, marketing, transport, and sale of food have had a highly detrimental impact on dietary patterns across the globe, with a widespread shift toward increased intake of fast foods and sugar-sweetened beverages (Adair and Popkin, 2005). In the West, dietary patterns are commonly high in saturated fats and refined sugar, with nutrient-poor and energy-dense foods contributing approximately 30% of the daily intakes of US adults (Kant, 2000). A comprehensive review of data from the recurrent National Health and Nutrition Examination

Surveys in the United States concluded that only one in 10 Americans has a "good" diet (Briefel and Johnson, 2004). Although slight improvements have been detected in the dietary intakes of sugar and fats in recent years, intakes of nutrient- and fiber-rich vegetables and whole grains remain far lower than recommended (Bowman et al., 2014). Moreover, compared with wealthier areas, the urban built environment of those living in low socioeconomic status neighborhoods promotes unhealthy food consumption, with more fast food outlets and convenience stores and associated advertising of unhealthy food products than wealthier areas (Larson et al., 2009), leading to pronounced health inequalities.

Equally, changes in economic conditions in developing economies, including increased income, trade liberalization, and globalization, as well as increased penetration of processed food industries, have led to profound shifts in habitual dietary patterns away from traditional diets higher in plant foods rich in fiber and nutrients toward patterns characterized by manufactured food products higher in saturated fat, sugar, salt, and refined carbohydrates and foods of animal origin. As a result, there is now a far greater burden of poor health and mortality from NCDs than from undernutrition and infectious diseases in Latin America, North Africa, the Middle East, South East and East Asia, and the Pacific Rim (Popkin, 2002). Indeed, more than three-quarters of all nutrition-related chronic diseases occur in developing countries (Popkin and Du, 2003). As one example, consumption of whole-grain cereals and vegetables decreased in China between 1989 and 1997 whereas the consumption of meat, meat products, and plant oils increased (Popkin and Du, 2003). This represents a shift away from carbohydrates to fats as the dominant energy source and was reflected in a concurrent increase in the prevalence of overweight individuals and obesity in China (Popkin and Du, 2003). Likewise, Indian data from 1987 to 1988 and from 1999 to 2000 showed a decrease in the consumption of rice and wheat, while whole milk and egg consumption increased, as did consumption of biscuits, salted snacks, prepared sweets, edible oils, and sugar (Food and Agriculture Organization, 2004). Alongside these changes were declines in the intake of fruit and vegetables. In particular, consumption of processed foods and ready-to-eat foods were observed to increase with income. Concordant with these changes, in 1999 one-third of men and half of women in the middle classes in India were obese.

When considering changes in dietary patterns over recent decades, it is also worth making a comparison with the composition of our ancestors' diets. It is estimated that dietary intakes of micronutrients for early humans may have been up to 10 times that of modern humans because of the composition of wild plant foods known to be consumed by hunter-gatherers (Brand-Miller and Holt, 1998); carbohydrate consumption was almost exclusively derived from fruits and vegetables (Eaton and Eaton, 2000). In comparison, contemporary Americans obtain 72% of their total dietary energy from dairy products, cereals, refined sugars, refined vegetable oils, and alcohol (Cordain et al., 2005). Furthermore, the high potassium-to-sodium ratios and high fiber intakes known to characterize Paleolithic diets are the inverse of contemporary Western diets (Cordain et al., 2005).

Although there was wide variation in dietary regimens for Stone Agers, preagricultural humans consumed more animal protein than current Westerners (Eaton and Eaton, 2000). A meta-analysis of dietary studies of hunter-gatherers reported that animal foods provided approximately 65% of energy intakes for early humans (Cordain et al., 2002). However, this did not appear to adversely affect CVD risk factors because of the different lipid profiles of the foods consumed; in contrast to intensively farmed cattle, wild game contain high levels of monounsaturated fatty acids as well as long-chain polyunsaturated fatty acids (PUFAs). In concert with higher intakes of plant foods and lower intakes of sodium, as well as much higher levels of physical activity, this pattern of consumption served to inhibit the development of CVD (Cordain et al., 2002). In support of this, intervention studies performed in indigenous Australian populations have reported a pronounced reduction in risk factors for CVD, as well as metabolic abnormalities associated with diabetes, after reversion to a traditional hunter-gatherer diet containing substantial quantities of red meat from wild animals (O'Dea, 1984; O'Dea and Sinclair, 1985). Reflecting these findings, nutritional studies of contemporary hunter-gathers have reported high plasma concentrations of folate and vitamin B_{12} (Metz et al., 1971).

Another important aspect of the shift in habitual diets globally is that of an increase in refined carbohydrate consumption. The consumption of caloric sweeteners, which include high fructose corn syrup and a wide range of other monosaccharides (glucose and fructose) and disaccharides (sucrose and saccharose), has increased significantly across the globe (Popkin and Nielsen, 2003), largely because of the proliferation of processed foods that have these sweeteners added to them. An analysis of exposure data from 52 countries, performed at Harvard University, demonstrated that raised blood glucose accounts for 21% of ischemic heart disease and 13% of stroke mortality worldwide (Danaei et al., 2006). Of note, higher-than-optimal blood glucose concentrations were associated with a higher risk of mortality than full-blown diabetes (Danaei et al., 2006). This underscores the deleterious impact of these dietary changes on a global scale.

NUTRIENTS AND MENTAL HEALTH

Although there has long been interest in the idea that diet is related to mental health, before 2009, scientific data were scarce and the existing literature focused primarily on individual nutrients or foods—particularly fish and the long-chain omega-3 polyunsaturated fatty acids (n-3 PUFAs). Estimates from studies examining Paleolithic nutrition and extant hunter-gatherer populations suggest that humans evolved to consume a diet consisting of an omega-6 to omega-3 ratio of 1–2:1 (Eaton and Konner, 1985). This compares to Western ratios of between 10 and 20:1 (Simopoulos, 2001). Several lines of evidence indicate that these changes in fatty acid consumption may have had a detrimental impact on mental health.

In one of the first studies in this field, Hibbeln (1998) suggested that substantial cross-national variation in prevalence rates of depression may be, in part, a function of a demonstrated, strong, inverse correlation between national levels of fish consumption and national depression prevalence rates across nine countries. In a similar study (Hibbeln, 2002), postpartum depression was inversely associated with docosahexaenoic acid (DHA) concentrations in breast milk in a multinational comparison of 16 countries, whereas a strong inverse relationship also existed between postpartum depression and fish consumption across 22 countries. Likewise, in another cross-national comparison (Noaghiul and Hibbeln, 2003), higher national seafood consumption was associated with lower prevalence rates of bipolar spectrum disorders. To test the hypothesis according to its proposed biological mechanisms, schizophrenia data were used as a control condition. Seafood consumption was not associated with national prevalence rates of schizophrenia in any analysis, supporting a specific relationship between n-3 PUFAs and mood disorders. Although these studies present findings that are supportive of the hypothesis of a relationship between n-3 PUFA consumption and depressive illness, the results must be viewed with caution. Clearly, a correlation between factors at the national level may be explained by a multitude of cultural, social, and economic factors that could not be controlled for in appropriate multivariate analyses. On the other hand, cross-national studies may provide a valuable perspective because the habitual consumption of a particular food group may be more stable over time at a population level than in that of individuals.

In several population studies, which allow for an assessment of possible confounding, low levels of fish and/or n-3 PUFA consumption are associated with increased depression (Appleton et al., 2007; Bountziouka et al., 2009; Colangelo et al., 2009; Silvers and Scott, 2002; Tanskanen et al., 2001; Timonen, et al., 2004), although some of these studies suggest nonlinear relationships (Jacka et al., 2013a; Sanchez-Villegas et al., 2007). However, trials of n-3 PUFA supplementation in depression have yielded equivocal results. One meta-analysis examining the effect of n-3 PUFA supplementation for depressed mood concluded that there was a small beneficial effect of treatment with n-3 PUFA compared with placebo, but that this benefit was restricted to those with major depressive disorder (MDD; Appleton et al., 2010). This may reflect an increased need for the long-chain omega-three fatty acids for those suffering major depression, in which the increased inflammation and accompanying oxidative stress commonly observed in major depression (Maes et al., 2011) results in increased lipid peroxidation and a reduction in lipid levels in neuronal membranes. On the other hand, another meta-analysis suggests that supplementation with n-3 PUFA formulations that are relatively higher in eicosapentaenoic acid (>60%) compared with DHA may be efficacious in treating depression (Lin et al., 2012). Another meta-analysis also concluded that n-3 PUFA as an adjunctive supplement improves bipolar depression but not mania (Sarris et al., 2012).

There are many other nutrients found in healthy foods that have also been related to mental health. Folate is found in abundance in vegetables, fruits, and salads, yet the intake of these foods is commonly less than recommended dietary intakes within populations. Clinical studies have long observed folate deficiency and low folate status in those with clinical depression, and low folate is also associated with depression in population studies (Morris et al., 2003), even in the presence of folate fortification (Ramos et al., 2004). Indeed, population studies are plentiful. In a study of middle-aged Finnish men, the odds of self-reported depression for those in the lowest tertile of folate intake were increased by nearly 50% after all adjustments (Tolmunen et al., 2003), whereas another prospective study in Finnish men reported that intakes of folate below the median were associated with a threefold increased risk of MDD over more than 10 years of follow-up (Tolmunen et al., 2004). Likewise, a study of 732 elderly Korean men reported that lower serum levels of folate and vitamin B_{12} and higher levels of homocysteine were all associated with an increased risk of clinically significant depression over the follow-up period (Kim et al., 2008), whereas a Japanese study reported that serum folate levels predicted depression risk over 3 years of follow-up in office workers (Nanri et al., 2012). Two cross-sectional, population-based studies also examined this relationship and found a significant, linear association of folate intake with depressive symptoms in Japanese men, but not women (Murakami et al., 2008), and an inverse relationship between folate intake and MDD in Australian women (Jacka et al., 2012b). A meta-analysis of case-control, population, and cohort studies confirmed the association between low folate status and depression (Gilbody et al., 2007), whereas a Cochrane review concluded that folate may be useful as an adjunctive treatment for depression, although it is still unclear as to whether supplementation will benefit those with low and normal levels of folate (Taylor et al., 2004).

Magnesium is another micronutrient that is found in abundance in healthy foods, such as fruits, vegetables, fish, legumes, and whole grains, and it is inversely associated with depression. A recent meta-analysis including data from nearly 20,000 participants reported a 1.34-fold increased risk of hypomagnesemia in those with depression (Cheungpasitporn et al., 2015); however, data from population studies focusing on dietary intakes are somewhat equivocal. Jacka et al. (2009) observed an inverse relationship between dietary magnesium intake and depression in a large sample of community-dwelling men and women in Norway that was independent of potentially confounding variables and reported similar inverse and independent relationships between magnesium intake and clinical depressive disorders in Australian women (Jacka et al., 2012b). In contrast, Derom et al. reported no relationship between magnesium intake and depression risk in the SUN Cohort study (Derom et al., 2012). Likewise, an inverse relationship between magnesium intake and depression in a large US study was only observed in younger people (Tarleton and Littenberg, 2015), with a positive relationship seen in older people. Barragan-Rodriguez et al. reported that magnesium supplementation was as effective as pharmacotherapy in treating depression in elderly diabetic patients with hypomagnesemia (Barragan-Rodriguez et al., 2008). However, magnesium was not found to alleviate symptoms of depression or anxiety in premenstrual women (Walker et al., 1998). Certainly, experimental studies support a role for magnesium in depression; in animals, a magnesium-deficient diet increases depression and anxiety-related behavior (Singewald et al., 2004), whereas magnesium treatment appears to improve such behaviors (Poleszak et al., 2004, 2005).

Zinc is another nutrient of particular interest in depressive illness. There have now been cross-sectional studies showing inverse relationships between the dietary intake of zinc and self-reported depression in pregnant women (Roy et al., 2011), female students (Amani et al., 2011), and a large representative sample of Australian women (Jacka et al., 2012b). In support of this finding, a recent study has also reported that women habitually consuming less than the recommended intake of red meat, a food rich in zinc, were more likely to be diagnosed with clinical depressive and/or anxiety disorders (Jacka et al., 2012a), although higher than recommended levels of intake were also associated with an increased likelihood of these illnesses. Low dietary zinc intake was also associated with increased risk of depression in older Australian men and women over time (Vashum et al., 2014). In a clinical context, low concentrations of zinc are commonly observed in patients with major depression (Swardfager et al., 2013) whereas zinc supplementation has been shown to enhance the efficacy of antidepressant therapy (Nowak et al., 2003a), with a systematic review supporting its use as an adjunctive therapy (Lai et al., 2011). There are also supportive data from animal studies suggesting that zinc may exert antidepressant effects (Nowak et al., 2003b). Thus further studies of zinc as a mono- and adjunctive therapy in depression may be warranted.

DIET QUALITY

It is important to recognize that magnesium, folate, zinc, and long-chain fatty acids are all components of a healthy diet, found primarily in foods such as leafy green vegetables, legumes, whole grains, lean red meat, and fish. As such it is likely that the apparent relationship between the consumption of these individual components of food and mental health is explained by the overall quality of an individual's habitual diet. As a response to this understanding, the new field of nutritional psychiatry has now, in concert with the wider field of nutrition research, moved away from examining individual nutrients toward an examination of the importance of whole diet in mental health. In this context there have now been many observational studies published in the last several years demonstrating cross-sectional and prospective relationships between diet quality and the common mental disorders in adults, adolescents, and children. In the first study to examine the relationship between dietary patterns and clinical mood and anxiety disorders, a dietary pattern comprising vegetables, fruit, beef, lamb, fish, and whole-grain foods was associated with a reduced likelihood of clinically diagnosed depressive and anxiety disorders, whereas a Western dietary pattern comprising processed and unhealthy foods was associated with an increased likelihood of psychological symptoms as well as MDD and dysthymia in Australian women. Increased a priori diet quality scores were also associated with reduced psychological symptoms (Jacka et al., 2010b). In this same cohort of women, increased scores on the same healthy dietary pattern were also associated with a halving in the odds for bipolar disorder whereas those with higher scores on the Western dietary pattern and glycemic load measures were more likely to have bipolar disorder (Jacka et al., 2011a). Associations between diet quality and mental health outcomes have also been reported in a study of more than 7000 adults in western Norway (Jacka et al., 2011c). A healthier diet, measured with an a priori diet quality score, was associated with a reduction in the odds ratios for depression and anxiety in women and with reduced odds for depression, but not anxiety, in men. Nanri et al. (2010) have also reported that middle-aged Japanese municipal employees who were in the highest tertile of healthy Japanese dietary pattern scores, characterized by higher intakes of vegetables, fruit, soy products, and mushrooms, were significantly less likely to be depressed than those in the lowest tertile, although there was no discernible relationship between unhealthy food intake and depression. In the United States, a healthier diet was associated with reduced depressive symptoms cross-sectionally, including after adjustment for race, gender, age, education, and income (Kuczmarski et al., 2010). Conversely, an increased consumption of high-calorie sweet foods was associated with increased depressive symptoms in more than 4500 middle-aged US women (Jeffery et al., 2009). In the same study, an increased intake of low-calorie foods (eg, green salads, roast chicken, baked fish, low-fat milk, and cold cereals) was associated with reduced depressive symptoms, independent of age, race, body mass index (BMI), and education.

There are many prospective studies that have also shed light on this topic. In Spain, Sanchez-Villegas et al. (2009) demonstrated an inverse association between the level of adherence to a Mediterranean dietary pattern (MDP) and the risk for incident depression over time in more than 10,000 middle-aged university graduates. This association existed before and after controlling for a comprehensive range of potentially confounding factors, including sociodemographic, anthropometric, and lifestyle factors; other health behaviors; and medical history. Of course, depression itself may cause poor dietary choices, which may in turn worsen an existing condition. Thus many of the prospective studies have conducted sensitivity analyses to investigate the "reverse causality" hypothesis. In the SUN Cohort study the authors attempted to refute reverse causality as an explanatory factor by repeating analyses after excluding participants who reported depression in the first 2 years of follow-up, as well as examining depression at or before the baseline assessment as an exposure, with adherence to the MDP as the outcome variable (Sanchez-Villegas et al., 2009). In fact, the relationship of diet to MDP adherence was strengthened rather than diminished after removing participants with incipient depression whereas there was no observable relationship between earlier depression and adherence to the MDP. A study undertaken in the ongoing Whitehall II cohort study also found an increased risk for incident depression over 5 years in people consuming a Western-style diet pattern as well as a reduced risk for those eating a "whole-foods" diet pattern (Akbaraly et al., 2009). These authors also excluded those identified with depression at baseline and reanalyzed the data, examining depression at an early time point as a predictor of diet quality at the next follow-up. Once again, results of these analyses did not support depression as a predictor of poor dietary behavior. Indeed, a recent Australian study explicitly addressed the reverse causality hypothesis and found—contrary to expectations—that individuals who had previously experienced depression had better diets on average than those who had no such history of depression (Jacka et al., 2015). Such data suggest that the relationship between depressive symptoms and dietary changes may not be straightforward.

Another important consideration in these observational studies is the possibility that other factors explain the association between diet and mental health. Given that socioeconomic position is consistently related to both poorer quality diet (Galobardes et al., 2001; Henderson et al., 2002) and risk for depression (Butterworth et al., 2012), there is no doubt that factors such as educational level, social disadvantage, and occupation are plausible explanations for the relationships observed between diet and depression. Although most previous studies in this field have included appropriate measures in their analyses and largely excluded them as explanatory variables, it is inevitable that the tools used to measure such factors will be imperfect and unable to fully capture the construct of socioeconomic circumstances. One recent study did attempt to address this issue and constructed a comprehensive variable that encompassed labor force status, occupation, educational attainment, income, welfare dependency, financial hardship, and childhood disadvantage. Although this construct did explain the cross-sectional relationship between unhealthy diet and depression observed in older Australian adults in this study, it did not fully explain the prospective associations seen between dietary patterns and mental health over time in this group (Jacka et al., 2014).

Thus the hypothesis that diet is related to common mental disorders, particularly depression, is supported by studies in a wide range of countries and cultures as diverse as Spain, Norway, China, the United States, Japan, Australia, and many others. Reflecting this, a recent systematic review and meta-analysis, including results from 13 observational studies, concluded that a healthy diet is significantly associated with a reduced odds for depression (odds ratio: 0.84; 95% confidence interval [CI]: 0.76, 0.92; $P<0.001$) (Lai et al., 2013). Likewise, a meta-analysis of 22 studies investigating the protective effects of adherence to a Mediterranean-style diet on brain diseases demonstrated that higher adherence was associated with a reduced risk for depression (relative risk$=0.68$, 95% CI: 0.54–0.86) as well as cognitive decline (Psaltopoulou et al., 2013).

At the other end of the age spectrum, diet quality is also associated with mental health in adolescents and children. In an Australian study, a lower consumption of a healthy diet and increased consumption of unhealthy and processed foods were independently associated with increased odds for self-reported symptomatic depression in more than 7000 young adolescents (Jacka et al., 2010a). For those adolescents in the highest category of "healthy" diet scores, the likelihood of depression was nearly halved compared with those in the lowest category, whereas for those in the highest quintile of "unhealthy" diet score, the likelihood of depression was increased by nearly 80% compared with the lowest quintile. These relationships demonstrated a dietary intake-response pattern observed before and after adjustment for a wide range of potential confounding factors, including sociodemographic factors, health and dieting behaviors, and familial environment (Jacka et al., 2010a). Jacka et al. (2011b) also examined approximately 3000 Australian adolescents and found that diet quality was cross-sectionally and prospectively associated with adolescent mental health . In this study, improvements in diet quality were mirrored by improvements in mental health whereas reductions in diet quality were associated with declining psychological functioning. Another Australian study reported that adolescents with a dietary pattern higher in take-away foods, red meat, and sweets exhibited higher levels of internalizing and externalizing behaviors, which are markers of mental health status (Oddy et al., 2009). However, there was no relationship observed between a healthy dietary pattern and such behaviors. Another study, in Chinese adolescents, showed inverse relationships between higher scores on a traditional dietary pattern, comprising whole grains, vegetables, fruit, rice, and soya products, and depression and anxiety as well as positive relationships between both an unhealthy snacking dietary pattern and a high meat dietary pattern and depression and anxiety (Weng et al., 2012). In Norway a high consumption of unhealthy foods was associated with increased odds for behavioral problems in adolescents whereas both fruit and fish consumption were associated with fewer behavioral problems (Overby and Hoigaard, 2012), although there was no relationship between vegetable consumption and behavior. Likewise, a German study reported that an increased intake of confectionery was associated with increased emotional symptoms in children compared with low intake whereas a higher diet quality score was associated with lower odds for emotional symptoms after adjustment for variables such as sociodemographic characteristics, BMI, physical activity, television viewing, and computer use (Kohlboeck et al., 2012).

Another important consideration is that of the possible impact of nutrition in very early life and its relationship to the risk for mental health problems in children. Early-life exposures appear to potently influence child behavioral, emotional, and learning outcomes (Lewis et al., 2014). Therefore a better understanding of this critical developmental period is of immense importance in identifying early-life risk factors that are modifiable, such as diet, to support prevention efforts. In this context there are important data from a very large Norwegian cohort study indicating that unhealthy maternal diet during pregnancy, as well as both healthy and unhealthy dietary patterns during the first years of life, are associated with the risk for mental health problems in young children (Jacka et al., 2013b). In this study there was evidence suggesting consistently great effects of unhealthy diets on children's emotional and behavioral outcomes compared with the possible effects of insufficient healthy food intake. This study has now received support from two further gold standard cohort studies. In the Generation R study in the Netherlands, a lower level of adherence to a healthy MDP and higher adherence to an unhealthy Dutch dietary pattern in pregnancy were independently related to emotional-behavioral dysregulation in children in their early years (Steenweg-de Graaff et al., 2014). Likewise, studies conducted using data from the Avon Longitudinal Study of Parents and Children in the United Kingdom have reported relationships between maternal dietary patterns and both cognition and emotional-behavioral dysregulation in children (Barker et al., 2013; Pina-Camacho et al., 2014).

Reflecting the new data in this field, a systematic review concluded that an increased consumption of unhealthy, sugary, and fat-rich foods is related to increased risk of psychological symptomatology in children and adolescents (O'Neil et al., 2014). Given that most mental health problems develop by age 25, and that diet is a modifiable environmental exposure for the entire population, these new data in children and adolescents have important public health implications. Taken together with the studies in adults, this nascent but compelling evidence base indicates that the global changes in dietary habits are likely to be influencing the prevalence of common mental disorders.

INTERVENTION STUDIES

This new body of observational data is notable for the relative consistency of the reported relationships and the observed effect sizes. Inverse relationships between diet quality and mental health have now been reported across a multitude of countries, from children through to the elderly, in men and women, and utilizing a wide range of mental health and dietary measures. However, although there is one trial currently underway (O'Neil et al., 2013), so far there have been no published studies that have specifically sought to answer the question "If I improve my diet, will I feel less depressed?". This is an increasingly common question in clinical practice and the general community, and it remains unanswered to date, representing a serious gap in our knowledge base. A systematic review examined the data from dietary interventions that have examined mental health outcomes in various populations and concluded that, although data from depressed samples are currently lacking, there is some evidence suggesting a positive impact of dietary improvement on depression (Opie et al., 2014).

It is also worth noting the new data from two intervention studies that support dietary improvement as a means to prevent the incidence of depression. In the large PREDIMED study, older individuals randomized to an MDP compared with a low-fat diet tended to be less likely to develop depression over the period of the intervention, and this relationship was particularly pronounced for those individuals with type 2 diabetes (Sanchez-Villegas et al., 2013). Those in the Mediterranean diet groups also demonstrated improved cognition compared with controls (Martinez-Lapiscina et al., 2013). Another US study reported that dietary counseling was as effective as psychotherapy in reducing the rate of transition from subsyndromal to clinical depression in older adults (Stahl et al., 2014). Although these two studies must be regarded as preliminary evidence given the lack of statistical power in the PREDIMED study and the lack of a control group in the US intervention, they do give rise to some optimism regarding the potential of dietary interventions to prevent depression.

CLINICAL APPLICATIONS

This new literature provides face validity for the role of nutritional factors in the genesis and management of depression. Although the nascent evidence base consists primarily of reports from observational studies, the data largely fulfill the Bradford

Hill criteria for causality (Jacka et al., 2012c) and are consistent and compelling. Moreover, although there is currently a dearth of evidence regarding the efficacy of dietary modulation to treat depression, it is clear that diet has a major impact on comorbid physical disorders that are disproportionally more common in people with depression, such as cardiovascular disorders and diabetes. This suggests that policy, public health, and clinical actions taken to improve diet should have benefits for mental health (Jacka et al., 2012c), with the precautionary principle supporting such actions.

It is critical that we now gain a detailed understanding of the pathophysiological pathways that mediate this relationship to develop targeted interventions. These are thus far unknown. Chronic low-grade inflammation, with accompanying oxidative stress, is a common feature of virtually all mental disorders, as well as the somatic disorders with which mental disorders are so commonly comorbid. This indicates a central role for immune system dysfunction in mental illness (Berk et al., 2013). Related to this is the new knowledge regarding the human gut microbiome as a core driver of immune functioning and the development of the brain and the metabolic and innate immune system during early life. Indeed, emerging data from experimental and human studies now suggest that the gut is a key pathway by which environmental factors, such as poor diet, sedentary behavior, and stress, influence the immune system and host health, with downstream effects on the risk for mental, as well as physical, disorders. This highlights the urgent need to elucidate the role of diet in the bidirectional communication within this axis and the development of new preventive and therapeutic interventions for these disorders based on modification of diet, the gut microbiome, and immune function.

REFERENCES

Adair, L.S., Popkin, B.M., 2005. Are child eating patterns being transformed globally? Obes. Res. 13, 1281–1299.

Akbaraly, T.N., Brunner, E.J., Ferrie, J.E., Marmot, M.G., Kivimaki, M., Singh-Manoux, A., 2009. Dietary pattern and depressive symptoms in middle age. Br. J. Psychiatry 195, 408–413.

Amani, R., Saeidi, S., Nazari, Z., Nematpour, S., 2011. Correlation between dietary zinc intakes and its serum levels with depression scales in young female students. Biol. Trace Elem. Res. 137, 150–158.

Appleton, K.M., Rogers, P.J., Ness, A.R., 2010. Updated systematic review and meta-analysis of the effects of n-3 long-chain polyunsaturated fatty acids on depressed mood. Am. J. Clin. Nutr. 91, 757–770.

Appleton, K.M., Woodside, J.V., Yarnell, J.W., Arveiler, D., Haas, B., Amouyel, P., Montaye, M., Ferrieres, J., Ruidavets, J.B., Ducimetiere, P., Bingham, A., Evans, A., 2007. Depressed mood and dietary fish intake: direct relationship or indirect relationship as a result of diet and lifestyle? J. Affect Disord. 104, 217–223.

Barker, E.D., Kirkham, N., Ng, J., Jensen, S.K., 2013. Prenatal maternal depression symptoms and nutrition, and child cognitive function. Br. J. Psychiatry 203, 417–421.

Barragan-Rodriguez, L., Rodriguez-Moran, M., Guerrero-Romero, F., 2008. Efficacy and safety of oral magnesium supplementation in the treatment of depression in the elderly with type 2 diabetes: a randomized, equivalent trial. Magnes. Res. Off. Organ Int. Soc. Dev. Res. Magnes. 21, 218–223.

Berk, M., Williams, L.J., Jacka, F., O'Neil, A., Pasco, J.A., Moylan, S., Allen, N.B., Stuart, A.L., Hayley, A.C., Byrne, M.L., Maes, M., 2013. So depression is an inflammatory disease, but where does the inflammation come from? BMC Med. 11, 200.

Bloom, D.E., Cafiero, E.T., Jane-Llopis, E., Abrahams-Gessel, S., Bloom, L.R., Fathima, S., Fiegl, A.B., 2011. The Global Economic Burden of Non-communicable Diseases: A Report by the World Economic Forum and the Harvard School of Public Health.

Bountziouka, V., Polychronopoulos, E., Zeimbekis, A., Papavenetiou, E., Ladoukaki, E., Papairakleous, N., Gotsis, E., Metallinos, G., Lionis, C., Panagiotakos, D., 2009. Long-term fish intake is associated with less severe depressive symptoms among elderly men and women: the MEDIS (MEDiterranean ISlands Elderly) epidemiological study. J. Aging Health 21, 864–880.

Bowman, S., Friday, J., Thoerig, R., Clemens, J., Moshfegh, A., 2014. Americans consume less added sugars and solid fats and consume more whole grains and oils: changes from 2003–04 to 2009–10. FASEB J. 28, 369.2.

Brand-Miller, J.C., Holt, S.H., 1998. Australian aboriginal plant foods: a consideration of their nutritional composition and health implications. Nutr. Res. Rev. 11, 5–23.

Briefel, R.R., Johnson, C.L., 2004. Secular trends in dietary intake in the United States. Annu. Rev. Nutr. 24, 401–431.

Butterworth, P., Olesen, S.C., Leach, L.S., 2012. The role of hardship in the association between socio-economic position and depression. Aust. N. Z. J. Psychiatry 46, 364–373.

Cheungpasitporn, W., Thongprayoon, C., Mao, M.A., Srivali, N., Ungprasert, P., Varothai, N., Sanguankeo, A., Kittanamongkolchai, W., Erickson, S.B., 2015. Hypomagnesaemia linked to depression: a systematic review and meta-analysis. Intern. Med. J. 45, 436–440.

Colangelo, L.A., He, K., Whooley, M.A., Daviglus, M.L., Liu, K., 2009. Higher dietary intake of long-chain omega-3 polyunsaturated fatty acids is inversely associated with depressive symptoms in women. Nutrition 25 (10).

Collishaw, S., Maughan, B., Goodman, R., Pickles, A., 2004. Time trends in adolescent mental health. J. Child Psychol. Psychiatry 45, 1350–1362.

Cordain, L., Eaton, S.B., Miller, J.B., Mann, N., Hill, K., 2002. The paradoxical nature of hunter-gatherer diets: meat-based, yet non-atherogenic. Eur. J. Clin. Nutr. 56 (Suppl. 1), S42–S52.

Cordain, L., Eaton, S.B., Sebastian, A., Mann, N., Lindeberg, S., Watkins, B.A., O'Keefe, J.H., Brand-Miller, J., 2005. Origins and evolution of the Western diet: health implications for the 21st century. Am. J. Clin. Nutr. 81, 341–354.

Danaei, G., Lawes, C.M., Vander Hoorn, S., Murray, C.J., Ezzati, M., 2006. Global and regional mortality from ischaemic heart disease and stroke attributable to higher-than-optimum blood glucose concentration: comparative risk assessment. Lancet 368, 1651–1659.

Derom, M.L., Martinez-Gonzalez, M.A., Sayon-Orea Mdel, C., Bes-Rastrollo, M., Beunza, J.J., Sanchez-Villegas, A., 2012. Magnesium intake is not related to depression risk in Spanish university graduates. J. Nutr. 142, 1053–1059.

Eaton, S.B., Eaton 3rd, S.B., 2000. Paleolithic versus modern diets–selected pathophysiological implications. Eur. J. Nutr. 39, 67–70.

Eaton, S.B., Konner, M., 1985. Paleolithic nutrition. A consideration of its nature and current implications. N. Engl. J. Med. 312, 283–289.

Fu, T.S., Lee, C.S., Gunnell, D., Lee, W.C., Cheng, A.T., 2013. Changing trends in the prevalence of common mental disorders in Taiwan: a 20-year repeated cross-sectional survey. Lancet 381, 235–241.

Food and Agriculture Organization (FAO), 2004. Globalization of food systems in developing countries: impact on food security and nutrition. FAO Food Nutr. 83.

Galobardes, B., Morabia, A., Bernstein, M.S., 2001. Diet and socioeconomic position: does the use of different indicators matter? Int. J. Epidemiol. 30, 334–340.

Gilbody, S., Lightfoot, T., Sheldon, T., 2007. Is low folate a risk factor for depression? A meta-analysis and exploration of heterogeneity. J. Epidemiol. Community Health 61, 631–637.

Henderson, L., Gregory, J., Swan, G., 2002. The National Diet and Nutrition Survey: Adults Aged 19–64 Years: Types and Quantities of Foods Consumed. HMSO, London.

Hibbeln, J.R., 1998. Fish consumption and major depression. Lancet 351, 1213.

Hibbeln, J.R., 2002. Seafood consumption, the DHA content of mothers' milk and prevalence rates of postpartum depression: a cross-national, ecological analysis. J. Affect. Disord. 69, 15–29.

Jacka, F., Kremer, P., Leslie, E., Berk, M., Patton, G., Toumbourou, J., Williams, J., 2010a. Associations between diet quality and depressed mood in adolescents: results from the Australian healthy neighbourhoods study. Aust. N. Z. J. Psychiatry 44, 435–442.

Jacka, F., Pasco, J., Mykletun, A., Williams, L., Hodge, A., O'Reilly, S., et al., 2010b. Association of Western and traditional diets with depression and anxiety in women. Am. J. Psychiatry 167, 305–311.

Jacka, F.N., Pasco, J.A., Mykletun, A., Williams, L.J., Nicholson, G.C., Kotowicz, M.A., Berk, M., 2011a. Diet quality in bipolar disorder in a population-based sample of women. J. Affect. Disord. 129, 332–337.

Jacka, F.N., Pasco, J.A., Williams, L.J., Mann, N., Hodge, A., Brazionis, L., Berk, M., 2012a. Red meat consumption and mood and anxiety disorders. Psychother. Psychosom. 81, 196–198.

Jacka, F.N., Cherbuin, N., Anstey, K.J., Butterworth, P., 2014. Dietary patterns and depressive symptoms over time: examining the relationships with socioeconomic position, health behaviors and cardiovascular risk. PLoS One 9, e87657.

Jacka, F.N., Cherbuin, N., Anstey, K.J., Butterworth, P., 2015. Does reverse causality explain the relationship between diet and depression? J. Affect. Disord. 175, 248–250.

Jacka, F.N., Kremer, P.J., Berk, M., de Silva-Sanigorski, A.M., Moodie, M., Leslie, E.R., Pasco, J.A., Swinburn, B.A., 2011b. A prospective study of diet quality and mental health in adolescents. PLoS One 6, e24805.

Jacka, F.N., Maes, M., Pasco, J.A., Williams, L.J., Berk, M., 2012b. Nutrient intakes and the common mental disorders in women. J. Affect. Disord. 141, 79–85.

Jacka, F.N., Mykletun, A., Berk, M., 2012c. Moving towards a population health approach to the primary prevention of common mental disorders. BMC Med. 10, 149.

Jacka, F.N., Mykletun, A., Berk, M., Bjelland, I., Tell, G.S., 2011c. The association between habitual diet quality and the common mental disorders in community-dwelling adults: the Hordaland health study. Psychosom. Med. 73, 483–490.

Jacka, F.N., Overland, S., Stewart, R., Tell, G.S., Bjelland, I., Mykletun, A., 2009. Association between magnesium intake and depression and anxiety in community-dwelling adults: the Hordaland health study. Aust. N. Z. J. Psychiatry 43, 45–52.

Jacka, F.N., Pasco, J.A., Williams, L.J., Meyer, B.J., Digger, R., Berk, M., 2013a. Dietary intake of fish and PUFA, and clinical depressive and anxiety disorders in women. Br. J. Nutr. 109, 2059–2066.

Jacka, F.N., Ystrom, E., Brantsaeter, A.L., Karevold, E., Roth, C., Haugen, M., Meltzer, H.M., Schjolberg, S., Berk, M., 2013b. Maternal and early postnatal nutrition and mental health of offspring by age 5 years: a prospective cohort study. J. Am. Acad. Child Adolesc. Psychiatry 52, 1038–1047.

Jeffery, R.W., Linde, J.A., Simon, G.E., Ludman, E.J., Rohde, P., Ichikawa, L.E., Finch, E.A., 2009. Reported food choices in older women in relation to body mass index and depressive symptoms. Appetite 52, 238–240.

Kant, A.K., 2000. Consumption of energy-dense, nutrient-poor foods by adult Americans: nutritional and health implications. The Third National Health and Nutrition Examination Survey, 1988–1994. Am. J. Clin. Nutr. 72, 929–936.

Kim, J.M., Stewart, R., Kim, S.W., Yang, S.J., Shin, I.S., Yoon, J.S., 2008. Predictive value of folate, vitamin B12 and homocysteine levels in late-life depression. Br. J. Psychiatry 192, 268–274.

Kohlboeck, G., Sausenthaler, S., Standl, M., Koletzko, S., Bauer, C., von Berg, A., Berdel, D., KrÃmer, U., Schaaf, B., Lehmann, I., Herbarth, O., Heinrich, J., 2012. Food intake, diet quality and behavioral problems in children: results from the GINI-plus/LISA-plus studies. Ann. Nutr. Metab. 60, 247–256.

Kuczmarski, M.F., Cremer Sees, A., Hotchkiss, L., Cotugna, N., Evans, M.K., Zonderman, A.B., 2010. Higher healthy eating index-2005 scores associated with reduced symptoms of depression in an urban population: findings from the Healthy Aging in Neighborhoods of Diversity across the Life Span (HANDLS) study. J. Am. Diet. Assoc. 110, 383–389.

Lai, J., Moxey, A., Nowak, G., Vashum, K., Bailey, K., McEvoy, M., 2011. The efficacy of zinc supplementation in depression: systematic review of randomised controlled trials. J. Affect Disord. 136 (1–2).

Lai, J.S., Hiles, S., Bisquera, A., Hure, A.J., McEvoy, M., Attia, J., 2013. A systematic review and meta-analysis of dietary patterns and depression in community-dwelling adults. Am. J. Clin. Nutr. 99, 181–197.

Larson, N.I., Story, M.T., Nelson, M.C., 2009. Neighborhood environments: disparities in access to healthy foods in the United States. Am. J. Prev. Med. 36, 74–81.

Lewis, A.J., Galbally, M., Gannon, T., Symeonides, C., 2014. Early life programming as a target for prevention of child and adolescent mental disorders. BMC Med. 12.

Lin, P.Y., Mischoulon, D., Freeman, M.P., Matsuoka, Y., Hibbeln, J., Belmaker, R.H., Su, K.P., 2012. Are omega-3 fatty acids antidepressants or just mood-improving agents? The effect depends upon diagnosis, supplement preparation, and severity of depression. Mol. Psychiatry 17, 1161–1163. author reply 1163–1167.

Maes, M., Galecki, P., Chang, Y.S., Berk, M., 2011. A review on the oxidative and nitrosative stress (O&NS) pathways in major depression and their possible contribution to the (neuro) degenerative processes in that illness. Prog. Neuropsychopharmacol. Biol. Psychiatry 35, 676–692.

Martinez-Lapiscina, E.H., Clavero, P., Toledo, E., Estruch, R., Salas-Salvado, J., San Julian, B., Sanchez-Tainta, A., Ros, E., Valls-Pedret, C., Martinez-Gonzalez, M.A., 2013. Mediterranean diet improves cognition: the PREDIMED-NAVARRA randomised trial. J. Neurol. Neurosurg. Psychiatry 84, 1318–1325.

Maughan, B., Collishaw, S., Meltzer, H., Goodman, R., 2008. Recent trends in UK child and adolescent mental health. Soc. Psychiatry Psychiatr. Epidemiol. 43, 305–310.

Metz, J., Hart, D., Harpending, H.C., 1971. Iron, folate, and vitamin B12 nutrition in a hunter-gatherer people: a study of the Kung Bushmen. Am. J. Clin. Nutr. 24, 229–242.

Morris, M.S., Fava, M., Jacques, P.F., Selhub, J., Rosenberg, I.H., 2003. Depression and folate status in the United States population. Psychother. Psychosom. 72, 80–87.

Murakami, K., Mizoue, T., Sasaki, S., Ohta, M., Sato, M., Matsushita, Y., Mishima, N., 2008. Dietary intake of folate, other B vitamins, and omega-3 polyunsaturated fatty acids in relation to depressive symptoms in Japanese adults. Nutrition 24, 140–147.

Murray, C.J., Vos, T., Lozano, R., Naghavi, M., Flaxman, A.D., Michaud, C., Ezzati, M., Shibuya, K., Salomon, J.A., Abdalla, S., Aboyans, V., Abraham, J., Ackerman, I., Aggarwal, R., Ahn, S.Y., Ali, M.K., Alvarado, M., Anderson, H.R., Anderson, L.M., Andrews, K.G., Atkinson, C., Baddour, L.M., Bahalim, A.N., Barker-Collo, S., Barrero, L.H., Bartels, D.H., Basanez, M.G., Baxter, A., Bell, M.L., Benjamin, E.J., Bennett, D., Bernabe, E., Bhalla, K., Bhandari, B., Bikbov, B., Bin Abdulhak, A., Birbeck, G., Black, J.A., Blencowe, H., Blore, J.D., Blyth, F., Bolliger, I., Bonaventure, A., Boufous, S., Bourne, R., Boussinesq, M., Braithwaite, T., Brayne, C., Bridgett, L., Brooker, S., Brooks, P., Brugha, T.S., Bryan-Hancock, C., Bucello, C., Buchbinder, R., Buckle, G., Budke, C.M., Burch, M., Burney, P., Burstein, R., Calabria, B., Campbell, B., Canter, C.E., Carabin, H., Carapetis, J., Carmona, L., Cella, C., Charlson, F., Chen, H., Cheng, A.T., Chou, D., Chugh, S.S., Coffeng, L.E., Colan, S.D., Colquhoun, S., Colson, K.E., Condon, J., Connor, M.D., Cooper, L.T., Corriere, M., Cortinovis, M., de Vaccaro, K.C., Couser, W., Cowie, B.C., Criqui, M.H., Cross, M., Dabhadkar, K.C., Dahiya, M., Dahodwala, N., Damsere-Derry, J., Danaei, G., Davis, A., De Leo, D., Degenhardt, L., Dellavalle, R., Delossantos, A., Denenberg, J., Derrett, S., Des Jarlais, D.C., Dharmaratne, S.D., Dherani, M., Diaz-Torne, C., Dolk, H., Dorsey, E.R., Driscoll, T., Duber, H., Ebel, B., Edmond, K., Elbaz, A., Ali, S.E., Erskine, H., Erwin, P.J., Espindola, P., Ewoigbokhan, S.E., Farzadfar, F., Feigin, V., Felson, D.T., Ferrari, A., Ferri, C.P., Fevre, E.M., Finucane, M.M., Flaxman, S., Flood, L., Foreman, K., Forouzanfar, M.H., Fowkes, F.G., Fransen, M., Freeman, M.K., Gabbe, B.J., Gabriel, S.E., Gakidou, E., Ganatra, H.A., Garcia, B., Gaspari, F., Gillum, R.F., Gmel, G., Gonzalez-Medina, D., Gosselin, R., Grainger, R., Grant, B., Groeger, J., Guillemin, F., Gunnell, D., Gupta, R., Haagsma, J., Hagan, H., Halasa, Y.A., Hall, W., Haring, D., Haro, J.M., Harrison, J.E., Havmoeller, R., Hay, R.J., Higashi, H., Hill, C., Hoen, B., Hoffman, H., Hotez, P.J., Hoy, D., Huang, J.J., Ibeanusi, S.E., Jacobsen, K.H., James, S.L., Jarvis, D., Jasrasaria, R., Jayaraman, S., Johns, N., Jonas, J.B., Karthikeyan, G., Kassebaum, N., Kawakami, N., Keren, A., Khoo, J.P., King, C.H., Knowlton, L.M., Kobusingye, O., Koranteng, A., Krishnamurthi, R., Laden, F., Lalloo, R., Laslett, L.L., Lathlean, T., Leasher, J.L., Lee, Y.Y., Leigh, J., Levinson, D., Lim, S.S., Limb, E., Lin, J.K., Lipnick, M., Lipshultz, S.E., Liu, W., Loane, M., Ohno, S.L., Lyons, R., Mabweijano, J., MacIntyre, M.F., Malekzadeh, R., Mallinger, L., Manivannan, S., Marcenes, W., March, L., Margolis, D.J., Marks, G.B., Marks, R., Matsumori, A., Matzopoulos, R., Mayosi, B.M., McAnulty, J.H., McDermott, M.M., McGill, N., McGrath, J., Medina-Mora, M.E., Meltzer, M., Mensah, G.A., Merriman, T.R., Meyer, A.C., Miglioli, V., Miller, M., Miller, T.R., Mitchell, P.B., Mock, C., Mocumbi, A.O., Moffitt, T.E., Mokdad, A.A., Monasta, L., Montico, M., Moradi-Lakeh, M., Moran, A., Morawska, L., Mori, R., Murdoch, M.E., Mwaniki, M.K., Naidoo, K., Nair, M.N., Naldi, L., Narayan, K.M., Nelson, P.K., Nelson, R.G., Nevitt, M.C., Newton, C.R., Nolte, S., Norman, P., Norman, R., O'Donnell, M., O'Hanlon, S., Olives, C., Omer, S.B., Ortblad, K., Osborne, R., Ozgediz, D., Page, A., Pahari, B., Pandian, J.D., Rivero, A.P., Patten, S.B., Pearce, N., Padilla, R.P., Perez-Ruiz, F., Perico, N., Pesudovs, K., Phillips, D., Phillips, M.R., Pierce, K., Pion, S., Polanczyk, G.V., Polinder, S., Pope 3rd, C.A., Popova, S., Porrini, E., Pourmalek, F., Prince, M., Pullan, R.L., Ramaiah, K.D., Ranganathan, D., Razavi, H., Regan, M., Rehm, J.T., Rein, D.B., Remuzzi, G., Richardson, K., Rivara, F.P., Roberts, T., Robinson, C., De Leon, F.R., Ronfani, L.,

Room, R., Rosenfeld, L.C., Rushton, L., Sacco, R.L., Saha, S., Sampson, U., Sanchez-Riera, L., Sanman, E., Schwebel, D.C., Scott, J.G., Segui-Gomez, M., Shahraz, S., Shepard, D.S., Shin, H., Shivakoti, R., Singh, D., Singh, G.M., Singh, J.A., Singleton, J., Sleet, D.A., Sliwa, K., Smith, E., Smith, J.L., Stapelberg, N.J., Steer, A., Steiner, T., Stolk, W.A., Stovner, L.J., Sudfeld, C., Syed, S., Tamburlini, G., Tavakkoli, M., Taylor, H.R., Taylor, J.A., Taylor, W.J., Thomas, B., Thomson, W.M., Thurston, G.D., Tleyjeh, I.M., Tonelli, M., Towbin, J.A., Truelsen, T., Tsilimbaris, M.K., Ubeda, C., Undurraga, E.A., van der Werf, M.J., van Os, J., Vavilala, M.S., Venketasubramanian, N., Wang, M., Wang, W., Watt, K., Weatherall, D.J., Weinstock, M.A., Weintraub, R., Weisskopf, M.G., Weissman, M.M., White, R.A., Whiteford, H., Wiebe, N., Wiersma, S.T., Wilkinson, J.D., Williams, H.C., Williams, S.R., Witt, E., Wolfe, F., Woolf, A.D., Wulf, S., Yeh, P.H., Zaidi, A.K., Zheng, Z.J., Zonies, D., Lopez, A.D., 2013. Disability-adjusted life years (DALYs) for 291 diseases and injuries in 21 regions, 1990–2010: a systematic analysis for the Global Burden of Disease Study 2010. Lancet 380, 2197–2223.

Nanri, A., Hayabuchi, H., Ohta, M., Sato, M., Mishima, N., Mizoue, T., 2012. Serum folate and depressive symptoms among Japanese men and women: a cross-sectional and prospective study. Psychiatry Res.

Nanri, A., Kimura, Y., Matsushita, Y., Ohta, M., Sato, M., Mishima, N., Sasaki, S., Mizoue, T., 2010. Dietary patterns and depressive symptoms among Japanese men and women. Eur. J. Clin. Nutr. 64, 832–839.

Noaghiul, S., Hibbeln, J.R., 2003. Cross-national comparisons of seafood consumption and rates of bipolar disorders. Am. J. Psychiatry 160, 2222–2227.

Nowak, G., Siwek, M., Dudek, D., Zieba, A., Pilc, A., 2003a. Effect of zinc supplementation on antidepressant therapy in unipolar depression: a preliminary placebo-controlled study. Pol. J. Pharmacol. 55, 1143–1147.

Nowak, G., Szewczyk, B., Wieronska, J.M., Branski, P., Palucha, A., Pilc, A., Sadlik, K., Piekoszewski, W., 2003b. Antidepressant-like effects of acute and chronic treatment with zinc in forced swim test and olfactory bulbectomy model in rats. Brain Res. Bull. 61, 159–164.

O'Dea, K., 1984. Marked improvement in carbohydrate and lipid metabolism in diabetic Australian aborigines after temporary reversion to traditional lifestyle. Diabetes 33, 596–603.

O'Dea, K., Sinclair, A.J., 1985. The effects of low-fat diets rich in arachidonic acid on the composition of plasma fatty acids and bleeding time in Australian aborigines. J. Nutr. Sci. Vitaminol. (Tokyo) 31, 441–453.

O'Donnell, M., Anderson, D., Morgan, V.A., Nassar, N., Leonard, H.M., Stanley, F.J., 2013. Trends in pre-existing mental health disorders among parents of infants born in Western Australia from 1990 to 2005. Med. J. Aust. 198, 485–488.

O'Neil, A., Berk, M., Itsiopoulos, C., Castle, D., Opie, R., Pizzinga, J., Brazionis, L., Hodge, A., Mihalopoulos, C., Chatterton, M.L., Dean, O.M., Jacka, F.N., 2013. A randomised, controlled trial of a dietary intervention for adults with major depression (the "SMILES" trial): study protocol. BMC Psychiatry 13.

O'Neil, A., Quirk, S.E., Housden, S., Brennan, S.L., Williams, L.J., Pasco, J.A., Berk, M., Jacka, F.N., 2014. Relationship between diet and mental health in children and adolescents: a systematic review. Am. J. Public Health 104, e31–e42.

Oddy, W.H., Robinson, M., Ambrosini, G.L., O'Sullivan, T.A., de Klerk, N.H., Beilin, L.J., Silburn, S.R., Zubrick, S.R., Stanley, F.J., 2009. The association between dietary patterns and mental health in early adolescence. Prev. Med. 49, 39–44.

Opie, R.S., O'Neil, A., Itsiopoulos, C., Jacka, F.N., 2014. The impact of whole-of-diet interventions on depression and anxiety: a systematic review of randomised controlled trials. Public Health Nutr. 1–20.

Overby, N., Hoigaard, R., 2012. Diet and behavioral problems at school in Norwegian adolescents. Food Nutr. Res. 56.

Pina-Camacho, L., Jensen, S., Gaysina, D., Barker, E.D., 2014. Maternal depression symptoms, unhealthy diet and child emotional–behavioural dysregulation. Eur. Neuropsychopharmacol. 24, S716–S717.

Poleszak, E., Szewczyk, B., Kedzierska, E., Wlaz, P., Pilc, A., Nowak, G., 2004. Antidepressant- and anxiolytic-like activity of magnesium in mice. Pharmacol. Biochem. Behav. 78, 7–12.

Poleszak, E., Wlaz, P., Kedzierska, E., Radziwon-Zaleska, M., Pilc, A., Fidecka, S., Nowak, G., 2005. Effects of acute and chronic treatment with magnesium in the forced swim test in rats. Pharmacol. Rep. 57, 654–658.

Popkin, B.M., 2002. The shift in stages of the nutrition transition in the developing world differs from past experiences! Public Health Nutr. 5, 205–214.

Popkin, B.M., Du, S., 2003. Dynamics of the nutrition transition toward the animal foods sector in China and its implications: a worried perspective. J. Nutr. 133, 3898S–3906S.

Popkin, B.M., Nielsen, S.J., 2003. The sweetening of the world's diet. Obes. Res. 11, 1325–1332.

Psaltopoulou, T., Sergentanis, T.N., Panagiotakos, D.B., Sergentanis, I.N., Kosti, R., Scarmeas, N., 2013. Mediterranean diet, stroke, cognitive impairment, and depression: a meta-analysis. Ann. Neurol. 74, 580–591.

Ramos, M.I., Allen, L.H., Haan, M.N., Green, R., Miller, J.W., 2004. Plasma folate concentrations are associated with depressive symptoms in elderly Latina women despite folic acid fortification. Am. J. Clin. Nutr. 80, 1024–1028.

Roy, A., Evers, S.E., Avison, W.R., Campbell, M.K., 2011. Higher zinc intake buffers the impact of stress on depressive symptoms in pregnancy. Nutr. Res. 30, 695–704.

Sanchez-Villegas, A., Delgado-Rodriguez, M., Alonso, A., Schlatter, J., Lahortiga, F., Majem, L.S., Martinez-Gonzalez, M.A., 2009. Association of the Mediterranean dietary pattern with the incidence of depression: the Seguimiento Universidad de Navarra/University of Navarra follow-up (SUN) cohort. Arch. Gen. Psychiatry 66, 1090–1098.

Sanchez-Villegas, A., Henriquez, P., Figueiras, A., Ortuno, F., Lahortiga, F., Martinez-Gonzalez, M.A., 2007. Long chain omega-3 fatty acids intake, fish consumption and mental disorders in the SUN cohort study. Eur. J. Nutr. 46, 337–346.

Sanchez-Villegas, A., Martinez-Gonzalez, M.A., Estruch, R., Salas-Salvado, J., Corella, D., Covas, M.I., Aros, F., Romaguera, D., Gomez-Gracia, E., Lapetra, J., Pinto, X., Martinez, J.A., Lamuela-Raventos, R.M., Ros, E., Gea, A., Warnberg, J., Serra-Majem, L., 2013. Mediterranean dietary pattern and depression: the PREDIMED randomized trial. BMC Med. 11, 208.

Sarris, J., Mischoulon, D., Schweitzer, I., 2012. Omega-3 for bipolar disorder: meta-analyses of use in mania and bipolar depression. J. Clin. Psychiatry 73, 81–86.

Silvers, K.M., Scott, K.M., 2002. Fish consumption and self-reported physical and mental health status. Public Health Nutr. 5, 427–431.

Simopoulos, A.P., 2001. n-3 fatty acids and human health: defining strategies for public policy. Lipids 36 (Suppl.), S83–S89.

Singewald, N., Sinner, C., Hetzenauer, A., Sartori, S.B., Murck, H., 2004. Magnesium-deficient diet alters depression- and anxiety-related behavior in mice–influence of desipramine and *Hypericum perforatum* extract. Neuropharmacology 47, 1189–1197.

Stahl, S.T., Albert, S.M., Dew, M.A., Lockovich, M.H., Reynolds 3rd, C.F., 2014. Coaching in healthy dietary practices in at-risk older adults: a case of indicated depression prevention. Am. J. Psychiatry 171, 499–505.

Steenweg-de Graaff, J., Tiemeier, H., Steegers-Theunissen, R.P., Hofman, A., Jaddoe, V.W., Verhulst, F.C., Roza, S.J., 2014. Maternal dietary patterns during pregnancy and child internalising and externalising problems. The Generation R Study. Clin. Nutr. 33, 115–121.

Swardfager, W., Herrmann, N., Mazereeuw, G., Goldberger, K., Harimoto, T., Lanctot, K.L., 2013. Zinc in depression: a meta-analysis. Biol. Psychiatry 74, 872–878.

Swinburn, B.A., Sacks, G., Hall, K.D., McPherson, K., Finegood, D.T., Moodie, M.L., Gortmaker, S.L., 2011. The global obesity pandemic: shaped by global drivers and local environments. Lancet 378, 804–814.

Tanskanen, A., Hibbeln, J.R., Tuomilehto, J., Uutela, A., Haukkala, A., Viinamaki, H., Lehtonen, J., Vartiainen, E., 2001. Fish consumption and depressive symptoms in the general population in Finland. Psychiatr. Serv. 52, 529–531.

Tarleton, E.K., Littenberg, B., 2015. Magnesium intake and depression in adults. J. Am. Board Fam. Med. 28, 249–256.

Taylor, M.J., Carney, S.M., Goodwin, G.M., Geddes, J.R., 2004. Folate for depressive disorders: systematic review and meta-analysis of randomized controlled trials. J. Psychopharmacol. 18, 251–256.

Timonen, M., Horrobin, D., Jokelainen, J., Laitinen, J., Herva, A., Rasanen, P., 2004. Fish consumption and depression: the Northern Finland 1966 birth cohort study. J. Affect. Disord. 82, 447–452.

Tolmunen, T., Hintikka, J., Ruusunen, A., Voutilainen, S., Tanskanen, A., Valkonen, V.P., Viinamaki, H., Kaplan, G.A., Salonen, J.T., 2004. Dietary folate and the risk of depression in Finnish middle-aged men. A prospective follow-up study. Psychother. Psychosom. 73, 334–339.

Tolmunen, T., Voutilainen, S., Hintikka, J., Rissanen, T., Tanskanen, A., Viinamaki, H., Kaplan, G.A., Salonen, J.T., 2003. Dietary folate and depressive symptoms are associated in middle-aged Finnish men. J. Nutr. 133, 3233–3236.

Twenge, J.M., Gentile, B., DeWall, C.N., Ma, D., Lacefield, K., Schurtz, D.R., 2010. Birth cohort increases in psychopathology among young Americans, 1938–2007: a cross-temporal meta-analysis of the MMPI. Clin. Psychol. Rev. 30, 145–154.

Vashum, K.P., McEvoy, M., Milton, A.H., McElduff, P., Hure, A., Byles, J., Attia, J., 2014. Dietary zinc is associated with a lower incidence of depression: findings from two Australian cohorts. J. Affect. Disord. 166, 249–257.

World Health Organization (WHO), 2011. Global Status Report on Noncommunicable Diseases 2010.

Walker, A.F., De Souza, M.C., Vickers, M.F., Abeyasekera, S., Collins, M.L., Trinca, L.A., 1998. Magnesium supplementation alleviates premenstrual symptoms of fluid retention. J. Women's Health Off. Publ. Soc. Adv. Women's Health Res. 7, 1157–1165.

Weng, T.T., Hao, J.H., Qian, Q.W., Cao, H., Fu, J.L., Sun, Y., Huang, L., Tao, F.B., 2012. Is there any relationship between dietary patterns and depression and anxiety in Chinese adolescents? Public Health Nutr. 15, 673–682.

Importance of the Microbiota in Early Life and Influence on Future Health

E.F. Verdu, C.L. Hayes

McMaster University, Farncombe Family Digestive Health Research Institute, Division of Gastroenterology, Hamilton, ON, Canada

S.M. O' Mahony

University College Cork, Department of Anatomy and Neuroscience, Cork, Ireland; University College Cork, APC Microbiome Institute, Cork, Ireland

INTRODUCTION

Just as in other mammals humans harbor enormous quantities of commensal microorganisms on the external and internal surfaces of our bodies. Within a particular habitat, for example, in the gut, the collection of these commensals is referred to as microbiota, the collective genome being termed the microbiome (Collins et al., 2012; Cryan and Dinan, 2012). Within our gut a unique combination of different populations of organisms exists. These are mainly bacteria but also archaea, viruses, and protozoa—roughly approximating 3–10 times the number of human cells (Blaser and Webb, 2014). With the advent of metagenomic high-throughput platforms, a better understanding of the composition of a healthy human gut microbiome has been achieved, albeit quite likely that multiple, individual-specific, "healthy" compositional states exist (Clarke et al., 2014a). The gastrointestinal (GI) microbiota is quickly being recognized as a vital player in health and disease. A well-balanced microbial community within the gut is known to confer many health benefits on the host, whilst many GI (Verdu, 2012; Clarke et al., 2014b; De Palma et al., 2014a; Galipeau and Verdu, 2014; Moloney et al., 2014; Verdu et al., 2015) and extra-GI diseases (Cryan and O'Mahony, 2011; Bercik et al., 2012; Desbonnet et al., 2014; Burokas et al., 2015; Gulden et al., 2015; Lopez-Cepero and Palacios, 2015; Melli et al., 2015) are associated with dysbiosis. The origin and development of a "healthy" gut microbiota starts in early life, which is designated as an important neurodevelopmental time window. This provides an opportunity for the colonizing microbiota to influence immature systems, such as the central nervous system (CNS), and can permanently impact host health and well-being. This is abetted by the bidirectional communication system, the microbiota–gut–brain axis, which includes the stress axis, the immune system, and neuronal elements such as the vagus nerve (Cryan and O'Mahony, 2011; De Palma et al., 2014b). During early life this axis is also developing and, is, in itself, open to modification by the gut microbiota (Sudo et al., 2004; O'Mahony et al., 2014). Stress during early life is known to be a predisposing factor for psychiatric disease in adulthood (Lupien et al., 2009) and has long-term effects on the colonization of the gut (O'Mahony et al., 2009). Conversely, disruption of the microbiota in early life, or its absence, leads to altered pain sensitivity (Amaral et al., 2008; O'Mahony et al., 2009), development of inflammatory bowel disease (IBD) (Shaw et al., 2010), asthma (Canova et al., 2015; Pitter et al., 2015), diabetes (Candon et al., 2015), and obesity (Saari et al., 2015). In this chapter we focus on the importance of the microbiota that colonize the GI tract in early life and events that can affect which bacteria take up residence (Fig. 9.1). We consider the systems that

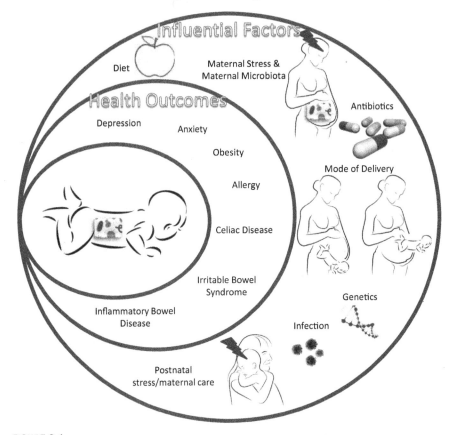

FIGURE 9.1

Some of the potential factors that can influence the colonization of the infant gut in early life. It is now apparent that these factors can have an impact both pre- and postnatally. Disruption of colonization by these factors can have long-term impacts on the future health of the child.

are concomitantly developing and ones that can be permanently affected by the pattern of colonization events. We highlight disorders that are associated with aberrant microbiota composition and microbiota–gut–brain axis signaling. Finally, we integrate these findings to define the implications for future health from a preventative, diagnostic, and therapeutic perspective.

THE DEVELOPING MICROBIOTA IN EARLY LIFE
PRENATAL MICROBIOTA COLONIZATION

Whilst the microbiota changes and evolves throughout the life span (Borre et al., 2014b; O'Mahony et al., 2015), here, we focus largely on the early life period. Previously held convictions that the fetus and intrauterine environment was sterile are now being challenged (El Aidy et al., 2013; Funkhouser and Bordenstein, 2013). Evidence put forward in support of this proposition include the demonstration that bacteria can be isolated from the meconium of healthy neonates (Jimenez et al., 2008), potentially as a result of prenatal colonization (Mshvildadze and Neu, 2010). A uterine source for these meconium-derived bacterial strains is suggested in part by studies indicating a microbial presence in amniotic fluid during preterm labor (DiGiulio et al., 2008). It is equally plausible, given the time delay between birth and meconium production, that the source of such bacteria is the mother's own microbiota. However, maternal infection cannot be eliminated as the amniotic source (Matamoros et al., 2013). Spontaneously released meconium, obtained from preterm babies, during the first three weeks of life, contained a specific microbiota that differs from those observed in early fecal samples (Moles et al., 2013). Firmicutes predominated in meconium while Proteobacteria was abundant in feces (Moles et al., 2013). In animal studies, genetically labeled *Enterococcus faecium* was detected in the amniotic fluid of pregnant rats and in the meconium of the offspring delivered via caesarean section following oral administration during pregnancy (Jimenez et al., 2008). These data suggest that maternal microbial transmission in mammals occurs during pregnancy and lactation. The placenta may be permissible to this translocation as Lactobaccillus and Bifidobacteria DNA were isolated from the placenta following delivery; however, there were no viable cells (Satokari et al., 2009). Moreover, a unique microbiome has been identified within the placenta that appears to correlate with the oral cavity population of the mother (Aagaard et al., 2014). Several bacterial species, including *Enterococcus*, *Streptococcus*, *Staphylococcus*, and *Propionibacterium*, have also been isolated from umbilical cord blood (Jimenez et al., 2008). These data suggest that this element may also be involved in the translocation of bacteria. The implications of prenatal microbiota transfer on the developing fetus and on future health are not yet known. Given that essential modulatory systems develop in utero, this period presents as an important influential opportunity for microbiota–host interactions. To date, the most explicit preclinical example of a prenatal role for the microbiome relates to development of the blood–brain barrier, which has been shown to be altered in germ-free animals (Braniste et al., 2014).

Despite the growing appreciation that the prenatal environment may not be sterile, it is still, nonetheless, accepted that the developing fetus is largely protected from bacterial infections (Costello et al., 2012).

Both the vaginal (Aagaard et al., 2012; Romero et al., 2014; Mueller et al., 2015a) and intestinal microbiota (Koren et al., 2012; Mueller et al., 2015a) undergo extensive remodeling over the course of pregnancy. As yet it is not known if there is transfer from these sites to the fetus prenatally. Specific changes include a decrease in proinflammatory Proteobacteria from the first to the third trimester and an increase in anti-inflammatory *Faecalibacterium prausnitzii* (Koren et al., 2012; Mueller et al., 2015a). Moreover, bacteria superior at energy harvesting are enriched during pregnancy to presumably support the growth of both mother and baby (Koren et al., 2012; Mueller et al., 2015a). The maintenance of the optimum microbial balance during pregnancy is essential to the successful inoculation of the baby during delivery; hence any situation likely to perturb the maternal microbiota, such as stress or antibiotic administration, has the potential to influence optimal vertical transmission to the baby.

It has been demonstrated that maternal stress, measured by reported stress or elevated cortisol levels, is associated with a differential gut microbiota in infant offspring (Zijlmans et al., 2015). This colonization pattern was related to infant GI symptoms and allergic reactions. Maternal prenatal stress impacts on the microbiota that will essentially colonize the infant during birth, thereby helping to shape future development (Jasarevic et al., 2015a,b). Indeed, a recent study has shown that prenatal stress in mice led to decreased maternal vaginal *Lactobacillus*, which subsequently resulted in decreased transmission of this bacterium to offspring (Jasarevic et al., 2015a). These results identify the vaginal microbiota as a novel factor by which prenatal stress may contribute to reprogramming of the developing baby with possible implications for future health and well-being. Moreover, we have recently shown that prenatal stress induced long-lasting alterations in the intestinal microbiota in adult offspring (Golubeva et al., 2015). In particular, the relative abundance of distinct bacteria genera significantly correlated with certain physiological parameters and the responsiveness of the stress axis. Hence, seeding the neonatal gut with a suboptimal microbiota can lead to long-lasting effects on overall future health. Of clinical relevance, intrapartum antibiotic use is associated with decreased bacterial diversity of the baby's first stool and lower abundance of beneficial bacteria (O'Neil et al., 2014), the long-term impact of which remains unexplored. The influence of prenatal events on the gut microbiota and subsequent impact on future health is coming to the fore, but more research is needed in order to realize the full impact.

FACTORS AFFECTING POSTNATAL MICROBIAL COLONIZATION

Environmental influences over microbiota development are substantial. Microbial nurturing and environmental conditions give rise to both a tailoring of the microbiota and a progressive sequence of dominant flora as the child matures as well as determining health outcomes (Clarke et al., 2014a; Moloney et al., 2014). Studies indicate that the initial GI microbial community composition is determined by delivery mode and that this maternally influenced microbial signature can last from months to years (Jakobsson et al., 2013; Clarke et al., 2014a) and influences health outcomes (Parfrey and Knight, 2012; Relman, 2012). Furthermore, infants born vaginally initially harbor a subject-specific microbiota dominated by lactic acid bacteria, for example, *Lactobacillus* spp. characteristic of their mother's vaginal and fecal microbiota (Dominguez-Bello et al., 2010; Vaishampayan et al., 2010). Whilst the initial microbial residents in babies born by caesarean section also exhibit features of maternal transmission, they tend to resemble the skin microbiota (Dominguez-Bello et al., 2010; Mueller et al., 2015b) and to be devoid of, or low in, *Bifidobacteria* spp. (Penders et al., 2006; Biasucci et al., 2008). Environmental sources from the hospital environment can also influence the initial microbiota of caesarean section–delivered infants (Dominguez-Bello et al., 2010). It also appears that alterations in bacterial richness and diversity associated with caesarean section delivery are accentuated by elective procedures (Azad et al., 2013). As a consequence of caesarean section delivery, decreased microbiota diversity and delay in colonization with beneficial *Bifidobacteria* spp. and *Bacteroidetes* persists for the first two years of life and is associated with reduced Th1 immune responses (Jakobsson et al., 2013). Importantly, however, infants delivered by caesarean section do eventually match up to their vaginally delivered counterparts in terms of stability and diversity of their adult microbiota (Maynard et al., 2012). However, more studies are necessary to assess the full implications of being born via caesarean section, the impact of altered initial colonization in vulnerable individuals, and the development of disorders in later life. Of note, preterm birth is associated with a considerably different GI microbiota profile than that observed in full-term counterparts (Barrett et al., 2013) and correlates with delays in development.

ENVIRONMENTAL INFLUENCES ON EARLY LIFE MICROBIOTA
Nutrition

A key element in shaping the microbiota in early life relates to nutritional factors. There is an increased abundance of certain *Bifidobacterium* spp., which thrive on human milk oligosaccharides (Zivkovic et al., 2011), in infants who are exclusively breastfed (Costello et al., 2012). Human milk microbiota also appears to be a direct source of *Bifidobacteria* and *Lactobacillus* in addition to its prebiotic properties (Fernandez et al., 2013). Moreover, the bacteria contained in breast milk has been noted to vary from colostrum to late lactation, by gestational age, maternal health status, and delivery mode (Khodayar-Pardo et al., 2014; O'Neil et al., 2014; Mueller et al., 2015a). The microbiota of formula-fed infants appear to have an increased diversity and a high abundance of coliforms, *Bacteroides* and *Clostridium difficile* (Penders et al., 2006; Azad et al., 2013). Moreover, a modest increase in both verbal and nonverbal IQ scores in breast-fed individuals has also been noted (Christakis, 2013). Collectively these studies perhaps indicate that particular microbes may impact on brain development and potentially future health. Maternal nutrition may also play a role in this context with some of the reported benefits at three years of age being most pronounced in infants whose mothers consumed more than two portions of fish per week while breast-feeding (Belfort et al., 2013).

Stress

Stress, the effects of which are predominantly mediated through the hypothalamic-pituitary-adrenal (HPA) axis, has long been known to influence the composition of the gut microbiota (Tannock and Savage, 1974). However, this influence is now more widely acknowledged; in particular, stress in early life significantly alters the microbiota in adulthood (O'Mahony et al., 2009). Hence, events during early life capable of activating the stress axis can potentially impact the developing microbiota in the neonatal period and vice versa. This could ultimately lead to dysbiosis in the GI tract and an inappropriate stress response persisting into adulthood.

Early Life Antibiotic Use and Germ-Free Environment

Early life antibiotic treatment is common practice (Vangay et al., 2015) with epidemiological studies highlighting associations between antibiotic use in early infancy and occurrence of diseases such as diabetes (Candon et al., 2015), obesity (Saari et al., 2015), asthma (Pitter et al., 2015), celiac disease (Canova et al., 2015), and IBD (Shaw et al., 2010). Longitudinal studies have demonstrated profound short- and long-term effects of antibiotics on the diversity and composition of the microbiota (Rodriguez et al., 2015). For example, neonatal antibiotic usage reduces the diversity of the *Bifidobacterium* spp. and *Bacteroides* (Hussey et al., 2011; Johnson and Versalovic, 2012). There are also some recent indications that an adult-like stable and diverse microbiota might not be acquired until adolescence, which, if confirmed, greatly extends the time window during which the microbiota can influence health outcomes (Agans et al., 2011). Germ-free mice provide a valuable model in which to assess the impact of growing up without a microbiota (Williams, 2014) and have proven useful as tools in which to assess the impact of the microbiota on CNS function (Collins et al., 2012; Farmer et al., 2014; Dinan et al., 2015; Stilling et al., 2015; Zhou and Foster, 2015; Stilling et al., 2016). Such work extends to behaviors relevant to mood, cognition, pain, and social interaction (Burokas et al., 2015). It is clear that the postnatal period is a dynamic phase of microbial development during which time there is a great deal of potential for this ecosystem to impact other concomitantly developing systems.

IMPACT OF EARLY LIFE MICROBIOTA ON THE DEVELOPMENT OF KEY HOST HOMEOSTATIC MECHANISMS
HOW IS INTESTINAL BARRIER DEVELOPMENT SHAPED BY THE MICROBIOTA?

The intestinal barrier is the host's first line of defense against luminal pathogens and toxins and yet must permit tolerance toward the commensal microbiota. At birth, however, the intestinal barrier is physiologically and morphologically immature. Upon colonization the intestinal barrier undergoes changes in order to cope with microbial interactions in order to reach a homeostatic state that maintains gut function and provides protection to the host thereby avoiding aberrant immune activation and inflammation (Fig. 9.2). Barrier changes induced by colonization have been studied using germ-free animal models and have focused on the impact of commensal microbiota on immune parameters of barrier maturation (El Aidy et al., 2012). Within days

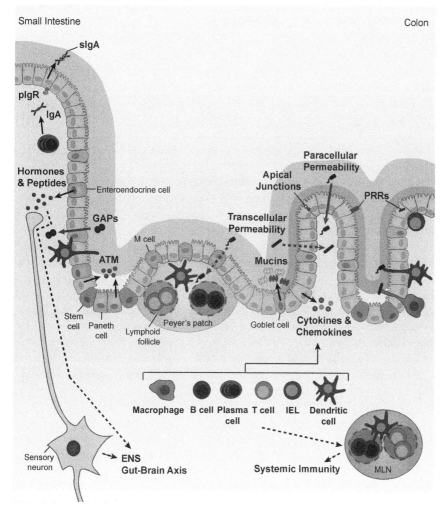

FIGURE 9.2

The intestinal barrier is the host's first line of defense against luminal pathogens and toxins, but must permit tolerance toward the commensal microbiota and environmental antigens while allowing passage of water, electrolytes, and nutrients. To facilitate these various functions, the intestinal barrier is composed of a semipermeable epithelial and mucus barrier that uses adaptive and innate immune features to limit translocation of pathogens and harmful antigens, and elicit measured immune responses when appropriate.

of conventionalization (colonization with mouse specific-pathogen-free (SPF) microbiota), the structure of the mucosa in germ-free mice is altered. Specifically, crypts elongate, small intestine villi shorten, cellular infiltration increases, the lamina propria expands, and differentiation of enterocytes into Paneth cells and enteroendocrine cells increases (Smith et al., 2007; El Aidy et al., 2012). Mucin expression, mucus layer thickness, and the proportion of sialylated to sulfated mucins also increase following colonization (Linden et al., 2008; Petersson et al., 2011; El Aidy et al., 2012; Frantz et al., 2012; Larsson et al., 2012). However, these changes to the mucus layer are dependent on the type of bacteria and their metabolic products. For example, colonization with the short-chain fatty acid (SCFA)-producer, *Bacteroides thetaiotaomicron* results in normal mucus layer development. However, when combined with an acetate consumer and butyrate producer, *Faecalibacterium prausnitzii*, the extent of the mucus layer changes are attenuated (Wrzosek et al., 2013). Furthermore, both luminal lipopolysaccharide and peptidoglycan can increase mucus thickness independently, demonstrating that bacterial antigen signaling alone can alter the mucus layer (Petersson et al., 2011).

Innate immune aspects of the barrier develop by day four postconventionalization of germ-free mice and include increased expression of pattern recognition receptors (PRRs) as well as secretion of antimicrobial peptides (Vaishnava et al., 2008; Gaboriau-Routhiau et al., 2009; Vaishnava et al., 2011; El Aidy et al., 2012; Frantz et al., 2012). The induction of antimicrobial peptide production is also influenced by the type and complexity of the microbiota, with studies showing that colonization of germ-free mice with SPF microbiota leads to greater MyD88/TRIFF-mediated RegIII-γ expression in the colon compared to the eight-strain altered Schaedler flora (Natividad and Verdu, 2013). Furthermore, monocolonization with the probiotic *Bifidobacterium breve* induced higher RegIII-γ expression than *Escherichia coli* JM83 (Natividad et al., 2013).

Intestinal permeability is a function of the intestinal barrier that must be carefully regulated in order to facilitate nutrient absorption and passage of electrolytes without permitting bacterial infiltration. Although luminal contents are taken up through enterocyte endocytosis in the small intestine, 97% of proteins undergo lysosomal degradation preventing transcellular trafficking of intact proteins (Heyman et al., 1986; Fujita et al., 1990). However, transcellular passage of intact proteins is transiently increased at days three and four after birth in the small intestine and coincides with translocation of live bacteria to mesenteric lymph nodes (MLNs) and spleen in *Morganella morganii* monocolonized mice (Heyman et al., 1986; Shroff et al., 1995). Given that maternal immunoglobulins from breast milk can undergo retrograde transcytosis by binding to apical neonatal Fc receptors (nFcR) on enterocytes (Simister and Rees, 1985), transiently increased transcellular permeability is an important mechanism for luminal antigen sampling and early life protection. On the other hand, paracellular permeability to large molecules is regulated by the structural integrity of tight junction and adherens junction protein complexes between adjacent epithelial cells. Compared to conventionally raised mice, both ileum adherens and tight junctions of germ-free mice are shorter in size, and expression of integral tight junction proteins is decreased (Kozakova et al., 2015). Translocation of live bacteria to the MLNs and spleen diminishes within one to three weeks of conventionalization and monocolonization of germ-free mice (Berg and Garlington, 1979; Shroff and Cebra, 1995). This may be due to immune maturation since the decline in bacterial translocation coincides with production of microbe-specific IgA in *Morganella morganii* monocolonized mice (Berg and Garlington, 1979; Shroff and Cebra, 1995).

Recently, goblet cell-associated antigen passages (GAPs) have been described. These allow translocation of antigens from the lumen to the lamina propria following muscarinic acetylcholine receptor 4 activation (McDole et al., 2012; Knoop et al., 2015). GAPs form in the adult small intestine but are inhibited in the colon by bacterial stimulation of MyD88 signaling under steady-state conditions, indicating region-specific regulation by the microbiota. It is unknown whether molecules pass through goblet cells themselves or paracellularly. Colonic goblet cells of young mice have higher incidence of endocytosis compared to adults, suggesting GAP antigen uptake may be higher during early colonization if endocytosis is involved (Colony and Specian, 1987).

Together these findings suggest microbial colonization impacts intestinal barrier maturation, although the influence of different microbial communities remains largely unknown. Since impaired barrier defenses and permeability regulation are associated with a number of GI and psychological disorders, determining if barrier dysfunction originates from early life colonizing microbiota-induced alterations may further elucidate disease pathogenesis.

IMMUNE DEVELOPMENT

Colonization studies have demonstrated microbial stimulation is required for maturation of lymphoid structures (Smith et al., 2007). Germ-free mice have immature isolated lymphoid follicles (ILFs), small Peyer's patches that lack germinal centers, and an absence of distinct T and B cell follicles in MLNs and spleen. However, these mature following colonization (Adachi et al., 1997; Bouskra et al., 2008). Maturation of ILFs is impaired in the absence of nucleotide-binding oligomerization domain-containing protein (NOD) 2. Toll-like receptor (TLR) signaling is completely attenuated without NOD1 signaling to recruit T and B cells (Bouskra et al., 2008). Moreover, the *Bacteroides fragilis* product, polysaccharide A (PSA), can stimulate expansion of spleen lymphocyte follicles (Mazmanian et al., 2005). Microbial stimulation, often through MyD88 signaling, is required to induce site-specific expansion and maturation of innate immune cells and is directly related to the level of microbiota complexity (Williams et al., 2006; Fujiwara et al., 2008; Balmer et al., 2014). Following colonization the capacity of spleen dendritic cells (DCs) and macrophages to produce proinflammatory cytokines and prime natural killer (NK) cells is enhanced and gut chemokine CX3C receptor 1 positive cell sampling of luminal antigens increases (Chieppa et al., 2006; Niess and Adler, 2010; Ganal et al., 2012). Over the first two weeks of colonization systemic neutrophil levels rise to compensate for microbial exposure and prevent septic bacterial infections; this is inhibited by perinatal antibiotic-induced microbiota depletion (Bandeira et al., 1990; Deshmukh et al., 2014). Following colonization intraepithelial lymphocyte (IEL) populations increase, particularly αβ T cell receptor-bearing cells, although maintenance of IEL populations is dependent upon stimulation of the aryl hydrocarbon receptor by dietary ligands (Li et al., 2011). Furthermore, MyD88 signaling in small intestinal epithelial cells leads to production of the bactericidal lectins, RegIIIγ and RegIIIβ, by γδ IELs, thus preventing bacterial translocation to the spleen (Ismail et al., 2011). Therefore, the microbiota stimulates expansion and maturation of innate immune cells.

Colonization also greatly influences development of adaptive immunity altering the abundance, phenotype, and function of T and B cells. Adaptive immune presence is observed by day eight in the colon and day 16 in the small intestine of conventionalized mice when a balance between pro- and anti-inflammatory responses is induced (Williams et al., 2006; Gaboriau-Routhiau et al., 2009; El Aidy et al., 2012). However, specific members of the microbiota can influence T cell induction and dictate the balance between effector and regulatory T cells following colonization. Bacteria belonging to Firmicutes, particularly the *Clostridia* class, are instrumental in inducing balanced T cell responses (Gaboriau-Routhiau et al., 2009; Atarashi et al., 2011, 2013; Chung et al., 2012; Atarashi et al., 2013). Colonization with microbiota low in Firmicutes leads to augmented T helper (Th)17 cells in the colon and this can be reversed by supplementation with Lachnospiraceae and Ruminococcaceae (Natividad et al., 2015). *Clostridium* clusters IV and XIVa, as well as *B. fragilis* PSA, stimulate expansion of interleukin (IL)10 expressing regulatory T cells (Tregs), whereas segmented filamentous bacteria (SFB) induce Th17 cells (Mazmanian et al., 2005; Ivanov et al., 2009; Round and Mazmanian, 2010; Atarashi et al., 2011; Geuking et al., 2011; Lathrop et al., 2011; Round et al., 2011; Atarashi et al., 2013). However, in the spleen, PSA induces Th1 differentiation, indicating different compartmental responses to microbial stimulation (Round and Mazmanian, 2010). Colonization of germ-free mice with human microbiota or SFB fails to elicit the same level of adaptive immune maturation seen in conventionalized mice. However, cohousing human microbiota colonized, or "humanized," mice with conventionalized mice that harbor SFB normalizes effector T cell levels in the gut but not Tregs (Chung et al., 2012). Germ-free mice have low amounts of invariant NK (iNK) T cells in the spleen and liver but high amounts in the colon (Wei et al., 2010; Olszak et al., 2012). Colonization with iNK T cell antigen-bearing *Sphingomonas* rapidly increases spleen and liver iNK T cell numbers and induces maturation and responsiveness to antigens, which is not observed with iNK T cell antigen lacking *E. coli* colonization (Wei et al., 2010; Wingender et al., 2012).

B cells are present in the spleen and intestinal lamina propria prior to birth, but require microbial signals for class switching and augmented antibody production in the spleen and Peyer's patches as well as antibody secretion into the gut lumen (Hansson et al., 2011). Furthermore, the presence of B cells in Peyer's patches and MLN diminishes without ongoing bacterial exposure, suggesting continual microbial stimulation is required for maintenance of germinal center B cell populations (Hapfelmeier et al., 2010). Low numbers of IgM-containing cells are present in the

MLN by day six of life in human infants and by day 12 IgM- and IgA-containing cells that are observed in the colon (Perkkio and Savilahti, 1980). In the small intestine, an abundance of IgA-secreting cells is observed by day 14 following mono-colonization with *E. coli* (Hapfelmeier et al., 2010). Following microbiota-driven MyD88 activation, epithelial cell expression of polymeric immunoglobulin receptor and sIgA transcytosis is increased (Frantz et al., 2012). The microbiota also affects the microbial specificity of sIgA produced (Shroff et al., 1995; Hapfelmeier et al., 2010; Lecuyer et al., 2014). Thus, microbiota drives B cell maturation and antibody production and influences IgA specificity.

The importance of early life microbiota is further demonstrated when evaluating immune development in germ-free mice colonized at older ages. Colonization at three weeks of age alters the relative abundances of systemic immune cells and cytokines and generates a proinflammatory bias of MLN cells (Hansen et al., 2012). Mice colonized in adulthood have higher colon iNK T cell accumulation and sustained expression of proinflammatory immune-related genes in the jejunum and colon, 77% of which have been linked to Crohn's disease in genome-wide association studies (Olszak et al., 2012; El Aidy et al., 2013). Therefore, delayed colonization can bias immune responses to be proinflammatory, further connecting early life microbiota disruption to development of inflammatory disorders later in life.

An important aspect of mucosal immunity is the ability to mount immune responses toward pathogens and toxins, but to also remain tolerant toward commensal microbes and environmental antigens. Following colonization establishment of oral tolerance toward the microbiota involves adaptation of both innate and adaptive immunity. During the first two weeks of life intestinal epithelial cells are transiently desensitized to TLR4 stimulation, protecting intestinal epithelial cells from induction of inflammation (Chassin et al., 2010). Conversely, following caesarean delivery, TLR4 desensitization does not occur, suggesting that mode of colonization, or colonizing microbiota, may be important factors in establishment of tolerance and homeostasis (Lotz et al., 2006). Furthermore, activation of MyD88 signaling inhibits trafficking of lumenal antigens to the MLN and induction of proinflammatory immune responses, suggesting that commensal bacteria themselves may promote tolerance (Diehl et al., 2013). Thus, it is clear that the microbiota drives development of the immune system and establishment of oral tolerance. Moreover, the presence or absence of specific bacteria can impact the balance between proinflammatory and regulatory responses. However, further work is needed to characterize the effects of different complex microbial communities on immune maturation and how this relates to susceptibility to disease.

DEVELOPMENT OF THE HYPOTHALAMIC-PITUITARY-ADRENAL AXIS AND STRESS RESPONSE

The brain–gut–microbiota axis is a bidirectional communication pathway between the central nervous system and the GI tract and encompasses neural, immune, and endocrine pathways (Cryan and O'Mahony, 2011; Bercik et al., 2012; De Palma et al., 2014b; Dinan et al., 2015). Perturbation of this axis results in alterations in the stress response and behavior and has been implicated in various disease states (Bonaz and Bernstein, 2013; Moloney et al., 2014; Borre et al., 2014a; Mayer et al., 2014; De Palma et al., in revision).

The appropriate development of the HPA stress axis determines the ability of an individual to cope and adapt to stressors. The stress hyporesponsive period occurs during the first two weeks of life in the rodent, with the majority of stressors evoking a subnormal response from the axis (Lupien et al., 2009). There is also evidence that this period also exists in humans and is thought to extend throughout childhood (Raabe and Spengler, 2013). It is also thought that this hyporesponsive period may have evolved to protect the rapidly developing child from the influence of elevated glucocorticoids (Raabe and Spengler, 2013). Early life stressors are associated with increased anxiety and depressive-like behaviors as well as GI disorders associated with a stress component (Lupien et al., 2009; O'Mahony et al., 2011). Given the influence of stress on the gut–brain axis (Grenham et al., 2011), appropriate development of the stress axis is essential to the balanced functioning of the gut–brain axis.

HEALTH OUTCOMES RELATED TO PERTURBATION OF THE INTESTINAL MICROBIOTA IN EARLY LIFE

Defects in intestinal barrier integrity, immune surveillance, and the stress responses can be detrimental to host health. A number of disorders are associated with altered neonatal colonization that may impact intestinal barrier and immune maturation, the gut–brain axis, and, therefore, may ultimately contribute to development of GI and psychological disorders.

DISORDERS OF THE GUT

Inflammatory Bowel Disease

Altered colonization is associated with increased susceptibility to IBD. Delivery by caesarean section and childhood antibiotic use are both associated with increased risk of IBD, although some studies report only an association with Crohn's disease, a higher prevalence specifically being reported in males exposed to antibiotics (Bager et al., 2012; Virta et al., 2012; Li et al., 2014; Ungaro et al., 2014; Sevelsted et al., 2015). Ulcerative colitis (UC), on the other hand, is associated with a decrease in Firmicutes and induces expansion of Th17 cells in the colon following colonization, the effects of which can be reversed by Lachnospiraceae and Ruminococcaceae supplementation suggesting that a lack of colonizing Firmicutes contributes to Th17-driven inflammation (Jiang et al., 2014; Natividad et al., 2015). Invariant NK T cells have also been implicated in the pathogenesis of UC. In particular, the mucosal accumulation of iNK T diminishes when colonization occurs in the neonatal period (Olszak et al., 2012). Therefore, altered colonization patterns may affect immune maturation, leading to a proinflammatory environment associated with IBD. Thus, dysbiosis and microbial dysfunction are observed in IBD pathogenesis with potential origins, in part, potentially lying in early life colonization patterns.

Celiac Disease

Celiac disease (CD) is a chronic inflammatory disorder of the small intestine resulting from intolerance to gluten in genetically susceptible hosts. Major histocompatibility class (MHC) II alleles, HLA-DQ2 and HLA-DQ8, confer susceptibility to CD due to their affinity for gluten peptides that are deamidated in the lamina propria by host tissue transglutaminase 2 (TG2) (Shan et al., 2002; Bergseng et al., 2005). Although the risk alleles HLA-DQ2 and HLA-DQ8 have been identified, only a small subset of these individuals develop CD, which suggests that the environment also influences CD pathogenesis (Verdu et al., 2015). Despite suggestions that early life gluten exposure and breast-feeding practices may impact CD risk (Ivarsson et al., 2000; Sellitto et al., 2012), recent clinical studies have not confirmed a protective effect of breast-feeding or age of gluten introduction in high-risk children (Jansen et al., 2014; Lionetti et al., 2014; Vriezinga et al., 2014; Sevelsted et al., 2015). It remains to be determined whether an alteration in the microbiota is a modifier of CD risk, in particular in subjects with low- or moderate-genetic risk. However, disruption to the microbiota in early life has been implicated in CD pathogenesis. Early antibiotic use has been associated with the emergence of CD (Marild et al., 2013; Canova et al., 2014), whilst other studies indicate that delivery mode is also influential, although not all studies support this link (Decker et al., 2010; Marild et al., 2013; Emilsson et al., 2015). Furthermore, infants at high risk of developing CD exhibit dysbiosis (De Palma et al., 2012; Sellitto et al., 2012). Moreover, NOD-DQ8 mice with microbiota lacking pathobionts and Proteobacteria (altered Schaedler flora, ASF) exhibit reduced sensitivity to gluten-induced immunopathology compared to conventional mice that harbor potentially opportunistic Proteobacteria (Verdu et al., 2015). Moreover, supplementation of ASF colonized mice with *E. coli* ENT CAI:5 isolated from CD patients reverts the protective effect of colonization. On the other hand, germ-free status is associated with an increased sensitivity to gluten likely related to the lack of immune maturation induced by commensal microbes (Verdu et al., 2015). Thus microbiota structure can either ameliorate or enhance immune responses to gluten in NOD-DQ8 mice.

DISORDERS OF THE BRAIN AND NERVOUS SYSTEM

Anxiety and Depression

Studies using germ-free mice have robustly and reproducibly shown that they are less anxious than their conventionally colonized counterparts (Sudo et al., 2004; Diaz Heijtz et al., 2011; Neufeld et al., 2011; Clarke et al., 2013), while a normo-anxious state can be reinstated by the introduction of a microbiota during critical early life time windows (Clarke et al., 2013). Depression as with other psychiatric disorders has been associated with stress in early life (Chen and Baram, 2015). Recently, increased fecal levels of Enterobacteriaceae and *Alistipes* and reduced levels of *Faecalibacterium* were noted in patients with major depressive disorder compared to healthy controls (Jiang et al., 2015). *Alistipes* species are indole positive, affecting the serotonin precursor tryptophan, while *Faecalibacterium* has anti-inflammatory properties (Jiang et al., 2015). We and others have shown that maternal separation, a form of early life stress, impacts on the gut microbiota in this animal model (O'Mahony et al., 2009; Dinan and Cryan, 2013; Park et al., 2013). Bailey and Coe (1999) investigated the stability of the indigenous microflora before and after maternal separation in rhesus monkeys and demonstrated a significant decrease in fecal bacteria, in particular of *Lactobacilli*, three days after separation, which correlated with stress-indicative behaviors and susceptibility to opportunistic bacterial infection. These results suggest that stress during this vulnerable period of microbiota development leads to gut–brain axis dysfunction and ultimately may increase vulnerability to disease. Despite the etiology of depression being associated with both early life stress and an altered gut microbiota, it is still unclear as to whether there is an interaction between the two.

Obesity

Administration of antibiotics during pregnancy is associated with an increased risk of obesity (Mueller et al., 2015b). Obesity itself is linked to an altered gut microbiota characterized by an altered *Firmicutes:Bacteroidetes* ratio relative to lean individuals (Schele et al., 2015). Hence, there is the possibility that prenatal microbiota manipulation can have long-term effects on the health of the infant including the propensity to gain weight. There are indications that caesarean section delivery influences adiposity and might be linked to an increased risk for both childhood and adult obesity (Goldani et al., 2011; Huh et al., 2012; Mesquita et al., 2013). Although an altered microbiota could precede the development of obesity, a causal relationship is still far from certain. Dietary factors, host physiology alterations later in life, and maternal obesity during pregnancy are also important considerations (Sirimi and Goulis, 2010; Flint, 2012). Hypothalamic dysfunction has also been implicated in this regard (Schellekens et al., 2012). Moreover breast-feeding, which confers a "healthier" microbial balance in babies, is associated with a reduced risk of obesity in both childhood and adulthood (Ejlerskov et al., 2015; Krenz-Niedbala et al., 2015).

Autism Spectrum Disorders

Autism spectrum disorders have also been linked to an abnormal composition of the gut microbiome (de Theije et al., 2011; Mulle et al., 2013). A preclinical study assessing the impact of maternal infection on both the gut and the brain in the offspring determined that maternal immune activation leads to altered gut microbiota, gut barrier function, and behavioral alterations indicative of autistic-like behavior (Hsiao et al., 2013). Furthermore, the impact of maternal infection on the function of the microbiota–gut–brain axis was reversed by the administration of *B. fragilis* to the offspring.

CONCLUDING REMARKS

We have considered how the gut microbiota in early life sculpts the development and maturation of key host regulatory systems, disruption of which may predispose to disease in an individual. Proof of principle studies in germ-free animals have clearly demonstrated a multidimensional impact of growing up without a microbiota. Domains affected by early life colonization include those relevant to GI and mental health as well as pain disorders and obesity. There is substantial overlap between the emergence of these disorders and distortions of the gut microbiome in early life. The restorative options that can be considered to counteract early life microbiome alterations and promote a return to a "healthy" microbiome composition have been well cataloged (Salazar et al., 2014; Mueller et al., 2015a). The tools at our disposal include precision nutritional strategies, such as probiotic and prebiotic supplementation, as well as increased efforts to encourage breast-feeding and limit caesarean section delivery to appropriate medically indicated circumstances. Future developments in this emerging field are not without their challenges, not least whether preclinical data will translate to the clinic. In any case, it is no longer sufficient to consider the host without regard to the microbiome. As our appreciation of early life microbiota grows, the potential for effective and earlier interventions for disease prevention is a tangible prospect. Translating this potential is undoubtedly a challenge but also an extremely worthwhile multidisciplinary venture.

REFERENCES

Aagaard, K., Ma, J., Antony, K.M., Ganu, R., Petrosino, J., Versalovic, J., 2014. The placenta harbors a unique microbiome. Sci. Transl. Med. 6, 237–265.

Aagaard, K., Riehle, K., Ma, J., Segata, N., Mistretta, T.A., Coarfa, C., Raza, S., Rosenbaum, S., Van den Veyver, I., Milosavljevic, A., Gevers, D., Huttenhower, C., Petrosino, J., Versalovic, J., 2012. A metagenomic approach to characterization of the vaginal microbiome signature in pregnancy. PLoS One 7, e36466.

Adachi, S., Yoshida, H., Kataoka, H., Nishikawa, S., 1997. Three distinctive steps in Peyer's patch formation of murine embryo. Int. Immunol. 9, 507–514.

Agans, R., Rigsbee, L., Kenche, H., Michail, S., Khamis, H.J., Paliy, O., 2011. Distal gut microbiota of adolescent children is different from that of adults. FEMS Microbiol. Ecol. 77, 404–412.

Amaral, F.A., Sachs, D., Costa, V.V., Fagundes, C.T., Cisalpino, D., Cunha, T.M., Ferreira, S.H., Cunha, F.Q., Silva, T.A., Nicoli, J.R., Vieira, L.Q., Souza, D.G., Teixeira, M.M., 2008. Commensal microbiota is fundamental for the development of inflammatory pain. Proc. Natl. Acad. Sci. U.S.A. 105, 2193–2197.

Atarashi, K., Tanoue, T., Oshima, K., Suda, W., Nagano, Y., Nishikawa, H., Fukuda, S., Saito, T., Narushima, S., Hase, K., Kim, S., Fritz, J.V., Wilmes, P., Ueha, S., Matsushima, K., Ohno, H., Olle, B., Sakaguchi, S., Taniguchi, T., Morita, H., Hattori, M., Honda, K., 2013. Treg induction by a rationally selected mixture of *Clostridia* strains from the human microbiota. Nature 500, 232–236.

Atarashi, K., Tanoue, T., Shima, T., Imaoka, A., Kuwahara, T., Momose, Y., Cheng, G., Yamasaki, S., Saito, T., Ohba, Y., Taniguchi, T., Takeda, K., Hori, S., Ivanov II, Umesaki, Y., Itoh, K., Honda, K., 2011. Induction of colonic regulatory T cells by indigenous *Clostridium* species. Science 331, 337–341.

Azad, M.B., Konya, T., Maughan, H., Guttman, D.S., Field, C.J., Chari, R.S., Sears, M.R., Becker, A.B., Scott, J.A., Kozyrskyj, A.L., Investigators, C.S., 2013. Gut microbiota of healthy Canadian infants: profiles by mode of delivery and infant diet at 4 months. CMAJ 185, 385–394.

Bager, P., Simonsen, J., Nielsen, N.M., Frisch, M., 2012. Cesarean section and offspring's risk of inflammatory bowel disease: a national cohort study. Inflamm. Bowel Dis. 18, 857–862.

Bailey, M.T., Coe C.L., 1999. Maternal separation disrupts the integrity of the intestinal microflora in infant rhesus monkeys. Dev. Pyschobiol. 35, 146–155.

Balmer, M.L., Schurch, C.M., Saito, Y., Geuking, M.B., Li, H., Cuenca, M., Kovtonyuk, L.V., McCoy, K.D., Hapfelmeier, S., Ochsenbein, A.F., Manz, M.G., Slack, E., Macpherson, A.J., 2014. Microbiota-derived compounds drive steady-state granulopoiesis via MyD88/TICAM signaling. J. Immunol. 193, 5273–5283.

Bandeira, A., Mota-Santos, T., Itohara, S., Degermann, S., Heusser, C., Tonegawa, S., Coutinho, A., 1990. Localization of gamma/delta T cells to the intestinal epithelium is independent of normal microbial colonization. J. Exp. Med. 172, 239–244.

Barrett, E., Guinane, C.M., Ryan, C.A., Dempsey, E.M., Murphy, B.P., O'Toole, P.W., Fitzgerald, G.F., Cotter, P.D., Ross, R.P., Stanton, C., 2013. Microbiota diversity and stability of the preterm neonatal ileum and colon of two infants. Microbiologyopen 2, 215–225.

Belfort, M.B., Rifas-Shiman, S.L., Kleinman, K.P., Guthrie, L.B., Bellinger, D.C., Taveras, E.M., Gillman, M.W., Oken, E., 2013. Infant feeding and childhood cognition at ages 3 and 7 years: effects of breastfeeding duration and exclusivity. JAMA Pediatr. 167, 836–844.

Bercik, P., Collins, S.M., Verdu, E.F., 2012. Microbes and the gut-brain axis. Neurogastroenterology Motil. 24, 405–413.

Berg, R.D., Garlington, A.W., 1979. Translocation of certain indigenous bacteria from the gastrointestinal tract to the mesenteric lymph nodes and other organs in a gnotobiotic mouse model. Infect. Immun. 23, 403–411.

Bergseng, E., Xia, J., Kim, C.Y., Khosla, C., Sollid, L.M., 2005. Main chain hydrogen bond interactions in the binding of proline-rich gluten peptides to the celiac disease-associated HLA-DQ2 molecule. J. Biol. Chem. 280, 21791–21796.

Biasucci, G., Benenati, B., Morelli, L., Bessi, E., Boehm, G., 2008. Cesarean delivery may affect the early biodiversity of intestinal bacteria. J. Nutr. 138, 1796S–1800S.

Blaser, M.J., Webb, G.F., 2014. Host demise as a beneficial function of indigenous microbiota in human hosts. mBio 5.

Bonaz, B.L., Bernstein, C.N., 2013. Brain-gut interactions in inflammatory bowel disease. Gastroenterology 144, 36–49.

Borre, Y.E., Moloney, R.D., Clarke, G., Dinan, T.G., Cryan, J.F., 2014a. The impact of microbiota on brain and behavior: mechanisms & therapeutic potential. Adv. Exp. Med. Biol. 817, 373–403.

Borre, Y.E., O'Keeffe, G.W., Clarke, G., Stanton, C., Dinan, T.G., Cryan, J.F., 2014b. Microbiota and neurodevelopmental windows: implications for brain disorders. Trends Mol. Med. 20, 509–518.

Bouskra, D., Brezillon, C., Berard, M., Werts, C., Varona, R., Boneca, I.G., Eberl, G., 2008. Lymphoid tissue genesis induced by commensals through NOD1 regulates intestinal homeostasis. Nature 456, 507–510.

Braniste, V., Al-Asmakh, M., Kowal, C., Anuar, F., Abbaspour, A., Toth, M., Korecka, A., Bakocevic, N., Ng, L.G., Kundu, P., Gulyas, B., Halldin, C., Hultenby, K., Nilsson, H., Hebert, H., Volpe, B.T., Diamond, B., Pettersson, S., 2014. The gut microbiota influences blood–brain barrier permeability in mice. Sci. Transl. Med. 6, 263ra158.

Burokas, A., Moloney, R.D., Dinan, T.G., Cryan, J.F., 2015. Microbiota regulation of the mammalian gut-brain axis. Adv. Appl. Microbiol. 91, 1–62.

Candon, S., Perez-Arroyo, A., Marquet, C., Valette, F., Foray, A.P., Pelletier, B., Milani, C., Ventura, M., Bach, J.F., Chatenoud, L., 2015. Antibiotics in early life alter the gut microbiome and increase disease incidence in a spontaneous mouse model of autoimmune insulin-dependent diabetes. PLoS One 10, e0125448.

Canova, C., Pitter, G., Ludvigsson, J.F., Romor, P., Zanier, L., Zanotti, R., Simonato, L., 2015. Coeliac disease and asthma association in children: the role of antibiotic consumption. Eur. Respir. J. 46, 115–122.

Canova, C., Zabeo, V., Pitter, G., Romor, P., Baldovin, T., Zanotti, R., Simonato, L., 2014. Association of maternal education, early infections, and antibiotic use with celiac disease: a population-based birth cohort study in northeastern Italy. Am. J. Epidemiol. 180, 76–85.

Chassin, C., Kocur, M., Pott, J., Duerr, C.U., Gutle, D., Lotz, M., Hornef, M.W., 2010. miR-146a mediates protective innate immune tolerance in the neonate intestine. Cell Host Microbe 8, 358–368.

Chen, Y., Baram, T.Z., 2015. Towards understanding how early-life stress re-programs cognitive and emotional brain networks. Neuropsychopharmacol. http://dx.doi.org/10.1038/npp.2015.181.

Chieppa, M., Rescigno, M., Huang, A.Y., Germain, R.N., 2006. Dynamic imaging of dendritic cell extension into the small bowel lumen in response to epithelial cell TLR engagement. J. Exp. Med. 203, 2841–2852.

Christakis, D.A., 2013. Breastfeeding and cognition: can IQ tip the scale? JAMA Pediatr. 167, 796–797.

Chung, H., Pamp, S.J., Hill, J.A., Surana, N.K., Edelman, S.M., Troy, E.B., Reading, N.C., Villablanca, E.J., Wang, S., Mora, J.R., Umesaki, Y., Mathis, D., Benoist, C., Relman, D.A., Kasper, D.L., 2012. Gut immune maturation depends on colonization with a host-specific microbiota. Cell 149, 1578–1593.

Clarke, G., Grenham, S., Scully, P., Fitzgerald, P., Moloney, R.D., Shanahan, F., Dinan, T.G., Cryan, J.F., 2013. The microbiome-gut-brain axis during early life regulates the hippocampal serotonergic system in a sex-dependent manner. Mol. Psychiatry 18, 666–673.

Clarke, G., O'Mahony, S.M., Dinan, T.G., Cryan, J.F., 2014a. Priming for health: gut microbiota acquired in early life regulates physiology, brain and behaviour. Acta Paediatr. 103, 812–819.

Clarke, G., Stilling, R.M., Kennedy, P.J., Stanton, C., Cryan, J.F., Dinan, T.G., 2014b. Minireview: gut microbiota: the neglected endocrine organ. Mol. Endocrinol. 28, 1221–1238.

Collins, S.M., Surette, M., Bercik, P., 2012. The interplay between the intestinal microbiota and the brain. Nat. Rev. Microbiol. 10, 735–742.

Colony, P.C., Specian, R.D., 1987. Endocytosis and vesicular traffic in fetal and adult colonic goblet cells. Anat. Rec. 218, 365–372.

Costello, E.K., Stagaman, K., Dethlefsen, L., Bohannan, B.J., Relman, D.A., 2012. The application of ecological theory toward an understanding of the human microbiome. Science 336, 1255–1262.

Cryan, J.F., Dinan, T.G., 2012. Mind-altering microorganisms: the impact of the gut microbiota on brain and behaviour. Nat. Rev. Neurosci. 13, 701–712.

Cryan, J.F., O'Mahony, S.M., 2011. The microbiome-gut-brain axis: from bowel to behavior. Neurogastroenterology Motil. 23, 187–192.

De Palma, G., Capilla, A., Nova, E., Castillejo, G., Varea, V., Pozo, T., Garrote, J.A., Polanco, I., Lopez, A., Ribes-Koninckx, C., Marcos, A., Garcia-Novo, M.D., Calvo, C., Ortigosa, L., Pena-Quintana, L., Palau, F., Sanz, Y., 2012. Influence of milk-feeding type and genetic risk of developing coeliac disease on intestinal microbiota of infants: the PROFICEL study. PLoS One 7, e30791.

De Palma, G., Collins, S.M., Bercik, P., 2014a. The microbiota-gut-brain axis in functional gastrointestinal disorders. Gut Microbe. 5, 419–429.

De Palma, G., Collins, S.M., Bercik, P., Verdu, E.F., 2014b. The microbiota-gut-brain axis in gastrointestinal disorders: stressed bugs, stressed brain or both? J. Physiol. 592, 2989–2997.

De Palma, G., Lynch, M.D.J., Lu, J., Dang, V.T., Deng, Y., Jury, J., Umeh, G., Miranda, P., Pigrau, M., Sidani, S., McLean, P.G., Moreno-Hagelsieb, G., Surrette, M.G., Bergonzelli, G.E., Verdu, E.F., Britz-McKibbin, P., Neufield, J.D., Collins, S.M., Bercik, P. Functional impact of IBS microbiota on the gut-brain axis. Sci. Transl. Med. 5, 419–429.

Decker, E., Engelmann, G., Findeisen, A., Gerner, P., Laass, M., Ney, D., Posovszky, C., Hoy, L., Hornef, M.W., 2010. Cesarean delivery is associated with celiac disease but not inflammatory bowel disease in children. Pediatrics 125, e1433–e1440.

Desbonnet, L., Clarke, G., Shanahan, F., Dinan, T.G., Cryan, J.F., 2014. Microbiota is essential for social development in the mouse. Mol. Psychiatry 19, 146–148.

Deshmukh, H.S., Liu, Y., Menkiti, O.R., Mei, J., Dai, N., O'Leary, C.E., Oliver, P.M., Kolls, J.K., Weiser, J.N., Worthen, G.S., 2014. The microbiota regulates neutrophil homeostasis and host resistance to *Escherichia coli* K1 sepsis in neonatal mice. Nat. Med. 20, 524–530.

Diaz Heijtz, R., Wang, S., Anuar, F., Qian, Y., Bjorkholm, B., Samuelsson, A., Hibberd, M.L., Forssberg, H., Pettersson, S., 2011. Normal gut microbiota modulates brain development and behavior. Proc. Natl. Acad. Sci. U.S.A. 108, 3047–3052.

Diehl, G.E., Longman, R.S., Zhang, J.X., Breart, B., Galan, C., Cuesta, A., Schwab, S.R., Littman, D.R., 2013. Microbiota restricts trafficking of bacteria to mesenteric lymph nodes by CX(3)CR1(hi) cells. Nature 494, 116–120.

DiGiulio, D.B., Romero, R., Amogan, H.P., Kusanovic, J.P., Bik, E.M., Gotsch, F., Kim, C.J., Erez, O., Edwin, S., Relman, D.A., 2008. Microbial prevalence, diversity and abundance in amniotic fluid during preterm labor: a molecular and culture-based investigation. PLoS One 3, e3056.

Dinan, T.G., Cryan, J.F., 2013. Melancholic microbes: a link between gut microbiota and depression? Neurogastroenterology Motil. 25, 713–719.

Dinan, T.G., Stilling, R.M., Stanton, C., Cryan, J.F., 2015. Collective unconscious: how gut microbes shape human behavior. J. Psychiatr. Res. 63, 1–9.

Dominguez-Bello, M.G., Costello, E.K., Contreras, M., Magris, M., Hidalgo, G., Fierer, N., Knight, R., 2010. Delivery mode shapes the acquisition and structure of the initial microbiota across multiple body habitats in newborns. Proc. Natl. Acad. Sci. U.S.A. 107, 11971–11975.

Ejlerskov, K.T., Christensen, L.B., Ritz, C., Jensen, S.M., Molgaard, C., Michaelsen, K.F., 2015. The impact of early growth patterns and infant feeding on body composition at 3 years of age. Br. J. Nutr. 1–12.

El Aidy, S., Hooiveld, G., Tremaroli, V., Backhed, F., Kleerebezem, M., 2013. The gut microbiota and mucosal homeostasis: colonized at birth or at adulthood, does it matter? Gut Microbe. 4, 118–124.

El Aidy, S., van Baarlen, P., Derrien, M., Lindenbergh-Kortleve, D.J., Hooiveld, G., Levenez, F., Dore, J., Dekker, J., Samsom, J.N., Nieuwenhuis, E.E., Kleerebezem, M., 2012. Temporal and spatial interplay of microbiota and intestinal mucosa drive establishment of immune homeostasis in conventionalized mice. Mucosal Immunol. 5, 567–579.

Emilsson, L., Magnus, M.C., Stordal, K., 2015. Perinatal risk factors for development of celiac disease in children, based on the prospective Norwegian mother and child cohort study. Clin. Gastroenterol. Hepatol. 13, 921–927.

Farmer, A.D., Randall, H.A., Aziz, Q., 2014. It's a gut feeling: how the gut microbiota affects the state of mind. J. Physiol. 592, 2981–2988.

Fernandez, L., Langa, S., Martin, V., Maldonado, A., Jimenez, E., Martin, R., Rodriguez, J.M., 2013. The human milk microbiota: origin and potential roles in health and disease. Pharmacol. Res. 69, 1–10.

Flint, H.J., 2012. The impact of nutrition on the human microbiome. Nutr. Rev. 70 (Suppl. 1), S10–S13.

Frantz, A.L., Rogier, E.W., Weber, C.R., Shen, L., Cohen, D.A., Fenton, L.A., Bruno, M.E., Kaetzel, C.S., 2012. Targeted deletion of MyD88 in intestinal epithelial cells results in compromised antibacterial immunity associated with downregulation of polymeric immunoglobulin receptor, mucin-2, and antibacterial peptides. Mucosal Immunol. 5, 501–512.

Fujita, M., Reinhart, F., Neutra, M., 1990. Convergence of apical and basolateral endocytic pathways at apical late endosomes in absorptive cells of suckling rat ileum in vivo. J. Cell Sci. 97 (Pt 2), 385–394.

Fujiwara, D., Wei, B., Presley, L.L., Brewer, S., McPherson, M., Lewinski, M.A., Borneman, J., Braun, J., 2008. Systemic control of plasmacytoid dendritic cells by CD8+ T cells and commensal microbiota. J. Immunol. 180, 5843–5852.

Funkhouser, L.J., Bordenstein, S.R., 2013. Mom knows best: the universality of maternal microbial transmission. PLoS Biol. 11, e1001631.

Gaboriau-Routhiau, V., Rakotobe, S., Lecuyer, E., Mulder, I., Lan, A., Bridonneau, C., Rochet, V., Pisi, A., De Paepe, M., Brandi, G., Eberl, G., Snel, J., Kelly, D., Cerf-Bensussan, N., 2009. The key role of segmented filamentous bacteria in the coordinated maturation of gut helper T cell responses. Immunity 31, 677–689.

Galipeau, H.J., Verdu, E.F., 2014. Gut microbes and adverse food reactions: focus on gluten related disorders. Gut Microbe. 5, 594–605.

Ganal, S.C., Sanos, S.L., Kallfass, C., Oberle, K., Johner, C., Kirschning, C., Lienenklaus, S., Weiss, S., Staeheli, P., Aichele, P., Diefenbach, A., 2012. Priming of natural killer cells by nonmucosal mononuclear phagocytes requires instructive signals from commensal microbiota. Immunity 37, 171–186.

Geuking, M.B., Cahenzli, J., Lawson, M.A., Ng, D.C., Slack, E., Hapfelmeier, S., McCoy, K.D., Macpherson, A.J., 2011. Intestinal bacterial colonization induces mutualistic regulatory T cell responses. Immunity 34, 794–806.

Goldani, H.A., Bettiol, H., Barbieri, M.A., Silva, A.A., Agranonik, M., Morais, M.B., Goldani, M.Z., 2011. Cesarean delivery is associated with an increased risk of obesity in adulthood in a Brazilian birth cohort study. Am. J. Clin. Nutr. 93, 1344–1347.

Golubeva, A.V., Crampton, S., Desbonnet, L., Edge, D., O'Sullivan, O., Lomasney, K.W., Zhdanov, A.V., Crispie, F., Moloney, R.D., Borre, Y.E., Cotter, P.D., Hyland, N.P., O'Halloran, K.D., Dinan, T.G., O'Keeffe, G.W., Cryan, J.F., 2015. Prenatal stress-induced alterations in major physiological systems correlate with gut microbiota composition in adulthood. Psychoneuroendocrinology 60, 58–74.

Grenham, S., Clarke, G., Cryan, J.F., Dinan, T.G., 2011. Brain-gut-microbe communication in health and disease. Front. Physiol. 2, 94.

Gulden, E., Wong, F.S., Wen, L., 2015. The gut microbiota and type 1 diabetes. Clin. Immunol. 159 (2), 143–153.

Hansen, C.H., Nielsen, D.S., Kverka, M., Zakostelska, Z., Klimesova, K., Hudcovic, T., Tlaskalova-Hogenova, H., Hansen, A.K., 2012. Patterns of early gut colonization shape future immune responses of the host. PLoS One 7, e34043.

Hansson, J., Bosco, N., Favre, L., Raymond, F., Oliveira, M., Metairon, S., Mansourian, R., Blum, S., Kussmann, M., Benyacoub, J., 2011. Influence of gut microbiota on mouse B2 B cell ontogeny and function. Mol. Immunol. 48, 1091–1101.

Hapfelmeier, S., Lawson, M.A., Slack, E., Kirundi, J.K., Stoel, M., Heikenwalder, M., Cahenzli, J., Velykoredko, Y., Balmer, M.L., Endt, K., Geuking, M.B., Curtiss 3rd, R., McCoy, K.D., Macpherson, A.J., 2010. Reversible microbial colonization of germ-free mice reveals the dynamics of IgA immune responses. Science 328, 1705–1709.

Heyman, M., Crain-Denoyelle, A.M., Corthier, G., Morgat, J.L., Desjeux, J.F., 1986. Postnatal development of protein absorption in conventional and germ-free mice. Am. J. Physiol. 251, G326–G331.

Hsiao, E.Y., McBride, S.W., Hsien, S., Sharon, G., Hyde, E.R., McCue, T., Codelli, J.A., Chow, J., Reisman, S.E., Petrosino, J.F., Patterson, P.H., Mazmanian, S.K., 2013. Microbiota modulate behavioral and physiological abnormalities associated with neurodevelopmental disorders. Cell 155, 1451–1463.

Huh, S.Y., Rifas-Shiman, S.L., Zera, C.A., Edwards, J.W., Oken, E., Weiss, S.T., Gillman, M.W., 2012. Delivery by caesarean section and risk of obesity in preschool age children: a prospective cohort study. Arch. Dis. Childhood 97, 610–616.

Hussey, S., Wall, R., Gruffman, E., O'Sullivan, L., Ryan, C.A., Murphy, B., Fitzgerald, G., Stanton, C., Ross, R.P., 2011. Parenteral antibiotics reduce *Bifidobacteria* colonization and diversity in neonates. Int. J. Microbiol. 2011.

Ismail, A.S., Severson, K.M., Vaishnava, S., Behrendt, C.L., Yu, X., Benjamin, J.L., Ruhn, K.A., Hou, B., DeFranco, A.L., Yarovinsky, F., Hooper, L.V., 2011. Gammadelta intraepithelial lymphocytes are essential mediators of host-microbial homeostasis at the intestinal mucosal surface. Proc. Natl. Acad. Sci. U.S.A. 108, 8743–8748.

Ivanov II, Atarashi, K., Manel, N., Brodie, E.L., Shima, T., Karaoz, U., Wei, D., Goldfarb, K.C., Santee, C.A., Lynch, S.V., Tanoue, T., Imaoka, A., Itoh, K., Takeda, K., Umesaki, Y., Honda, K., Littman, D.R., 2009. Induction of intestinal Th17 cells by segmented filamentous bacteria. Cell 139, 485–498.

Ivarsson, A., Persson, L.A., Nystrom, L., Ascher, H., Cavell, B., Danielsson, L., Dannaeus, A., Lindberg, T., Lindquist, B., Stenhammar, L., Hernell, O., 2000. Epidemic of coeliac disease in Swedish children. Acta Paediatr. 89, 165–171.

Jakobsson, H.E., Abrahamsson, T.R., Jenmalm, M.C., Harris, K., Quince, C., Jernberg, C., Bjorksten, B., Engstrand, L., Andersson, A.F., 2013. Decreased gut microbiota diversity, delayed *Bacteroidetes* colonisation and reduced Th1 responses in infants delivered by caesarean section. Gut. http://dx.doi.org/10.1136/gutjnl-2012-303249.

Jansen, M.A., Tromp II, Kiefte-de Jong, J.C., Jaddoe, V.W., Hofman, A., Escher, J.C., Hooijkaas, H., Moll, H.A., 2014. Infant feeding and anti-tissue transglutaminase antibody concentrations in the generation R study. Am. J. Clin. Nutr. 100, 1095–1101.

Jasarevic, E., Howerton, C.L., Howard, C.D., Bale, T.L., 2015a. Alterations in the vaginal microbiome by maternal stress are associated with metabolic reprogramming of the offspring gut and brain. Endocrinology 156 (9), 3265–3276. http://dx.doi.org/10.1210/en.2015-1177.

Jasarevic, E., Rodgers, A.B., Bale, T.L., 2015b. A novel role for maternal stress and microbial transmission in early life programming and neurodevelopment. Neurobiol. Stress 1, 81–88.

Jiang, H., Ling, Z., Zhang, Y., Mao, H., Ma, Z., Yin, Y., Wang, W., Tang, W., Tan, Z., Shi, J., Li, L., Ruan, B., 2015. Altered fecal microbiota composition in patients with major depressive disorder. Brain Behav. Immun. 48, 186–194.

Jiang, W., Su, J., Zhang, X., Cheng, X., Zhou, J., Shi, R., Zhang, H., 2014. Elevated levels of Th17 cells and Th17-related cytokines are associated with disease activity in patients with inflammatory bowel disease. Inflamm. Res. 63, 943–950.

Jimenez, E., Marin, M.L., Martin, R., Odriozola, J.M., Olivares, M., Xaus, J., Fernandez, L., Rodriguez, J.M., 2008. Is meconium from healthy newborns actually sterile? Res. Microbiol. 159, 187–193.

Johnson, C.L., Versalovic, J., 2012. The human microbiome and its potential importance to pediatrics. Pediatrics 129, 950–960.

Khodayar-Pardo, P., Mira-Pascual, L., Collado, M.C., Martinez-Costa, C., 2014. Impact of lactation stage, gestational age and mode of delivery on breast milk microbiota. J. Perinatol. 34, 599–605.

Knoop, K.A., McDonald, K.G., McCrate, S., McDole, J.R., Newberry, R.D., 2015. Microbial sensing by goblet cells controls immune surveillance of luminal antigens in the colon. Mucosal Immunol. 8, 198–210.

Koren, O., Goodrich, J.K., Cullender, T.C., Spor, A., Laitinen, K., Backhed, H.K., Gonzalez, A., Werner, J.J., Angenent, L.T., Knight, R., Backhed, F., Isolauri, E., Salminen, S., Ley, R.E., 2012. Host remodeling of the gut microbiome and metabolic changes during pregnancy. Cell 150, 470–480.

Kozakova, H., Schwarzer, M., Tuckova, L., Srutkova, D., Czarnowska, E., Rosiak, I., Hudcovic, T., Schabussova, I., Hermanova, P., Zakostelska, Z., Aleksandrzak-Piekarczyk, T., Koryszewska-Baginska, A., Tlaskalova-Hogenova, H., Cukrowska, B., 2015. Colonization of germ-free mice with a mixture of three lactobacillus strains enhances the integrity of gut mucosa and ameliorates allergic sensitization. Cell Mol. Immunol. http://dx.doi.org/10.1038/cmi.2015.09.

Krenz-Niedbala, M., Koscinski, K., Puch, E.A., Zelent, A., Breborowicz, A., 2015. Is the relationship between breastfeeding and childhood risk of asthma and obesity mediated by infant antibiotic treatment? Breastfeed Med. 10 (6), 326–333.

Larsson, E., Tremaroli, V., Lee, Y.S., Koren, O., Nookaew, I., Fricker, A., Nielsen, J., Ley, R.E., Backhed, F., 2012. Analysis of gut microbial regulation of host gene expression along the length of the gut and regulation of gut microbial ecology through MyD88. Gut 61, 1124–1131.

Lathrop, S.K., Bloom, S.M., Rao, S.M., Nutsch, K., Lio, C.W., Santacruz, N., Peterson, D.A., Stappenbeck, T.S., Hsieh, C.S., 2011. Peripheral education of the immune system by colonic commensal microbiota. Nature 478, 250–254.

Lecuyer, E., Rakotobe, S., Lengline-Garnier, H., Lebreton, C., Picard, M., Juste, C., Fritzen, R., Eberl, G., McCoy, K.D., Macpherson, A.J., Reynaud, C.A., Cerf-Bensussan, N., Gaboriau-Routhiau, V., 2014. Segmented filamentous bacterium uses secondary and tertiary lymphoid tissues to induce gut IgA and specific T helper 17 cell responses. Immunity 40, 608–620.

Li, Y., Innocentin, S., Withers, D.R., Roberts, N.A., Gallagher, A.R., Grigorieva, E.F., Wilhelm, C., Veldhoen, M., 2011. Exogenous stimuli maintain intraepithelial lymphocytes via aryl hydrocarbon receptor activation. Cell 147, 629–640.

Li, Y., Tian, Y., Zhu, W., Gong, J., Gu, L., Zhang, W., Guo, Z., Li, N., Li, J., 2014. Cesarean delivery and risk of inflammatory bowel disease: a systematic review and meta-analysis. Scand. J. Gastroenterol. 49, 834–844.

Linden, S.K., Sutton, P., Karlsson, N.G., Korolik, V., McGuckin, M.A., 2008. Mucins in the mucosal barrier to infection. Mucosal Immunol. 1, 183–197.

Lionetti, E., Castellaneta, S., Francavilla, R., Pulvirenti, A., Tonutti, E., Amarri, S., Barbato, M., Barbera, C., Barera, G., Bellantoni, A., Castellano, E., Guariso, G., Limongelli, M.G., Pellegrino, S., Polloni, C., Ughi, C., Zuin, G., Fasano, A., Catassi, C., Weaning, S.W.G., Risk, C.D., 2014. Introduction of gluten, HLA status, and the risk of celiac disease in children. N. Engl. J. Med. 371, 1295–1303.

Lopez-Cepero, A.A., Palacios, C., 2015. Association of the intestinal microbiota and obesity. P R Health Sci. J. 34, 60–64.

Lotz, M., Gutle, D., Walther, S., Menard, S., Bogdan, C., Hornef, M.W., 2006. Postnatal acquisition of endotoxin tolerance in intestinal epithelial cells. J. Exp. Med. 203, 973–984.

Lupien, S.J., McEwen, B.S., Gunnar, M.R., Heim, C., 2009. Effects of stress throughout the lifespan on the brain, behaviour and cognition. Nat. Rev. Neurosci. 10, 434–445.

Marild, K., Ye, W., Lebwohl, B., Green, P.H., Blaser, M.J., Card, T., Ludvigsson, J.F., 2013. Antibiotic exposure and the development of coeliac disease: a nationwide case-control study. BMC Gastroenterol. 13, 109.

Matamoros, S., Gras-Leguen, C., Le Vacon, F., Potel, G., de La Cochetiere, M.F., 2013. Development of intestinal microbiota in infants and its impact on health. Trends Microbiol. 21, 167–173.

Mayer, E.A., Knight, R., Mazmanian, S.K., Cryan, J.F., 2014. Gut Microbe. Brain Paradigm Shift Neurosci. 34, 15490–15496.

Maynard, C.L., Elson, C.O., Hatton, R.D., Weaver, C.T., 2012. Reciprocal interactions of the intestinal microbiota and immune system. Nature 489, 231–241.

Mazmanian, S.K., Liu, C.H., Tzianabos, A.O., Kasper, D.L., 2005. An immunomodulatory molecule of symbiotic bacteria directs maturation of the host immune system. Cell 122, 107–118.

McDole, J.R., Wheeler, L.W., McDonald, K.G., Wang, B., Konjufca, V., Knoop, K.A., Newberry, R.D., Miller, M.J., 2012. Goblet cells deliver luminal antigen to CD103+ dendritic cells in the small intestine. Nature 483, 345–349.

Melli, L.C., do Carmo-Rodrigues, M.S., Araujo-Filho, H.B., Sole, D., de Morais, M.B., 2015. Intestinal microbiota and allergic diseases: a systematic review. Allergol. Immunopathol. (Madr.). http://dx.doi.org/10.1016/j.aller.2015.01.013.

Mesquita, D.N., Barbieri, M.A., Goldani, H.A., Cardoso, V.C., Goldani, M.Z., Kac, G., Silva, A.A., Bettiol, H., 2013. Cesarean section is associated with increased peripheral and central adiposity in young adulthood: cohort study. PLoS One 8, e66827.

Moles, L., Gomez, M., Heilig, H., Bustos, G., Fuentes, S., de Vos, W., Fernandez, L., Rodriguez, J.M., Jimenez, E., 2013. Bacterial diversity in meconium of preterm neonates and evolution of their fecal microbiota during the first month of life. PLoS One 8, e66986.

Moloney, R.D., Desbonnet, L., Clarke, G., Dinan, T.G., Cryan, J.F., 2014. The microbiome: stress, health and disease. Mamm. Genome 25, 49–74.

Mshvildadze, M., Neu, J., 2010. The infant intestinal microbiome: friend or foe? Early Hum. Dev. 86 (Suppl. 1), 67–71.

Mueller, N.T., Bakacs, E., Combellick, J., Grigoryan, Z., Dominguez-Bello, M.G., 2015a. The infant microbiome development: mom matters. Trends Mol. Med. 21, 109–117.

Mueller, N.T., Whyatt, R., Hoepner, L., Oberfield, S., Dominguez-Bello, M.G., Widen, E.M., Hassoun, A., Perera, F., Rundle, A., 2015b. Prenatal exposure to antibiotics, cesarean section and risk of childhood obesity. Int. J. Obes. (Lond.) 39, 665–670.

Mulle, J.G., Sharp, W.G., Cubells, J.F., 2013. The gut microbiome: a new frontier in autism research. Curr. Psychiatry Rep. 15, 337.

Natividad, J.M., Hayes, C.L., Motta, J.P., Jury, J., Galipeau, H.J., Philip, V., Garcia-Rodenas, C.L., Kiyama, H., Bercik, P., Verdu, E.F., 2013. Differential induction of antimicrobial REGIII by the intestinal microbiota and *Bifidobacterium breve* NCC2950. Appl. Environ. Microbiol. 79, 7745–7754.

Natividad, J.M., Pinto-Sanchez, M.I., Galipeau, H.J., Jury, J., Jordana, M., Reinisch, W., Collins, S.M., Bercik, P., Surette, M.G., Allen-Vercoe, E., Verdu, E.F., 2015. Ecobiotherapy rich in firmicutes decreases susceptibility to colitis in a humanized gnotobiotic mouse model. Inflamm. Bowel Dis. 21 (8), 1883–1893.

Natividad, J.M., Verdu, E.F., 2013. Modulation of intestinal barrier by intestinal microbiota: pathological and therapeutic implications. Pharmacol. Res. 69, 42–51.

Neufeld, K.M., Kang, N., Bienenstock, J., Foster, J.A., 2011. Reduced anxiety-like behavior and central neurochemical change in germ-free mice. Neurogastroenterology Motil. 23, 255–264, e119.

Niess, J.H., Adler, G., 2010. Enteric flora expands gut lamina propria CX3CR1[+] dendritic cells supporting inflammatory immune responses under normal and inflammatory conditions. J. Immunol. 184, 2026–2037.

O'Mahony, S.M., Clarke, G., Borre, Y.E., Dinan, T.G., Cryan, J.F., 2015. Serotonin, tryptophan metabolism and the brain-gut-microbiome axis. Behav. Brain Res. 277, 32–48.

O'Mahony, S.M., Felice, V.D., Nally, K., Savignac, H.M., Claesson, M.J., Scully, P., Woznicki, J., Hyland, N.P., Shanahan, F., Quigley, E.M., Marchesi, J.R., O'Toole, P.W., Dinan, T.G., Cryan, J.F., 2014. Disturbance of the gut microbiota in early-life selectively affects visceral pain in adulthood without impacting cognitive or anxiety-related behaviors in male rats. Neuroscience 277, 885–901.

O'Mahony, S.M., Hyland, N.P., Dinan, T.G., Cryan, J.F., 2011. Maternal separation as a model of brain-gut axis dysfunction. Psychopharmacology 214, 71–88.

O'Mahony, S.M., Marchesi, J.R., Scully, P., Codling, C., Ceolho, A.M., Quigley, E.M., Cryan, J.F., Dinan, T.G., 2009. Early life stress alters behavior, immunity, and microbiota in rats: implications for irritable bowel syndrome and psychiatric illnesses. Biol. Psychiatry 65, 263–267.

O'Neil, A., Itsiopoulos, C., Skouteris, H., Opie, R.S., McPhie, S., Hill, B., Jacka, F.N., 2014. Preventing mental health problems in offspring by targeting dietary intake of pregnant women. BMC Med. 12, 208.

Olszak, T., An, D., Zeissig, S., Vera, M.P., Richter, J., Franke, A., Glickman, J.N., Siebert, R., Baron, R.M., Kasper, D.L., Blumberg, R.S., 2012. Microbial exposure during early life has persistent effects on natural killer T cell function. Science 336, 489–493.

Parfrey, L.W., Knight, R., 2012. Spatial and temporal variability of the human microbiota. Clin. Microbiol. Infect. 18 (Suppl. 4), 8–11.

Park, A.J., Collins, J., Blennerhassett, P.A., Ghia, J.E., Verdu, E.F., Bercik, P., Collins, S.M., 2013. Altered colonic function and microbiota profile in a mouse model of chronic depression. Neurogastroenterology Motil. 25, 733-e575.

Penders, J., Thijs, C., Vink, C., Stelma, F.F., Snijders, B., Kummeling, I., van den Brandt, P.A., Stobberingh, E.E., 2006. Factors influencing the composition of the intestinal microbiota in early infancy. Pediatrics 118, 511–521.

Perkkio, M., Savilahti, E., 1980. Time of appearance of immunoglobulin-containing cells in the mucosa of the neonatal intestine. Pediatr. Res. 14, 953–955.

Petersson, J., Schreiber, O., Hansson, G.C., Gendler, S.J., Velcich, A., Lundberg, J.O., Roos, S., Holm, L., Phillipson, M., 2011. Importance and regulation of the colonic mucus barrier in a mouse model of colitis. Am. J. Physiol. Gastrointest. Liver Physiol. 300, G327–G333.

Pitter, G., Ludvigsson, J.F., Romor, P., Zanier, L., Zanotti, R., Simonato, L., Canova, C., 2015. Antibiotic exposure in the first year of life and later treated asthma, a population based birth cohort study of 143,000 children. Eur. J. Epidemiol. 31, 85–94.

Raabe, F.J., Spengler, D., 2013. Epigenetic risk factors in PTSD and depression. Front. Psychiatry 4, 80.

Relman, D.A., 2012. The human microbiome: ecosystem resilience and health. Nutr. Rev. 70 (Suppl. 1), S2–S9.

Rodriguez, J.M., Murphy, K., Stanton, C., Ross, R.P., Kober, O.I., Juge, N., Avershina, E., Rudi, K., Narbad, A., Jenmalm, M.C., Marchesi, J.R., Collado, M.C., 2015. The composition of the gut microbiota throughout life, with an emphasis on early life. Microb. Ecol. Health Dis. 26, 26050.

Romero, R., Hassan, S.S., Gajer, P., Tarca, A.L., Fadrosh, D.W., Bieda, J., Chaemsaithong, P., Miranda, J., Chaiworapongsa, T., Ravel, J., 2014. The vaginal microbiota of pregnant women who subsequently have spontaneous preterm labor and delivery and those with a normal delivery at term. Microbiome 2, 18.

Round, J.L., Lee, S.M., Li, J., Tran, G., Jabri, B., Chatila, T.A., Mazmanian, S.K., 2011. The toll-like receptor 2 pathway establishes colonization by a commensal of the human microbiota. Science 332, 974–977.

Round, J.L., Mazmanian, S.K., 2010. Inducible Foxp3+ regulatory T-cell development by a commensal bacterium of the intestinal microbiota. Proc. Natl. Acad. Sci. U.S.A. 107, 12204–12209.

Saari, A., Virta, L.J., Sankilampi, U., Dunkel, L., Saxen, H., 2015. Antibiotic exposure in infancy and risk of being overweight in the first 24 months of life. Pediatrics 135, 617–626.

Salazar, N., Arboleya, S., Valdes, L., Stanton, C., Ross, P., Ruiz, L., Gueimonde, M., de Los Reyes-Gavilan, C.G., 2014. The human intestinal microbiome at extreme ages of life. Dietary intervention as a way to counteract alterations. Front. Genet. 5, 406.

Satokari, R., Gronroos, T., Laitinen, K., Salminen, S., Isolauri, E., 2009. *Bifidobacterium* and *Lactobacillus* DNA in the human placenta. Lett. Appl. Microbiol. 48, 8–12.

Schele, E., Grahnemo, L., Anesten, F., Hallen, A., Backhed, F., Jansson, J.O., 2015. Regulation of body fat mass by the gut microbiota: possible mediation by the brain. Peptides 00094–00097.

Schellekens, H., Finger, B.C., Dinan, T.G., Cryan, J.F., 2012. Ghrelin signalling and obesity: at the interface of stress, mood and food reward. Pharmacol. Ther. 135, 316–326.

Sellitto, M., Bai, G., Serena, G., Fricke, W.F., Sturgeon, C., Gajer, P., White, J.R., Koenig, S.S., Sakamoto, J., Boothe, D., Gicquelais, R., Kryszak, D., Puppa, E., Catassi, C., Ravel, J., Fasano, A., 2012. Proof of concept of microbiome-metabolome analysis and delayed gluten exposure on celiac disease autoimmunity in genetically at-risk infants. PLoS One 7, e33387.

Sevelsted, A., Stokholm, J., Bonnelykke, K., Bisgaard, H., 2015. Cesarean section and chronic immune disorders. Pediatrics 135, e92–e98.

Shan, L., Molberg, O., Parrot, I., Hausch, F., Filiz, F., Gray, G.M., Sollid, L.M., Khosla, C., 2002. Structural basis for gluten intolerance in celiac sprue. Science 297, 2275–2279.

Shaw, S.Y., Blanchard, J.F., Bernstein, C.N., 2010. Association between the use of antibiotics in the first year of life and pediatric inflammatory bowel disease. Am. J. Gastroenterol. 105, 2687–2692.

Shroff, K.E., Cebra, J.J., 1995. Development of mucosal humoral immune responses in germ-free (GF) mice. Adv. Exp. Med. Biol. 371A, 441–446.

Shroff, K.E., Meslin, K., Cebra, J.J., 1995. Commensal enteric bacteria engender a self-limiting humoral mucosal immune response while permanently colonizing the gut. Infect. Immun. 63, 3904–3913.

Simister, N.E., Rees, A.R., 1985. Isolation and characterization of an Fc receptor from neonatal rat small intestine. Eur. J. Immunol. 15, 733–738.

Sirimi, N., Goulis, D.G., 2010. Obesity in pregnancy. Hormones (Athens) 9, 299–306.

Smith, K., McCoy, K.D., Macpherson, A.J., 2007. Use of axenic animals in studying the adaptation of mammals to their commensal intestinal microbiota. Semin. Immunol. 19, 59–69.

Stilling, R.M., Dinan, T.G., Cryan, J.F., 2016. The brain's geppetto-microbes as puppeteers of neural function and behaviour? J. Neurovirol. 22, 14–21.

Stilling, R.M., Ryan, F.J., Hoban, A.E., Shanahan, F., Clarke, G., Claesson, M.J., Dinan, T.G., Cryan, J.F., 2015. Microbes & neurodevelopment–absence of microbiota during early life increases activity-related transcriptional pathways in the amygdala. Brain Behav. Immun. 50, 209–220.

Sudo, N., Chida, Y., Aiba, Y., Sonoda, J., Oyama, N., Yu, X.N., Kubo, C., Koga, Y., 2004. Postnatal microbial colonization programs the hypothalamic-pituitary-adrenal system for stress response in mice. J. Physiol. 558, 263–275.

Tannock, G.W., Savage, D.C., 1974. Influences of dietary and environmental stress on microbial populations in the murine gastrointestinal tract. Infect. Immun. 9, 591–598.

de Theije, C.G., Wu, J., da Silva, S.L., Kamphuis, P.J., Garssen, J., Korte, S.M., Kraneveld, A.D., 2011. Pathways underlying the gut-to-brain connection in autism spectrum disorders as future targets for disease management. Eur. J. Pharmacol. 668 (Suppl. 1), S70–S80.

Ungaro, R., Bernstein, C.N., Gearry, R., Hviid, A., Kolho, K.L., Kronman, M.P., Shaw, S., Van Kruiningen, H., Colombel, J.F., Atreja, A., 2014. Antibiotics associated with increased risk of new-onset Crohn's disease but not ulcerative colitis: a meta-analysis. Am. J. Gastroenterol. 109, 1728–1738.

Vaishampayan, P.A., Kuehl, J.V., Froula, J.L., Morgan, J.L., Ochman, H., Francino, M.P., 2010. Comparative metagenomics and population dynamics of the gut microbiota in mother and infant. Genome Biol. Evol. 2, 53–66.

Vaishnava, S., Behrendt, C.L., Ismail, A.S., Eckmann, L., Hooper, L.V., 2008. Paneth cells directly sense gut commensals and maintain homeostasis at the intestinal host-microbial interface. Proc. Natl. Acad. Sci. U.S.A. 105, 20858–20863.

Vaishnava, S., Yamamoto, M., Severson, K.M., Ruhn, K.A., Yu, X., Koren, O., Ley, R., Wakeland, E.K., Hooper, L.V., 2011. The antibacterial lectin RegIIIgamma promotes the spatial segregation of microbiota and host in the intestine. Science 334, 255–258.

Vangay, P., Ward, T., Gerber, J.S., Knights, D., 2015. Antibiotics, pediatric dysbiosis, and disease. Cell Host Microbe 17, 553–564.

Verdu, E.F., 2012. Differences in intestinal microbial composition in children with IBS-what does it all mean? Am. J. Gastroenterol. 107, 1752–1754.

Verdu, E.F., Galipeau, H.J., Jabri, B., 2015. Novel players in coeliac disease pathogenesis: role of the gut microbiota. Nat. Rev. Gastroenterol. Hepatol. 12 (9), 497–506.

Virta, L., Auvinen, A., Helenius, H., Huovinen, P., Kolho, K.L., 2012. Association of repeated exposure to antibiotics with the development of pediatric Crohn's disease–a nationwide, register-based finnish case-control study. Am. J. Epidemiol. 175, 775–784.

Vriezinga, S.L., Auricchio, R., Bravi, E., Castillejo, G., Chmielewska, A., Crespo Escobar, P., Kolacek, S., Koletzko, S., Korponay-Szabo, I.R., Mummert, E., Polanco, I., Putter, H., Ribes-Koninckx, C., Shamir, R., Szajewska, H., Werkstetter, K., Greco, L., Gyimesi, J., Hartman, C., Hogen Esch, C., Hopman, E., Ivarsson, A., Koltai, T., Koning, F., Martinez-Ojinaga, E., te Marvelde, C., Pavic, A., Romanos, J., Stoopman, E., Villanacci, V., Wijmenga, C., Troncone, R., Mearin, M.L., 2014. Randomized feeding intervention in infants at high risk for celiac disease. N. Engl. J. Med. 371, 1304–1315.

Wei, B., Wingender, G., Fujiwara, D., Chen, D.Y., McPherson, M., Brewer, S., Borneman, J., Kronenberg, M., Braun, J., 2010. Commensal microbiota and CD8[+] T cells shape the formation of invariant NKT cells. J. Immunol. 184, 1218–1226.

Williams, A.M., Probert, C.S., Stepankova, R., Tlaskalova-Hogenova, H., Phillips, A., Bland, P.W., 2006. Effects of microflora on the neonatal development of gut mucosal T cells and myeloid cells in the mouse. Immunology 119, 470–478.

Williams, S.C., 2014. Gnotobiotics. Proc. Natl. Acad. Sci. U.S.A. 111, 1661.

Wingender, G., Stepniak, D., Krebs, P., Lin, L., McBride, S., Wei, B., Braun, J., Mazmanian, S.K., Kronenberg, M., 2012. Intestinal microbes affect phenotypes and functions of invariant natural killer T cells in mice. Gastroenterology 143, 418–428.

Wrzosek, L., Miquel, S., Noordine, M.L., Bouet, S., Joncquel Chevalier-Curt, M., Robert, V., Philippe, C., Bridonneau, C., Cherbuy, C., Robbe-Masselot, C., Langella, P., Thomas, M., 2013. *Bacteroides thetaiotaomicron* and *Faecalibacterium prausnitzii* influence the production of mucus glycans and the development of goblet cells in the colonic epithelium of a gnotobiotic model rodent. BMC Biol. 11, 61.

Zhou, L., Foster, J.A., 2015. Psychobiotics and the gut-brain axis: in the pursuit of happiness. Neuropsychiatric Dis. Treat. 11, 715–723.

Zijlmans, M.A., Korpela, K., Riksen-Walraven, J.M., de Vos, W.M., de Weerth, C., 2015. Maternal prenatal stress is associated with the infant intestinal microbiota. Psychoneuroendocrinology 53, 233–245.

Zivkovic, A.M., German, J.B., Lebrilla, C.B., Mills, D.A., 2011. Human milk glycobiome and its impact on the infant gastrointestinal microbiota. Proc. Natl. Acad. Sci. U.S.A. 108 (Suppl. 1), 4653–4658.

The Microbiome in Aging: Impact on Health and Wellbeing

10

M.C. Neto

University College Cork, School of Microbiology, Cork, Ireland

P.W. O'Toole

University College Cork, School of Microbiology, Cork, Ireland; University College Cork, APC Microbiome Institute, Cork, Ireland

INTRODUCTION

The population of the world is rapidly aging. Improvements in sanitation, medical care, and nutrition have contributed to a significant increase in the average lifespan of most citizens in developed countries. This demographic trend will continue throughout the 21st century as it spreads to the developing countries (Maijó et al., 2014), creating pressures on health-care systems and social structures. The World Health Organization estimated that the number of individuals aged 60 years or older will nearly triple, increasing from approximately 650 million in 2005 to almost 2 billion by 2050 (United Nations, 2005). By 2045–50, life expectancy is expected to reach 83 years in developed countries and 75 years in the less developed regions of the world (United Nations, 2013).

A comprehensive understanding of the physiology of aging is required to inform effective public health strategies aimed at improving the health and quality of life of older adults, ensuring that they stay active and independent for longer and potentially increasing their longevity while delaying their need for long-term care. Elucidating the cellular mechanisms of the natural aging process and the forces that operate on it will also identify what lifestyle changes, dietary choices, and medical interventions can have the greatest impact for healthier aging (Cusack and O'Toole, 2013).

The human gut microbiome has emerged in the last decade as a major contributor to metabolic and immunological functions in the human body. Alterations in the adult gut microbiota have been linked to inflammatory and metabolic disorders including inflammatory bowel disease (IBD; Shanahan, 2012), irritable bowel syndrome (IBS; Kassinen et al., 2007), type 2 diabetes (T2D; Qin et al., 2012), obesity (Le Chatelier et al., 2013), and colorectal cancer (Louis et al., 2014). As the results from studies focused on particular aspects of the human microbiome accumulate, a clearer picture of what drives these shifts will hopefully emerge. This should permit the

The Gut-Brain Axis. http://dx.doi.org/10.1016/B978-0-12-802304-4.00010-4

development of recommendations for the maintenance of a health-promoting microbial ecosystem and inform potential manipulations of these microbial communities
to reverse disease and promote recovery to full health. Therefore understanding the
role that the human microbiota plays in aging and how it can be harnessed to delay
aging-related health loss is essential and has emerged as a new area of study that we
review here.

GENERAL FEATURES OF THE MICROBIOTA
MICROBIOTA THROUGHOUT LIFE

Humans live in association with immense populations of bacteria, archaea, viruses,
and bacteriophages—collectively called the human microbiome—and fungi
(Hoffmann et al., 2013) that have coevolved with the human host to perform several
functions that affect physiology and metabolism (DiBaise et al., 2012).

In the womb, babies live in essentially sterile conditions (Aagaard et al., 2014).
During and after birth infants became inoculated with maternal and environmental
microbes. Facultative anaerobes such as enterococci and enterobacteria are typically
the first colonizers, followed by strict anaerobes such as *Bifidobacterium*, *Bacteroides* spp., and *Clostridium* once the initial oxygen is depleted (Adlerberth and Wold,
2009; Walsh et al., 2014). However, this succession process can vary greatly depending on the delivery mode and feeding regime, with vaginally delivered babies acquiring a gut microbiota resembling the maternal vaginal microbial community whereas
C-section-born babies are colonized mostly by the bacteria on the maternal skin and
in the environment (Dominguez-Bello et al., 2010; Ursell et al., 2013). Whether
babies are breast fed or not also affects the bacteria that will proliferate and establish themselves in the infant gut. Bifidobacteria predominate in the gut of breast-fed
babies whereas bottle-fed babies tend to present a more diverse microbial population
(Duncan and Flint, 2013). This initial bacterial colonization and establishment of a
healthy intestinal microbiota is essential for the neonatal immune system to develop
and mature (Walker and Iyengar, 2014), and its absence is hypothesized to contribute
to later development of asthma, allergies, type I diabetes, and other autoimmune
disorders (Kelly et al., 2007; Voreades et al., 2014). Animals bred under germ-free
conditions have immature immune systems and greater susceptibility to infection,
increased nutritional requirements, and structural and functional deficiencies compared with their conventionally raised counterparts (Smith et al., 2007).

As a result of the introduction of solid foods, the microbiota of the infant diversi-
fies, reflected in increased abundance of *Firmicutes*, and by 2–3 years of age resembles that of an adult (De Filippo et al., 2010; Bergström et al., 2014). The intestinal
microbiota of a healthy adult is relatively stable over time (Claesson et al., 2011),
with high interindividual variability but sharing a common set of metabolic capabilities (Tap et al., 2009). The microbiome, the term given to the combined genomes of
these microorganisms, has been estimated to contain 150 times more genes than the

human genome (Qin et al., 2010). In this mutualistic ecosystem, the human gut offers the microbiota a constant supply of nutrients whereas the microbes provide their host with energy through the fermentation of indigestible dietary components, fundamental vitamins via microbial biosynthesis, and protection from pathogen colonization as a result of competition for resources (Lozupone et al., 2012; Flint et al., 2012).

Throughout the length of the gut, different regions harbor distinct microbial communities that are adapted to local conditions such as tissue structure, host secretions, pH, and oxygen concentration. The small intestine, with its short transit time, excretion of digestive enzymes, and high bile salt concentrations provides a relatively challenging environment for colonizing microbes whereas the large intestine with longer transit times, more neutral pH, and lower oxygen concentrations allows thriving of a larger microbial community dominated by obligate anaerobic bacteria (Zoetendal et al., 2012). The small intestine microbiota consists mainly of facultative anaerobes such as gram-positive streptococci, lactobacilli, and enterococci and gram-negative *Proteobacteria* and *Bacteroides* whereas the microbiota of the large intestine of a healthy adult is composed primarily of the bacterial phyla *Bacteroidetes* and *Firmicutes*, with smaller proportions of *Proteobacteria*, *Actinobacteria*, *Fusobacteria*, and *Verrucomicrobia* (Eckburg et al., 2005; Zhang et al., 2014). Despite the recognition of this regional compositional difference, most studies focus on the distal part of the large intestine and characterize the easily accessible fecal-derived populations as proxy.

The microbial communities of the large intestine of a healthy adult possess a wide range of metabolic capabilities and live in a situation of constant microbial interaction and interspecies cross-feeding by which the various groups of bacteria cooperate to degrade the available nondigestible dietary substrates and endogenous secretions to extract from them the maximum energetic yield possible. The carbohydrates that escape digestion by the host enzymes (mainly dietary fibers including resistant starch, nonstarch polysaccharides, and nondigestible oligosaccharides) enter the proximal colon and are fermented by obligate anaerobic bacteria to form short-chain fatty acids (SCFAs) such as acetate, propionate, and butyrate; other metabolites such as pyruvate, lactate, and ethanol; and gases such as hydrogen, carbon dioxide, methane, and hydrogen sulfide (Flint et al., 2012). SCFAs inhibit pathogens by lowering the intestinal pH; increasing the absorption of ions such as calcium, magnesium, and iron; modulating intestinal motility; and suppressing inflammation (Tiihonen et al., 2010). Saccharolytic bacteria in human feces belong predominantly to the genera *Bifidobacterium*, *Ruminococcus*, *Eubacterium*, *Lactobacillus*, and *Clostridium* (Scheid et al., 2013). Acetate and propionate are absorbed into the bloodstream and travel to the liver, where hepatocytes assimilate acetate through lipogenesis and propionate through gluconeogenesis (Conterno et al., 2011; Hosseini et al., 2011). Butyrate is a major energy substrate for the colonic epithelium, which helps regulate cell growth and differentiation (Chung et al., 1985; Pryde et al., 2002). *Coprococcus* sp., *Roseburia* sp., *Roseburia intestinalis*, and *Faecalibacterium prausnitzii* are some of the species of butyrate-producing bacteria isolated from human fecal samples (Duncan et al., 2002). In addition to carbohydrates, residual protein, peptides, and amino acids also reach the colon (Moco and Ross, 2015). Most microbial protein degradation occurs in the distal colon where the pH is favorable for the growth of proteolytic bacteria (Walker et al., 2005; Walsch et al., 2014). Proteolytic bacteria in human feces consist primarily of *Bacteroides* and *Propionibacterium*, with lower numbers of the genera *Streptococcus*, *Clostridium*, *Bacillus*, and *Staphylococcus* (MacFarlane et al., 1986). High-level protein fermentation can lead to increased levels of branched fatty acids, ammonia, phenols, and sulfides, which are absorbed into the host as well as excreted, and are regarded as harmful for health, leading to disease states such as colon cancer and ulcerative colitis (Windey et al., 2012). Therefore a diet rich in nondigestible carbohydrates is recommended to counteract this tendency and shift the gut fermentation toward saccharolytic activity (Sanchez et al., 2009). The gut microbiota also contributes to the micronutrients available to the human host by producing essential B vitamins such as folate, riboflavin, vitamin B12, and vitamin K (O'Connor et al., 2014). In addition, certain bacterial species play a role in peptide and amino acid metabolism, and there are several different bacterial species that can metabolize aromatic amino acids (eg, tryptophan; Duncan and Flint, 2013). Furthermore, some species such as *Bacteroides thetaiotaomicron* and *Akkermansia muciniphila* specialize in feeding on the mucin layer secreted by the goblet cells in the intestine (Alcock et al., 2014).

MICROBIOME RICHNESS

Metagenomic population analysis has shown that although there is considerable interindividual variability in the presence and absence of the bacterial species found in the gastrointestinal tract across space and time (Gill et al., 2006; Costello et al., 2009), certain bacterial populations are shared among groups of humans (Arumugam et al., 2011) that may be required for the appropriate functioning of the gut (Tremaroli and Bäckhed, 2012). Because of its dynamic nature, influenced by genetics, diet, metabolism, age, geography, antibiotic treatment, and even stress, the microbiota profile of an individual might be a good reflection of his/her environmental history and could contribute to individual differences in risk of illness, disease course, and response to treatment (Foster and Neufeld, 2013).

Tap et al. (2009) investigated the presence of a set of bacterial species common to the fecal microbiota of healthy individuals. The identification of 66 operational taxonomic units (OTUs) present in more than 50% of individuals in a study cohort of 17 healthy adults living in France or the Netherlands included members of the genera *Faecalibacterium*, *Ruminococcus*, *Eubacterium*, *Dorea*, *Bacteroides*, *Alistipes*, and *Bifidobacterium*. Comparing this bacterial "phylogenetic core" against core OTUs present in fecal samples of healthy individuals from four other studies in other countries (Eckburg et al., 2005; Gill et al., 2006; Manichanh et al., 2006; Li et al., 2008), they identified 24 common core OTUs, all belonging to the phylum *Firmicutes*. Their results led them to hypothesize that although the microbiota composition is host specific, the healthy human microbiota phylogenetic core may be realistically represented by approximately 50 bacterial species that support a conserved set of metabolic functions. Addressing a similar question, Qin et al. (2010) looked at the commonalities and differences between the microbiota of different individuals by analyzing fecal samples of 124 healthy, overweight, and obese adults, as well as IBD patients, from Denmark and Spain. They reported that the entire cohort harbored between 1000 and 1150 prevalent bacterial species and that each individual had at least 160 such species, of which 18 were shared between all individuals and 75 were common to more than 50% of individuals.

Arumugam et al. (2011) set out to specifically investigate the gut microbiome diversity across different populations (Danish, French, Italian, Spanish, Japanese, and American). The authors grouped individuals into discrete clusters called *entero-types*, based on the abundances of key bacterial genera in their gut microbiota, which seemed to be independent of nationality, age, sex, or body mass index (Wu et al., 2011). They identified three such enterotypes enriched in the genera *Bacteroides*, *Prevotella*, or *Ruminococcus* that they hypothesized to focus on different routes for the extraction of energy from the fermentable substrates available in the colon (Arumugam et al., 2011; Koren et al., 2013). Although most studies agree with the *Bacteroides* and *Prevotella* groupings, which have been associated with protein/animal fat–rich and plant-based fiber-rich diets, respectively, there is less support for the third group (Wu et al., 2011; Luzopone et al., 2012; Bergström et al., 2014; Voreades et al., 2014). Wu et al. (2011) studied whether a short-term change in diet could affect change in microbiota composition by giving either a high-fat/low-fiber or a low-fat/high-fiber diet to 10 individuals over a 10-day period. Although microbiome composition changes were detected within 24h of the start of the intervention, enterotype stability remained constant throughout, leading the authors to conclude that enterotypes are associated with long-term diet.

HOW HABITUAL DIET MODULATES MICROBIOTA DIVERSITY

Diet appears to be one of the main modulators of gut microbiota composition. In recent years metagenomic studies comparing the gut microbiome of nonindustrialized rural communities from Africa and South America with those of industrialized Western communities from Europe and North America have revealed specific gut microbiome adaptations to their respective diets and lifestyles (De Filippo et al., 2010; Yatsunenko et al., 2012; Ou et al., 2013; Schnorr et al., 2014). Individual members of the microbiota, and particular associations of those, have been shown to be highly dependent on certain dietary components (Alcock et al., 2014). *Bacteroides plebeius*, found in Japanese but not in American individuals, is an example of such a specialist microbe. It acquired genes for porphyranases, agarases, and associated proteins by horizontal gene transfer that allow it to degrade seaweed polysaccharides, an important element of the diet of its host (Hehemann et al., 2010). The adults of a Tanzanian hunter-gatherer tribe, the Hadza, have been recently shown to be completely deficient in *Bifidobacterium*, which typically composes 1%–10% of the gut microbial population of a Western adult. It was hypothesized that this might result from an absence of dairy products and contact with livestock in their lifestyle, which needs to be confirmed by identifying bifidobacteria in their breast-fed infants (Schnorr et al., 2014). David et al. (2014) examined whether consumption of a plant-based diet, high in fiber but low in fat and protein, or an animal-based diet, high in fat and protein but low in fiber, for 5 days could alter the gut microbiota of 10 American volunteers in a rapid diet-specific manner. On the phylogenetic level the animal-based diet resulted in an increased abundance of bile-tolerant microorganisms (*Alistipes*, *Bilophila*, and *Bacteroides*) and decreased levels of bacteria that metabolize dietary plant polysaccharides from the phylum *Firmicutes* (*Roseburia*, *Eubacterium rectale*, and *Ruminococcus bromii*). Furthermore, metabolite analysis revealed that the animal-based diet resulted in significantly lower levels of products of carbohydrate fermentation, higher concentrations of products of amino acid biosynthesis and fermentation, an increased expression of β-lactamase genes, and an increased microbial metabolism of bile acids. The authors concluded from these results that the gut microbiota is able to adjust quickly to alterations in diet.

Wu et al. (2014) compared the gut microbiota metabolite production between 15 vegans and 16 omnivores living in an urban Western environment to investigate the effects of diet on the gut microbiota and the host metabolome. Although having elevated levels of vitamins and other plant-based products in their plasma, reflecting the higher intake of plant carbohydrates, the vegan subject metabolome presented no increase in SCFA or methane production in comparison to the omnivore metabolome. Also, there were no significant differences in the composition of the gut microbiota between the groups. The authors proposed that residence in Westernized societies might lead to loss of certain "keystone species" able to extract higher amounts of SCFAs from a plant-based diet, as was found in inhabitants of a rural village in Burkina Faso (De Filippo et al., 2010). This is supported by the finding that although vegans in the study were phytoestrogen consumers, only 40% of them had detectable amounts of equol in their plasma.

To study the temporal relationships among food intake, gut microbiota profile, and metabolic and inflammatory phenotype, Cotillard et al. (2013) conducted a dietary intervention in which 38 obese and 11 overweight French individuals were given a 6-week energy-restricted high-protein diet followed by a 6-week weight-maintenance diet. According to their quantitative metagenomic approach, they found a bimodal distribution of bacterial gene numbers and identified 18 low-gene count (LGC) individuals and 27 high-gene count (HGC) individuals. Increased gene richness was associated with a significant decrease in adiposity measures, circulating cholesterol, and inflammation. Because only the LGC group responded to the diet change with an increase in gene richness, the authors proposed that gene richness might help predict the efficacy of dietary interventions in overweight and obese individuals.

In a similar study, Le Chatelier et al. (2013) compared the microbial gene richness in fecal samples of 123 nonobese and 169 obese Danish individuals. Twenty-three percent (23%) of the individuals in this population had low bacterial richness. At the phylum level, LGC individuals had higher populations of *Proteobacteria* and *Bacteroidetes* whereas HGC individuals had increased abundance of *Verrumicrobia*,

Actinobacteria, and *Euryarchaeota*. At the species level, *Bacteroides* and *Ruminococcus gnavus* was more prevalent in LGC individuals whereas *F. prausnitzii* was more frequent in HGC individuals. At the functional level, LGC individuals had increased potential to manage oxidative stress and degrade mucus, decreased potential to reduce hydrogen and produce methane, and a lower abundance of butyrate-producing bacteria. The authors propose that an imbalance in bacterial species with potential pro- and anti-inflammatory properties may trigger the low-grade inflammation and insulin resistance associated with obesity. Qin et al. (2012) used shotgun sequencing to analyze the gut microbiota of 345 Chinese T2D patients and nondiabetic individuals. Patients with T2D presented a reduction in the abundance of butyrate-producing bacteria, including *E. rectale*, *F. prausnitzii*, and *R. intestinalis*; an increase in the abundance of opportunistic pathogens, such as *Bacteroides caccae*, *Clostridium ramosum*, and *Escherichia coli*; and an increased potential for sulfate reduction and for oxidative stress resistance. The authors suggested that T2D pathophysiology might be associated with a "functional dysbiosis" rather than with the presence or lack of a specific microbial species.

Microbial symbiosis is a ubiquitous aspect of life, and these interactions certainly played a central role in the evolutionary success of higher organisms. Having a diverse microbial component contributing to an increased energy extraction potential from the available resources has facilitated species survival by ensuring that they can evolve, adapt, and respond to environmental stressors as and when they occur. Together with antibiotic therapy, diet is a main modulator of microbiota composition, and, while a diverse diet can contribute to microbiota richness, the continued consumption of a nutritionally narrow diet, poor in fiber and rich in fat, such as the Western diet, can lead to shifts in the human gut microbiota and reduction of its functional capabilities. Over time this reduction in diversity, reflected in lower gene count and lower SCFA production, can impair the functional redundancy of the microbial communities in the human gut, affect its cross-feeding networks, produce metabolic stress, elicit inflammation, and contribute to disease (Thorburn et al., 2014). It can be argued that, if sustained, the associated loss in key species or functional groups that have evolved with the human population over millennia might be irreversible and may have unpredictable consequences for generations to come. On the other hand, as characterization of different populations are completed, it becomes clear that there is no single, stable microbiota state that is conducive to health and that many alternative states are possible and probably ideally suited to different individual determinants and circumstances likely to change throughout life (Lahti et al., 2014).

MICROBIOTA IN THE ELDERLY
CHANGES DURING AGING

Aging is a complex multifactorial process characterized by the progressive functional decline of the principal physiological systems accompanied by the development of age (Weinert and Timiras, 2003; Rampelli et al., 2013b; Calçada et al., 2014). These physiological changes, together with modifications in lifestyle, nutritional behavior, and host immune system function, lead to inevitable alterations at the level of the human gut microbiota (Biagi et al., 2010). Here we overview some of the physiological changes that occur during aging, including changes of immune system function and studies published to date that focused on the microbiota of elderly individuals. Reviews of the different aspects of aging from changes in diet and lifestyle; to markers of organ and cognitive health; to the microbiota in the elderly; immunosenescence, inflamm-aging, and epigenetic markers of aging can be found in volumes 136–137 of the publication *Mechanisms of Ageing and Development* released in March–April 2014 in the context of the launching of the European intervention project NU-AGE.

Many age-related factors such as changes in socioeconomic status, mobility, and physical and mental health may affect the dietary patterns of the elderly (Meydani, 2001). The increase in thresholds for taste and smell and the diminished masticatory function, as a consequence of teeth and muscle mass loss that occur during aging (Newton et al., 1993; Boyce and Shone, 2006), can result in food tasting flat and uninteresting and lead to a selection of a narrower and less nutritionally balanced diet. As a general rule in the westernized countries studied, the more dependent, frail, and removed from the community an aged individual is, the more likely it is that they will be consuming a highly caloric fat-rich diet with reduced variety and fiber consumption (Claesson et al., 2012). Even with a balanced diet, the decrease in the production of gastric acid that frequently arises in the elderly is associated with a decreased absorption of various micronutrients such as iron, folate, calcium, and vitamins K and B12 (Saltzman and Russell, 1998). At the same time, this increase in colonic pH might allow an increase in the abundance of less beneficial groups in the microbiota as a slightly acidic pH favors the growth of beneficial commensal bacteria (Duncan and Flint, 2013). Other major problems in old age are changes in anorectal physiology and fecal impaction, resulting in constipation and longer transit times (Firth and Prather, 2002). A diminished sensation of thirst also adds to an impaired water balance in the body and slower bowel movements (Kenney and Chiu, 2001). In addition to causing discomfort, this also leads to longer retention of bacterial matter and an increase in bacterial protein fermentation and undesirable putrefactive processes in the gut (Macfarlane et al., 1989; Woodmansey, 2007).

IMMUNOSENESCENCE AND INFLAMM-AGING

Early in life, both the innate immune system, that patrols the mucosal barrier, and the adaptive immune system, that downregulates the immune response in the presence of harmless stimuli or upregulates it in response to invasion of the epithelium, develop through exposure to antigens of the commensal bacteria in the gut (Sommer and Bäckhed, 2013). Under normal circumstances in a healthy adult, the bacterial load in direct contact with the intestinal epithelia is kept low by a fine-tuned mechanism of immune tolerance and immune response (Magrone and Jirillo, 2013).

Immunosenescence (ie, the decreased effectiveness of the immune response brought on by the advancement of age) is one of the main causes for increased disease susceptibility in the elderly. Only a detailed understanding of how different immune cells become senescent will permit the design of efficient interventional strategies to prevent age-related immune degradation and potentially induce immune rejuvenation (Boraschi and Italiani, 2014). Our current understanding of immunosenescence points toward a reduction in immune function because of a cumulative dysfunction throughout the various steps involved in immune tolerance and response rather than one particular step in the process being cut. At the base of it lies a decline in naïve T cell production in the thymus and reduced B cell production in the bone marrow (Miller and Kelsoe, 1995), combined with a decreased diversity in the naïve lymphocytes that are produced (Naylor et al., 2005). In addition, the naïve T and B cells produced are less responsive to the antigens presented to them, and even when they do get activated and proliferate they do so to a lesser extent (Li et al., 2012). Furthermore, the dendritic cells and other antigen-presenting cell precursors become less effective with age at picking up and presenting antigens to these naïve cells (Panda et al., 2010). While in a healthy adult a dynamic balance is kept between the pool of naïve lymphocytes and the pool of effector and memory cells, in the elderly the memory cells accumulated over a lifetime take up the space needed for the storage of new naïve T and B cells (reviewed by Brunner et al., 2011). Even the antibodies produced by older B cells are commonly of low affinity, providing less efficient protection (Eaton et al., 2004). Collectively, immunosenescence leads to impaired responses to immune challenges, especially when encountering new antigens. Extrinsic factors such as oxidative stress and long-term exposure to antigen due to persistent viral infections can also contribute to immune dysfunction (High et al., 2012).

Inflamm-aging—a state of chronic low-grade systemic inflammation—induced and maintained by elevation of circulating acute-phase proteins and proinflammatory cytokines, is another hallmark of aging (Franceschi, 2007; Bacalani et al., 2014). This immunologically fragile state leaves the older individual more susceptible not just to infection but also to the development of major age-related chronic diseases such as autoimmune disease and cancer (Vadasz et al., 2013). Frailer elderly individuals have significantly higher levels of markers of inflammation in their serum such as tumor necrosis factor (TNF)-α, interleukin (IL)-6, IL-8, and C-reactive protein (CRP) (De Martinis et al., 2006; Claesson et al., 2012). Interestingly, it has been proposed that centenarians, individuals that managed to extend their lifespan, are able to counteract the damaging effects of inflamm-aging by activating various antiinflammatory markers, such as IL-10 and TNF-β1, thus protecting themselves from an otherwise proinflammatory profile (Larbi et al., 2008; Müller et al., 2013). In addition to immunosenescence and inflamm-aging, the aging of the endocrine system, mitochondrial dysfunction, and microRNA dysregulation have recently been explored as causes for age-related health deterioration (Vitale et al., 2013). The roles played by commensal bacteria in the development of the immune system and the programs of immunosenescence and inflamm-aging in the elderly have been reviewed by Brestoff and Artis (2013) and by Maijó et al. (2014), respectively.

MICROBIOME COMPOSITION IN THE ELDERLY

Recent studies have examined the microbiota composition changes in aging considering their possible consequences for the health of the elderly, yet their scope is still relatively limited. Studies in the 1990s started investigating the composition of the gut microbiota of elderly individuals through culture-dependent and biochemical methods, which were complemented in the following decades by fluorescence in situ hybridization (FISH) and quantitative real-time polymerase chain reaction (qPCR) methods. More recently, phylogenetic microarray Human Intestinal Tract Chip (HITChip), 16S rRNA pyrosequencing, and shotgun sequencing were performed aiming at an in-depth description of the elderly gut microbiome and its capabilities. Despite this increase in data, the results of many of these studies are conflicting, which can be attributable to experimental and study design differences between them. Care must be taken in comparing the results across studies as the use of different DNA extraction methods, comparative analysis tools, and particularities of the study populations themselves can contribute to variation and introduction of unintended bias. For example, some culture-dependent studies have reported an overestimation of bifidobacteria levels with culture compared with FISH (Langendijk et al., 1995; Sghir et al., 1998; Doré et al., 1998; Hopkins et al., 2002). On the other hand, less aggressive and less efficient DNA extraction methods might lead to underestimation of *Bacteroidetes* spp. or *Actinobacteria* numbers seen with some culture-independent methods (Salonen et al., 2010). Some 16S rRNA universal primers have also been shown to have a bias against high GC bacteria (Farris and Olson, 2007). In addition, they can be designed to amplify different regions of the gene, which can itself exist in multiple copies per bacteria (Riesenfeld et al., 2004), and they cannot discriminate between active or damaged members of the bacterial community (Maurice et al., 2013). Although the maturation of high-throughput sequencing technologies has allowed the study of greater number of samples per group, initial phylogenetic and functional studies suffered from small sample size because of cost limitations, as occurs these days with metabolomic studies. Parameters such as the age range used to define the elderly study group, the geographic area studied, the diet and physical and mental health state of the subjects, and their exposure to antibiotics and other drugs have to be considered as possible confounding factors. A summarized selection of these studies is presented in Table 10.1.

Extensive interindividual variation in the composition of the intestinal microbiota of subjects aged 65 or older at the genus and species level was found when compared to healthy adults (Claesson et al., 2011). In addition, despite a maintenance in the number of total anaerobes (Woodmansey et al., 2004), a decline in microbiota diversity is repeatedly described in the elderly (O'Toole and Claesson, 2010), with reduced numbers of bifidobacteria and other beneficial bacteria and an increase in *Enterobacteriaceae* and other facultative anaerobes (Woodmansey et al., 2007). An increase in the relative abundance of *Bacteroidetes* and a decrease in the relative abundance of *Firmicutes* was equally observed in elderly adults (>65 years; Claesson et al., 2011).

Table 10.1 Selected Studies of the Human Gut Microbiota of the Elderly

References	Aim	Sample Size	Profiling Method	Major Findings in the Elderly Group
Hopkins et al. (2002), Hopkins and Macfarlane (2002)	Assess bacterial species diversity in the human feces with respect to age and *C. difficile* infection.	5 healthy elderly people (67–88 years) and 4 elderly patients diagnosed with CDAD (68–73 years).	Culture-dependent methods; FISH	High interindividual variation ↓Bifidobacteria Elderly patients with CDAD: ↓species diversity, ↑facultative anaerobes.
He et al. (2003), Harmsen et al. (2002)	Increase knowledge on the gut microbiota of elderly people.	11 healthy adults (20–55 years) and 15 healthy elderly volunteers (>75 years).	DGGE; qPCR	↑*Enterobacteriaceae*, ↑*Eubacterium cylindroides* group and ↑*Lactobacillus*/*Enterococcus* group. ↓*Bacteroides*/*Prevotella*, ↓*E. rectale*/ *C. coccoides*, and ↓*Faecalibacterium* groups.
Woodmansey et al. (2004)	Characterize major groups of fecal bacteria in healthy young adults, in healthy elderly people, and in hospitalized elderly patients receiving antibiotics.	12 healthy adults (19–35 years), 6 healthy elderly people (67–75 years), and 10 elderly hospitalized patients receiving antibiotics (73–101 years).	Culture-dependent method	↓*Bacteroides*, ↓bifidobacteria alterations in the dominant clostridial species. ↓Species diversity ↓amylolytic activities ↓SCFA concentrations ↑facultative anaerobes. ↑Proteolytic bacteria specifically in the antibiotic-treated elderly group.
Bartosch et al. (2004)	Monitor various bacterial groups in stool samples obtained from elderly individuals.	Three groups of elderly: 35 free-living (63–90 years), 21 hospitalized antibiotic users (65–100 years), and 38 hospitalized nonusers (66–103 years).	qPCR	Both groups of hospitalized elderly showed lower total bacterial levels, which was further reduced in antibiotic users.
van Tongeren et al. (2005)	Study the relationship between fecal microbiota composition and frailty in the elderly.	23 elderly volunteers (70–100 years), divided into low-frailty (n = 13) and high-frailty (n = 10) groups.	FISH	No differences between the low-frailty group and healthy adults. High-frailty elderly: ↓*Lactobacilli*, ↓*Bacteroides*/*Prevotella*, ↓*E. rectale*/ *C. coccoides*, ↓*F. prausnitzii*, ↑*Ruminococcus*, ↑*Atopobium*.
Mueller et al. (2006)	Compare intestinal microbiota composition in adults and elderly across four European locations.	230 fecal samples in total from two age groups: 20–50 years (n = 85) and >60 years (n = 145).	FISH	Marked country-age variation (particularly microbiota composition and abundance of bifidobacteria). ↑*Enterobacteria* in all elderly.
Tiihonen et al. (2008)	Compare effect of aging with and without NSAID on gastrointestinal microbiology and immunology.	14 young adults (21–39 years), 29 elderly NSAID users (70–88 years), and 26 elderly NSAID nonusers (68–84 years).	FISH; qPCR	Both elderly groups: ↑aerobes. Elderly NSAID users: ↓*C. coccoides*/ *Eubacterium rectale*, ↓SCFA, ↓butyric acid, ↓propionic acid, ↓isocapronic acid, and ↓prostaglandin E2.

Continued

Table 10.1 Selected Studies of the Human Gut Microbiota of the Elderly—cont'd

References	Aim	Sample Size	Profiling Method	Major Findings in the Elderly Group
Zwielehner et al. (2009)	Look for aging-related shifts in diversity and composition of the fecal microbiota.	17 healthy adults (18–31 years) and 17 hospitalized elderly (78–94 years) at three different time points two days apart.	DGGE; qPCR	Institutionalized elderly: ↓microbiota diversity, ↑Bacteroides, ↓bifidobacteria, and ↓Clostridium cluster IV.
Mariat et al. (2009)	Study age-related changes in intestinal microbiota composition.	21 healthy adults (25–45 years) and 20 elderly subjects (70–90 years).	qPCR	↑E. coli ↓Firmicutes/Bacteroidetes ratio (10.9 in elderly and 0.6 in adults).
Mäkivuokko et al. (2010)	Compare the intestinal microbial communities of elderly NSAID users and nonusers with the ones of healthy adults.	9 healthy adults (21–39 years), 9 elderly NSAID users (77–85 years), and 9 elderly NSAID nonusers (70–83 years).	Clone-based sequencing of full-length 16S rRNA amplicons; %G + C profiling	Both elderly groups: ↑Firmicutes, particularly Clostridium XIVa, ↓Bacteroidetes. Elderly NSAID users: ↑total microbe numbers compared with elderly NSAID nonusers.
Biagi et al. (2010)	Explore age-related differences in gut microbiota and inflammatory status among Italian young adults, elderly, and centenarians.	20 young adults (25–40 years), 43 elderly (59–78), and 21 centenarians (99–104 years).	qPCR and HITChip	Core fecal microbiota across age groups was constituted mainly of Bacteroides and Firmicutes, predominantly Clostridium clusters XIVa and IV. Centenarians: ↓microbiota diversity, ↑facultative anaerobes, ↓Clostridium XIVa, ↑IL-6, ↑IL-8, ↑IL-1a, and ↑TNF-α levels.
Claesson et al. (2011)	Investigate the composition and variability of the gut microbiota in an Irish elderly cohort.	9 young subjects (28–46 years), 61 elderly subjects (65–96 years), including 43 receiving antibiotics.	16S rRNA 454 sequencing	Both elderly groups: ↑interindividual variability, ↑Bacteroidetes/Firmicutes ratio variability, ↑Clostridia cluster IV (including Faecalibacterium spp.), ↓Clostridia cluster XIVa. Elderly antibiotic users: ↑Bacteroidetes, ↑Bacteroidetes/Firmicutes ratio.

Table 10.1 Selected Studies of the Human Gut Microbiota of the Elderly—cont'd

References	Aim	Sample Size	Profiling Method	Major Findings in the Elderly Group
Claesson et al. (2012)	Investigate links among diet, environment, health, and intestinal microbiota in an Irish elderly cohort.	13 young adult (mean 36 years) and 178 elderly subjects (64–102 years), stratified by residence setting into community-dwelling (n = 83), day-hospital (n = 20), rehabilitation (n = 15), and long-term residential care (n = 60).	16S rRNA 454 sequencing	Community-dwelling fecal microbiota: "low-fat/high-fiber" or a "moderate fat/high-fiber" diet, ↑Firmicutes. Long-stay fecal microbiota: "moderate fat/low-fiber" or "high-fat/low-fiber" diet, ↑Bacteroidetes.
Rea et al. (2012)	Examine the carriage rate of C. difficile as a function of fecal microbiota composition in elderly subjects.	273 elderly subjects, stratified by residence setting into community-dwelling (n = 123), day-hospital (n = 43), rehabilitation (n = 48), and long-term residential care (n = 103).	16S rRNA 454 sequencing	C. difficile carriage rates for community, outpatients, rehabilitation, and long-stay were 1.6, 9.5, 8, and 13%, respectively. CDAD patients and patients from whom C. difficile R027 was isolated had a marked reduction in microbial diversity.
Rampelli et al. (2013b)	Investigate the contribution of the gut metagenome to human longevity.	One young adult (38 years), 5 elderly (59–75 years), and 3 centenarians (99–102 years).	Shotgun sequencing and metabolomics	Elderly (vs. adults); ↓saccharolytic potential, ↑proteolytic functions, ↑pathobionts. Centenarians: ↓genes for SCFA production, ↓genes for aromatic amino acid biosynthesis.
Collino et al. (2013)	Identify the molecular footprints of longevity by using metabolomics plus intestinal microbiota composition.	21 young adults (24–40 years), 283 elderly, and 143 centenarians (99–111 years).	¹H-NMR profiling in urine and LC-MS/MS approaches in serum	Centenarians: remodeling of lipid, amino acid metabolism, and gut microbiota functionality, including alteration of specific glycerophospholipids and sphingolipids, ↓tryptophan and ↑extraction of PAG and PCS through urine.

%G + C, guanine-cytosine content; CDAD, C. difficile-associated diarrhea; DGGE, denaturing gradient gel electrophoresis; FISH, fluorescence in situ hybridization; HITChip, human intestinal tract chip; LC-MS/MS, liquid chromatography–tandem mass spectrometry; ¹H-NMR, hydrogen-1 nuclear magnetic resonance; IL, interleukin; NSAID, nonsteroidal antiinflammatory drugs; PAG, phenylacetylglutamine; PCS, p-cresol sulfate; qPCR, quantitative polymerase chain reaction; rRNA, ribosomal ribonucleic acid; SCFA, short-chain fatty acid; TNF-α, tumor necrosis factor-α

Van Tongeren et al. (2005) applied FISH to compare the microbiota composition in fecal samples of Dutch elderly persons with low and high frailty scores. Individuals with high frailty scores had lower numbers of lactobacilli, *F. prausnitzii*, and bacteria from the *Bacteroides/Prevotella* group as well as higher numbers of *Enterobacteriaceae*. qPCR was used by Mariat et al. (2009) to quantify major bacterial groups in fecal samples of French infants, adults, and elderly subjects (70–90 years). Elderly subjects in this study exhibited high levels of *E. coli* and *Bacteroidetes* and the *Firmicutes/Bacteroidetes* ratio was observed to evolve during the different life stages from 0.4 to 10.9 to 0.6.

To compare the intestinal microbiota composition across geographic regions, adult and elderly individuals (>60 years) from four locations in France, Germany, Italy, and Sweden were recruited to take part in a study by Mueller et al. (2006). FISH coupled with flow cytometry was performed, and marked country-age interactions were observed for the German and Italian study groups. Although levels of bifidobacteria were higher in the Italian study population than in any other study group, independent of age, the levels of enterobacteria were found to be higher in the elderly across all countries. Although an age-related reduction in *F. prausnitzii* was noted, their numbers remained significantly higher in the Swedish volunteers when compared with the other nationalities. These variations in the microbiota composition between the elderly populations from these different countries underline the potential influence of many external factors in the determination of the microbiota composition and indicate that care must be taken when comparing results from geographically distinct communities.

The ELDERMET consortium founded in 2007 (http://eldermet.ucc.ie) was established to investigate the composition of the intestinal microbiota specific to the elderly Irish population (>65 years) as a determinant and indicator of health. Claesson et al. (2011) characterized by 16S rRNA amplicon sequencing the fecal microbiota of 161 of these elderly individuals in comparison to younger controls at time-zero plus a 3-month repeat for 26 of them. The interindividual variability observed in the elderly group was extremely high with *Bacteroidetes* overall dominating followed by *Firmicutes*. Some individuals presented high numbers of *Proteobacteria* or of representatives of the phylum *Actinobacteria*. Considerable variation in the proportion of the total number of reads for *Clostridium* clusters IV and XIVa predominated among the elderly and the young subjects, respectively. Overall, the elderly subjects had much higher abundance of *Faecalibacterium* spp. Among the elderly, antibiotic users had a significant increase in the relative abundance of *Bacteroidetes* with decreases in the relative abundance of *Firmicutes* and *Proteobacteria*. The repeat sample microbiota compositional differences were greater between individuals than within individuals over time.

Our group then investigated links among diet, environment, health, and microbiota by determining the fecal microbiota composition of 178 Irish elderly people stratified by residence location. The diet differed among groups, with community-dwelling elderly having mostly a healthier low to moderate fat/high-fiber diet (enriched in plant-based foods) and elderly in long-term residential care having a less healthy predominantly high-fat/low-fiber diet (enriched in animal products and sugars). The results suggested that diet composition determines the composition of the microbiota and that a more diverse diet promotes a more diverse gut microbiota from phylogenetic and functional points of view. Elderly people in long-term residential care had a higher proportion of phylum *Bacteroidetes* compared with community-dwelling elderly with a higher proportion of phylum *Firmicutes*. The transition from health to frailty was accompanied by a loss in *Prevotella* and *Ruminococcus* co-abundance groups (CAGs) and an increase in *Alistipes* and *Oscillibacter* CAGs. Other factors associating with this transition were weight loss, reduction in calf circumference, poor Barthel index scores (measure of activity and independence), and poor functional independence measure scores. An analysis of the fecal water metabolites separated community from long-stay subjects with the long-stay subjects having higher levels of carbohydrates and lipids and the community subjects having higher levels of the SCFAs butyrate, acetate, and propionate. Subjects in long-term residential care and in rehabilitation also had significantly higher levels of serum inflammatory markers such as TNF-α, IL-6, IL-8, and CRP than community-dwelling elderly, which significantly correlated with the microbiota. The study made a complete case for the microbiota-related acceleration of aging-related health deterioration and a starting point for the use of dietary interventions for the modulation of the microbiota for the promotion of healthier aging (Claesson et al., 2012).

Biagi et al. (2010) used HITChip and qPCR of 16S rRNA of specific bacterial groups to explore the age-related differences in the gut microbiota composition among Italian young adults, elderly, and centenarians. This was the first study to narrow the range of age of the elderly group (59–78 years) and to include an additional group of extremely old individuals (99–104 years). The microbial composition and diversity of the gut ecosystem of the elderly was highly similar to that of the young adults (25–40 years) but differed significantly from that of the centenarians, indicating that an aged gut microbiota may only occur after age 70–75 years. The centenarian microbiota presented a rearrangement in the *Firmicutes* population with a decrease in *Clostridium* cluster XIVa and a change in the elements of the *Clostridium* cluster IV. The centenarian microbiota was particularly characterized by a reduction in health-associated genera such as *Faecalibacterium*, *Eubacterium*, *Roseburia*, *Bifidobacterium*, and *Lactobacillus* together with an enrichment in facultative anaerobes such as *Proteobacteria*, a group containing many of the so-called pathobionts (eg, *Escherichia* and *Streptococcus*), elements of the microbial community that might in situations of microbiota instability behave as opportunistic pathogens. Likely in tandem with this proliferation of pathobionts, an increase in proinflammatory cytokines IL-6 and IL-8 was observed in the peripheral blood of this very old group.

In a collaboration with our metagenomics platform, Rampelli et al. (2013b) applied an Illumina shotgun sequencing approach to analyze a subset of this group of individuals (three centenarians, five elderly people, and one 38-year-old control) to characterize the intestinal bacterial coding capacities in the elderly gut and coupled this with the analysis of urine metabolomics. Reduced abundance was found for genes involved in SCFA production and for aromatic amino acid biosynthesis (tryptophan and phenylalanine) in the centenarians. As in previous studies, centenarian gut microbiota was found to be enriched in pathobionts. Overall there was a decrease in the saccharolytic potential in the elderly, whereas proteolytic functions were more abundant than in the intestinal metagenome of younger adults.

Collino et al. (2013) used a metabonomic and lipidomic profiling strategy to investigate the metabolic phenotype in this population of Italian centenarian, elderly, and adult individuals and cross-referenced it with the intestinal microbiota composition available for a subset of the study population. Mass spectrometry profiling of blood serum revealed a reduction in tryptophan concentration with age as well as a remodeling of the lipidome associated with extended longevity with decreased concentration in sphingomyelins and specific glycerophospholipids in centenarians. It is interesting to note that tryptophan is an amino acid that forms the substrate for the biosynthesis of serotonin (Fitzgerald et al., 2008), a neurotransmitter involved in regulating mood and gastrointestinal tract secretion, motility, and perception (Clarke et al., 2009). Depletion of tryptophan has been reported in IBS, anxiety, and depression (Fitzgerald et al., 2008). Indoleamine 2,3-dioxygenase (IDO) is an interferon-γ-induced enzyme involved in catabolizing tryptophan to kynurenine, which has been shown to be increased in nonagenarians compared with young individuals (Pertovaara et al., 2006). Therefore a chronic low-grade inflammatory state, a fundamental characteristic of aging, might induce IDO, leading to tryptophan degradation to kynurenine. Limited tryptophan availability in the elderly as observed in the centenarians of this study might lead to decreased serotonin biosynthesis and over time, increased susceptibility to neuropsychiatric disorders (Capuron et al., 2011). It is also proposed by the authors that the lipidome alterations observed with increased longevity may reflect a response of the centenarian body to the accumulating oxidative and chronic inflammatory stress associated with their extremely old phenotype. The elderly individuals in this study were further split by familial longevity into offspring of centenarians and offspring of non-long–lived parents. In the offspring of centenarians, the concentrations of specific lysophosphatidylcholines, glycerophospholipids, and the amino acids serine and phenylalanine were significantly higher than in the other group. Urine nuclear magnetic resonance profiles displayed increased levels of phenylacetylglutamine, *p*-cresol-sulfate, and 2-hydroxybenzoate in centenarians compared with elderly, hypothesized to be due to age-related changes in the composition of the gut bacteria such as a decrease in the abundance of several butyrate-producing bacteria from the *Clostridium* cluster XIVa and an increase in the abundance of *Proteobacteria*.

Other microbial populations may play an important role in shaping the elderly gut microbiome but are at this point largely understudied. Two species of Archaea, *Methanobrevibacter smithii* and *Metanophaera stadtmanae*, have been reported to account for approximately 1% of the microbiome in the general population and both numbers and diversity increase with age (Mihajlovski et al., 2010; Biagi et al., 2010; O'Connor et al., 2014). *Methanomassiliicoccus luminyensis* has recently also been isolated from a fecal specimen collected from an 86-year-old healthy man in France (Dridi et al., 2012). The resulting increase in methane in the colon was suggested to contribute to slower transit times by influencing smooth muscle contractility

(Pimentel et al., 2006; Duncan and Flint, 2013). To the best of our knowledge no study has been published to date investigating the virome in the elderly population. As established by Qin et al. (2010), approximately 5% of the coding capacity of the microbiome belongs to bacteriophage sequences. It would be interesting to investigate intestinal bacteriophage composition in old age (Dalmasso et al., 2014) and understand the role that these entities play in shaping the bacterial populations in health and disease.

In summary, the gut microbiome of the elderly populations studied was characterized by reduced diversity when compared with the microbiome of healthy adults, with a decrease in bifidobacteria and other groups with antiinflammatory properties together with an increase in facultative anaerobes. In terms of metabolism, there seems to be a reduction in colonic SCFA production and amino acid biosynthetic capabilities. By splitting the study population into elderly and centenarians, it became evident that an age-related shift in gut microbiota composition and function may only occur after age 70–75 years. Further studies will lead to the identification of alternative healthy microbial stable states in the elderly and define parameters to aim for.

PRESSURES ON THE AGING MICROBIOME

More than 75% of people over 65 years of age take one or more prescription drugs (Chrischillers et al., 1992; Tiihonen et al., 2010). Therefore it is important to understand how these can affect the elderly nutritional status (Genser, 2008; Biagi et al., 2012), gut microbiota function, and how the microbiota might interfere with the intended drug effect via altered turnover in the aging body. Various examples have emerged recently in which the human gastrointestinal microbiome affects drug therapeutic efficacy and/or toxicity. Haiser et al. (2013) recently published a study of the inactivation of the cardiac drug digoxin by the gut bacterium *Actinobacterium Eggerthella lenta*. More studies like this are needed before we fully understand the impact of the microbiota on the compounds that are prescribed to the elderly often in numbers and for prolonged lengths of time.

Elderly subjects are frequently treated with antibiotics. Broad-spectrum antibiotic therapy affects not only the target pathogenic bacterium but also the wider intestinal microbiota as a whole, leading to perturbations of the commensal flora and decreasing its colonization resistance (O'Sullivan et al., 2013). As mentioned before, this can have numerous unappreciated consequences. Even after cessation of an antibiotic course, up to one-third of the bacterial diversity lost might not be recovered (Dethlefsen et al., 2008). Particularly, hospitalization and antibiotic use reduces the abundance of members of the *Bacteroides-Prevotella* group (Bartosch et al., 2004) while producing shifts in the group's composition and reducing the *Bifidobacterium* spp., *Desulfovibrio* spp., *Clostridium* spp., and *Faecalibacterium* spp. populations (Jernberg et al., 2010). The dangers of a low diversity gut ecosystem are epitomized by *Clostridium difficile*-associated diarrhea (CDAD) after antibiotic therapy. Colonization of a susceptible gut by a virulent strain of *C. difficile*–producing toxins and shedding spores can lead to a wide array of illnesses from mild diarrhea to fulminant relapsing diarrhea and pseudomembranous colitis that may be extremely difficult to eradicate despite repeated courses of antibiotics (Rea et al., 2012). *C. difficile* is an important nosocomial pathogen among the elderly with carriage rates in hospitals up to 20% (Karlström et al., 1998). Fecal transplantation, a procedure in which an individual with a severe dysbiotic gut receives a fecal microbiota transplant from a healthy donor to restore diversity and a state of health, has emerged as an extremely effective method for fighting CDAD in cases of recurrent *C. difficile* infection (CDI; Fuentes et al., 2014).

PROBIOTICS, PREBIOTICS AND OTHER MODULATORS OF THE MICROBES IN THE ELDERLY

NU-AGE is a European Union-funded project (FP7) that is currently testing whether a 1-year Mediterranean whole diet is able to lower inflamm-aging in subjects aged 65–79 years across five European countries (http://www.nu-age.eu/). An exhaustive characterization of the volunteers' cognitive and cardiovascular function, bone density, muscle mass, and digestive and immune health will be complemented by an interdisciplinary molecular approach with metagenomic, transcriptomic, metabolomics, and epigenetic profiles (Santoro et al., 2014). This study will allow the development of a predictive model for inflamm-aging–based nutrition in the elderly that might then be applied to other longevity-extending diets such as the Okinawa diet (Willcox et al., 2014) that might be adopted in other parts of the world.

Probiotics have recently been redefined as "live microorganisms that, when administered in adequate amounts, confer a health benefit on the host" (Hill et al., 2014). They can contribute to prevent gut colonization by pathogenic microorganisms through producing inhibitory substances, blocking adhesion sites, competing for resources, and stimulating host immunity. Some might also contribute to increase the diversity of beneficial bacteria and therefore the resilience of the ecosystem as a whole. Prebiotics are typically nondigestible dietary fiber compounds added to the diet that pass undigested through the small intestine and stimulate the growth and/or activity of beneficial bacteria in the gastrointestinal microbiota (Gibson and Roberfroid, 1995; Slavin, 2013). These can be fructooligosaccharides (FOS), galactooligosaccharides (GOS), mannanoligosaccharides, xylooligosaccharides (XOS), polysaccharides (eg, inulin), sugar alcohols (eg, lactitol), or sources of fiber such as wheat bran and linseed. Some fruits and vegetables such as tomato, banana, artichoke, onion, garlic, and soybean are also rich in these components (Al-Sheraji et al., 2013). In the elderly, prebiotics aim to stimulate the growth of bifidobacteria and other health-promoting bacteria and their antiinflammatory products, aim to reduce transit time, and aid probiotics in modulating the immune system. More recent studies have used a synbiotic approach, the complementary use of a prebiotic in conjunction with one or more probiotic strains. Some studies selected to illustrate the effect of probiotics, prebiotics, and synbiotics on the human gut microbiota and the immune system of the elderly are presented in Table 10.2.

Table 10.2 Selected Studies Showing the Effect of Probiotics, Prebiotics, and Synbiotics on the Human Gut Microbiota of the Elderly

References	Aim	Study Design	Population	Age (Years)	Intervention	Key Findings in Treatment(s) Group
Kleesen et al. (1997)	Examine the effects of lactose or inulin on the bowel function of constipated elderly patients.	Randomized, double-blind, parallel study.	$n=10$ (prebiotic inulin) $n=15$ (lactose)	76.4 (mean)	Inulin at 20 g/day (days 1–8) and then at 40 g/day (days 12–19).	↑Bifidobacteria ↓Enterobacteria ↓Enterococci ↑Laxative effect
Chung et al. (2007)	Evaluate the effects of XOS on the intestinal microbiota and gastrointestinal function of the elderly.	Crossover study.	$n=9$ (placebo) $n=13$ (prebiotic)	79.8±6.6 77.5±6.7	XOS (4 g/day) or sucrose (placebo) for 3 weeks followed by a 3-week washout period.	↑Bifidobacteria ↑Fecal moisture ↓Colonic pH
Ahmed et al. (2007)	Determine the effect of 3 different doses of *B. lactis* HN019 (DR10TM) on the intestinal flora of elderly human subjects.	Double-blind, randomized, placebo-controlled study.	$n=20$ (placebo) $n=20$ (low dose) $n=20$ (medium dose) $n=20$ (high dose)	≥60	Reconstituted skimmed milk with or without *B. lactis* HN019 at different levels [6.5 × 10⁷ CFU/day [low], 1.0 × 10⁹ CFU/day [medium], and 5 × 10⁹ CFU/day [high]] for 4 weeks.	All treatment groups: ↑bifidobacteria ↑lactobacilli ↑enterococci ↓enterobacteria
Pitkala et al. (2007)	Study whether a fermented oat drink with 2 selected *B. longum* strains influences bowel movements among elderly nursing home residents.	Double-blind, randomized, placebo-controlled study.	$n=67$ (placebo) $n=56$ (*B. longum*) $n=86$ (*B. lactis*)	65–102 65–99 61–99	Fermented oat drink with *B. longum* 46 and 2C, commercial fermented oat drink with *B. lactis* Bb12 or pasteurized fermented oat drink without viable bacteria daily for 7 months.	Both treatment groups: ↑bowel movements
Vulevic et al. (2008)	Examine the effect of a prebiotic GOS mixture on immune function and fecal microbiota composition in healthy elderly subjects.	Randomized, double-blind, placebo-controlled, crossover study.	$n=44$ (crossover)	69.3±4	GOS mixture (5.5 g/day) or placebo for 10 weeks followed by a 4-week washout period and then the other treatment for 10 weeks.	↑Bifidobacteria ↑*Lactobacillus*/*Enterococcus* spp. ↑*C. coccoides/E. rectale* ↓*C. histolyticum* ↓*E. coli* ↓*Desulfovibrio* spp. ↓IL-1β, IL-6, TNF-α ↑IL-10

Continued

Table 10.2 Selected Studies Showing the Effect of Probiotics, Prebiotics, and Synbiotics on the Human Gut Microbiota of the Elderly—cont'd

References	Aim	Study Design	Population	Age (Years)	Intervention	Key Findings in Treatment(s) Group
An et al. (2010)	Investigate the efficacy of a LAB supplement in the management of nursing home residents suffering from chronic constipation.	Intervention study.	n = 19 (probiotic)	77.1 ± 10.1	LAB twice a day for 2 weeks.	↑LAB ↓Tryptophanase activity ↓Urease activity ↑Frequency of defacation (not statistically significant).
Guillemard et al. (2010)	Assess the effect of consumption of a fermented dairy product containing L. casei DN-114 001 on the resistance to CIDs in a population of elderly volunteers.	Multicentric, double-blind, placebo-controlled study.	n = 434 (placebo) n = 430 (probiotic)	69–95	Fermented dairy drink (Actimel) with or without L. casei DN-114001 daily during a 3-month winter period.	↑L. casei ↓Average duration of gastrointestinal and common respiratory infections.
Walton et al. (2011)	Study if GOS benefits individuals of 50 years and older, through modulation of fecal microbiota.	Randomized, double-blind, placebo-controlled, crossover study. Parallel three-stage culture systems using fecal inocula.	n = 37	≥50	Juice (placebo) consumed for 3 weeks followed by GOS in juice (4 g/day) consumed twice daily for 3 weeks.	↑Bifidobacteria in vivo and in vitro ↑Butyrate in vitro No change in fecal water genotoxicity.
Zaharoni et al. (2011)	Determine the impact of probiotics on the prevention of problems with bowel movement, malnutrition, and infection.	Double-blind, randomized, placebo-controlled study.	Hospitalized elderly patients: n = 101 (placebo) n = 114 (probiotic)	75.7 ± 8.6 76.4 ± 8.5	VSL#3 (8 strains of Bifidobacteria sp., Lactobacillus sp., and S. thermophiles) or placebo for 45 days.	↓Diarrhea ↓Laxative use More pronounced among participants aged ≥80 years.

Table 10.2 Selected Studies Showing the Effect of Probiotics, Prebiotics, and Synbiotics on the Human Gut Microbiota of the Elderly—cont'd

References	Aim	Study Design	Population	Age (Years)	Intervention	Key Findings in Treatment(s) Group
Rampelli et al. (2013a)	Evaluate whether a probiotics-containing biscuit modulates the intestinal microbiota in the elderly.	Randomized, double-blind, placebo-controlled trial.	n=32 split into placebo and probiotic	71–88	Biscuit containing *B. longum* Bar33 and *L. helveticus* Bar13 for 30 days.	↓*Clostridium* cluster XI, ↓*C. difficile*, ↓*C. perfringens*, ↓*E. faecium* ↓*Campylobacter*
Maneerat et al. (2013)	Enquire whether GOS, *B. lactis* Bi-07 (Bi-07) or a combination has an impact on immune function and the gut microbiota in healthy elderly adults.	Randomized, double-blind, placebo-controlled, crossover trial.	n=9 (placebo) n=8 (probiotic) n=9 (prebiotic) n=10 (synbiotic)	63.0 (mean) 64.6 (mean) 70.7 (mean) 70.5 (mean)	Prebiotic GOS (8 g/day) or probiotic Bi-07 or both Bi-07 and GOS or maltodextrin (placebo) for 3-week periods separated by 4-week washout periods.	Bi-07: ↑phagocytic activity of monocytes and granulocytes.
Kondo et al. (2013)	Investigate the effects of *B. longum* BB536 on the health management of elderly patients receiving enteral feeding.	Two double-blind, placebo-controlled trials.	n=32 (placebo) n=37 (BB536-L) n=33 (BB536-H)	83.9±7.5 84.4±6.8 84.4±10.1	*B. longum* BB536-L or BB536-H powders (2.5×10¹⁰ and 5×10¹⁰CFUs, respectively) or placebo for 16weeks.	BB536: ↑bifidobacteria ↑normally formed stools BB536-L: ↑defecation frequency.

CFUs, *colony forming units*; GOS, *galactooligosaccharide*; FOS, *fructooligosaccharide*; IL, *interleukin*; TNF-α, *tumor necrosis factor α*; XOS, *xylooligosaccharide*; LAB, *lactic acid bacteria*; CIDs, *common infectious diseases*.

In a study by Bouhnik et al. (2007), the ingestion of FOS in the elderly increased the abundance of bifidobacteria and lactobacilli and decreased the abundance of enterobacteria compared with controls. Roberfroid et al. (1998) suggested that independent of the dose of FOS, the increase in abundance of bifidobacteria is limited to an extent by the initial bifidobacteria proportion in the gut microbiota. However, in another study elderly nursing home residents had their diet supplemented with a fermented oat drink containing probiotic *Bifidobacterium longum* 46 and *B. longum* 2C or a nonfermented placebo oat drink for 6 months, and the levels of bifidobacteria were significantly increased by the intervention, with diversity increased beyond the strains included in the supplement, which remained elevated until at least 2 months into the washout period (Lahtinen et al., 2009). Biscuits containing the probiotics *B. longum* Bar33 and *Lactobacillus helveticus* Bar13 given by Rampelli et al. (2013a) to a cohort of Italian elderly for 1 month reduced the age-related increase in the opportunistic pathogens *Clostridium* cluster XI, *C. difficile*, *Clostridium perfringens*, *Enterococcus faecium* and the enteropathogenic genus *Campylobacter*. The administration for 2 weeks of the probiotic *Lactobacillus acidophilus* NCFM together with the prebiotic lactitol in healthy elderly taking nonsteroidal antiinflammatory drugs halted the drug-induced reduction in both the *Blautia coccoides-E. rectale* bacterial group levels and in the *Clostridium* cluster XIVab levels (Björklund et al., 2012). The strict anaerobe *Faecalibacterium prausnitzii*, one of the most abundant bacteria in the human intestinal microbiota of healthy adults, is a butyrate-producer with proven antiinflammatory capabilities and an example of a potential good target for the development of an efficacious probiotic. However, because of its oxygen-sensitivity nature, formulation efforts are still underway to make it available as such (Khan et al., 2014).

A common problem in the elderly is reduced bowel function because of a combination of reduced physical activity, reduced fiber consumption and reduced water intake together with reduced intestinal motility (Tiihonen et al., 2010). In one study supplementation with 4 g of XOS per day for 3 weeks significantly increased the population of bifidobacteria and the fecal moisture content while decreasing the fecal pH value (Chung et al., 2007). Inulin was also shown to exhibit a laxative effect (Kleesen et al., 1997). Drinking a fermented oat drink with two selected *B. longum* strains also had a positive effect on the defecation frequency in elderly nursing home residents (Pitkala et al., 2007).

Vulenic et al. (2008) administered GOS to healthy elderly subjects and observed an increase in beneficial bacteria *Bifidobacterium* spp., *Lactobacillus/Enterococcus* spp., and *Clostridium coccoides/E. rectale* and a decrease in the abundance of *Bacteroides* spp., *Clostridium hystolyticum*, and *E. coli* (Scheid et al., 2013). In addition, an increase in natural killer (NK) cell activity and production of antiinflammatory cytokines, together with a decrease in the production of the proinflammatory cytokines IL-6, IL-1β, and TNF-α, was noted in the treatment group. In another study of hospitalized elderly patients, consumption of FOS led to an increase in bifidobacteria and the percentage of T lymphocytes and a decrease in the expression of IL-6 (Guigoz et al., 2002). Ouwehand et al. (2008) administered two *B. longum* strains or a commercial probiotic *Bifidobacterium lactis* Bb-12 to institutionalized elderly in Finland for 6 months and observed a reduction in the regulatory cytokine IL-10 and the proinflammatory cytokine TNF-α. Consumption of *B. lactis* Bi-07 was given together with GOS to a healthy elderly population and was shown to improve the phagocytic activity of monocytes and granulocytes (Maneerat et al., 2013).

Because of immunosenescence, the immune system of older people displays reduced response to vaccination (Boraschi and Italiani, 2014). Studies investigated whether the intake of prebiotics preceding influenza and pneumococcus vaccination had any effect on immune function in the elderly. A trial with oligofructan consumption for 28 weeks showed no change in immunological parameters (Bunout et al., 2002) whereas another that used a diet supplemented with FOS and *Lactobacillus paracasei* showed an increased T cell proportion and NK cell activity after 4 months of supplementation in comparison with controls plus a self-reported reduction in infections (Bunout et al., 2004).

The gut–brain axis and the involvement of the intestinal microbiome in cognitive function in elderly people have only now begun to be investigated, but this seems a promising field for dietary, probiotic, and prebiotic intervention. In an aging rat model, treatment with VLS#3, a probiotic mixture containing eight gram-positive bacterial strains (*Bifidobacterium*, *Lactobacillus*, and *Streptococcus*), led to consistent changes in microbiota composition with increases in *Actinobacteria* and *Bacteroidetes* abundance. This was accompanied by an attenuated age-related deficit in long-term potentiation positively affecting brain function (Distrutti et al., 2014). In the elderly, polyphenol-rich foods in the Mediterranean diet such as olive oil and red wine have been associated with better cognitive function in subjects at high cardiovascular risk (Valls-Pedret et al., 2012). In another study, polyphenols were shown to have antiinflammatory properties in vitro and in vivo, with stimulation of regulatory T cells and decrease in local IL-1β and TNF-α levels in the elderly (Magrone and Jirillo, 2013). As mentioned earlier, tryptophan levels have been shown to decrease with age with potential effects on mental health in the elderly (Collino et al., 2013). Bravo et al. (2013) have successfully used a tryptophan-enriched cereal supplement to improve nocturnal sleep, melatonin, serotonin, and total antioxidant capacity levels and mood in elderly humans.

Subjects with active CDAD or a history of CDAD harbor lower numbers of *Faecalibacterium* spp. and *Bifidobacterium* levels than healthy subjects (Rea et al., 2012), and various probiotic formulations have been tested to promote growth of these and other health-promoting groups in an attempt to increase microbiota diversity and create a gut environment less susceptible to recurrence. Hickson et al. (2007) reported a reduction in CDAD incidence in hospitalized elderly taking antibiotics, with lower prevalence of *C. difficile* toxin and presentation of diarrhea, in elderly treated a with probiotic drink containing *Lactobacillus casei*, *Lactobacillus bulgaricus*, and *Streptococcus thermophilus*. Thuricin CD produced by *Bacillus thuringiensis* has been described as an effective therapy against *C. difficile* without affecting microbiota diversity in a distal colon model (Rea et al., 2011; Walsch et al., 2014), which could be an interesting alternative therapy for CDAD in the elderly. Lakshminarayanan et al. (2013) isolated and characterized 13 bacteriocin-producing strains from fecal samples of 266 elderly Irish subjects that might potentially be used for their probiotic potential as modulators of the gut ecosystem and inhibitors of pathogens.

Fecal transplants have emerged as a second-line therapy for recurrent CDI with cure achieved in 89.5% of elderly individuals (60–101 years) at 2 months to 5 years follow-up, with sustained microbiota diversity increase correlating with clinical remission (Burke and Lamont, 2013). A recent study proposed the use of a stool substitute composed of 33 different intestinal bacteria isolated in pure culture from a single healthy donor to treat recurrent CDI. A pilot on two elderly patients resulted in recovery from CDI with sustained increased diversity in the microbial profile at 24 weeks postprocedure, in spite of one of the patients going through several courses of antibiotics for other unrelated infections (Petrof et al., 2013a).

FUTURE PERSPECTIVES

As discussed, probiotics, prebiotics, and synbiotics have been developed that beneficially affect, to at least some degree, the gut microbiota composition in the elderly, modulate gut metabolism, and reduce inflammation. Where these therapies are insufficient because the microbial communities have suffered from continuous perturbation, fecal transplants or stool substitutes have been effective in restoring intestinal health. A follow-on from a stool substitute would be the use of microbial ecosystem therapeutics, whole bacterial communities derived from the human gastrointestinal tract designed to seed unhealthy gut environments with healthy, resilient, and robust microbial communities (Petrof et al., 2013b). Artificial microbial consortia composed of intestinal bacteria cultured from particularly healthy elderly individuals and therefore particularly suited to an elderly population could become an interesting alternative to current approaches to effectively modulate and restore microbial diversity in the elderly gut. In addition to bifidobacteria and lactobacilli usually stimulated by the current approaches, it would then be possible to increase the proportion of other health-promoting microbes such as the butyrate-producing genera *Coprococcus*, *Roseburia*, and *Butyricicoccus* in the elderly gut, the groups most closely associated with the community-dwelling elderly group in the study by Claesson et al. (2012). Other bacterial products such as polysaccharide A, a bacterial molecule with antiinflammatory effects isolated from the gut bacteria *Bacteroides fragilis*, which has been shown to boost regulatory T cell function and to prevent and treat IBD and multiple sclerosis in animal models (Ochoa-Repáraz et al., 2010), might be interesting to address immunosenescence and inflamm-aging. At some point in the future when the human microbial ecosystems and the forces that shape them are better understood, bacteriophages might become important tools for the active modulation of the human gut microbiota (Dalmasso et al., 2014).

Large longitudinal studies will be required to draw a clear picture of confounding factors such as genetics, diet, metabolism, age, geography, antibiotic and other treatments, as well as standardized sample collection, processing, and analysis methods. Stronger randomized, double-blind, placebo-controlled studies of microbiome modulation strategies, including prebiotics, probiotics, and dietary interventions, will test the actual value of these new tools. Furthermore, human and animal studies, informed by metabolomics, will clarify the set of functional capabilities that a healthy human microbial ecosystem requires; how that varies across age, genetics, and living circumstances; and the mechanisms that lead to dysbiosis and how to prevent it or bring it back into mutualistic balance (Foster and Neufeld, 2013). These studies will permit the characterization of responders and nonresponders to these therapies so that approaches can be tailored to individual circumstances and needs.

Focused research will also be required to isolate and characterize more representatives of the human gut microbiota, either through co-cultivation or with single-cell sequencing technologies. Integration of the metagenomic data obtained with metatranscriptomic, metaproteomics, and metabolomics will certainly contribute to an ecosystem view of the microbiota and its many potential health states. Studies investigating the microbiota of elderly individuals at different stages of frailty in humanized mouse models such as the one used by Turnbaugh et al. (2008) or studies focusing on the molecular mechanisms of aging itself using invertebrate model systems such as the fruit fly *Drosophila melanogaster* (Broderick et al., 2014) and the nematode worm *Caenorhabditis elegans* (Cabreiro and Gems, 2013) will increase our understanding of the underlying mechanisms of aging. Further mechanistic studies on the individual components of the microbiota and their products in the elderly and how they can be harnessed to counter the stresses of aging will certainly in the long term lead to healthier aging and improve the tools available to the medical profession today.

REFERENCES

Aagaard, K., Ma, J., Antony, K.M., Ganu, R., Petrosino, J., Versalovic, J., 2014. The placenta harbors a unique microbiome. Sci. Transl. Med. 6 (237), ra65. http://dx.doi.org/10.1126/scitranslmed.3008599.

Adlerberth, I., Wold, A.E., 2009. Establishment of the gut microbiota in Western infants. Acta Paediatr. Int. J. Paediatr. 98 (2), 229–238. http://dx.doi.org/10.1111/j.1651-2227.2008.01060.x.

Ahmed, M., Prasad, J., Gill, H., Stevenson, L., Gopal, P., 2007. Impact of consumption of different levels of *Bifidobacterium lactis* HN019 on the intestinal microflora of elderly human subjects. J. Nutr. Health Aging 11, 26–31.

Alcock, J., Maley, C.C., Aktipis, C.A., 2014. Is eating behavior manipulated by the gastrointestinal microbiota? Evolutionary pressures and potential mechanisms. Bioessays 36 (10), 940–949. http://dx.doi.org/10.1002/bies.201400071.

Al-Sheraji, S.H., Ismail, A., Manap, M.Y., Mustafa, S., Yusof, R.M., Hassan, F.A., 2013. Prebiotics as functional foods: a review. J. Funct. Foods 5 (4), 1542–1553. http://dx.doi.org/10.1016/j.jff.2013.08.009.

An, H.M., Baek, E.H., Jang, S., Lee, D.K., Kim, M.J., Kim, J.R., Lee, K.O., Park, J.G., Ha, N.J., 2010. Efficacy of Lactic Acid Bacteria (LAB) supplement in management of constipation among nursing home residents. Nutr. J. 9 (5). http://dx.doi.org/10.1186/1475-2891-9-5.

Arumugam, M., Raes, J., Pelletier, E., Le Paslier, D., Yamada, T., Mende, D.R., Fernandes, G.R., Tap, J., Bruls, T., Batto, J.-M., Bertalan, M., Borruel, N., Casellas, F., Fernandez, L., Gautier, L., Hansen, T., Hattori, M., Hayashi, T., Kleerebezem, M., Kurokawa, K., Leclerc, M., Levenez, F., Manichanh, C., Nielsen, H.B., Nielsen, T., Pons, N., Poulain, J., Qin, J., Sicheritz-Ponten, T., Tims, S., Torrents, D., Ugarte, E., Zoetendal, E.G., Wang, J., Guarner, F., Pedersen, O., de Vos, W.M., Brunak, S., Doré, J., Antolín, M., Artiguenave, F., Blottiere, H.M., Almeida, M., Brechot, C., Cara, C., Chervaux, C., Cultrone, A., Delorme, C., Denariaz, G., Dervyn, R., Foerstner, K.U., Friss, C., van de Guchte, M., Guedon, E., Haimet, F., Huber, W., van Hylckama-Vlieg, J., Jamet, A., Juste, C., Kaci, G., Knol, J., Lakhdari, O., Layec, S., Le Roux, K., Maguin, E., Mérieux, A., Melo Minardi, R., M'rini, C., Muller, J., Oozeer, R., Parkhill, J., Renault, P., Rescigno, M., Sanchez, N., Sunagawa, S., Torrejon, A., Turner, K., Vandemeulebrouck, G., Varela, E., Winogradsky, Y., Zeller, G., Weissenbach, J., Ehrlich, S.D., Bork, P., 2011. Enterotypes of the human gut microbiome. Nature 473, 174–180. http://dx.doi.org/10.1038/nature10187.

Bacalini, M.G., Friso, S., Olivieri, F., Pirazzini, C., Giuliani, C., Capri, M., Santoro, A., Franceschi, C., Garagnani, P., 2014. Present and future of anti-ageing epigenetic diets. Mech. Ageing Dev. 136-137, 101–115. http://dx.doi.org/10.1016/j.mad.2013.12.006.

Bartosch, S., Fite, A., Macfarlane, G.T., McMurdo, M.E.T., 2004. Characterization of bacterial communities in feces from healthy elderly volunteers and hospitalized elderly patients by using real-time PCR and effects of antibiotic treatment on the fecal microbiota. Appl. Environ. Microbiol. 70, 3575–3581. http://dx.doi.org/10.1128/AEM.70.6.3575-3581.2004.

Bergström, A., Skov, T.H., Bahl, M.I., Roager, H.M., Christensen, L.B., Ejlerskov, K.T., Mølgaard, C., Michaelsen, K.F., Licht, T.R., 2014. Establishment of intestinal microbiota during early life: a longitudinal, explorative study of a large cohort of Danish infants. Appl. Environ. Microbiol. 80, 2889–2900. http://dx.doi.org/10.1128/AEM.00342-14.

Biagi, E., Candela, M., Fairweather-Tait, S., Franceschi, C., Brigidi, P., 2012. Ageing of the human metaorganism: the microbial counterpart. Age 34, 247–267. http://dx.doi.org/10.1007/s11357-011-9217-5.

Biagi, E., Nylund, L., Candela, M., Ostan, R., Bucci, L., Pini, E., Nikkïla, J., Monti, D., Satokari, R., Franceschi, C., Brigidi, P., De Vos, W., 2010. Through ageing, and beyond: gut microbiota and inflammatory status in seniors and centenarians. PLoS One 5, e10667. http://dx.doi.org/10.1371/journal.pone.0010667.

Björklund, M., Ouwehand, A.C., Forssten, S.D., Nikkilä, J., Tiihonen, K., Rautonen, N., Lahtinen, S.J., 2012. Gut microbiota of healthy elderly NSAID users is selectively modified with the administration of *Lactobacillus acidophilus* NCFM and lactitol. Age 34, 987–999. http://dx.doi.org/10.1007/s11357-011-9294-5.

Boraschi, D., Italiani, P., 2014. Immunosenescence and vaccine failure in the elderly: strategies for improving response. Immunol. Lett. 162, 346–353. http://dx.doi.org/10.1016/j.imlet.2014.06.006.

Bouhnik, Y., Achour, L., Paineau, D., Riottot, M., Attar, A., Bornet, F., 2007. Four-week short chain fructo-oligosaccharides ingestion leads to increasing fecal bifidobacteria and cholesterol excretion in healthy elderly volunteers. Nutr. J. 6 (42). http://dx.doi.org/10.1186/1475-2891-6-42.

Boyce, J.M., Shone, G.R., 2006. Effects of ageing on smell and taste. Postgrad. Med. J. 82, 239–241. http://dx.doi.org/10.1136/pgmj.2005.039453.

Bravo, R., Matito, S., Cubero, J., Paredes, S.D., Franco, L., Rivero, M., Rodriguez, A.B., Barriga, C., 2013. Tryptophan-enriched cereal intake improves nocturnal sleep, melatonin, serotonin, and total antioxidant capacity levels and mood in elderly humans. Age 35, 1277–1285. http://dx.doi.org/10.1007/s11357-012-9419-5.

Brestoff, J.R., Artis, D., 2013. Commensal bacteria at the interface of host metabolism and the immune system. Nat. Immunol. 14, 676–684. http://dx.doi.org/10.1038/ni.2640.

Broderick, N.A., Buchon, N., Lemaitre, B., 2014. Microbiota-induced changes in *Drosophila melanogaster* host gene expression and gut morphology. MBio 5 (3), e01117–14. http://dx.doi.org/10.1128/mBio.01117-14.

Brunner, S., Herndler-Brandstetter, D., Weinberger, B., Grubeck-Loebenstein, B., 2011. Persistent viral infections and immune aging. Ageing Res. Rev. 10 (3), 362–369. http://dx.doi.org/10.1016/j.arr.2010.08.003.

Bunout, D., Barrera, G., Hirsch, S., Gattas, V., de la Maza, M.P., Haschke, F., Steenhout, P., Klassen, P., Hager, C., Avendano, M., Petermann, M., Munoz, C., 2004. Effects of a nutritional supplement on the immune response and cytokine production in free-living Chilean elderly. J. Parenter. Enter. Nutr. 28, 348–354. http://dx.doi.org/10.1177/0148607104028005348.

Bunout, D., Hirsch, S., de la Maza, M.P., Munoz, C., Haschke, F., Steenhout, P., Klassen, P., Barrera, G., Gattas, V., Petermann, M., 2002. Effects of prebiotics on the immune response to vaccination in the elderly. J. Parenter. Enter. Nutr. 26, 372–376. http://dx.doi.org/10.1177/0148607102026006372.

Burke, K.E., Lamont, J.T., 2013. Fecal transplantation for recurrent *Clostridium difficile* infection in older adults: a review. J. Am. Geriatr. Soc. 61 (8), 1394–1398. http://dx.doi.org/10.1111/jgs.12378.

Cabreiro, F., Gems, D., 2013. Worms need microbes too: microbiota, health and aging in *Caenorhabditis elegans*. EMBO Mol. Med. 5, 1300–1310. http://dx.doi.org/10.1002/emmm.201100972.

Calçada, D., Vianello, D., Giampieri, E., Sala, C., Castellani, G., de Graaf, A., Kremer, B., van Ommen, B., Feskens, E., Santoro, A., Franceschi, C., Bouwman, J., 2014. The role of low-grade inflammation and metabolic flexibility in aging and nutritional modulation thereof: a systems biology approach. Mech. Ageing Dev. 136-137, 138–147. http://dx.doi.org/10.1016/j.mad.2014.01.004.

Capuron, L., Schroecksnadel, S., Féart, C., Aubert, A., Higueret, D., Barberger-Gateau, P., Layé, S., Fuchs, D., 2011. Chronic low-grade inflammation in elderly persons is associated with altered tryptophan and tyrosine metabolism: role in neuropsychiatric symptoms. Biol. Psychiatry 70, 175–182. http://dx.doi.org/10.1016/j.biopsych.2010.12.006.

Chrischilles, E.A., Foley, D.J., Wallace, R.B., Lemke, J.H., Semla, T.P., Hanlon, J.T., Glynn, R.J., Ostfeld, A.M., Guralnik, J.M., 1992. Use of medications by persons 65 and over: data from the established populations for epidemiologic studies of the elderly. J. Gerontol. 47, M137–M144.

Chung, Y.C., Hsu, C.K., Ko, C.Y., Chan, Y.C., 2007. Dietary intake of xylooligosaccharides improves the intestinal microbiota, fecal moisture, and pH value in the elderly. Nutr. Res. 27, 756–761. http://dx.doi.org/10.1016/j.nutres.2007.09.014.

Chung, Y.S., Song, I.S., Erickson, R.H., Sleisenger, M.H., Kim, Y.S., 1985. Effect of growth and sodium butyrate on brush border membrane-associated hydrolases in human colorectal cancer cell lines. Cancer Res. 45, 2976–2982.

Claesson, M.J., Cusack, S., O'Sullivan, O., Greene-Diniz, R., de Weerd, H., Flannery, E., Marchesi, J.R., Falush, D., Dinan, T., Fitzgerald, G., Stanton, C., van Sinderen, D., O'Connor, M., Harnedy, N., O'Connor, K., Henry, C., O'Mahony, D., Fitzgerald, A.P., Shanahan, F., Twomey, C., Hill, C., Ross, R.P., O'Toole, P.W., 2011. Composition, variability, and temporal stability of the intestinal microbiota of the elderly. Proc. Natl. Acad. Sci. U.S.A 108 (Suppl. 1), 4586–4591. http://dx.doi.org/10.1073/pnas.1000097107.

Claesson, M.J., Jeffery, I.B., Conde, S., Power, S.E., O'Connor, E.M., Cusack, S., Harris, H.M.B., Coakley, M., Lakshminarayanan, B., O'Sullivan, O., Fitzgerald, G.F., Deane, J., O'Connor, M., Harnedy, N., O'Connor, K., O'Mahony, D., van Sinderen, D., Wallace, M., Brennan, L., Stanton, C., Marchesi, J.R., Fitzgerald, A.P., Shanahan, F., Hill, C., Ross, R.P., O'Toole, P.W., 2012. Gut microbiota composition correlates with diet and health in the elderly. Nature 488, 178–184. http://dx.doi.org/10.1038/nature11319.

Clarke, G., Fitzgerald, P., Cryan, J.F., Cassidy, E.M., Quigley, E.M., Dinan, T.G., 2009. Tryptophan degradation in irritable bowel syndrome: evidence of indoleamine 2,3-dioxygenase activation in a male cohort. BMC Gastroenterol. 9 (6). http://dx.doi.org/10.1186/1471-230X-9-6.

Collino, S., Montoliu, I., Martin, F.P.J., Scherer, M., Mari, D., Salvioli, S., Bucci, L., Ostan, R., Monti, D., Biagi, E., Brigidi, P., Franceschi, C., Rezzi, S., 2013. Metabolic signatures of extreme longevity in northern Italian centenarians reveal a complex remodeling of lipids, amino acids, and gut microbiota metabolism. PLoS One 8 (8). http://dx.doi.org/10.1371/journal.pone.0056564.

Conterno, L., Fava, F., Viola, R., Tuohy, K.M., 2011. Obesity and the gut microbiota: does up-regulating colonic fermentation protect against obesity and metabolic disease? Genes Nutr. 6 (3), 241–260. http://dx.doi.org/10.1007/s12263-011-0230-1.

Costello, E.K., Lauber, C.L., Hamady, M., Fierer, N., Gordon, J.I., Knight, R., 2009. Bacterial community variation in human body habitats across space and time. Science 326, 1694–1697. http://dx.doi.org/10.1126/science.1177486.

Cotillard, A., Kennedy, S.P., Kong, L.C., Prifti, E., Pons, N., Le Chatelier, E., Almeida, M., Quinquis, B., Levenez, F., Galleron, N., Gougis, S., Rizkalla, S., Batto, J.-M., Renault, P., Doré, J., Zucker, J.-D., Clément, K., Ehrlich, S.D., 2013. Dietary intervention impact on gut microbial gene richness. Nature 500, 585–588. http://dx.doi.org/10.1038/nature12480.

Cusack, S., O'Toole, P.W., 2013. Challenges and implications for biomedical research and intervention studies in older populations: insights from the ELDERMET study. Gerontology 59 (2), 114–121. http://dx.doi.org/10.1159/000343158.

Dalmasso, M., Hill, C., Ross, R.P., 2014. Exploiting gut bacteriophages for human health. Trends Microbiol. 22 (7), 399–405. http://dx.doi.org/10.1016/j.tim.2014.02.010.

David, L.A., Maurice, C.F., Carmody, R.N., Gootenberg, D.B., Button, J.E., Wolfe, B.E., Ling, A.V., Devlin, A.S., Varma, Y., Fischbach, M.A., Biddinger, S.B., Dutton, R.J., Turnbaugh, P.J., 2014. Diet rapidly and reproducibly alters the human gut microbiome. Nature 505, 559–563. http://dx.doi.org/10.1038/nature12820.

De Filippo, C., Cavalieri, D., Di Paola, M., Ramazzotti, M., Poullet, J.B., Massart, S., Collini, S., Pieraccini, G., Lionetti, P., 2010. Impact of diet in shaping gut microbiota revealed by a comparative study in children from Europe and rural Africa. Proc. Natl. Acad. Sci. U.S.A. 107, 14691–14696. http://dx.doi.org/10.1073/pnas.1005963107.

De Martinis, M., Franceschi, C., Monti, D., Ginaldi, L., 2006. Inflammation markers predicting frailty and mortality in the elderly. Exp. Mol. Pathol. 80 (3), 219–227. http://dx.doi.org/10.1016/j.yexmp.2005.11.004.

Dethlefsen, L., Huse, S., Sogin, M.L., Relman, D.A., 2008. The pervasive effects of an antibiotic on the human gut microbiota, as revealed by deep 16s rRNA sequencing. PLoS Biol. 6, 2383–2400. http://dx.doi.org/10.1371/journal.pbio.0060280.

DiBaise, J.K., Frank, D.N., Mathur, R., 2012. Impact of the gut microbiota on the development of obesity: current concepts. Am. J. Gastroenterol. 1, 22–27. http://dx.doi.org/10.1038/ajgsup.2012.5.

Distrutti, E., O'Reilly, J.-A., McDonald, C., Cipriani, S., Renga, B., Lynch, M.A., Fiorucci, S., 2014. Modulation of intestinal microbiota by the probiotic VSL#3 resets brain gene expression and ameliorates the age-related deficit in LTP. PLoS One 9, e106503. http://dx.doi.org/10.1371/journal.pone.0106503.

Dominguez-Bello, M.G., Costello, E.K., Contreras, M., Magris, M., Hidalgo, G., Fierer, N., Knight, R., 2010. Delivery mode shapes the acquisition and structure of the initial microbiota across multiple body habitats in newborns. Proc. Natl. Acad. Sci. U.S.A. 107, 11971–11975. http://dx.doi.org/10.1073/pnas.1002601107.

Doré, J., Sghir, A., Hannequart-Gramet, G., Corthier, G., Pochart, P., 1998. Design and evaluation of a 16S rRNA-targeted oligonucleotide probe for specific detection and quantitation of human faecal *Bacteroides* populations. Syst. Appl. Microbiol. 21, 65–71. http://dx.doi.org/10.1016/S0723-2020(98)80009-X.

Dridi, B., Fardeau, M.L., Ollivier, B., Raoult, D., Drancourt, M., 2012. *Methanomassiliicoccus luminyensis* gen. nov., sp. nov., a methanogenic archaeon isolated from human faeces. Int. J. Syst. Evol. Microbiol. 62, 1902–1907. http://dx.doi.org/10.1099/ijs.0.033712-0.

Duncan, S.H., Barcenilla, A., Stewart, C.S., Pryde, S.E., Flint, H.J., 2002. Acetate utilization and butyryl coenzyme A (CoA): acetate-CoA transferase in butyrate-producing bacteria from the human large intestine. Appl. Environ. Microbiol. 68, 5186–5190. http://dx.doi.org/10.1128/AEM.68.10.5186-5190.2002.

Duncan, S.H., Flint, H.J., 2013. Probiotics and prebiotics and health in ageing populations. Maturitas 75, 44–50. http://dx.doi.org/10.1016/j.maturitas.2013.02.004.

Eaton, S.M., Burns, E.M., Kusser, K., Randall, T.D., Haynes, L., 2004. Age-related defects in CD4 T cell cognate helper function lead to reductions in humoral responses. J. Exp. Med. 200, 1613–1622. http://dx.doi.org/10.1084/jem.20041395.

Eckburg, P.B., Bik, E.M., Bernstein, C.N., Purdom, E., Dethlefsen, L., Sargent, M., Gill, S.R., Nelson, K.E., Relman, D.A., 2005. Diversity of the human intestinal microbial flora. Science 308, 1635–1638. http://dx.doi.org/10.1126/science.1110591.

Farris, M.H., Olson, J.B., 2007. Detection of *Actinobacteria* cultivated from environmental samples reveals bias in universal primers. Lett. Appl. Microbiol. 45, 376–381. http://dx.doi.org/10.1111/j.1472-765X.2007.02198.x.

Firth, M., Prather, C.M., 2002. Gastrointestinal motility problems in the elderly patient. Gastroenterology 122, 1688–1700. http://dx.doi.org/10.1053/gast.2002.33566.

Fitzgerald, P., Cassidy Eugene, M., Clarke, G., Scully, P., Barry, S., Quigley Eamonn, M.M., Shanahan, F., Cryan, J., Dinan Timothy, G., 2008. Tryptophan catabolism in females with irritable bowel syndrome: relationship to interferon-gamma, severity of symptoms and psychiatric co-morbidity. Neurogastroenterol. Motil. 20, 1291–1297. http://dx.doi.org/10.1111/j.1365-2982.2008.01195.x.

Flint, H.J., Scott, K.P., Louis, P., Duncan, S.H., 2012. The role of the gut microbiota in nutrition and health. Nat. Rev. Gastroenterol. Hepatol. 9, 577–589. http://dx.doi.org/10.1038/nrgastro.2012.156.

Foster, J.A., McVey Neufeld, K.A., 2013. Gut-brain axis: how the microbiome influences anxiety and depression. Trends Neurosci. 36 (5), 305–312. http://dx.doi.org/10.1016/j.tins.2013.01.005.

Franceschi, C., 2007. Inflammaging as a major characteristic of old people: can it be prevented or cured? Nutr. Rev. 65 (12 Pt 2), S173–S176. http://dx.doi.org/10.1111/j.1753-4887.2007.tb00358.x.

Fuentes, S., van Nood, E., Tims, S., Heikamp-de Jong, I., Ter Braak, C.J., Keller, J.J., Zoetendal, E.G., de Vos, W.M., 2014. Reset of a critically disturbed microbial ecosystem: faecal transplant in recurrent *Clostridium difficile* infection. ISME J. 8, 1621–1633. http://dx.doi.org/10.1038/ismej.2014.13.

Genser, D., 2008. Food and drug interaction: consequences for the nutrition/health status. Ann. Nutr. Metab. 52 (Suppl. 1), 29–32. http://dx.doi.org/10.1159/000115345.

Gibson, G.R., Roberfroid, M.B., 1995. Dietary modulation of the human colonic microbiota: introducing the concept of prebiotics. J. Nutr. 125, 1401–1412. http://dx.doi.org/10.1079/NRR200479.

Gill, S.R., Pop, M., Deboy, R.T., Eckburg, P.B., Turnbaugh, P.J., Samuel, B.S., Gordon, J.I., Relman, D.A., Fraser-Liggett, C.M., Nelson, K.E., 2006. Metagenomic analysis of the human distal gut microbiome. Science 312, 1355–1359. http://dx.doi.org/10.1126/science.1124234.

Guigoz, Y., Rochat, F., Perruisseau-Carrier, G., Rochat, I., Schiffrin, E.J., 2002. Effects of oligosaccharide on the faecal flora and non-specific immune system in elderly people. Nutr. Res. 22, 13–25. http://dx.doi.org/10.1016/S0271-5317(01)00354-2.

Guillemard, E., Tondu, F., Lacoin, F., Schrezenmeir, J., 2010. Consumption of a fermented dairy product containing the probiotic *Lactobacillus casei* DN-114 001 reduces the duration of respiratory infections in the elderly in a randomised controlled trial. Br. J. Nutr. 103, 58–68.

Haiser, H.J., Gootenberg, D.B., Chatman, K., Sirasani, G., Balskus, E.P., Turnbaugh, P.J., 2013. Predicting and manipulating cardiac drug inactivation by the human gut bacterium *Eggerthella lenta*. Science 341, 295–298. http://dx.doi.org/10.1126/science.1235872.

Harmsen, H.J.M., Raangs, G.C., He, T., Degener, J.E., Welling, G.W., 2002. Extensive set of 16S rRNA-based probes for detection of bacteria in human feces. Appl. Environ. Microbiol. 68, 2982–2990. http://dx.doi.org/10.1128/AEM.68.6.2982-2990.2002.

He, T., Harmsen, H., Raangs, G., Welling, G., 2003. Composition of faecal microbiota of elderly people. Microb. Ecol. Health Dis. 15 (4), 153–159. http://dx.doi.org/10.1080/08910600310020505.

Hehemann, J.-H., Correc, G., Barbeyron, T., Helbert, W., Czjzek, M., Michel, G., 2010. Transfer of carbohydrate-active enzymes from marine bacteria to Japanese gut microbiota. Nature 464, 908–912. http://dx.doi.org/10.1038/nature08937.

Hickson, M., D'Souza, A.L., Muthu, N., Rogers, T.R., Want, S., Rajkumar, C., Bulpitt, C.J., 2007. Use of probiotic *Lactobacillus* preparation to prevent diarrhoea associated with antibiotics: randomised double blind placebo controlled trial. BMJ 335 (80). http://dx.doi.org/10.1136/bmj.39231.599815.55.

High, K.P., Akbar, A.N., Nikolich-Zugich, J., 2012. Translational research in immune senescence: assessing the relevance of current models. Semin. Immunol. 24 (5), 373–382. http://dx.doi.org/10.1016/j.smim.2012.04.007.

Hill, C., Guarner, F., Reid, G., Gibson, G.R., Merenstein, D.J., Pot, B., Morelli, L., Canani, R.B., Flint, H.J., Salminen, S., Calder, P.C., Sanders, M.E., 2014. Expert consensus document: the International Scientific Association for Probiotics and Prebiotics consensus statement on the scope and appropriate use of the term probiotic. Nat. Rev. Gastroenterol. Hepatol. 11, 506–514. http://dx.doi.org/10.1038/nrgastro.2014.66.

Hoffmann, C., Dollive, S., Grunberg, S., Chen, J., Li, H., Wu, G.D., Lewis, J.D., Bushman, F.D., 2013. Archaea and fungi of the human gut microbiome: correlations with diet and bacterial residents. PLoS One 8 (6), e66019. http://dx.doi.org/10.1371/journal.pone.0066019.

Hopkins, M.J., Macfarlane, G.T., 2002. Changes in predominant bacterial populations in human faeces with age and with *Clostridium difficile* infection. J. Med. Microbiol. 51, 448–454.

Hopkins, M.J., Sharp, R., Macfarlane, G.T., 2002. Variation in human intestinal microbiota with age. Dig. Liver Dis. 34 (Suppl. 2), S12–S18. http://dx.doi.org/10.1016/S1590-8658 (02)80157-8.

Hosseini, E., Grootaert, C., Verstraete, W., Van de Wiele, T., 2011. Propionate as a health-promoting microbial metabolite in the human gut. Nutr. Rev. 69, 245–258. http://dx.doi.org/10.1111/j.1753-4887.2011.00388.x.

Jernberg, C., Lofmark, S., Edlund, C., Jansson, J., 2010. Long-term impacts of antibiotic exposure on the human intestinal microbiota. Microbiology-Sgm 156, 3216–3223. http://dx.doi.org/10.1099/mic.0.040618-0.

Karlström, O., Fryklund, B., Tullus, K., Burman, L.G., 1998. A prospective nationwide study of *Clostridium difficile*-associated diarrhea in Sweden. The Swedish *C. difficile* Study Group. Clin. Infect. Dis. 26, 141–145.

Kassinen, A., Krogius-Kurikka, L., Mäkivuokko, H., Rinttilä, T., Paulin, L., Corander, J., Malinen, E., Apajalahti, J., Palva, A., 2007. The fecal microbiota of irritable bowel syndrome patients differs significantly from that of healthy subjects. Gastroenterology 133, 24–33. http://dx.doi.org/10.1053/j.gastro.2007.04.005.

Kelly, D., King, T., Aminov, R., 2007. Importance of microbial colonization of the gut in early life to the development of immunity. Mutat. Res. – Fundam. Mol. Mech. Mutagen 622, 58–69. http://dx.doi.org/10.1016/j.mrfmmm.2007.03.011.

Kenney, W.L., Chiu, P., 2001. Influence of age on thirst and fluid intake. Med. Sci. Sports Exerc. 33 (9), 1524–1532. http://dx.doi.org/10.1097/00005768-200109000-00016.

Khan, M.T., Van Dijl, J.M., Harmsen, H.J.M., 2014. Antioxidants keep the potentially probiotic but highly oxygen-sensitive human gut bacterium *Faecalibacterium prausnitzii* alive at ambient air. PLoS One 9 (5), e96097. http://dx.doi.org/10.1371/journal.pone.0096097.

Kleessen, B., Sykura, B., Zunft, H.J., Blaut, M., 1997. Effects of inulin and lactose on fecal microflora, microbial activity, and bowel habit in elderly constipated persons. Am. J. Clin. Nutr. 65, 1397–1402. http://dx.doi.org/10.3109/09637486.2010.527323.

Kondo, J., Xiao, J.Z., Shirahata, A., Baba, M., Abe, A., Ogawa, K., Shimoda, T., 2013. Modulatory effects of *Bifidobacterium longum* BB536 on defecation in elderly patients receiving enteral feeding. World J. Gastroenterol. 19, 2162–2170. http://dx.doi.org/10.3748/wjg.v19.i14.2162.

Koren, O., Knights, D., Gonzalez, A., Waldron, L., Segata, N., Knight, R., Huttenhower, C., Ley, R.E., 2013. A guide to enterotypes across the human body: meta-analysis of microbial community structures in human microbiome datasets. PLoS Comput. Biol. 9 (1), e1002863. http://dx.doi.org/10.1371/journal.pcbi.1002863.

Lahti, L., Salojärvi, J., Salonen, A., Scheffer, M., de Vos, W.M., 2014. Tipping elements in the human intestinal ecosystem. Nat. Commun. 5 (4344). http://dx.doi.org/10.1038/ncomms5344.

Lahtinen, S.J., Tammela, L., Korpela, J., Parhiala, R., Ahokoski, H., Mykkänen, H., Salminen, S.J., 2009. Probiotics modulate the *Bifidobacterium* microbiota of elderly nursing home residents. Age 31, 59–66. http://dx.doi.org/10.1007/s11357-008-9081-0.

Lakshminarayanan, B., Guinane, C.M., O'Connor, P.M., Coakley, M., Hill, C., Stanton, C., O'Toole, P.W., Ross, R.P., 2013. Isolation and characterization of bacteriocin-producing bacteria from the intestinal microbiota of elderly Irish subjects. J. Appl. Microbiol. 114, 886–898. http://dx.doi.org/10.1111/jam.12085.

Langendijk, P.S., Schut, F., Jansen, G.J., Raangs, G.C., Kamphuis, G.R., Wilkinson, M.H.F., Welling, G.W., 1995. Quantitative fluorescence in situ hybridization of *Bifidobacterium* spp. with genus-specific 16S rRNA-targeted probes and its application in fecal samples. Appl. Environ. Microbiol. 61, 3069–3075.

Larbi, A., Franceschi, C., Mazzatti, D., Solana, R., Wikby, A., Pawelec, G., 2008. Aging of the immune system as a prognostic factor for human longevity. Physiology 23, 64–74. http://dx.doi.org/10.1152/physiol.00040.2007.

Le Chatelier, E., Nielsen, T., Qin, J., Prifti, E., Hildebrand, F., Falony, G., Almeida, M., Arumugam, M., Batto, J.-M., Kennedy, S., Leonard, P., Li, J., Burgdorf, K., Grarup, N., Jørgensen, T., Brandslund, I., Nielsen, H.B., Juncker, A.S., Bertalan, M., Levenez, F., Pons, N., Rasmussen, S., Sunagawa, S., Tap, J., Tims, S., Zoetendal, E.G., Brunak, S., Clément, K., Doré, J., Kleerebezem, M., Kristiansen, K., Renault, P., Sicheritz-Ponten, T., de Vos, W.M., Zucker, J.-D., Raes, J., Hansen, T., Bork, P., Wang, J., Ehrlich, S.D., Pedersen, O., 2013. Richness of human gut microbiome correlates with metabolic markers. Nature 500, 541–546. http://dx.doi.org/10.1038/nature12506.

Li, G., Smithey, M.J., Rudd, B.D., Nikolich-Žugich, J., 2012. Age-associated alterations in CD8α+ dendritic cells impair CD8 T-cell expansion in response to an intracellular bacterium. Aging Cell 11, 968–977. http://dx.doi.org/10.1111/j.1474-9726.2012.00867.x.

Li, M., Wang, B., Zhang, M., Rantalainen, M., Wang, S., Zhou, H., Zhang, Y., Shen, J., Pang, X., Zhang, M., Wei, H., Chen, Y., Lu, H., Zuo, J., Su, M., Qiu, Y., Jia, W., Xiao, C., Smith, L.M., Yang, S., Holmes, E., Tang, H., Zhao, G., Nicholson, J.K., Li, L., Zhao, L., 2008. Symbiotic gut microbes modulate human metabolic phenotypes. Proc. Natl. Acad. Sci. U.S.A. 105, 2117–2122. http://dx.doi.org/10.1073/pnas.0712038105.

Louis, P., Hold, G.L., Flint, H.J., 2014. The gut microbiota, bacterial metabolites and colorectal cancer. Nat. Rev. Micro. 12, 661–672. http://dx.doi.org/10.1038/nrmicro3344.

Lozupone, C.A., Stombaugh, J.I., Gordon, J.I., Jansson, J.K., Knight, R., 2012. Diversity, stability and resilience of the human gut microbiota. Nature 489, 220–230. http://dx.doi.org/10.1038/nature11550.

Macfarlane, G.T., Cummings, J.H., Allison, C., 1986. Protein degradation by human intestinal bacteria. J. Gen. Microbiol. 132, 1647–1656. http://dx.doi.org/10.1099/00221287-132-6-1647.

Macfarlane, G.T., Hay, S., Gibson, G.R., 1989. Influence of mucin on glycosidase, protease and arylamidase activities of human gut bacteria grown in a 3-stage continuous culture system. J. Appl. Bacteriol. 66, 407–417.

Magrone, T., Jirillo, E., 2013. The interaction between gut microbiota and age-related changes in immune function and inflammation. Immun. Ageing 10 (31). http://dx.doi.org/10.1186/1742-4933-10-31.

Maijó, M., Clements, S.J., Ivory, K., Nicoletti, C., Carding, S.R., 2014. Nutrition, diet and immunosenescence. Mech. Ageing Dev. 136–137, 116–128. http://dx.doi.org/10.1016/j.mad.2013.12.003.

Mäkivuokko, H., Tiihonen, K., Tynkkynen, S., Paulin, L., Rautonen, N., 2010. The effect of age and non-steroidal anti-inflammatory drugs on human intestinal microbiota composition. Br. J. Nutr. 103, 227–234. http://dx.doi.org/10.1017/S0007114509991553.

Maneerat, S., Lehtinen, M.J., Childs, C.E., Forssten, S.D., Alhoniemi, E., Tiphaine, M., Yaqoob, P., Ouwehand, A.C., Rastall, R.A., 2013. Consumption of *Bifidobacterium lactis* Bi-07 by healthy elderly adults enhances phagocytic activity of monocytes and granulocytes. J. Nutr. Sci. 3 (e4). http://dx.doi.org/10.1017/jns.2013.31.

Manichanh, C., Rigottier-Gois, L., Bonnaud, E., Gloux, K., Pelletier, E., Frangeul, L., Nalin, R., Jarrin, C., Chardon, P., Marteau, P., Roca, J., Dore, J., 2006. Reduced diversity of faecal microbiota in Crohn's disease revealed by a metagenomic approach. Gut 55, 205–211. http://dx.doi.org/10.1136/gut.2005.073817.

Mariat, D., Firmesse, O., Levenez, F., Guimarães, V., Sokol, H., Doré, J., Corthier, G., Furet, J.-P., 2009. The *Firmicutes/Bacteroidetes* ratio of the human microbiota changes with age. BMC Microbiol. 9 (123). http://dx.doi.org/10.1186/1471-2180-9-123.

Maurice, C.F., Haiser, H.J., Turnbaugh, P.J., 2013. Xenobiotics shape the physiology and gene expression of the active human gut microbiome. Cell 152, 39–50. http://dx.doi.org/10.1016/j.cell.2012.10.052.

Meydani, M., 2001. Nutrition interventions in aging and age-associated disease. Ann. N.Y. Acad. Sci. 928, 226–235. http://dx.doi.org/10.1111/j.1749-6632.2001.tb05652.x.

Mihajlovski, A., Doré, J., Levenez, F., Alric, M., Brugère, J.F., 2010. Molecular evaluation of the human gut methanogenic archaeal microbiota reveals an age-associated increase of the diversity. Environ. Microbiol. Rep. 2, 272–280. http://dx.doi.org/10.1111/j.1758-2229.2009.00116.x.

Miller, C., Kelsoe, G., 1995. Ig VH hypermutation is absent in the germinal centers of aged mice. J. Immunol. 155, 3377–3384.

Moco, S., Ross, A., 2015. Can we use metabolomics to understand changes to gut microbiota populations and function? A nutritional perspective. In: Kochhar, S., Martin, F.-P. (Eds.), Metabonomics and Gut Microbiota in Nutrition and Disease, Chapter 5, Molecular and Integrative Toxicology. Springer, London, pp. 83–108. http://dx.doi.org/10.1007/978-1-4471-6539-2_5.

Mueller, S., Saunier, K., Hanisch, C., Norin, E., Alm, L., Midtvedt, T., Cresci, A., Silvi, S., Orpianesi, C., Verdenelli, M.C., Clavel, T., Koebnick, C., Zunft, H.J.F., Doré, J., Blaut, M., 2006. Differences in fecal microbiota in different European study populations in relation to age, gender, and country: a cross-sectional study. Appl. Environ. Microbiol. 72, 1027–1033. http://dx.doi.org/10.1128/AEM.72.2.1027-1033.2006.

Müller, L., Fülöp, T., Pawelec, G., 2013. Immunosenescence in vertebrates and invertebrates. Immun. Ageing 10 (12). http://dx.doi.org/10.1186/1742-4933-10-12.

Naylor, K., Li, G., Vallejo, A.N., Lee, W.-W., Koetz, K., Bryl, E., Witkowski, J., Fulbright, J., Weyand, C.M., Goronzy, J.J., 2005. The influence of age on T cell generation and TCR diversity. J. Immunol. 174, 7446–7452. http://dx.doi.org/10.4049/jimmunol.174.11.7446.

Newton, J.P., Yemm, R., Abel, R.W., Menhinick, S., 1993. Changes in human jaw muscles with age and dental state. Gerodontology 10, 16–22.

O'Connor, E.M., O'Herlihy, E.A., O'Toole, P.W., 2014. Gut microbiota in older subjects: variation, health consequences and dietary intervention prospects. Proc. Nutr. Soc. 73 (4), 441–451. http://dx.doi.org/10.1017/S0029665114000597.

O'Sullivan, Ó., Coakley, M., Lakshminarayanan, B., Conde, S., Claesson, M.J., Cusack, S., Fitzgerald, A.P., O'Toole, P.W., Stanton, C., Ross, R.P., 2013. Alterations in intestinal microbiota of elderly Irish subjects post-antibiotic therapy. J. Antimicrob. Chemother. 68, 214–221. http://dx.doi.org/10.1093/jac/dks348.

O'Toole, P.W., Claesson, M.J., 2010. Gut microbiota: changes throughout the lifespan from infancy to elderly. Int. Dairy J. 20 (4), 281–291. http://dx.doi.org/10.1016/j.idairyj.2009.11.010.

Ochoa-Repáraz, J., Mielcarz, D.W., Wang, Y., Begum-Haque, S., Dasgupta, S., Kasper, D.L., Kasper, L.H., 2010. A polysaccharide from the human commensal *Bacteroides fragilis* protects against CNS demyelinating disease. Mucosal Immunol. 3, 487–495. http://dx.doi.org/10.1038/mi.2010.29.

Ou, J., Carbonero, F., Zoetendal, E.G., DeLany, J.P., Wang, M., Newton, K., Gaskins, H.R., O'Keefe, S.J.D., 2013. Diet, microbiota, and microbial metabolites in colon cancer risk in rural Africans and African Americans. Am. J. Clin. Nutr. 98, 111–120. http://dx.doi.org/10.3945/ajcn.112.056689.

Ouwehand, A.C., Bergsma, N., Parhiala, R., Lahtinen, S., Gueimonde, M., Finne-Soveri, H., Strandberg, T., Pitkälä, K., Salminen, S., 2008. *Bifidobacterium* microbiota and parameters of immune function in elderly subjects. FEMS Immunol. Med. Microbiol. 53, 18–25. http://dx.doi.org/10.1111/j.1574-695X.2008.00392.x.

Panda, A., Qian, F., Mohanty, S., van Duin, D., Newman, F.K., Zhang, L., Chen, S., Towle, V., Belshe, R.B., Fikrig, E., Allore, H.G., Montgomery, R.R., Shaw, A.C., 2010. Age-associated decrease in TLR function in primary human dendritic cells predicts influenza vaccine response. J. Immunol. 184, 2518–2527. http://dx.doi.org/10.4049/jimmunol.0901022.

Pertovaara, M., Raitala, A., Lehtimäki, T., Karhunen, P.J., Oja, S.S., Jylhä, M., Hervonen, A., Hurme, M., 2006. Indoleamine 2,3-dioxygenase activity in nonagenarians is markedly increased and predicts mortality. Mech. Ageing Dev. 127, 497–499. http://dx.doi.org/10.1016/j.mad.2006.01.020.

Petrof, E.O., Gloor, G.B., Vanner, S.J., Weese, S.J., Carter, D., Daigneault, M.C., Brown, E.M., Schroeter, K., Allen-Vercoe, E., 2013a. Stool substitute transplant therapy for the eradication of *Clostridium difficile* infection: "RePOOPulating" the gut. Microbiome 1 (3). http://dx.doi.org/10.1186/2049-2618-1-3.

Petrof, E.O., Claud, E.C., Gloor, G.B., Allen-Vercoe, E., 2013b. Microbial ecosystems therapeutics: a new paradigm in medicine? Benef. Microbes 4, 53–65. http://dx.doi.org/10.3920/BM2012.0039.

Pimentel, M., Lin, H.C., Enayati, P., van den Burg, B., Lee, H.-R., Chen, J.H., Park, S., Kong, Y., Conklin, J., 2006. Methane, a gas produced by enteric bacteria, slows intestinal transit and augments small intestinal contractile activity. Am. J. Physiol. Gastrointest. Liver Physiol. 290, G1089–G1095. http://dx.doi.org/10.1152/ajpgi.00574.2004.

Pitkala, K.H., Strandberg, T.E., Finne Soveri, U.H., Ouwehand, A.C., Poussa, T., Salminen, S., 2007. Fermented cereal with specific bifidobacteria normalizes bowel movements in elderly nursing home residents. A randomized, controlled trial. J. Nutr. Health Aging 11, 305–311.

Pryde, S.E., Duncan, S.H., Hold, G.L., Stewart, C.S., Flint, H.J., 2002. The microbiology of butyrate formation in the human colon. FEMS Microbiol. Lett. 217 (2), 133–139. http://dx.doi.org/10.1016/S0378-1097(02)01106-0.

Qin, J., Li, R., Raes, J., Arumugam, M., Burgdorf, K.S., Manichanh, C., Nielsen, T., Pons, N., Levenez, F., Yamada, T., Mende, D.R., Li, J., Xu, J., Li, S., Li, D., Cao, J., Wang, B., Liang, H., Zheng, H., Xie, Y., Tap, J., Lepage, P., Bertalan, M., Batto, J.-M., Hansen, T., Le Paslier, D., Linneberg, A., Nielsen, H.B., Pelletier, E., Renault, P., Sicheritz-Ponten, T., Turner, K., Zhu, H., Yu, C., Li, S., Jian, M., Zhou, Y., Li, Y., Zhang, X., Li, S., Qin, N., Yang, H., Wang, J., Brunak, S., Doré, J., Guarner, F., Kristiansen, K., Pedersen, O., Parkhill, J., Weissenbach, J., Antolin, M., Artiguenave, F., Blottiere, H., Borruel, N., Bruls, T., Casellas, F., Chervaux, C., Cultrone, A., Delorme, C., Denariaz, G., Dervyn, R., Forte, M., Friss, C., van de Guchte, M., Guedon, E., Haimet, F., Jamet, A., Juste, C., Kaci, G., Kleerebezem, M., Knol, J., Kristensen, M., Layec, S., Le Roux, K., Leclerc, M., Maguin, E., Melo Minardi, R., Oozeer, R., Rescigno, M., Sanchez, N., Tims, S., Torrejon, T., Varela, E., de Vos, W., Winogradsky, Y., Zoetendal, E., Bork, P., Ehrlich, S.D., Wang, J., 2010. A human gut microbial gene catalogue established by metagenomic sequencing. Nature 464, 59–65. http://dx.doi.org/10.1038/nature08821.

Qin, J., Li, Y., Cai, Z., Li, S., Zhu, J., Zhang, F., Liang, S., Zhang, W., Guan, Y., Shen, D., Peng, Y., Zhang, D., Jie, Z., Wu, W., Qin, Y., Xue, W., Li, J., Han, L., Lu, D., Wu, P., Dai, Y., Sun, X., Li, Z., Tang, A., Zhong, S., Li, X., Chen, W., Xu, R., Wang, M., Feng, Q., Gong, M., Yu, J., Zhang, Y., Zhang, M., Hansen, T., Sanchez, G., Raes, J., Falony, G., Okuda, S.,

Almeida, M., LeChatelier, E., Renault, P., Pons, N., Batto, J.-M., Zhang, Z., Chen, H., Yang, R., Zheng, W., Li, S., Yang, H., Wang, J., Ehrlich, S.D., Nielsen, R., Pedersen, O., Kristiansen, K., Wang, J., 2012. A metagenome-wide association study of gut microbiota in type 2 diabetes. Nature 490, 55–60. http://dx.doi.org/10.1038/nature11450.

Rampelli, S., Candela, M., Severgnini, M., Biagi, E., Turroni, S., Roselli, M., Carnevali, P., Donini, L., Brigidi, P., 2013a. A probiotics-containing biscuit modulates the intestinal microbiota in the elderly. J. Nutr. Health Aging 17 (2), 166–172. http://dx.doi.org/10.1007/s12603-012-0372-x.

Rampelli, S., Candela, M., Turroni, S., Biagi, E., Collino, S., Toole, P.W.O., Brigidi, P., 2013b. Functional metagenomic profiling of intestinal microbiome in extreme ageing. Aging 5 (12), 902–912.

Rea, M.C., Dobson, A., O'Sullivan, O., Crispie, F., Fouhy, F., Cotter, P.D., Shanahan, F., Kiely, B., Hill, C., Ross, R.P., 2011. Effect of broad- and narrow-spectrum antimicrobials on *Clostridium difficile* and microbial diversity in a model of the distal colon. Proc. Natl. Acad. Sci. U.S.A. 108 (Suppl. 1), 4639–4644. http://dx.doi.org/10.1073/pnas.1001224107.

Rea, M.C., O'Sullivan, O., Shanahan, F., O'Toole, P.W., Stanton, C., Ross, R.P., Hill, C., 2012. *Clostridium difficile* carriage in elderly subjects and associated changes in the intestinal microbiota. J. Clin. Microbiol. 50, 867–875. http://dx.doi.org/10.1128/JCM.05176-11.

Riesenfeld, C.S., Schloss, P.D., Handelsman, J., 2004. Metagenomics: genomic analysis of microbial communities. Annu. Rev. Genet. 38, 525–552. http://dx.doi.org/10.1146/annurev.genet.38.072902.091216.

Roberfroid, M.B., Van Loo, J.A., Gibson, G.R., 1998. The bifidogenic nature of chicory inulin and its hydrolysis products. J. Nutr. 128, 11–19. http://dx.doi.org/10.1038/ejcn.2009.64.

Salonen, A., Nikkilä, J., Jalanka-Tuovinen, J., Immonen, O., Rajilić-Stojanović, M., Kekkonen, R.A., Palva, A., de Vos, W.M., 2010. Comparative analysis of fecal DNA extraction methods with phylogenetic microarray: effective recovery of bacterial and archaeal DNA using mechanical cell lysis. J. Microbiol. Methods 81 (2), 127–134. http://dx.doi.org/10.1016/j.mimet.2010.02.007.

Saltzman, J.R., Russell, R.M., 1998. The aging gut: nutritional issues. Gastroenterol. Clin. North Am. 27 (2), 309–324. http://dx.doi.org/10.1016/S0889-8553(05)70005-4.

Sanchez, J.I., Marzorati, M., Grootaert, C., Baran, M., Van Craeyveld, V., Courtin, C.M., Broekaert, W.F., Delcour, J.A., Verstraete, W., Van De Wiele, T., 2009. Arabinoxylan-oligosaccharides (AXOS) affect the protein/carbohydrate fermentation balance and microbial population dynamics of the Simulator of Human Intestinal Microbial Ecosystem. Microb. Biotechnol. 2, 101–113. http://dx.doi.org/10.1111/j.1751-7915.2008.00064.x.

Santoro, A., Brigidi, P., Gonos, E.S., Bohr, V.A., Franceschi, C., 2014. Mediterranean diet and inflammaging in the elderly: the European project NU-AGE. Preface. Mech. Ageing Dev. 136-137, 1–2. http://dx.doi.org/10.1016/j.mad.2014.01.006.

Scheid, M.M.A., Moreno, Y.M.F., Maróstica Junior, M.R., Pastore, G.M., 2013. Effect of prebiotics on the health of the elderly. Food Res. Int. 3 (1), 57–60. http://dx.doi.org/10.1016/j.foodres.2013.04.003.

Schnorr, S.L., Candela, M., Rampelli, S., Centanni, M., Consolandi, C., Basaglia, G., Turroni, S., Biagi, E., Peano, C., Severgnini, M., Fiori, J., Gotti, R., De Bellis, G., Luiselli, D., Brigidi, P., Mabulla, A., Marlowe, F., Henry, A.G., Crittenden, A.N., 2014. Gut microbiome of the Hadza hunter-gatherers. Nat. Commun. 5 (3654). http://dx.doi.org/10.1038/ncomms4654.

Sghir, A., Chow, J.M., Mackie, R.I., 1998. Continuous culture selection of bifidobacteria and lactobacilli from human faecal samples using fructooligosaccharide as selective substrate. J. Appl. Microbiol. 85, 769–777. http://dx.doi.org/10.1111/j.1365-2672.1998.00590.x.

Shanahan, F., 2012. The microbiota in inflammatory bowel disease: friend, bystander, and sometime-villain. Nutr. Rev. 70 (Suppl. 1), S31–S37. http://dx.doi.org/10.1111/j.1753-4887.2012.00502.x.

Slavin, J., 2013. Fiber and prebiotics: mechanisms and health benefits. Nutrients 5 (4), 1417–1435. http://dx.doi.org/10.3390/nu5041417.

Smith, K., McCoy, K.D., Macpherson, A.J., 2007. Use of axenic animals in studying the adaptation of mammals to their commensal intestinal microbiota. Semin. Immunol. 9 (2), 59–69. http://dx.doi.org/10.1016/j.smim.2006.10.002.

Sommer, F., Bäckhed, F., 2013. The gut microbiota–masters of host development and physiology. Nat. Rev. Microbiol. 11, 227–238. http://dx.doi.org/10.1038/nrmicro2974.

Tap, J., Mondot, S., Levenez, F., Pelletier, E., Caron, C., Furet, J.P., Ugarte, E., Muñoz-Tamayo, R., Paslier, D.L.E., Nalin, R., Dore, J., Leclerc, M., 2009. Towards the human intestinal microbiota phylogenetic core. Environ. Microbiol. 11, 2574–2584. http://dx.doi.org/10.1111/j.1462-2920.2009.01982.x.

Thorburn, A.N., Macia, L., Mackay, C.R., 2014. Diet, metabolites, and "western-lifestyle" inflammatory diseases. Immunity 40 (6), 833–842. http://dx.doi.org/10.1016/j.immuni.2014.05.014.

Tiihonen, K., Ouwehand, A.C., Rautonen, N., 2010. Human intestinal microbiota and healthy ageing. Ageing Res. Rev. 9 (2), 107–116. http://dx.doi.org/10.1016/j.arr.2009.10.004.

Tiihonen, K., Tynkkynen, S., Ouwehand, A., Ahlroos, T., Rautonen, N., 2008. The effect of ageing with and without non-steroidal anti-inflammatory drugs on gastrointestinal microbiology and immunology. Br. J. Nutr. 100, 130–137. http://dx.doi.org/10.1017/S000711450888871X.

Tremaroli, V., Bäckhed, F., 2012. Functional interactions between the gut microbiota and host metabolism. Nature 489, 242–249. http://dx.doi.org/10.1038/nature11552.

Turnbaugh, P.J., Bäckhed, F., Fulton, L., Gordon, J.I., 2008. Diet-induced obesity is linked to marked but reversible alterations in the mouse distal gut microbiome. Cell Host Microbe 3, 213–223. http://dx.doi.org/10.1016/j.chom.2008.02.015.

United Nations, Department of Economic and Social Affairs, P.D., 2005. World Population Prospects: The 2004 Revision. New York. doi:ST/ESA/SER.A/246.

United Nations, Department of Economic and Social Affairs, P.D., 2013. World Population Ageing 2013, 2013, ST/ESA/SER.A/348.

Ursell, L.K., Van Treuren, W., Metcalf, J.L., Pirrung, M., Gewirtz, A., Knight, R., 2013. Replenishing our defensive microbes. BioEssays 35, 810–817. http://dx.doi.org/10.1002/bies.201300018.

Vadasz, Z., Haj, T., Kessel, A., Toubi, E., 2013. Age-related autoimmunity. BMC Med. 11 (94). http://dx.doi.org/10.1186/1741-7015-11-94.

Valls-Pedret, C., Lamuela-Raventós, R.M., Medina-Remón, A., Quintana, M., Corella, D., Pintó, X., Martínez-González, M.Á., Estruch, R., Ros, E., 2012. Polyphenol-rich foods in the Mediterranean diet are associated with better cognitive function in elderly subjects at high cardiovascular risk. J. Alzheimers Dis. 29, 773–782. http://dx.doi.org/10.3233/JAD-2012-111799.

Van Tongeren, S.P., Slaets, J.P.J., Harmsen, H.J.M., Welling, G.W., 2005. Fecal microbiota composition and frailty. Appl. Environ. Microbiol. 71, 6438–6442. http://dx.doi.org/10.1128/AEM.71.10.6438-6442.2005.

Vitale, G., Salvioli, S., Franceschi, C., 2013. Oxidative stress and the ageing endocrine system. Nat. Rev. Endocrinol. 9, 228–240. http://dx.doi.org/10.1038/nrendo.2013.29.

Voreades, N., Kozil, A., Weir, T., 2014. Diet and the development of the human intestinal microbiome. Front. Microbiol. 5 (494). http://dx.doi.org/10.3389/fmicb.2014.00494.

Vulevic, J., Drakoularakou, A., Yaqoob, P., Tzortzis, G., Gibson, G.R., 2008. Modulation of the fecal microflora profile and immune function by a novel trans-galactooligosaccharide mixture (B-GOS) in healthy elderly volunteers. Am. J. Clin. Nutr. 88 (5), 1438–1446. http://dx.doi.org/10.3945/ajcn.2008.26242.

Walker, A.W., Duncan, S.H., Carol McWilliam Leitch, E., Child, M.W., Flint, H.J., 2005. pH and peptide supply can radically alter bacterial populations and short-chain fatty acid ratios within microbial communities from the human colon. Appl. Environ. Microbiol. 71, 3692–3700. http://dx.doi.org/10.1128/AEM.71.7.3692-3700.2005.

Walker, W.A., Iyengar, S.R., 2014. Breastmilk, microbiota and intestinal immune homeostasis. Pediatr. Res. http://dx.doi.org/10.1038/pr.2014.160.

Walsh, C.J., Guinane, C.M., O'Toole, P.W., Cotter, P.D., 2014. Beneficial modulation of the gut microbiota. FEBS Lett. 588 (22), 4120–4130. http://dx.doi.org/10.1016/j.febslet.2014.03.035.

Walton, G.E., van den Heuvel, E.G., Kosters, M.H., Rastall, R.A., Tuohy, K.M., Gibson, G.R., 2011. A randomised crossover study investigating the effects of galacto-oligosaccharides on the faecal microbiota in men and women over 50 years of age. Br. J. Nutr. 107 (10), 1466–1475. http://dx.doi.org/10.1017/S0007114511004697 [pii]\r10.1017/S0007114511004697.

Weinert, B.T., Timiras, P.S., 2003. Invited review: theories of aging. J. Appl. Physiol. 95, 1706–1716. http://dx.doi.org/10.1152/japplphysiol.00288.2003.

Willcox, D.C., Scapagnini, G., Willcox, B.J., 2014. Healthy aging diets other than the Mediterranean: a focus on the Okinawan diet. Mech. Ageing Dev. 136–137, 148–162. http://dx.doi.org/10.1016/j.mad.2014.01.002.

Windey, K., de Preter, V., Verbeke, K., 2012. Relevance of protein fermentation to gut health. Mol. Nutr. Food Res. 56 (1), 184–196. http://dx.doi.org/10.1002/mnfr.201100542.

Woodmansey, E.J., 2007. Intestinal bacteria and ageing. J. Appl. Microbiol. 102, 1178–1186. http://dx.doi.org/10.1111/j.1365-2672.2007.03400.x.

Woodmansey, E.J., McMurdo, M.E.T., Macfarlane, G.T., Macfarlane, S., 2004. Comparison of compositions and metabolic activities of fecal microbiotas in young adults and in antibiotic-treated and non-antibiotic-treated elderly subjects. Appl. Environ. Microbiol. 70, 6113–6122. http://dx.doi.org/10.1128/AEM.70.10.6113-6122.2004.

Wu, G.D., Chen, J., Hoffmann, C., Bittinger, K., Chen, Y.-Y., Keilbaugh, S.A., Bewtra, M., Knights, D., Walters, W.A., Knight, R., Sinha, R., Gilroy, E., Gupta, K., Baldassano, R., Nessel, L., Li, H., Bushman, F.D., Lewis, J.D., 2011. Linking long-term dietary patterns with gut microbial enterotypes. Science 334 (6052), 105–108. http://dx.doi.org/10.1126/science.1208344.

Wu, G.D., Compher, C., Chen, E.Z., Smith, S.A., Shah, R.D., Bittinger, K., Chehoud, C., Albenberg, L.G., Nessel, L., Gilroy, E., Star, J., Weljie, A.M., Flint, H.J., Metz, D.C., Bennett, M.J., Li, H., Bushman, F.D., Lewis, J.D., 2014. Comparative metabolomics in vegans and omnivores reveal constraints on diet-dependent gut microbiota metabolite production. Gut. http://dx.doi.org/10.1136/gutjnl-2014-308209.

Yatsunenko, T., Rey, F.E., Manary, M.J., Trehan, I., Dominguez-Bello, M.G., Contreras, M., Magris, M., Hidalgo, G., Baldassano, R.N., Anokhin, A.P., Heath, A.C., Warner, B., Reeder, J., Kuczynski, J., Caporaso, J.G., Lozupone, C.A., Lauber, C., Clemente, J.C., Knights, D., Knight, R., Gordon, J.I., 2012. Human gut microbiome viewed across age and geography. Nature 486, 222–227. http://dx.doi.org/10.1038/nature11053.

Zaharoni, H., Rimon, E., Vardi, H., Friger, M., Bolotin, A., Shahar, D.R., 2011. Probiotics improve bowel movements in hospitalized elderly patients – the PROAGE study. J. Nutr. Health Aging 15, 215–220. http://dx.doi.org/10.1007/s12603-010-0323-3.

Zhang, Z., Geng, J., Tang, X., Fan, H., Xu, J., Wen, X., Ma, Z.S., Shi, P., 2014. Spatial heterogeneity and co-occurrence patterns of human mucosal-associated intestinal microbiota. ISME J. 8, 881–893. http://dx.doi.org/10.1038/ismej.2013.185.

Zoetendal, E.G., Raes, J., van den Bogert, B., Arumugam, M., Booijink, C.C., Troost, F.J., Bork, P., Wels, M., de Vos, W.M., Kleerebezem, M., 2012. The human small intestinal microbiota is driven by rapid uptake and conversion of simple carbohydrates. ISME J. 6 (7), 1415–1426. http://dx.doi.org/10.1038/ismej.2011.212.

Zwielehner, J., Liszt, K., Handschur, M., Lassl, C., Lapin, A., Haslberger, A.G., 2009. Combined PCR-DGGE fingerprinting and quantitative-PCR indicates shifts in fecal population sizes and diversity of *Bacteroides*, bifidobacteria and *Clostridium* cluster IV in institutionalized elderly. Exp. Gerontol. 44, 440–446. http://dx.doi.org/10.1016/j.exger.2009.04.002.

Long-Term Implications of Antibiotic Use on Gut Health and Microbiota in Populations Including Patients With Cystic Fibrosis

11

J. Deane

Teagasc Food Research Centre, Cork, Ireland; University College Cork, Department of Medicine, Cork, Ireland

M.C. Rea

Teagasc Food Research Centre, Fermoy, Cork, Ireland; University College Cork, APC Microbiome Institute, Cork, Ireland

F. Fouhy

Teagasc Food Research Centre, Fermoy, Cork, Ireland

C. Stanton

Teagasc Food Research Centre, Fermoy, Cork, Ireland; University College Cork, APC Microbiome Institute, Cork, Ireland

R.P. Ross

University College Cork, APC Microbiome Institute, Cork, Ireland; University College Cork, College of Science, Engineering and Food Science, Cork, Ireland

B.J. Plant

University College Cork, Cork Cystic Fibrosis Centre, Cork University Hospital, Cork, Ireland; University College Cork, Department of Medicine, Cork, Ireland

INTRODUCTION

Since the discovery by Alexander Fleming of penicillin in 1929 and the subsequent journey of antibiotic research and discovery, antibiotics have revolutionized human health on a global scale. Antibiotic therapy can be acknowledged for a significant increase in life expectancy between 1944 and 1972, a period of intensive and successful antibiotic research (Cotter et al., 2012). However, the negative effects of antibiotic therapy are well documented, most notably antimicrobial resistance, which is now accepted as a global issue spanning medical, economic, and environmental fronts. The World Health Organization, Centers for Disease Control and Prevention (CDC), and European Center for Disease Prevention and Control consider multidrug-resistant (MDR) infections caused by antibiotic-resistant bacteria as an emergent global disease and a major threat to public health (Roca et al., 2015). However, this review will focus on the more pervasive effects of antibiotic therapy on the gut microbiome and the far-reaching effects on the health of the host. The antibiotic-mediated perturbations of the microbiome and disruption of related functionality is an area of much research. In recent years the collateral damage caused by antibiotic use has come into focus (Blaser, 2011). Antibiotic therapy can be likened to a war of attrition on the gut microbiota because subsequent rounds of therapy result in loss of diversity followed by incomplete recovery causing the bacterial population to shift from the initial assemblage. The control of infection through antibiotic use, while not diminishing its importance, has potentially devastating consequences downstream not only for the individual, as host-microbe interactions are disturbed, but also for society with the potential dissemination of MDR determinants. In this review we examine the literature regarding the effects of various families of antibiotics on the gut microbiota, discussing in particular issues with relevance to a cystic fibrosis (CF) cohort, such as MDR as a result of chronic antibiotic use, *Clostridium difficile*, and disruption of host-microbiota mutualistic relationships.

Perturbations of the gut microbiota can occur via many external environmental factors, but perhaps the most dramatic modulatory effects are seen with antibiotic use. The immediate impact of short-term antibiotic therapy on the gut microbiota is extensively investigated. However, longitudinal studies mapping the recovery of the microbiota in the aftermath are limited, with even greater gaps in our knowledge regarding the long-term effects of chronic antibiotic use on the gut microbiota. Studies focusing on short-term antibiotic use have demonstrated the profound and pervasive effects of the antibiotic, the resilience of the gut microbiota after treatment (Dethlefsen et al., 2008; Jernberg et al., 2007), and reduction of fecal bacterial load and diversity (Xu et al., 2014; Iapichino et al., 2008; Jakobsson et al., 2010). Others have demonstrated the differential effects of different classes of antibiotics on the gut microbiota and how the resultant assembly after antibiotic treatment may be influenced by mode of action (Perez-Cobas et al., 2013). It is widely reported that immediately after antibiotic treatment an increase in *Enterococcus* species (Iapichino et al., 2008) and a decrease in *Bifidobacteria, Clostridia, Desulfovibrio, Faecalibacterium* and *Bacteroides* species (Adamsson et al., 1999; Bartosch et al., 2004; Jernberg et al., 2007; O'Sullivan et al., 2013) is expected. Most microbiota recover after 4 weeks; however, a long-term persistence of expressed antibiotic resistance genes, particularly carried by *Enterococcus* species, after a short-term antibiotic treatment was noted up to 4 years posttreatment in some human studies (Jakobsson et al., 2010; Jernberg et al., 2007).

CF cohorts are ideal candidate groups to investigate the effects of antibiotic use on gut health and microbiota. CF is a monogenic disorder, thereby reducing confounding factors and so facilitating inferences regarding antibiotic effects on the gut microbiota. CF is a potentially life-threatening autosomal-recessive disorder affecting 70,000 individuals worldwide, with Ireland having the highest prevalence (~1100 patients) and incidence rates (1 in 1353; Farrell, 2008). It results from mutations in the cystic fibrosis transmembrane conductance regulator (CFTR) gene, located on the long arm of chromosome 7 (Collins, 1992), of which the most common is ΔF508 (a deletion of phenylalanine at codon 508). CFTR gene mutations result in defective chloride ion transport in the respiratory, hepatobiliary, gastrointestinal, reproductive tracts, and the pancreas (Quinton, 1990). The natural progression of CF is characterized by chronic lung function decline punctuated by recurrent periods of temporary worsening of symptoms, known as pulmonary exacerbations (Amadori et al., 2009; Flume et al., 2009). Prophylactic antibiotic therapy plays a pivotal role in treating CF patients; combating frequent lung infections, slowing the rate of lung function decline, and ultimately prolonging life. Indeed antibiotic discovery, amongst other therapeutic options, has significantly contributed to the increased life expectancy of CF sufferers, meaning many survive into their thirties and beyond whereas in the 1950s few lived to attend primary school. The increasing life expectancy of CF individuals presents further new therapeutic challenges (Plant et al., 2013). A global shifting pattern of antibiotic use is seen in antibiotic therapy for CF patients in which prophylaxis, maintenance, and chronic antibiotic therapy have been shown to improve clinical outcomes and survival (Moskowitz et al., 2008; Szaff et al., 1983).

Although the gut microbiota of CF patients is poorly documented, it can be assumed that intensive and frequent courses of antibiotics alter its diversity and function as a symbiotic partner with the host. Seventy percent of the immune system is harbored in the gastrointestinal tract, meaning perturbations in the microbiome at the very least will have implications for host immunity, but also for energy extraction efficiency from food, mental well-being, and colonization resistance against pathogenic microorganisms (Weiner, 2000; Faria and Weiner, 2005; Vighi et al., 2008). Defining and characterizing the gut microbiota of a CF population can provide information applicable to the wider medical community. A picture of the gut microbiota of CF patients as a unique entity that is a signature of the disease is emerging in recent research. The characteristic CF intestinal microbiome is thought to be as a result of a combination of factors including the CFTR malfunction itself, chronic antibiotic use, high-fat diet, pancreatic enzyme supplementation, and suppression of gastric acid (Bruzzese et al., 2014). The CF gut has been shown to have lower counts of lactic acid bacteria (LAB), *Clostridium* species, *Bifidobacterium* species, *Veillonella* species, and *Bacteroides-Prevotella* species, whereas Enterobacteriaceae counts were increased in the CF cohort (Duytchaever et al., 2011). As expected in a cohort with chronic antibiotic use, CF patients have been shown to have lower species richness, evenness, diversity, and reduced temporal stability of intestinal microbiota (Scanlan et al., 2012). In particular, the reduction of diversity and abundance of *Bifidobacterium* species (*Bifidobacterium longum, Bifidobacterium catenulatum, Bifidobacterium pseudocatenulatum*, and *Bifidobacterium adolescentis*), *Clostridium* cluster XIVa, and *Clostridium* cluster IV (*R. bromii* and *Faecalibacterium prausnitzii*) has been described (Duytschaever et al., 2013). Bifidobacterium species have a greater antimicrobial susceptibility to many antibiotics used in the treatment of CF pulmonary exacerbations and reduced adhesion capacity to inflamed mucosa (Lee and O'Sullivan, 2010; Russell et al., 2011), perhaps explaining their reduction in a CF cohort. Evidence from Madan et al. (2012) revealed a core lung-gut microbiota dominated by *Veillonella* and *Streptococcus*, with similarities between population fluctuations between the two sites. Furthermore, they show that select genera (*Roseburia, Dorea, Sporacetigenium, Coprococcus, Blautia, Enterococcus,* and *Escherichia*) of the gut microbiota precede bacterial populations found in the lung. Allelic variations of the CFTR gene have also been shown to have effects on the gut microbiota, with homozygous F508del and severe disease phenotype CF patients exhibiting greater dysbiotic fecal microbiota compared with heterozygous milder disease phenotype patients, a signature most likely reflective of reduced therapies (Schippa et al., 2013). It is hypothesized that imbalance of the intestinal microbiota of CF patients may be associated with causes, or aids, the progression of the disease and may be a predictor of expected outcomes after antibiotic therapy (Duytschaever et al., 2011).

ANTIBIOTICS USE AMONG PERSONS WITH CYSTIC FIBROSIS

Antibiotic regimens for CF patients currently follow one of the following strategies: a symptomatic regimen that is treatment of pulmonary exacerbation upon notice of acute symptoms (Elphick and Tan, 2005) or elective regimens that may comprise treatment of the chronic infection with intravenous, inhaled, and/or oral antibiotics at regular intervals to delay or prevent long-term deterioration in the absence of recent clinical deterioration (Høiby, 1993; Moskowitz et al., 2008). The latter elective regimens constitute chronic antibiotic usage or prophylaxis and have become routine practice to prevent or delay pulmonary exacerbations. CF patients typically undergo antibiotic treatment involving a combination of inhaled and oral therapies as well as potentially intravenous treatments from different mechanistic classes (eg, ceftazidime and tobramycin; Smyth et al., 2014; Flume et al., 2009). With the advent of efficient nebulization devices in the 1990s, inhaled antibiotics became the mainstay in CF therapy maintenance, enabling eradication of initial *Pseudomonas* infection (Ramsey et al., 1999; Pamukcu et al., 1995; Wall et al., 1983; Moskowitz et al., 2008; Gibson et al., 2003). Inhaled antibiotics result in greater concentrations arriving directly to the respiratory system secretions, local to the infection (Moskowitz et al., 2008). Nebulized/inhaled tobramycin, aztreonam, and colistin form the main therapeutic options for eradication and/or suppression of *Pseudomonas aeruginosa* in the lung (Döring et al., 2012). Nebulization duration is associated with a significant treatment burden on the patient and may result in poorer clinical outcomes because of reduced compliance with the treatment regimen (Sawicki and Tiddens, 2012). Advances in addressing patient treatment burden are seen with the emergence of portable dry powder formulations of tobramycin (TOBI podhaler) and colistimethate sodium (Colobreathe; Konstan et al., 2011; Schuster et al., 2013; Uttley et al., 2013). Rapid delivery systems for antibiotic therapies via portable inhalers significantly reduce treatment burden and increase adherence (Harrison et al., 2014).

The success of a particular antibiotic treatment regimen is assessed primarily by considering its efficacy at suppression or eradication of the infectious agents and subsequent improvement in lung function, measured as FEV_1 (Forced Expiratory

Volume in the first second). In addition to the need for hospitalization, the length of time until the requirement for additional antibiotics, the time to reoccurrence of pulmonary exacerbation, the number and severity of adverse events experienced by patients, and the convenience and patient satisfaction (hence ease of compliance) for the patient are factors considered.

THE MODULATORY EFFECTS OF SPECIFIC ANTIBIOTICS ON THE GUT MICROBIOTA (NON-CYSTIC FIBROSIS HOSTS)

The human gut microbiota is individual specific at the bacterial strain level (Turnbaugh and Gordon, 2009; Lozupone et al., 2012; Schloissnig et al., 2013). How antibiotic therapies interact and perturb the microbiota varies between individuals, with individuals on the same antibiotic, dose, and time showing varying effects, albeit similar trends (Perez-Cobas et al., 2013). Dethlefsen et al. (2008) showed not only interindividual variation in response to ciprofloxacin but also different responses of taxa. Grouping of metagenomic data from several individuals may mask individual perturbations. Therefore it is preferable to measure distance from baseline in each individual to reveal the true effect of the antibiotic treatment (Engelbrektson et al., 2006). Diet, genetics, and health status as well as the dynamics of the microbiota itself may contribute to stability within the intestinal microbiota, enabling some communities to have more resilience than others in response to antibiotic therapy (Perez-Cobas et al., 2013). This elaborate network fed by numerous variables presents a huge challenge when analyzing microbiota responses to antibiotic treatment. Countering the effect of the antibiotic is the resilience and stability of the microbiota. The balance of the microbiota to external pressures is mediated by host–microbe interactions, microbe–microbe interactions, and physiochemical factors (Edlund et al., 2000).

The effects of antibiotics on the gut microbiome are unique to each antibiotic and depend on several factors: the target spectra, the dose and duration, the method of administration and the pharmacokinetic and pharmacodynamic properties of the agent (incomplete absorption or secretion of intravenous antibiotics by bile or intestinal mucosa may result in higher concentrations in the intestine with greater ecological effects; Edlund et al., 2000; Jernberg et al., 2010; Adamsson et al., 1999). Disturbances may be assessed (1) qualitatively (emergence of novel bacteria types with resistance genes, plasmids, and transposons) or (2) quantitatively (changes in microbiota composition due to antibiotic pressures; Edlund et al., 2000). Broad-spectrum antibiotic treatments affect not only the aberrant pathogenic bacteria but also beneficial members of the gut community, reduce diversity and richness, and disturb the ecology of the gut (Jernberg et al., 2007; Dethlefsen and Relman, 2011; O' Sullivan et al., 2012). However, it remains a challenge to distinguish antibiotic effects on the gut microbiota from other confounding factors such as stress, diet and host genetics (Jernberg et al., 2010). The route of administration has implications for antibiotic-mediated disturbances in the gut microbiota because oral, inhaled and intravenous routes result in different concentrations in different sites (Liu and Derendorf, 2003; Liu et al., 2002).

The gut microbiota has a degree of resilience to antibiotic treatment, the strength of which may vary depending on which microorganisms form a given individual's microbiota, some conferring more stability than others. Recovery of gut microbiota is often rapid, ranging from 2 days (Dethlefsen and Relman, 2011) to 2 weeks (Ubeda et al., 2010); however, individual taxa have different recovery rates, some slower than others as seen with increased proportions of Lachnospiracaea and Clostridiacaea by Antonopoulos and colleagues (2009) 6 weeks posttreatment with cefoperazone. For many, recovery is often incomplete or partial (Dethlefsen and Relman, 2011). This resilience may be apparent in the first round of therapy, and it is in subsequent, repetitive or prolonged rounds of therapy that shifts in the microbiota may be seen (Perez-Cobas et al., 2013). The magnitude and rate of the response is primarily dictated by the initial microbial community, with some communities displaying a prolonged directional shift and others a more rapid response (Dethlefsen and Relman, 2011). Initial community composition could be an important indication of expected outcomes after antibiotic use, such as likelihood of pathogen overgrowth or development of antibiotic-associated diarrhea (AAD; De La Cochetiere et al., 2008; Ozaki et al., 2004). Although the gut microbiota is stable, it is never static. Its periodic variations within a normal range make it difficult to definitively attribute loss or gain of certain taxa to certain antibiotics. Dethlefsen and Relman (2011) explain that the long-term stability of the gut microbiota is maintained by restoring forces after external disturbances rather than rigidity or resistance to change. However, the restoring forces will not withstand repeated antibiotic courses, even in cases in which the microbiota has completely recovered after an initial antibiotic treatment.

Antibiotics families vary in mode of action and target specificity and therefore in the fingerprint they leave on the gut microbiota. Perez-Cobas et al. (2013) showed that the greatest influence on the microbiota is the antimicrobial effect and the mode of antibiotic action. At the compositional level, the mode of action exerts the greatest effect, although at the functional level the antimicrobial effect is the driving force (Perez-Cobas et al., 2013). The mode of action of the antimicrobial agent produces different effects on the gut community. O'Sullivan et al. (2013) noted a significantly greater reduction of *Bifidobacterium* species and significant differences in levels of *Anaerococcus*, *Denitrobacterium*, *Faecalibacterium*, *Lactonifactor*, and *Proteus* species in subjects receiving only a nucleic acid inhibitor compared with subjects on antibiotics with cell envelope mode of action, whereas subjects receiving only cell envelope antibiotics had significantly increased levels (10-fold) of *Lactobacillus* species and significant differences in levels of *Ascomycota* and *Elusimicrobia*. They concluded that cell envelope inhibitors had less impact on the intestinal microbiota than nucleic acid synthesis inhibitors. The effects are taxa specific with some more susceptible than others; however, signatures of antimicrobial classes can be seen in bacterial profiles after treatment, with individuals' diverse microbiota converging to similar compositions when administered the same antibiotic (Perez-Cobas et al., 2013; Jernberg et al., 2010; Antonopoulos et al., 2009). The selection of antibiotic should be based not only on the expected success of the antibiotic treatment but also on the level of ecological disturbances (Edlund et al., 2000). There is a lack of information detailing the effects of chronic usage of different antibiotic classes on the gut micro-biota. Here we discuss the signatures produced by short-term use of different antibi-otic classes, as shown in human studies, unless stated otherwise. See Table 11.1 for a summary of the effects of specific antibiotic classes on the intestinal microbiota.

Macrolides

Macrolides are so called because of their macrocyclic ring, which may be 14, 15, or 16 membered (Hamilton-Miller, 1992). They have a protein synthesis inhibitory mode of action. Macrolides have been shown to inhibit protein synthesis by caus-ing a dissociation of the peptidyl-tRNA from the ribosome (Tenson et al., 2003). Azithromycin has been shown to significantly improve quality of life in CF patients, reduce C-reactive protein levels, reduce the rate of lung function decline (FEV$_1$ mea-surements), reduce the number of respiratory exacerbations, and significantly reduce systemic inflammation (Saiman et al., 2003; Wolter et al., 2002). Azithromycin is chosen for macrolide therapy over other macrolides, such as erythromycin, because of less adverse effects on the gastrointestinal tract. Azithromycin is also known to have negative effects on the bacterial motility of *P. aeruginosa* through suppression of flagellin expression at subinhibitory concentrations (Kawamura-Sato et al., 2000). In a study of three adults presenting with gastric and duodenal ulcers, Jakobsson et al. (2010) showed the negative impact of Clarithromycin on members of the Acti-nobacteria phyla; significant reductions of *Escherichia coli*; suppression of *Bifido-bacterium*, *Lactobacillus*, and *Clostridium* species; and an increase in *Enterococcus*, *Enterobacter*, *Citrobacter*, *Klebsiella*, and *Pseudomonas* species. Clarithromycin has been shown to strongly suppress anaerobic populations in a study of healthy adults comparing Clarithromycin to a fluoroquinolone, moxifloxacin-based treat-ment regimen (Adamsson et al., 1999; Brismar et al., 1991; Edlund et al., 2000). This has important implications for total ecological disturbances because the anaero-bic population is mainly responsible for colonization resistance (Waaij, 1989; Hertz et al., 2014). Adamsson et al. (1999) also showed a significant qualitative change with an increase of resistant *Bacteroides* from 2% to 76% in a study of 30 adults with *Helicobacter pylori* infection. This indicates an antibiotic class with the ability for ecological disruption and promotion of resistant strains. This contrasts with the findings of Morotomi et al. (2011), which show that macrolide antibiotic treatments tended toward dominance of *Streptococcus* species and seemed to have less dramatic effects on the microbiota with samples remaining similar to healthy intestinal micro-biota in a study of 29 healthy adults (Morotomi et al., 2011).

β-Lactams

β-Lactams, encompassing cephalosporins, carbapenems, penicillins, monobactams, and cephamycins, are considered the most successful antibiotic class discovered (Lewis, 2013). β-Lactams form an important part of treatment of pulmonary exac-erbation for CF patients. Ceftazidime, meropenem, flucloxacillin, piperacillin/taxo-bactam, and aztreonam are all β-lactam therapies commonly used by CF patients. β-Lactams have a bactericidal mode of action that disrupts cell wall synthesis,

Table 11.1 Summary of the Effects of Specific Antibiotic Classes on the Intestinal Microbiota

Antibiotic Class	Specific Antibiotic Examples	Mode of Action	Gut Microbiota Effects	References
Aminoglycosides	Tobramycin	Bactericidal agents that inhibit protein synthesis by binding the 30S prokaryotic subunit.	Little in literature. Bifidobacteria are known to have innate resistance due to lack of cytochrome-mediated transport mechanism for aminoglycoside uptake.	Bryan et al. (1979)
Macrolides	Azithromycin, erythromycin, clarithromycin	Protein synthesis inhibitory mode of action by initiating a dissociation of the peptidyl-tRNA from the ribosome.	Clarithromycin has been shown to reduce Actinobacteria phyla, E. coli, bifidobacteria, lactobacilli, clostridia, and anaerobic populations and increase enterococci, Enterobacter, Citrobacter, Klebsiella, Pseudomonas, and resistant Bacteroides.	Jakobsson et al. (2010) Adamsson et al. (1999) Brismar et al. (1991) Edlund et al. (2000)
β-Lactams	Penicillin, ceftazidime, meropenem, flucloxacillin, coamoxiclav, piperacillin/ tazobactam, aztreonam	Bactericidal mode of action, disrupting cell wall synthesis, specifically in the final cross-linking stage of the peptidoglycan layer.	Increase of Bacteroides, Blautia, Faecalibacterium, Parabacteroides—most probably due to high rate of resistance in these genera. Significant reduction of anaerobic population.	Perez-Cobas et al. (2013) Monreal et al. (2005) Morotomi et al. (2011) Adamsson et al. (1999)
Lincosamides	Clindamycin	Bacteriostatic antimicrobial effect and protein synthesis mode of action.	Decreases in Bacteroides and Blautia. Increase in Enterobacteriaceae.	Perez-Cobas et al. (2013)
Fluoroquinolones	Moxifloxacin, ciprofloxacin	Inhibition of DNA gyrase and topoisomerase IV. Fluoroquinolones sequester these enzymes into a drug/enzyme/DNA complex that holds double-stranded DNA breaks together, blocking replication.	Decrease in Faecalibacterium, Bacteroides, enterococci, enterobacteria. Clostridia, Bifidobacteria, Lachnospiraceae, Ruminococcaceae, and Enterobacteriaceae.	Perez-Cobas et al. (2013) Dethlefsen and Relman (2011) Edlund et al. (2000)

Table 11.1 Summary of the Effects of Specific Antibiotic Classes on the Intestinal Microbiota—cont'd

Antibiotic Class	Specific Antibiotic Examples	Mode of Action	Gut Microbiota Effects	References
Polymyxins	Colistin sulfomethate	Induces changes to the permeability of the cell wall by binding anionic lipopolysaccharide molecules and displacing calcium and magnesium, leading to cell leakage and death.	Orally administered colistin is poorly absorbed in the gut; therefore it has little effect on the intestinal microbiota.	WHO (2006)
Nitroimidazoles	Metronidazole	Entering cell in inactive state, becoming activated in the bacterial cytoplasm through electron transfer of the nitro group of the drug to a cytotoxic state with DNA-binding capabilities.	Active against anaerobic bacteria. Decreases in Firmicutes and Bacteroidetes and increases in Enterobacteriaceae. Metronidazole concentration appears low in feces; therefore intestinal microbiota effects are minimal.	Rea et al. (2010) Sullivan et al. (2001)
Glycopeptides	Vancomycin	Interferes with glycosylation of the assembled peptidoglycan polymer after transport to the cell membrane.	Loss of *C. leptum*, *C. coccoides*, *C. symbiosum*, *P. luminescens*. Decrease in Firmicutes, Bacteroidetes, Clostridiaceae, Bacteroidaceae, Porphyromonadaceae, *Clostridium*, and *Odoribacter*. Increase in Proteobacteria, Enterobacteriaceae, Streptococcaceae, *Lactococcus*, *Sutterella*, and *Desulfovibrio*.	Rea et al. (2011) Yap et al. (2008) Murphy et al. (2013)

specifically the final cross-linking stage of the peptidoglycan layer (Page, 2012; Tipper, 1979; Strominger and Tipper, 1965). β-Lactams demonstrate broad-range activity against gram-negative and gram-positive bacteria (Holten and Onusko, 2000). Discovered in 1928 by Alexander Fleming, in 1940 penicillin was the first antibiotic to be produced in a large scale and is accredited with having saved millions of wounded during World War II. However, before its discovery the first β-lactamase was identified in 1940 in *E. coli* (Abraham and Chain, 1940), which was countered by the first β-lactamase inhibitor (clavulanic acid) in 1976. Clavulanic acid, along with amoxicillin, now forms part of Augmentin (Foulstone and Reading, 1982). After the first β-lactamase there have been many challenges to the success of β-lactams. Carbapenemases, classified as either molecular class B (metallo-β-lactamases), A, or D (serine carbapenemases, also known as oxacillinases) form three of the four known classes of β-lactamases (Miriagou et al., 2010). The host of specific carbapenemases varies depending on class. Metallo-β-lactamases are disseminated mainly in *P. aeruginosa*, but also *Acinetobacter baumanii, Enterobaceriaceae*, and *Klebsiella pneumonia* (Queenan and Bush, 2007, Walsh, 2008). *K. pneumonia* is the most common host of class A carbapenems (Queenan and Bush, 2007), although there have been reports of its occurrence in other species such as *Klebsiella oxytoca, Salmonella enterica, E. coli, Enterobacter* species, and *Pseudomonas* species (Queenan and Bush, 2007, Deshpande et al., 2006; Navon-Venezia et al., 2006; Villegas et al., 2007; Bennett et al., 2009). Oxacillinases (class D) are common in *A. baumanii* (Queenan and Bush, 2007). Most recently, the emergence of New Delhi metallo-β-lactamase-1 in 2008, which has since spread worldwide, has transformed mildly pathogenic bacteria into lethal MDR bacteria (Rolain et al., 2010). The prevalence of metallo-β-lactamases in *P. aeruginosa* is of significant clinical concern given the importance of *P. aeruginosa* in CF lung exacerbations. Metallo-β-lactamase–producing *P. aeruginosa* have shown an increase in the last 10 years and have been implicated in septicemia and pneumonia (Kouda et al., 2009; Gutiérrez et al., 2007; Pitout et al., 2007; Lagatolla et al., 2006). Extended spectrum β-lactamases (ESBLs) present another challenge to the treatment of gram-negative infections and are the main source of hospital- and community-acquired infections (Pitout and Laupland, 2008). Mainly arising in Enterobacteriaceae such as *E. coli* and *Klebsiella* species, ESBLs have plasmid encoded capability of hydrolyzing the β-lactam ring of the oxy-imino-cephalosporins (cefotaxime, ceftriaxone, and ceftazidime) and monobactams (aztreonam; Bush and Jacoby, 2010; Dortet et al., 2012). Cephamycins (cefoxitin) and carabapenems (imipenem and meropenem) retain their activity against ESBL-producing bacteria. Reassuringly, in some cases β-lactamase inhibitors such as clavulanic acid and tazobactam still have the ability to inhibit ESBLs (Bush and Jacoby, 2010).

Bacteroides, Blautia, and Faecalibacterium species have been shown to increase in a study of four adults after a single antibiotic treatment with β-lactams such as ampicillin, amoxicillin, cefazolin, and sulbactam (Perez-Cobas et al., 2013; Monreal et al., 2005). This bacterial profile has been shown to be associated with bactericidal agents but not bacteriostatic antimicrobials. The increase seen in the *Bacteroides* and *Parabacteroides* species may be explained by the presence of a high rate of β-lactamase-producing strains observed in these genera. In addition, high levels of *cfiA* gene identified suggest these strains act as reservoirs for antibiotic resistance genes and the common occurrence of *cepA* gene, which is responsible for production of cephalosporinases and penicillinases (Nakano et al., 2011; Wybo et al., 2007). Morotomi et al. (2011) also reported a dominance of *Enterococcus* genus after a single β-lactam antibiotic treatment. Adamsson et al. (1999) show that compared with a macrolide treatment (clarithromycin), a β-lactam treatment showed reduced, although still significant, ecological impact on the anaerobic populations and less emergence of resistant strains after treatment. The reduced disruption to anaerobic populations was also noted by Stark et al. (1993). In addition, Perez-Cobas et al. (2013) have demonstrated the metabolic effects of β-lactams in the alteration of bile acids, cholesterol, and hormones by intestinal bacteria. They showed a higher expression of genes related to energy metabolism during β-lactam treatment. This supports the hypothesis that long-term use of antibiotics undermines host-microbe mutualistic relationships.

Lincosamides

Clindamycin is a class of lincosamide antibiotics used to treat mainly anaerobic infections (Hedberg and Nord, 2002) with a bacteriostatic antimicrobial effect and a protein synthesis inhibitor mode of action. Resistance to clindamycin has increased significantly over the last two decades. Perez-Cobas et al. (2013) observed marked decreases in *Bacteroides* and *Blautia* genera immediately after administration; however, after 3 days a recovery of *Bacteroides* was observed, suggesting acquisition of resistance genes by these bacteria. They also noted that clindamycin induced an increase in Enterobacteriaceae compensating for loss of anaerobic bacteria. In comparison with other agents (fluoroquinolone or β-lactams) clindamycin was shown to result in a more variable and stronger effect on microbial community structure. Clindamycin has been shown to result in an increase in abundance of resistance genes, relative to other antibiotics such as moxifloxacin, amoxicillin, and cefazolin/ampicillin/sulbactam combination, mostly of the efflux pump class (Perez-Cobas et al., 2013).

Fluoroquinolones

Fluoroquinolones inhibit bacterial cell proliferation by inhibiting DNA gyrase and topoisomerase IV, both essential enzymes in bacterial DNA transcription and replication (Hooper, 2001). In addition to inhibiting these two enzymes, fluoroquinolones sequester these enzymes into a drug/enzyme/DNA complex that holds double-stranded DNA breaks together, blocking replication (Drlica, 1999). Treatment with different antibiotics from the fluoroquinolone class presents a similar initial response in the gut microbiota. Moxifloxacin showed a decrease in *Faecalibacterium* and *Bacteroides*, with ciprofloxacin showing similar effects with additional decreases seen in Lachnospiraceae and Ruminococcaceae (Perez-Cobas et al., 2013; Dethlefsen and Relman, 2011). Earlier fluoroquinolones such as ciprofloxacin, levofloxacin, norofloxacin, and orofloxacin target aerobic bacteria, mainly gram negatives, but similar to moxifloxacin, a methoxyquinolone, they result in a reduction in numbers of Enterobacteriaceae. Moxifloxacin has a wider reaching activity than the others with activity against respiratory pathogens, including β-lactamase–producing aerobic gram-positive cocci; *Haemophilus* and *Moraxella*; aerobic gram negatives; and intracellular and atypical microorganism such as *Legionella*, *Chlamydia*, and *Mycobacterium*. Moxifloxacin also has activity against gram-positive and gram-negative anaerobes. In a study looking at the effects of repeated courses of oral ciprofloxacin (500 mg twice daily for 5 days at 2- and 8-month time points in a 10-month study) and the disturbance to the gut microbiota in three subjects, Dethlefsen and Relman (2011) showed an almost complete return to the pre-ciprofloxacin state after the first treatment; however, after a second treatment the microbiota community composition was different from what it had been at the start of the study and appeared to be stable in its new state. Edlund et al. (2000) also showed significant decreases of enterococci, enterobacteria, bifidobacteria, and clostridia during moxifloxacin treatment (400 mg oral administration once daily for 7 days).

An interesting feature of fluoroquinolones is their ability to bind reversibly to bacteria and fecal material, resulting in reduced amounts of the drug in the intestine, translating to less disturbance of the total microbial intestinal population by fluoroquinolones (Edlund et al., 2000; Lidbeck et al., 1988). Because of this, moxifloxacin has a more targeted effect on the gut microbiota with more limited ecological disturbances (Edlund et al., 2000).

Polmyxins

Colistin sulfomethate is cyclopeptide, belonging to the family of polymyxins, which is produced by *Bacillus polymyxa* var. *colistinus* (Jeong et al., 2009; Storm et al., 1977). Colistin is mainly active against gram-negative organisms. Its mode of action involves inducing changes in the permeability of the cell wall by binding anionic lipopolysaccharide molecules and displacing calcium and magnesium, thus causing cell leakage and death (Jeong et al., 2009). Orally administered colistin is known to be poorly absorbed in the gastrointestinal tract, and studies show that when excreted it is bound to the fecal material (Eichenwald and McCracken, 1978). This may reduce the perturbation effect of the drug in vivo. Jeong et al. (2009) show that *E. coli* was the most susceptible to colistin. Colistin sulfomethate is one of the most frequently used antibiotics for treatment of exacerbations in CF patients. Early eradication of *Pseudomonas* infection with nebulized drug, aggressive treatment of acute exacerbations with intravenous therapy, and long-term suppressive maintenance therapy again nebulized are the three primary modes of usage in CF management. Colistin forms part of each of these (Littlewood et al., 2000). *P. aeruginosa* is known to frequently develop resistance to β-lactam antibiotics and aminoglycosides. However, thus far in vitro resistance of *Pseudomonas* species to colistin is rare, cementing its place as a useful treatment for pseudomonal infections for the foreseeable future. Wright et al. (2013) have shown using in vitro culture methods that antibiotics (ceftazadime, colistin, azithromycin, and tobramycin) at subinhibitory concentrations result in the phenotypic population diversification of *P. aeruginosa*. It is interesting to note that they demonstrated that ceftazadime and colistin contributed to more diversification than tobramycin and azithromycin. Diversification of the *P. aeruginosa* populations in the CF lung negatively affect antibiotic therapy success, leading to a chronic infection state and ultimately to progression of the disease. Whether this diversification pressure is also exerted on taxa in the gut has not been reported. Knowledge of differential diversification potential of antibiotics can contribute to more informed decisions for antibiotic selection in management and control of infection.

Nitrimidazoles

Metronidazole is the prototype of the nitroimidazole family and most widely used for treatment of anaerobic and protozoal infections (Lamp et al., 1999). Along with fidomoxacin and vancomycin, metronidazole is the mainstay of *C. difficile* treatment (Surawicz et al., 2013; Cornely et al., 2014), estimated to have colonized up to 50% of CF patients (Binkovitz et al., 1999; Bauer et al., 2014). Metronidazole is known to have activity against gram-negative (*Bacteroides fragilis*) and gram-positive (*C. difficile*) anaerobes (Lofmark et al., 2010). Metronidazole functions by entering the cell in its inactive or prodrug state, becoming activated in the bacterial cytoplasm through an electron transfer to the nitro group of the drug, or protozoa organelles, to a cytotoxic state with DNA-binding capabilities. Inhibition of DNA synthesis and DNA damage by oxidation leads to DNA degradation and cell death (Land and Johnson, 1999; Diniz et al., 2000; Lofmark et al., 2010). Its activity is limited to anaerobic bacteria because aerobes lack the appropriate transfer proteins, conferring them with intrinsic resistance to metronidazole (Reysset, 1996). Mechanisms of resistance to metronidazole are primarily based on either decreased uptake of the prodrug or reduced electron transfer capabilities (Land and Johnson, 1999). Nitroimidazole (*nim*) resistance genes encode an alternative reductase protein that converts nitroimidazole to a nontoxic derivative, thus avoiding DNA damage (Reysset, 1996; Leiros et al., 2004; Lofmark et al., 2010). Metronidazole resistance is generally low, although there have been reports of resistance in *Sutterella* species (Jousimies-Somer et al., 2002). *C. difficile* maintains its susceptibility to metronidazole with no significant clinical resistance observed (Lofmark et al., 2010; Terhes et al., 2014). In a study using high-throughput sequencing, Rea et al. (2011) demonstrated phylum (reduction of Firmicutes and Bacteriodetes and increase of Proteobacteria) and family (increasing Enterobacteriaceae) effects of administering metronidazole in a colonic model experiment. The concentration of metronidazole in feces is low as a result of efficient absorption; therefore alterations to the normal microbiota after metronidazole treatment are minimal (Sullivan et al., 2001). Nagy and Foldes (1991) propose a mechanism of inactivation of metronidazole by intestinal enterococci, thus reducing its effect on the gastrointestinal microbiota. The success of oral metronidazole in *Clostridium difficile* infection (CDI) treatment is a result of the elevated plasma serum levels that diffuse through the damaged intestinal mucosa of infected individuals with greater efficiency (Sullivan et al., 2001).

Glycopeptides

Glycopeptide antibiotics have an inhibitory mode of action on late-stage peptido-glycan polymer synthesis. Glycopeptide antibiotics interfere with glycosylation of the assembled peptidoglycan polymer after transport to the cell membrane (Reynolds, 1989). Vancomycin, teicoplanin, and most recently telvancin are the only glycopeptide antibiotics approved by the US Food and Drug Administration (FDA; Van Bambeke et al., 2004, Damodaran and Madhan, 2011). Glycopeptides are active against most gram-positive organisms but few gram-negative organisms. Vancomy-cin remains the first-line drug against methicillin-resistant *Staphylococcus aureus* (MRSA); however, emergence of resistance in enterococci and staphylococci has led to a restriction in the use of vancomycin as well as teicoplanin (Van Bambeke et al., 2004; Damodaran and Madhan, 2011). Yap and colleagues showed the dis-turbance effect of vancomycin on the gut microbiota in mice using a 2×100 mg/kg per day dose for 2 days. *Clostridium leptum*, *Clostridium coccoides*, *Cenarchaeum symbiosum*, and *Photorhabdus luminescens* were lost immediately after treatment, with subsequent rapid recovery of *C. leptum* and *C. coccoides*. In an environmentally controlled 24-h model distal colonic experiment, Rea et al. (2011) showed a decrease in the major phyla, Firmicutes and Bacteroidetes, and an increase in Proteobacteria after addition of $90 \mu M$ vancomycin at eight hourly intervals. The rapid proliferation of Enterobacteriaceae at the expense of other gram negatives and Firmicutes dur-ing vancomycin treatment is reported (Rea et al., 2011; Yap et al., 2008). In a diet-induced obesity mouse model administering 2 mg/day vancomycin for 20 weeks, Murphy et al. (2013) attributed the decrease in Firmicutes and Bacteroidetes at the phylum level to a decrease in Clostridaceae and Bacteroidaceae at the family level, respectively, and increasing Proteobacteriaceae was attributed to increasing Entero-bacteriaceae. At the family level they also noted decreases in Porphyromonadaeae and increases in Streptococcaceae and Desulfovibrionaceae, whereas at the genus level increases in *Lactococcus*, *Sutterella*, and *Desulfovibrio* and decreases in *Clos-tridium* and *Odoribacter* were observed.

Effects of Combination Therapy on Gut Microbiota

Combination or multidrug therapy often confers advantages over single drug therapy in terms of a wider range of targets, synergistic effects, reduction of MDR organisms, and reduction in total amount of antibiotic used; however, it incurs high costs, compli-cations for administration, and drug-related toxicity (Elphick and Tan, 2005; Perron et al., 2012; Gould and van der Meer, 2007). Taylor et al. (1993) reported that 80% of clinics had preference for combination therapy. Combinational antibiotic therapy poses challenges to identifying, quantifying, and comparing the specific effects of anti-biotic classes on the gut microbiota. At present, treatment of *P. aeruginosa* infection in patients with CF involves two to three antibiotics, demonstrating improved synergy (Zebouh et al., 2008; Hewer and Smyth, 2014). In general, this may include the use of inhaled antibiotics such as tobramycin and colistin (Littlewood and Macdonald, 1987, Ratjen et al., 2001), oral quinolones such as ciprofloxacin (Taccetti et al., 2005), and intravenous antibiotics usually involving a β-lactam antibiotic in combination with an aminoglycoside antibiotic (Döring et al., 2000, Hewer and Smyth, 2014). Combination therapies are a commonly used approach for biofilm management, with the rationale that multiple antibiotics, with a range of individual targets can combine to help suppress or eradicate the varying antagonistic phenotypes present in the biofilm (Barraud et al., 2013). Colistin is known to be active against bacterial cells with low metabolic activity whereas tetracycline and ciprofloxacin are known to be active against metabolically active cells (Pamp et al., 2008; Herrman et al., 2010).

Conclusive results yielding specific guidelines for treatment of pulmonary exacerbations and delaying chronic *P. aeruginosa* infection in CF patients have yet to be reached on whether combinational or monotherapy is more effective because of a lack of studies testing combinational therapy options versus monotherapy in a head-to-head manner with control for confounding factors. Of the studies available, it is difficult to unequivocally indicate which is the most effective because studies differ in length of administration of antibiotic, age, health status and history of patient cohort; differing times from detection to initiation of treatment; frequency of surveillance; markers of success; and statistical analysis. However, the current physician consensus infers a preference for combinational therapy for patients with CF (Elphick and Tan, 2005).

LONG-TERM ISSUES OF CHRONIC ANTIBIOTIC USE
MULTIDRUG RESISTANCE

Almost immediately after the introduction of the first antibiotics, a parallel emergence of resistance has inhibited their success (Davies and Davies, 2010). Most recently, a World Health Organization report on antimicrobial resistance (AMR) (2014) warns of the dangers of entering a postantibiotic era in which minor infections could emerge as life threatening diseases in the face of an AMR pandemic. MDR is a major public health issue facing the medical and wider community (Laxminarayan et al., 2013). In the European Union (EU), AMR is estimated to be responsible for 25,000 deaths each year, whereas health-care–related costs are estimated to be €0.9 billion with a further €1.5 billion expenditure on productivity losses (Rodier, 2011; Report EEJT, 2009). MDR is compromising our ability to manage infectious disease. Well-documented MDR organisms include *P. aeruginosa* and *Burkholderia cepacia* complex, as well as emerging methicillin-resistant *Stenotrophmonas maltophilia* and MRSA. MDR was responsible for 23,000 deaths in the United States in 2013, of which MRSA and *Streptococcus pneumoniae* were responsible for 11,000 and 7000 deaths, respectively (CDC, 2013). Antibiotic overuse and misuse is the driving force of the development of resistant organisms (Laxminarayan and Heymann, 2012). An empirical strategy of treatment based on expert consensus remains the mode of action on diagnosis of pulmonary exacerbation. This generalized treatment strategy inevitably contributes to the adverse effects of antibiotic overuse in terms of dose and time. This is compounded by the increase in age of the CF demographic

(Waters and Ratjen, 2006) globally (CFRI Annual report 2011; Davis, 2006; www. cff.org), with the ratio of adult CF patients to pediatrics increasing each year.

The human gastrointestinal tract is an environment where 10^{13}–10^{14} microorganisms are in constant interaction, providing an ideal situation for rapid dissemination of resistance genes between commensals and pathogens (Salyers et al., 2004; Davies, 1994). The human gut microbiota is now viewed as a reservoir where commensals and pathogens are in direct contact, thus facilitating the spread of resistance genes (Salyers et al., 2004; Sommer et al., 2009; Fouhy et al., 2014). Studies have established that the gut resistome is established in infancy, even in the absence of antibiotic therapy, growing and diversifying with age (Fouhy et al., 2014). In response to antibiotic therapy, resistance genes are expressed and selected, with strains carrying resistance proliferating, amplifying the resistance reservoir (Lu et al., 2014; Fouhy et al., 2014). In CF patients, or other groups on chronic antibiotic therapy, the resistome is likely to have increased capabilities. Whole genome sequencing has shown that lateral gene transfer and mobilizable elements that incorporate into various host bacteria are responsible for most resistance (Ochman et al., 2000). Transferable resistance genes may arise in commensals and through lateral gene transfer mechanisms spread to clinically relevant pathogenic strains. It is postulated that the gut microbiome may facilitate the acquisition of resistance by pathogenic strains (Sommer et al., 2009). Sommer et al. (2009) used a functional metagenomic approach to characterize the antibiotic resistome of two healthy unrelated humans who had not been treated with antibiotics for a least 1 year. Phylogenetic profiling of aerobically cultured strains from the gut microbiome showed they were primarily members of the Proteobacteria phyla and to a lesser extent Firmicutes and Actinobacteria. Resistance genes belonging to one of the following classes—tetracycline efflux pumps, two classes of aminoglycoside-modifying enzymes, and three classes of β-lactam–inactivating enzymes (TEM, AmpC, and CTX-M)—were detected. Characterizing the human gut resistome may increase understanding of the origin of the antibiotic resistance, ultimately addressing the MDR issue.

The expression and subsequent persistence of resistance genes ensuing antibiotic treatment varies depending on antibiotic class, duration, and dose strength of treatment. Persistence of resistance may be observed years after an antibiotic course. For instance, after a 5-day antibiotic treatment (500 mg twice daily) with ciprofloxacin, initial gut microbiota perturbations recover; however, resistance to the particular antibiotic is enriched and may be observed for months or even years afterwards (Dethlefsen et al., 2008). Likewise, Sjölund et al. (2003) showed that in three of five patients post-clarithromycin treatment, erythromycin resistance was present after 1 year and in one patient after 3 years. Jernberg et al. (2007) also showed the persistence of resistance genes (*ermF*, *ermG*, and *ermB*) after clindamycin treatment up to 2 years after a 7-day antibiotic treatment. Shoemaker et al. (2001) demonstrated that the presence of the *tetQ* gene has increased from 30% to 80% in all strains of *Bacteroides* as a result of conjugal gene transfer in the last three decades.

Some genera may contribute to multidrug resistance more than others by acting as a reservoir for mobilizable resistance determinants. *Bacteroides* and *Parabacteroides* species are mutualistic inhabitants of the gut performing many beneficial functions for the host, such as carbohydrate metabolism (Xu et al., 2003). *Bacteroides* form 25% of the adult human gut microbiota (Salyers, 1984) and have been implicated in many opportunistic infections, particularly *B. fragilis* (Wexler, 2007; Cao et al., 2014). They have an innate ability to produce β-lactamases such as cephalosporinases and penicillinases encoded by the *cepA* gene (Gutacker et al., 2000). Clindamycin resistance, encoded by the *ermF*, *ermB* or *ermG* genes or through efflux pumps, in *Bacteriodales* ranges from 10% to 42% and confers protection against macrolides, lincosamides, and stretogramin B (Wybo et al., 2007; Gupta et al., 2003; Nakano et al., 2011; Shoemaker et al., 2001; Pumbwe et al., 2007). In a study by Nakano and colleagues (2011), 53.5% of tested *Bacteroides* and *Parabacteroides* strains were tetracycline resistant, primarily because of the acquisition of the *tetQ* ribosome protection protein. The rise of resistance genes in predominating and functionally vital genera of the human gastrointestinal tract provide pathogens with increased opportunity for acquisition of many resistance determinants.

AMR rates are increasing and studies such as the SMART (Study for Monitoring Antimicrobial Resistance Trends), PROTEKT (Prospective Resistant Organism Tracking and Epidemiology for the Ketolide Telithromycin), and SENTRY (an international, longitudinal study on the susceptibility of pathogens sponsored by Bristol Meyers Squibb) seek to globally monitor and characterize AMR rates (Morrissey et al., 2013). The SMART study describes the increase in prevalence of ESBLs, conferring resistance to β-lactams, in Asia, Europe, Latin America, Middle East, North America, and the South Pacific. The study also reports the increasing resistance to fluoroquinolones, particularly in *P. aeruginosa* (increases from 22% to 33% were seen in North America). Macrolide resistance rates have also been shown to be increasing (Cresti et al., 2002). Recent studies have indicated this is due to the epidemic spread of *erm*B resistance genes among streptococcal populations and in particular *Streptococcus pyrogenes*, either by horizontal gene transfer or clonal expansion of resistant isolates after selective pressures of antibiotic treatment (Jakobsson et al., 2010). Sjölund et al. (2003) have reported the presence of macrolide-resistant enterococci after selection by clarithromycin and metronidazole.

Development of Opportunistic Pathogens and Antibiotic-Associated Diarrhea

Chronic antibiotic therapy results in significant alterations in the gut microbiota, creating opportunities for opportunistic pathogens, primarily *C. difficile*, to establish and proliferate. *C. difficile* is mostly a nosocomical infection of the elderly, but it can also be community acquired, affecting younger populations and adults. The CDC has linked *C. difficile* to 14,000 deaths in America (CDC, 2013). The European Center for Disease Control estimates that CDI costs the EU €3 billion per year (ECDC, 2015). Broad-spectrum antibiotic therapy has been associated with increased incidence of *C. difficile* and is identified as one of the most well-recognized risk factors for *C. difficile* and indeed recurrent and refractory CDI (Bartlett and Gerding, 2008; Diggs and Surawicz, 2009). Broad-spectrum antibiotics induce a dysbiotic gut microbiota, particularly among anaerobic populations, providing *C. difficile* with an opportunity to proliferate. Indeed, Owens et al. (2008) reported 94% of hospitalized patients with

CDI had received antibiotics before or during their hospital stay. *C. difficile* is responsible for 20–25% of AAD cases and 90–100% of pseudomembraneous colitis (Rea et al., 2010; Cramer et al., 2008). Ironically, antibiotic treatment of CDI perpetuates its proliferation, increasing strains resistant to vancomycin, particularly enterococci (Chang et al., 2008), lowering diversity and providing *C. difficile* with opportunity to proliferate. The association between ampicillin, cephalosporins, and fluoroquinolones and CDI is well recognized in the literature (Gerding, 2004; Sullivan et al., 2001). It is interesting to note that the emergence of particular antibiotics as risk factors for CDI has paralleled the frequency of that particular antibiotic class in general medical use. The increase of CDI was initially associated with clindamycin, which is the preferential treatment for various anaerobic, streptococcal, and *Staphylococcus* infections. Since the 1990s, the increase in the use of fluoroquinolones to treat various infections has precipitated these antibiotics in becoming risk factors for CDI and has contributed to the emergence of hypervirulent strains such as ribotype 027, which is characterized by fluoroquinolone resistance, binary toxin production, and increased toxin production due to a mutation in the *tcdC* gene (Pepin et al., 2005; Kuijper et al., 2008). Metronidazole and vancomycin have also been determined as risk factors for CDI. In cases in which antibiotics are necessary to treat concomitant infection, alternative antibiotics to those identified as CDI development risk factors should be used where possible. As expected, increased duration of antibiotic courses and antibiotic combination therapy are associated with increased risk of CDI (Owens et al., 2008). Not all antibiotics for CDI infection are associated with increased risk. Piperacillin in combination with tazobactam has shown considerable success in treatment of CDI but with less associated risk of increased development of infection or relapse (Owen et al., 2008). Vancomycin and, more recently, fidaxomicin (2011) are the only drugs approved by the FDA for CDI treatment. Fidaxomicin is particularly effective in treating recurrent CDI because it has less impact on the fecal microbiota, translating into a more resilient microbial assemblage after treatment. Fidaxomicin shows less risk of development of resistance than vancomycin in in vitro studies (Zar et al., 2007). Alternative therapies that may facilitate the reduction of antibiotics are necessary to treat CDI. These include fecal microbial transplant (FMT), which is an alternative therapy at conceptual stage with early pioneering case studies showing considerable success in patients with reoccurring symptomatic *C. difficile* (Petrof et al., 2013; Koenigsknecht and Young, 2013). Another alternative includes thuricin CD, a novel antimicrobial peptide (AMP) or bacteriocin produced by *Bacillus thuringiensis*, which has been patented as a CDI therapy (Rea et al., 2010). The potency of thuricin CD has been shown to be greater than vancomycin and in some cases greater than metronidazole. In addition, thuricin CD shows no antimicrobial activity against a range of commercially available probiotics, demonstrating its narrow substrate range (Rea et al., 2011).

Asymptomatic carriage of *C. difficile* in CF is well recognized; however, the mechanisms of protection against infection, but not colonization, are not fully understood. Carriage rates in healthy adults vary from 0% to 15% (Viscidi et al., 1981; Nakamura et al., 1981), compared with up to 50% in CF cohorts—a result of prophylaxis and frequent hospitalizations. However, unlike normal populations in which approximately 50% of colonized individuals develop CDI, or in more severe cases pseudomembranous colitis, development of response to *C. difficile* toxins is rare in CF patients (Kyne et al., 2000; Peach et al., 1986; Welkon et al., 1985). It is hypothesized that the unique microbial assemblage of CF patients with high levels of Enterbacteriaceae, lactobacilli, *Pseudomonas*, and *Staphylococcus* confers protection and resistance against *C. difficile* growth, but not colonization (Rolfe et al., 1981). Welkon et al. (1985) suggest an altered gut pH as a result of defective ion transport inhibits toxin production or degrades toxins, although there is no evidence to support this. Another possibility postulates that exposure to *C. difficile* at such an early age mediates an immune response that protects in later life (Welkon et al., 1985). The relatively low incidence of CDI despite high rates of toxigenic *C. difficile* colonization and antibiotic usage is an area of much needed research.

Metagenomic studies in cohorts with *Clostridium difficile*-associated diarrhea (CDAD) that have investigated microbiome shifts noted increases in *C. difficile* and Bacteroidetes, *C. coccoides*, *Eubacterium rectale*, *Ruminococcus gnavus*, and *Clostridium nexile* (Chang et al., 2008). It is interesting to note that the Bacteroidetes phylum seems to show a strong association with CDAD in several studies. Manges et al. (2010) show that low levels of Bacteroidetes are associated with CDAD. Tvede and Rask-Madsen (1989) demonstrate using bacteriotherapy experiments that the absence of *Bacteroides* species such as *Bacteroides ovatus*, *Bacteroides vulgaricus*, and *Bacteroides thetaiotaomicron* may result in recurring CDI whereas their abundance in the gut microbiota may afford protection against colonization and proliferation against *C. difficile*. Low Firmicutes and *Bacteroides* ratios, along with increasing facultative anaerobes, have been shown to be associated with *C. difficile* colonization in infants (Rousseau et al., 2011). Metagenomic studies of patients with CDI noted a decrease in alpha diversity at the DNA level (Chang et al., 2008; Knecht et al., 2014). However, Knecht et al. hypothesize that instead of a microbiota-wide compositional change, a loss of functionality of a single species may impair the resilience of the microbiota to *C. difficile* colonization. These functions may include short-chain fatty acids (SCFAs) or antimicrobial production, which may protect against *C. difficile* proliferation. Recent research by Knecht et al. (2014) indicates that Lachnospiraceae may be one such species in which low or high levels are associated with protection against or colonization with *C. difficile*.

Antibiotic substitutions for other options with less risk of CDI development associated may be effective (Vonberg et al., 2008). Further research into drug development is warranted to provide options that cause less disruption to the microbiota, consequently affording *C. difficile* less opportunity to proliferate.

Interference of Mutualistic Host–Microbe Interactions through Antibiotic-Induced Alteration of Gut Microbiome

The human intestinal microbiota develops a partnership with the host and is essential to health and functions such as nutrition, immunoregulation, metabolism, development, and pathogen resistance. With approximately 100 times more genes than the human genome, the gut microbiome lends us functional features we have not had to evolve ourselves (Backhed et al., 2005). Although the intestinal community does seem to have a level of taxonomic functional redundancy, antibiotic-mediated elimination or significant reduction of important members of the microbiota is likely to affect functionality and host physiology, particularly in the case of chronic antibiotic therapy (Perez-Cobas et al., 2013). Many key species of the human intestinal microbiota perform important functions; however, disruption of the core gut colonizers by antibiotic therapy may have a more profound effect on the functioning of the microbiota as a symbiotic partner of the host. Examples include *B. thetaiotaomicron*, a prominent mutualist in the intestinal microbiome, which has a genome-encoded capacity for carbohydrate metabolism far greater than the carbohydrate-metabolizing capabilities of our human genome (Shipman et al., 2000; Backhed et al., 2005). The gut microbiota also functions in regulation of bile acid and choline metabolism. The gut microbiota ecosystem comprises a dynamic network of functional interactions. As in any ecosystem, even targeted, or narrow-spectrum antibiotic effects will influence not only the target but also indirectly affect many interaction partners (Willing et al., 2011). Antibiotic therapy can induce host immunity effects through the loss of bacterial ligands, metabolites, and specific bacterial signals (Willing et al., 2011). Receptors involved in host immunity, such as toll-like receptors and NOD-like receptors are activated by specific bacterial ligands such as lipopolysaccarhide, lipoteichoic acid, flagellin, and peptidoglycan. The loss of specific bacterial ligands reduces immune signals (Wells et al., 2011). Metabolic profiles of antibiotic-treated mice show a reduction of SCFAs, with downstream reduction in the antiinflammatory effects of SCFAs as well as functions in regulation of cell proliferation, differentiation, growth, apoptosis, vasodilation, and wound healing (Yap et al., 2008; Millard et al., 2002; Leung et al., 2009; Bergman, 1990). Populations of bacteria have specific signals associated with them that may be lost after antibiotic treatment. In addition, many studies report reduced expression and secretion of AMPs, directly affecting first-line microbial defense (Meyer-Hoffert et al., 2008). Taken together, these factors result in a host more susceptible to pathogen insult (Willing et al., 2011).

The diversity of the human gut microbiota is the result of natural selection at the microbial level and the host level (Backhed et al., 2005). Diversity confers resilience to stress, such as antibiotic therapy, by harboring a diverse range of responses. This is known as the insurance hypothesis (Guarner, 2007). In general, low diversity correlates with poor health status (Lozupone et al., 2012; Claesson et al., 2012). This is one of the primary caveats of gut health and is demonstrated in infants, adults, and elderly populations. Many disease states have been associated with low-diversity microbiota signatures in recent years. Antibiotics as agents drive the microbiota to an altered assemblage through a gradual drift or dramatic shift, which may lead to the onset of microbiota-related diseases associated with less diversity, such as obesity (Turnbaugh et al., 2006), diabetes (Larsen et al., 2010), and inflammatory bowel disease (IBD; Dicksved et al., 2008). Turnbaugh et al. (2006) demonstrated that colonization of germ-free mice with "obese" microbiota resulted in development of obese phenotype and likewise in lean mice. Childhood antibiotic use and the resulting altered microbiota are potentially associated with asthma, atopic disease and obesity

(Marra et al., 2006; Noverr and Huffnagle, 2005). Low gut microbiota diversity in infants has been associated with eczema (Abrahamsson et al., 2012), particularly of the phylum Bacteroidetes and its genus *Bacteroides*. Indeed, in a study of 123 CF children, 59% presented with skin hypersensitivity allergy (Warner et al., 1976). Although not proposed by the authors at the time, low-diversity gut microbiota may have contributed to the hypersensitivity observed. The reduction of gut microbiota diversity after exposure to antibiotics is well documented. Antibiotic exposure may reduce overall diversity and/or diversity of select taxonomic groups, as seen by Jernberg et al. (2007) in a study of four patients exposed to 150 mg clindamycin 4 times daily. They observed an overall reduction in gut microbiota diversity but also a reduction in diversity of the *Bacteroides* community and emergence of clindamycin-resistant strains. In a study investigating the effects of ciprofloxacin (500 mg twice daily for 5 days) on the gut microbiota of adult patients, the abundance of one-third of bacterial taxa were reduced (Dethlefsen and Relman, 2011). Likewise, Rea et al. (2010) showed reduction of diversity after exposure to metronidazole and vancomycin in a human colonic model, mostly accounted for by the proportional increase of Enterobacteriaceae. However, despite the well-acknowledged effect of the lack of diversity on host health, the functional redundancy and resilience of the gut microbiota is also accepted. Indeed, Dethlefsen et al. (2008) have demonstrated that although the gut microbiota was disturbed after treatment with ciprofloxacin, they observed a continuity of microbial functions. It remains to be investigated whether the low-diversity microbiota disorders described could be the result of perturbations brought about by antibiotics alone or a combination of factors in which antibiotic therapy is perhaps the factor that tips the balance to a disease state.

The hygiene hypothesis is quoted frequently as an argument against sterilizing our environment and indeed our bodies through antibiotic use (Wills-Karp et al., 2001). The increasing incidence of autoimmune disorders such as asthma, eczema, celiac disease, and IBD may be related to disruption of normal host–microbe interactions by antibiotics (Guarner et al., 2006). Guarner hypothesizes that deficient exposure to mutualistic bacteria such as bifidobacteria and lactobacilli explains the increase of immunodysregulatory disorders in modern society. Guarner proposes the use of prebiotics and probiotics as a more favorable method of infection control.

MODULATION OF THE GUT MICROBIOTA
DIET

Diet has rapid and profound modulatory effects on the gut microbiota composition and functionality. Various diet types, including high-fat, high-sugar, "Western," and low-fat, polysaccharide-rich diets, have been associated with microbiota signatures differing at the compositional and functional gene level. Particular bacterial species have genetically encoded specific metabolic capabilities. The gut microbiota adapts to dietary intake to select bacterial populations with the genetic capabilities best suited for metabolism substrates of a given diet (Scott et al., 2008; Power et al., 2014). The rapid response of the gut microbiota to changes in diet has been demonstrated by studies in conventionalized germ-free mice. A change from a low-fat/plant-rich diet to a high fat and sugar/low plant polysaccharides "Western diet" showed changes in the gut microbiota within a single day, with increases in Firmicutes and decreases in Bacteroidetes (Turnbaugh et al., 2009). Hildebrandt et al. (2009) showed a similar rapid response in the gut microbiota to a dietary change (high-fat/low-fiber or low-fat/high-fiber) within 24 h. Most pertinent to CF are the effects of a high-fat diet on the gut microbiota composition. Dietary requirements for CF persons include 120–150% estimated average requirement of energy and 200% reference nutrient intake for protein (Littlewood and Macdonald., 1987; Pencharz and Durie., 1993). In addition, it is recommended that the CF total calorie intake should comprise 40% fat (White et al., 2004). The response of the gut microbiota to dietary fat is well documented. De Filippo et al. (2010) established the profound difference between the gut microbiota of European children on a typical Western diet (high fat, sugar, animal protein, and starch and low fiber content) and children in the African state of Burkina Faso, who consumed a predominantly vegetarian diet that was high in plant polysaccharides, starch, and fiber and low in animal protein and sugar. The Burkina Faso children had a lower abundance of Firmicutes and a higher abundance of Bacteroidetes genera (*Xylanibacter* and *Prevotella*), involving cellulose and xylan hydrolysis, enabling efficient energy extraction from their plant-rich diet. Indeed, a study by Wu et al. (2011) linked gut microbial enterotypes dominated by either *Bacteroides* or *Prevotella* with diets dominated by either protein and animal fat or carbohydrates along with low meat and dairy intake, respectively. A high-fat diet has been shown to influence a less diverse microbiota and a higher proportion of Bacteroidetes, *Parabacteroides*, *Eubacterium*, *Anaerotruncus*, *Lactonifactor*, and *Coprobacillus* in elderly subjects (Claesson et al., 2012). In the same study, community-dwelling subjects having a predominantly low to moderate fat intake had higher abundance of *Prevotella*, *Coprococcus*, and *Roseburia*. In addition to compositional microbial effects, a high-fat diet has been shown to result in a low-grade intestinal inflammatory state, which is a hallmark of CF (Arkan et al., 2005; Werlin et al., 2010).

Gastrointestinal manifestations of CF include exocrine pancreatic insufficiency (PI), steatorrhoea, intestinal inflammation, distal intestinal obstruction syndrome (DIOS) and cystic fibrosis–related diabetes (CFRD). PI occurs in 90% of CF patients, resulting in malabsorption of fat; protein; and fat-soluble vitamins A, D, E, and K and subsequent malnutrition (Fieker et al., 2011; Dodge and Turck, 2006). Undigested, unabsorbed dietary fat is excreted in stools, known as steatorrhoea (Somaraju and Solis-Moya, 2014) PI predisposes CF individuals to the onset of DIOS, an obstruction of fecal transit at the ileocecal junction (Somaraju and Solis-Moya, 2014). DIOS occurs in 10–20% of patients because of increased water absorption as a result of defective intestinal CFTR. CFRD occurs in approximately 2% of children, 19% of adolescents, and 40–50% of adults presenting with CF. CFRD, distinct from the type I and type II diabetes found in the general population (Stecenko and Moran, 2010) is associated with poorer pulmonary function and nutritional status (Koch et al., 2001;

Marshall et al., 2005). Although there is a paucity of information on how these gastrointestinal manifestations affect the intestinal microbiota, especially in the CF context, a microbiota response to such comorbidities is probable.

Positive Modulation of the Gut Microbiota

Positive modulation of the gut microbiota and host health can be achieved using probiotics, most commonly *Lactobacillus* or *Bifidobacterium* species. The beneficial effects of probiotics are perhaps more subtle than previously thought. Scientists are moving from a theory that probiotics alter total gut microbiome composition to a concept of prebiotics conferring a direct health benefit on the host (Power et al., 2014; Ouwehand et al., 2002). Thus far probiotics have been demonstrated to have therapeutic potential in treatment of AAD (Videlock and Cremonini, 2012; Hempel et al., 2012), CDI (Na and Kelly, 2011), IBD (Isaacs and Herfarth, 2008), and irritable bowel syndrome (Andersen and Baumgart, 2006). There have been preliminary but promising studies trialing administration of *Lactobacillus rhamnosus* GG (LGG) as a probiotic in pediatric CF cohorts. Bruzzese et al. (2004, 2014) showed the success of LGG in reducing intestinal inflammation as indicated by the noninvasive inflammatory markers nitric oxide and fecal calprotectin. The treated cohort also reported decreased abdominal pain. To further investigate the positive effects of LGG for the CF population, Bruzzese et al. (2007) investigated the effects of LGG administration on the rate of pulmonary exacerbation. They demonstrated a protective effect of LGG in children chronically infected with *Pseudomonas* and consequently a reduction in pulmonary exacerbations and increase in FEV_1. Weiss et al. (2010) showed a significant reduction in pulmonary exacerbations in children with CF infected with *P. aeruginosa* after administration of a probiotic cocktail containing *Lactobacillus acidophilus*, *Lactobacillus bulgaricus*, *Bifidobacterium bifidum*, and *Streptococcus thermophilus*; 90% of patients were also receiving azithromycin treatment at the time. The offsite effects of *Lactobacillus* species on *Pseudomonas* in the lung suggest a direct effect between the former and the latter, supported by earlier studies in mice in which LGG administration reduced *Pseudomonas* species, and *Lactobacillus plantarum* showed inhibitory activity toward *Pseudomonas* species (Valdez et al., 2005). Bruzzese et al. (2014) showed partial recovery of gut microbiota in CF children on antibiotic treatment who were subsequently treated with LGG with a significant increase of *Bacteroides* and a trend toward an increase in *F. prausnitzii*, a known antiinflammatory agent.

Probiotic strains with antibiotic tolerance may have application after or during antibiotic therapy. However, antibiotic tolerance in probiotic bacteria is generally associated with safety concerns by food safety authorities such as the European Food Safety Authority (EFSA) because of the risk of dissemination of resistance determinants from probiotics to commensal or pathogenic members of the gastrointestinal microbiota. Plasmid or mobile genetic element mediated resistance carried by many probiotic genera poses a serious safety issue (Sharma and Singh Saharan, 2014). In addition, there are issues for antibiotic–probiotic combination therapy and possible resulting antagonistic relationships that may exist. Increased bacterial load due to the presence of viable probiotics may reduce the potency of antibiotics. It has been shown that the potency of vancomycin decreases depending on the numbers of bacteria exposed (Udekwu et al., 2009). Probiotic-antibiotic combinations that preserve the potency of the antibiotic and the viability of the probiotic must be selected (Hammad and Shimamoto, 2010). Antibiotic-tolerant probiotic therapies remain at the conceptual stage because of difficulty in determining safety. However, the potential for application in a cohort with chronic antibiotic usage warrants further research into this novel area.

Knowledge of which microbiota community composition resists change more efficiently may be important in probiotic development. It may be possible to direct microbial communities toward a more resilient assemblage in individuals for whom chronic antibiotic use is necessary. In the future, probiotics may provide an adjunct therapy along with antibiotics for the treatment of CF symptoms. The possibility of reduction of antibiotics through use of alternative therapies, such as probiotics, is attractive to patients and clinicians.

FUTURE DIRECTIONS

Antimicrobial discovery has been in decline since the 1970s, and MDR is an increasingly serious threat to global public health. As an immediate response to MDR we can curb the inappropriate use and overuse of antibiotics, gain knowledge on antibiotic effects, and administer at doses that target aberrant bacteria while beneficial bacteria are preserved, all of which can help preserve and maintain the effectiveness of antibiotics for the next generation. In this age of high-throughput, next-generation sequencing technologies, it is imperative that we use the technologies available to us to tailor the antibiotics currently available to the individual instead of the "catch-all" broad-spectrum approach that has consequences on our antibiotic resources. CFMATTERS (Cystic Fibrosis Microbiome Derived Antimicrobial Therapy Trial in Exacerbations Results Stratified) is an EU-funded multicenter study currently examining this question in adult patients with CF (www.cfmatters.eu, https://clinicaltrials.gov/ct2/show/NCT02526004). Alternative additional strategies dealing with infection need to be brought from the bench to mainstream clinical practice. There have been several studies investigating the use of bacteriophage as a therapeutic to treat CF lung infection, particularly in treating *Pseudomonas* infection, but also *S. aureus* and *B. cepacia* (Brussow, 2012; Debarbieux et al., 2010; Alemayehu et al., 2012, Morello et al., 2011). Phage therapy is advantageous over antibiotic therapy because of its specificity to the target pathogen, its ability to replicate at the site of infection, and its ability to evolve along with bacterial populations that may develop resistance. Alemayehu et al. (2012) have demonstrated the efficacy of a phage cocktail (a myovirus (ϕNH-4) and a podovirus (ϕMR299-2)) to clear murine *Pseudomonas* lung infection. Furthermore, it has been shown that phage not only cleared *Pseudomonas* infection but also prevented infection when administered 24 h before infection, highlighting a potential role of phage in prophylaxis (Debarbieux et al., 2010; Morello et al., 2011).

Inhibition of *Pseudomonas* virulence and biofilm formation through disabling quorum sensing networks is another potential therapeutic approach for infection control. O'Loughlin et al. (2013) have demonstrated the utility of a quorum sensing inhibitory molecule (meta-bromo-thiolactone) to block pathogenesis by interacting with the two major quorum sensing systems Lux I/R. In addition they demonstrated the potential for preventative and curative treatment using meta-bromo-thiolactone. Further work is needed in these areas.

CONCLUSION

The collateral consequences of antibiotic therapy on the gut microbiota have been widely studied, and it is accepted that chronic and/or long-term antibiotic use has compositional and potentially functional effects on the gut microbiota. In a cohort with chronic antibiotic usage, such as CF, antibiotic resistance capabilities are expected to be high with consequences for subsequent antibiotic therapy. The long-term persistence of resistance genes in the gut microbiota in response to antibiotic therapy poses a concern for the clinical management of infection. Moving forward, tailored, individualized antibiotic strategies may prove critical along with additional options other than antibiotics. Phage therapy and targeting of quorum sensing networks may provide alternatives or adjunct therapies to antibiotic therapy in the future. Probiotics may be used as restorative agents to reintroduce depleted populations and maintain the gut microbiota ecosystem. In the interim, the medical community and wider society must endeavor to preserve our antibiotic resources through strategic and rational administration.

ACKNOWLEDGMENTS

The authors and their work are supported by the Science Foundation of Ireland (SFI)-funded Center for Science, Engineering and Technology; the APC Microbiome Institute; and in part by CFMATTERS. CFMATTERS has received funding from the EU's Seventh Framework Program (FP7/2007–2013) under grant agreement No. 603038.

REFERENCES

Abraham, E.P., Chain, E., 1940. An enzyme from bacteria able to destroy penicillin. 1988 July–August Rev. Infect. Dis. 10 (4), 677–678.

Abrahamsson, T.R., et al., 2012. Low diversity of the gut microbiota in infants with atopic eczema. J. Allergy. Clin. Immunol. 129 (2), 434–440, 440.e1–20.

Adamsson, I., Nord, C.E., Lundquist, P., et al., 1999. Comparative effects of omeprazole, amoxicillin plus metronidazole on the oral, gastric and intestinal microflora in *Helicobacter pylori*-infected patients. J. Antimicrob. Chemother. 44, 629–640.

Alemayehu, D., Casey, P.G., McAuliffe, O., Guinane, C.M., Martin, J.G., Shanahan, F., Coffey, A., Paul Ross, R., Hill, C., 2012. Bacteriophages φMR299-2 and φNH-4 can eliminate *Pseudomonas aeruginosa* in the murine lung and on cystic fibrosis lung airway cells. MBio 3 (2), e00029–12.

Amadori, A., et al., 2009. Recurrent exacerbations affect FEV(1) decline in adult patients with cystic fibrosis. Respir. Med. 103 (3), 407–413.

Andresen, V., Baumgart, D.C., 2006. Role of probiotics in the treatment of irritable bowel syndrome: potential mechanisms and current clinical evidence. Int. J. Probiotics Prebiotics 1 (1), 11.

Antonopoulos, D.A., et al., 2009. Reproducible community dynamics of the gastrointestinal microbiota following antibiotic perturbation. Infect. Immun. 77 (6), 2367–2375.

Arkan, M.C., Hevener, A.L., Greten, F.R., Maeda, S., Li, Z.W., Long, J.M., et al., 2005. IKK-β links inflammation to obesity-induced insulin resistance. Nat. Med. 11 (2), 191–198.

Bäckhed, F., Ley, R.E., Sonnenburg, J.L., Peterson, D.A., Gordon, J.I., 2005. Host-bacterial mutualism in the human intestine. Science 307 (5717), 1915–1920.

Barraud, N., et al., 2013. Mannitol enhances antibiotic sensitivity of persister bacteria in *Pseudomonas aeruginosa* biofilms. PLoS One 8 (12), e84220.

Bartlett, J.G., Gerding, D.N., 2008. Clinical recognition and diagnosis of *Clostridium difficile* infection. Clin. Infect. Dis. 46 (Suppl. 1), S12–S18.

Bartosch, S., Fite, A., Macfarlane, G.T., McMurdo, M.E., June 2004. Characterization of bacterial communities in feces from healthy elderly volunteers and hospitalized elderly patients by using real-time PCR and effects of antibiotic treatment on the fecal microbiota. Appl. Environ. Microbiol. 70 (6), 3575–3581.

Bauer, M.P., Farid, A., Bakker, M., Hoek, R.A.S., Kuijper, E.J., Dissel, J.T., 2014. Patients with cystic fibrosis have a high carriage rate of non-toxigenic *Clostridium difficile*. Clin. Microbiol. Infect. 20 (7), O446–O449.

Bennett, J.W., Herrera, M.L., Lewis, J.S., Wickes, B.W., Jorgensen, J.H., 2009. KPC-2-producing *Enterobacter cloacae* and *Pseudomonas putida* coinfection in a liver transplant recipient. Antimicrob. Agents Chemother. 53 (1), 292–294.

Bergman, E.N., 1990. Energy contributions of volatile fatty acids from the gastrointestinal tract in various species. Physiol. Rev. 70 (2), 567–590.

Binkovitz, L.A., Allen, E., Bloom, D., Long, F., Hammond, S., Buonomo, C., Donnelly, L.F., 1999. Atypical presentation of *Clostridium difficile* colitis in patients with cystic fibrosis. Am. J. Roentgenol. 172 (2), 517–521.

Blaser, M., 2011. Antibiotic overuse: stop the killing of beneficial bacteria. Nature 476 (7361), 393–394.

Brismar, B., et al., 1991. Comparative effects of clarithromycin and erythromycin on the normal intestinal microflora. Scand. J. Infect. Dis. 23 (5), 635–642.

Brüssow, H., 2012. Pseudomonas biofilms, cystic fibrosis, and phage: a silver lining? MBio 3 (2), e00061–12.

Bruzzese, E., et al., 2004. Intestinal inflammation is a frequent feature of cystic fibrosis and is reduced by probiotic administration. Aliment. Pharmacol. Ther. 20 (7), 813–819.

Bruzzese, E., et al., 2007. Effect of Lactobacillus GG supplementation on pulmonary exacerbations in patients with cystic fibrosis: a pilot study. Clin. Nutr. 26 (3), 322–328.

Bruzzese, E., et al., 2014. Disrupted intestinal microbiota and intestinal inflammation in children with cystic fibrosis and its restoration with Lactobacillus GG: a randomised clinical trial. PLoS One 9 (2), e87796.

Bryan, L.E., Kowand, S.K., Van Den Elzen, H.M., 1979. Mechanism of aminoglycoside antibiotic resistance in anaerobic bacteria: *Clostridium perfringens* and *Bacteroides fragilis*. Antimicrob. Agents Chemother 15 (1), 7–13.

Bush, K., Jacoby, G.A., 2010. Updated functional classification of β-lactamases. Antimicrob. Agents Chemother. 54 (3), 969–976.

Cao, Y., Rocha, E.R., Jeffrey Smith, C., 2014. Efficient utilization of complex N-linked glycans is a selective advantage for *Bacteroides fragilis* in extraintestinal infections. Proc. Nat. Acad. Sci. 111 (35), 12901–12906.

CDC, 2013. Antibiotic Resistance threats in the United States, 2013. Centre for Disease Control. GA, Atlanta. http://www.cdc.gov/drugresistance/threat-report-2013/.

CFRI Annual Report, 2011. http://www.cfri.ie/docs/annual_reports/CFRI2011.pdf.

Chang, J.Y., et al., 2008. Decreased diversity of the fecal microbiome in recurrent *Clostridium difficile*—associated diarrhea. J. Infect. Dis. 197 (3), 435–438.

Collins, F.S., May 8 , 1992. Cystic fibrosis: molecular biology and therapeutic implications. Science 256 (5058), 774–779.

Claesson, M.J., Jeffery, I.B., Conde, S., Power, S.E., O'Connor, E.M., Cusack, S., et al., 2012. Gut microbiota composition correlates with diet and health in the elderly. Nature 488 (7410), 178–184.

Cornely, O.A., Nathwani, D., Ivanescu, C., Odufowora-Sita, O., Retsa, P., Odeyemi, I.A., 2014. Clinical efficacy of fidaxomicin compared with vancomycin and metronidazole in *Clostridium difficile* infections: a meta-analysis and indirect treatment comparison. J. Antimicrob. Chemother. dku261.

Cotter, P.D., Stanton, C., Ross, R.P., Hill, C., 2012. The impact of antibiotics on the gut microbiota as revealed by high throughput DNA sequencing. Dis. Med. 13 (70), 193–199.

Cramer, J.P., Burchard, G.D., Lohse, A.W., 2008. Old dogmas and new perspectives in antibiotic-associated diarrhea. Medizinische Klinik (Munich, Germany: 1983) 103 (5), 325–338.

Cresti, S., et al., 2002. Resistance determinants and clonal diversity in group A streptococci collected during a period of increasing macrolide resistance. Antimicrob. Agents Chemother. 46 (6), 1816–1822.

Damodaran, S.E., Madhan, S., 2011. Telavancin: a novel lipoglycopeptide antibiotic. J. Pharmacol. Pharmacother. 2 (2), 135.

Davies, J., 1994. Inactivation of antibiotics and the dissemination of resistance genes. Science 264 (5157), 375–382.

Davies, J., Davies, D., 2010. Origins and evolution of antibiotic resistance. Microbiol. Mol. Biol. Rev. 74 (3), 417–433.

Davis, P.B., 2006. Cystic fibrosis since 1938. Am. J. Respir. Crit. Care Med. 173 (5), 475–482.

Debarbieux, L., Leduc, D., Maura, D., Morello, E., Criscuolo, A., Grossi, O., Balloy, V., Touqui, L., 2010. Bacteriophages can treat and prevent *Pseudomonas aeruginosa* lung infections. J. Infect. Dis. 201 (7), 1096–1104.

De Filippo, C., Cavalieri, D., Di Paola, M., Ramazzotti, M., Poullet, J.B., Massart, S., et al., 2010. Impact of diet in shaping gut microbiota revealed by a comparative study in children from Europe and rural Africa. Proc. Nat. Acad. Sci. 107 (33), 14691–14696.

De La Cochetière, M.-F., et al., 2008. Effect of antibiotic therapy on human fecal microbiota and the relation to the development of *Clostridium difficile*. Microb. Ecol. 56 (3), 395–402.

Deshpande, L.M., Rhomberg, P.R., Sader, H.S., Jones, R.N., 2006. Emergence of serine carbapenemases (KPC and SME) among clinical strains of Enterobacteriaceae isolated in the United States medical centers: report from the MYSTIC program (1999–2005). Diag. Microbiol. Infect. Dis. 56 (4), 367–372.

Dethlefsen, L., et al., 2008. The pervasive effects of an antibiotic on the human gut microbiota, as revealed by deep 16S rRNA sequencing. PLoS Biol. 6 (11), e280.

Dethlefsen, L., Relman, D.A., 2011. Incomplete recovery and individualised responses of the human distal gut microbiota to repeated antibiotic perturbation. PNAS 108, 4554–4561.

Dicksved, J., Halfvarson, J., Rosenquist, M., Järnerot, G., Tysk, C., Apajalahti, J., et al., 2008. Molecular analysis of the gut microbiota of identical twins with Crohn's disease. ISME J. 2 (7), 716–727.

Diggs, N.G., Surawicz, C.M., 2009. Evolving concepts in *Clostridium difficile* colitis. Curr. Gastroenterol. Rep. 11 (5), 400–405.

Diniz, C.G., Santos, S.G., Pestana, A.C.N., Farias, L.M., Carvalho, M.A.R., 2000. Chromosomal breakage in the *B. fragilis* group induced by metronidazole treatment. Anaerobe 6 (3), 149–153.

Dodge, J.A., Turck, D., 2006. Cystic fibrosis: nutritional consequences and management. Best Prac. Res. Clin. Gastroenterol. 20 (3), 531–546.

Döring, G., Conway, S.P., Heijerman, H.G.M., Hodson, M.E., Høiby, N., Smyth, A., et al., 2000. Antibiotic therapy against *Pseudomonas aeruginosa* in cystic fibrosis: a European consensus. Eur. Respir. J. 16 (4), 749–767.

Döring, G., Flume, P., Heijerman, H., Elborn, J.S., Consensus Study Group, 2012. Treatment of lung infection in patients with cystic fibrosis: current and future strategies. J. Cystic Fibrosis 11 (6), 461–479.

Dortet, L., Poirel, L., Nordmann, P., 2012. Rapid detection of carbapenemase-producing Pseudomonas species. J. Clin. Microbiol. 01597.

Drlica, K., 1999. Mechanism of fluoroquinolone action. Curr. Opin. Microbiol. 2 (5), 504–508.

Duytschaever, G., Huys, G., Bekaert, M., Boulanger, L., De Boeck, K., Vandamme, P., 2011. Cross-sectional and longitudinal comparisons of the predominant fecal microbiota compositions of a group of pediatric patients with cystic fibrosis and their healthy siblings. Appl. Environ. Microbiol. 77 (22), 8015–8024.

Duytschaever, G., Huys, G., Bekaert, M., Boulanger, L., De Boeck, K., Vandamme, P., 2013. Dysbiosis of bifidobacteria and Clostridium cluster XIVa in the cystic fibrosis fecal microbiota. J. Cystic Fibrosis 12 (3), 206–215.

ECDC, 2015. European Surveillance of Clostridium Difficile Infections. Surveillance Protocol Version 2.1. European Centre for Disease Prevention and Control, Stockholm.

Edlund, C., Beyer, G., Lode, H., et al., 2000. Comparative effects of moxifloxacin and clarithromycin on the normal intestinal microflora. Scand. J. Infect. Dis. 32, 81–85.

Eichenwald, H.F., McCracken, G.H., 1978. Antimicrobial therapy in infants and children: Part I. Review of antimicrobial agents. J. Pediatr 93 (3), 337–356.

Elphick, H.E., Tan, A.A., 2005. Single versus combination intravenous antibiotic therapy for people with cystic fibrosis. Cochrane Library CD002007.

Engelbrektson, A.L., et al., 2006. Analysis of treatment effects on the microbial ecology of the human intestine. FEMS Microbiol. Ecol. 57 (2), 239–250.

Faria, A.M., Weiner, H.L., 2005. Oral tolerance. Immunol. Rev. 206, 232–259.

Farrell, P.M., 2008. The prevalence of cystic fibrosis in the European Union. J. Cyst. Fibros 7 (5), 450–453.

Fieker, A., Philpott, J., Armand, M., 2011. Enzyme replacement therapy for pancreatic insufficiency: present and future. Clin. Exp. Gastroenterol. 4, 55.

Flume, P.A., Mogayzel Jr., P.J., Robinson, K.A., Goss, C.H., Rosenblatt, R.L., Kuhn, R.J., Marshall, B.C., 2009. Cystic fibrosis pulmonary guidelines: treatment of pulmonary exacerbations. Am. J. Respir. Crit. Care Med. 180 (9), 802–808.

Fouhy, F., Ogilvie, L.A., Jones, B.V., Ross, R.P., Ryan, A.C., et al., 2014. Identification of aminoglycoside and β-lactam resistance genes from within an infant gut functional metagenomic library. PLoS One 9 (9), e108016.

Foulstone, M., Reading, C., 1982. Assay of amoxicillin and clavulanic acid, the components of Augmentin, in biological fluids with high-performance liquid chromatography. Antimicrob. Agents Chemother. 22 (5), 753–762.

Gerding, D.N., 2004. Clindamycin, cephalosporins, fluoroquinolones, and *Clostridium difficile*–associated diarrhea: this is an antimicrobial resistance problem. Clin. Infect. Dis. 38 (5), 646–648.

Gibson, R.L., Burns, J.L., Ramsey, B.W., 2003. Pathophysiology and management of pulmonary infections in cystic fibrosis. Am. J. Respir. Crit. Care Med. 168 (8), 918–951.

Gould, I.M., van der Meer, J.W. (Eds.), 2007. Antibiotic Policies: Fighting Resistance. Springer.

Guarner, F., et al., 2006. Mechanisms of disease: the hygiene hypothesis revisited. Nat. Clin. Pract. Gastroenterol. Hepatol. 3 (5), 275–284.

Guarner, F., 2007. Hygiene, microbial diversity and immune regulation. Curr. Opin. Gastroenterol. 23 (6), 667–672.

Gupta, A., et al., 2003. A new *Bacteroides* conjugative transposon that carries an ermB gene. Appl. Environ. Microbiol. 69 (11), 6455–6463.

Gutacker, M., et al., 2000. Identification of two genetic groups in *Bacteroides fragilis* by multilocus enzyme electrophoresis: distribution of antibiotic resistance (cfiA, cepA) and enterotoxin (bft) encoding genes. Microbiology 146 (5), 1241–1254.

Gutiérrez, O., Juan, C., Cercenado, E., Navarro, F., Bouza, E., Coll, P., et al., 2007. Molecular epidemiology and mechanisms of carbapenem resistance in *Pseudomonas aeruginosa* isolates from Spanish hospitals. Antimicrob. Agents Chemother. 51 (12), 4329–4335.

Hamilton-Miller, J.M.T., 1992. In-vitro activities of 14-, 15- and 16-membered macrolides against gram-positive cocci. J. Antimicrob. Chemother. 29 (2), 141–147.

Hammad, A.M., Shimamoto, T., 2010. Towards a compatible probiotic–antibiotic combination therapy: assessment of antimicrobial resistance in the Japanese probiotics. J. Appl. Microbiol. 109 (4), 1349–1360.

Harrison, M.J., McCarthy, M., Fleming, C., Hickey, C., Shortt, C., Eustace, J.A., Murphy, D.M., Plant, B.J., 2014. Inhaled versus nebulised tobramycin: a real world comparison in adult cystic fibrosis (CF). J. Cystic Fibrosis 13 (6), 692–698.

Hedberg, M., Nord, C.E., 2002. Anaerobic Bacteria. Antimicrobial Therapy and Vaccines, second ed. Apple Tree Productions, New York, pp. 55–62.

Hempel, S., Newberry, S.J., Maher, A.R., Wang, Z., Miles, J.N., Shanman, R., et al., 2012. Probiotics for the prevention and treatment of antibiotic-associated diarrhea: a systematic review and meta-analysis. JAMA 307 (18), 1959–1969.

Herrmann, G., Yang, L., Wu, H., Song, Z., Wang, H., et al., 2010. Colistin-tobramycin combinations are superior to monotherapy concerning the killing of biofilm *Pseudomonas aeruginosa*. J. Infect. Dis. 202, 1585–1592. http://dx.doi.org/10.1086/656788. PubMed: 20942647.

Hertz, F.B., Løbner-Olesen, A., Frimodt-Møller, N., 2014. Antibiotic selection of *Escherichia coli* sequence type 131 in a mouse intestinal colonization model. Antimicrob. Agents Chemother. 58 (10), 6139–6144.

Hildebrandt, M.A., Hoffmann, C., Sherrill–Mix, S.A., Keilbaugh, S.A., Hamady, M., Chen, Y.Y., et al., 2009. High-fat diet determines the composition of the murine gut microbiome independently of obesity. Gastroenterology 137 (5), 1716–1724.

Høiby, N., 1993. Antibiotic therapy for chronic infection of Pseudomonas in the lung. Ann. Review Med. 44, 1–10.

Holten, K.B., Onusko, E.M., 2000. Appropriate prescribing of oral beta-lactam antibiotics. Am. Fam. Physician 62 (3), 611–620.

Hooper, D.C., 2001. Emerging mechanisms of fluoroquinolone resistance. Emerging Infect. Dis. 7 (2), 337.

Hewer, S.C.L., Smyth, A.R., 2014. Antibiotic strategies for eradicating *Pseudomonas aeruginosa* in people with cystic fibrosis. Cochrane Library. http://dx.doi.org/10.1002/14651858.

Iapichino, G., Callegari, M.L., Marzorati, S., Cigada, M., Corbella, D., Ferrari, S., Morelli, L., 2008. Impact of antibiotics on the gut microbiota of critically ill patients. J. Med. Microbiol. 57 (8), 1007–1014.

Isaacs, K., Herfarth, H., 2008. Role of probiotic therapy in IBD. Inflammation Bowel Dis. 14 (11), 1597–1605.

Jakobsson, H.E., et al., 2010. Short-term antibiotic treatment has differing long-term impacts on the human throat and gut microbiome. PLoS One 5 (3), e9836.

Jeong, S.H., et al., 2009. Risk assessment of ciprofloxacin, flavomycin, olaquindox and colistin sulfate based on microbiological impact on human gut biota. Regul. Toxicol. Pharmacol. 53 (3), 209–216.

Jernberg, C., et al., 2007. Long-term ecological impacts of antibiotic administration on the human intestinal microbiota. ISME J. 1 (1), 56–66.

Jernberg, C., et al., 2010. Long-term impacts of antibiotic exposure on the human intestinal microbiota. Microbiology 156 (Pt 11), 3216–3223.

Jousimies-Somer, H.R., Summanen, P., Citron, D.M., Baron, E.J., Wexler, H.M., Finegold, S.M., 2002. Anaerobic Bacteriology Manual. Star Publishing Company, Belmont California.

Kawamura-Sato, K., et al., 2000. Effect of subinhibitory concentrations of macrolides on expression of flagellin in *Pseudomonas aeruginosa* and *Proteus mirabilis*. Antimicrob. Agents Chemother. 44 (10), 2869–2872.

Knecht, H., et al., 2014. Effects of β-lactam antibiotics and fluoroquinolones on human gut microbiota in relation to *Clostridium difficile* associated diarrhea. PLoS One 9 (2), e89417.

Koch, C., Rainisio, M., Madessani, U., Harms, H.K., Hodson, M.E., Mastella, G., et al., 2001. Presence of cystic fibrosis-related diabetes mellitus is tightly linked to poor lung function in patients with cystic fibrosis: data from the European epidemiologic registry of cystic fibrosis. Pediatr. Pulmonol. 32 (5), 343–350.

Koenigsknecht, M.J., Young, V.B., 2013. Faecal microbiota transplantation for the treatment of recurrent *Clostridium difficile* infection: current promise and future needs. Curr. Opin. Gastroenterol. 29 (6), 628–632.

Konstan, M.W., Flume, P.A., Kappler, M., Chiron, R., Higgins, M., Brockhaus, F., et al., 2011. Safety, efficacy and convenience of tobramycin inhalation powder in cystic fibrosis patients: the EAGER trial. J. Cystic Fibrosis 10 (1), 54–61.

Kouda, S., Ohara, M., Onodera, M., Fujiue, Y., Sasaki, M., Kohara, T., et al., 2009. Increased prevalence and clonal dissemination of multidrug-resistant *Pseudomonas aeruginosa* with the blaIMP-1 gene cassette in Hiroshima. J. Antimicrob. Chemother. dkp142.

Kuijper, E.J., Barbut, F., Brazier, J.S., Kleinkauf, N., Eckmanns, T., Lambert, M.L., et al., 2008. Update of *Clostridium difficile* Infection due to PCR Ribotype 027 in Europe.

Kyne, L., Warny, M., Qamar, A., Kelly, C.P., 2000. Asymptomatic carriage of *Clostridium difficile* and serum levels of IgG antibody against toxin A. N. Engl. J. Med. 342, 390–397.

Lagatolla, C., Edalucci, E., Dolzani, L., Riccio, M.L., De Luca, F., Medessi, E., et al., 2006. Molecular evolution of metallo-β-lactamase-producing *Pseudomonas aeruginosa* in a nosocomial setting of high-level endemicity. J. Clin. Microbiol. 44 (7), 2348–2353.

Lamp, K.C., Freeman, C.D., Klutman, N.E., Lacy, M.K., 1999. Pharmacokinetics and pharmacodynamics of the nitroimidazole antimicrobials. Clin. Pharmacokinet. 36 (5), 353–373.

Land, K.M., Johnson, P.J., 1999. Molecular basis of metronidazole resistance in pathogenic bacteria and protozoa. Drug Resist. Updates 2 (5), 289–294.

Larsen, N., Vogensen, F.K., Van Den Berg, F.W., Nielsen, D.S., Andreasen, A.S., Pedersen, B.K., et al., 2010. Gut microbiota in human adults with type 2 diabetes differs from non-diabetic adults. PloS One 5 (2), e9085.

Laxminarayan, R., Heymann, D.L., 2012. Challenges of drug resistance in the developing world. BMJ 344, e1567.

Laxminarayan, R., Duse, A., Wattal, C., Zaidi, A.K., Wertheim, H.F., Sumpradit, N., et al., 2013. Antibiotic resistance—the need for global solutions. Lancet Infect. Dis. 13 (12), 1057–1098.

Lee, J.H., O'Sullivan, D.J., 2010. Genomic insights into bifidobacteria. Microbiol. Mol. Biol. Rev. 74 (3), 378–416.

Leiros, H.K.S., Kozielski-Stuhrmann, S., Kapp, U., Terradot, L., Leonard, G.A., McSweeney, S.M., 2004. Structural basis of 5-Nitroimidazole antibiotic resistance. The crystal structure of nimA from *Deinococcus radiodurans*. J. Biol. Chem. 279 (53), 55840–55849.

Leung, C.H., Lam, W., Ma, D.L., Gullen, E.A., Cheng, Y.C., 2009. Butyrate mediates nucleotide-binding and oligomerisation domain (NOD) 2-dependent mucosal immune responses against peptidoglycan. Eur. J. Immunol. 39 (12), 3529–3537.

Lewis, K., 2013. Platforms for antibiotic discovery. Nat. Rev. Drug Dis. 12 (5), 371–387.

Lidbeck, A., et al., 1988. Impact of *Lactobacillus acidophilus* on the normal intestinal microflora after administration of two antimicrobial agents. Infection 16 (6), 329–336.

Littlewood, J.M., MacDonald, A., 1987. Rationale of modern dietary recommendations in cystic fibrosis. J. Royal Soc. Med. 80 (Suppl. 15), 16.

Littlewood, J., et al., 2000. A ten year review of colomycin. Respir. Med. 94 (7), 632–640.

Liu, P., Müller, M., Derendorf, H., 2002. Rational dosing of antibiotics: the use of plasma concentrations versus tissue concentrations. Int. J. Antimicrob. Agents 19 (4), 285–290.

Liu, P., Derendorf, H., 2003. Antimicrobial tissue concentrations. Infect. Dis. Clin. North Am. 17 (3), 599–613.

Löfmark, S., Edlund, C., Nord, C.E., 2010. Metronidazole is still the drug of choice for treatment of anaerobic infections. Clin. Infect. Dis. 50 (Suppl. 1), S16–S23.

Lozupone, C.A., Stombaugh, J.I., Gordon, J.I., Jansson, J.K., Knight, R., 2012. Diversity, stability and resilience of the human gut microbiota. Nature 489 (7415), 220–230.

Lu, N., Hu, Y., Zhu, L., Yang, X., Yin, Y., Lei, F., et al., 2014. DNA Microarray Analysis Reveals that Antibiotic Resistance-gene Diversity in Human Gut Microbiota Is Age Related. Scientific Reports, p. 4.

Madan, J.C., Koestler, D.C., Stanton, B.A., Davidson, L., Moulton, L.A., Housman, M.L., et al., 2012. Serial analysis of the gut and respiratory microbiome in cystic fibrosis in infancy: interaction between intestinal and respiratory tracts and impact of nutritional exposures. mBio 3 (4), e00251–12.

Manges, A.R., Labbe, A., Loo, V.G., et al., 2010. Comparative metagenomic study of alterations to the intestinal microbiota and risk of nosocomial *Clostridium difficile*-associated disease. J. Infect. Dis. 202, 1877–1884.

Marshall, B.C., Butler, S.M., Stoddard, M., Moran, A.M., Liou, T.G., Morgan, W.J., 2005. Epidemiology of cystic fibrosis-related diabetes. J. Pediatr. 146 (5), 681–687.

Marra, F., Lynd, L., Coombes, M., Richardson, K., Legal, M., et al., 2006. Does antibiotic exposure during infancy lead to development of asthma?: A systematic review and metaanalysis. Chest 129, 610–618.

Meyer-Hoffert, U., Hornef, M.W., Henriques-Normark, B., Axelsson, L.G., Midtvedt, T., Pütsep, K., Andersson, M., 2008. Secreted enteric antimicrobial activity localises to the mucus surface layer. Gut 57 (6), 764–771.

Millard, A., Mertes, P.M., Ittelet, D., Villard, F., Jeannesson, P., Bernard, J., 2002. Butyrate affects differentiation, maturation and function of human monocyte-derived dendritic cells and macrophages. Clin. Exp. Immunol. 130 (2), 245–255.

Miriagou, V., Cornaglia, G., Edelstein, M., Galani, I., Giske, C.G., Gniadkowski, M., et al., 2010. Acquired carbapenemases in Gram-negative bacterial pathogens: detection and surveillance issues. Clin. Microbiol. Infect. 16 (2), 112–122.

Monreal, M.T.F.D., Pereira, P.C.M., Lopes, C.A.D.M., 2005. Intestinal microbiota of patients with bacterial infection of the respiratory tract treated with amoxicillin. Braz. J. Infect. Dis. 9 (4), 292–300.

Morello, E., Saussereau, E., Maura, D., Huerre, M., Touqui, L., Debarbieux, L., 2011. Pulmonary bacteriophage therapy on *Pseudomonas aeruginosa* cystic fibrosis strains: first steps towards treatment and prevention. PloS One 6 (2), e16963.

Morotomi, N., et al., 2011. Evaluation of intestinal microbiotas of healthy Japanese adults and effect of antibiotics using the 16S ribosomal RNA gene based clone library method. Biol. Pharm. Bull. 34 (7), 1011–1020.

Morrissey, I., Hackel, M., Badal, R., Bouchillon, S., Hawser, S., Biedenbach, D., 2013. A review of ten years of the study for monitoring antimicrobial resistance trends (SMART) from 2002 to 2011. Pharmaceuticals 6 (11), 1335–1346.

Moskowitz, S.M., et al., 2008. Shifting patterns of inhaled antibiotic use in cystic fibrosis. Pediatr. Pulmonol. 43 (9), 874–881.

Murphy, E.F., Cotter, P.D., Hogan, A., O'Sullivan, O., Joyce, A., Fouhy, F., et al., 2013. Divergent metabolic outcomes arising from targeted manipulation of the gut microbiota in diet-induced obesity. Gut 62 (2), 220–226.

Na, X., Kelly, C., 2011. Probiotics in *Clostridium difficile* infection. J. Clin. Gastroenterol. 45, S154–S158.

Nagy, E., Földes, J., 1991. Inactivation of metronidazole by *Enterococcus faecalis*. J. Antimicrob. Chemother. 27 (1), 63–70.

Nakamura, S., et al., 1981. Isolation of *Clostridium difficile* from the feces and the antibody in sera of young and elderly adults. Microbiol. Immunol. 25 (4), 345–351.

Nakano, V., et al., 2011. Antimicrobial resistance and prevalence of resistance genes in intestinal Bacteroidales strains. Clinics 66 (4), 543–547.

Navon-Venezia, S., Chmelnitsky, I., Leavitt, A., Schwaber, M.J., Schwartz, D., Carmeli, Y., 2006. Plasmid-mediated imipenem-hydrolyzing enzyme KPC-2 among multiple carbapenem-resistant *Escherichia coli* clones in Israel. Antimicrob. Agents Chemother. 50 (9), 3098–3101.

Noverr, M.C., Huffnagle, G.B., 2005. The 'microflora hypothesis' of allergic diseases. Clin. Exp. Allergy 35, 1511–1520.

Ochman, H., et al., 2000. Lateral gene transfer and the nature of bacterial innovation. Nature 405 (6784), 299–304.

O'Loughlin, C.T., Miller, L.C., Siryaporn, A., Drescher, K., Semmelhack, M.F., Bassler, B.L., 2013. A quorum-sensing inhibitor blocks *Pseudomonas aeruginosa* virulence and biofilm formation. Proc. Nat. Acad. Sci. 110 (44), 17981–17986.

O'Sullivan, Ó., Coakley, M., Lakshminarayanan, B., Conde, S., Claesson, M.J., Cusack, S., et al., 2012. Alterations in intestinal microbiota of elderly Irish subjects post-antibiotic therapy. J. Antimicrob. Chemother. http://dx.doi.org/10.1093/jac/dks348.

O'Sullivan, O., et al., 2013. Alterations in intestinal microbiota of elderly Irish subjects post-antibiotic therapy. J. Antimicrob. Chemother. 68 (1), 214–221.

Ouwehand, A.C., Salminen, S., Isolauri, E., 2002. Probiotics: an overview of beneficial effects. Antonie Van Leeuwenhoek 82 (1–4), 279–289.

Owens, R.C., et al., 2008. Antimicrobial-associated risk factors for *Clostridium difficile* infection. Clin. Infect. Dis. 46 (Suppl. 1), S19–S31.

Ozaki, E., et al., 2004. *Clostridium difficile* colonization in healthy adults: transient colonization and correlation with enterococcal colonization. J. Med. Microbiol. 53 (2), 167–172.

Page, M.G., 2012. Beta-lactam Antibiotics. Antibiotic Discovery and Development. Springer, pp. 79–117.

Pamp, S.J., Gjermansen, M., Johansen, H.K., Tolker-Nielsen, T., 2008. Tolerance to the antimicrobial peptide colistin in *Pseudomonas aeruginosa* biofilms is linked to metabolically active cells, and depends on the pmr and mexAB-oprM genes. Mol. Microbiol. 68, 223–240. http://dx.doi.org/10.1111/j.1365-2958.2008.06152.x. PubMed:18312276.

Pamukcu, A., Bush, A., Buchdahl, R., 1995. Effects of *Pseudomonas aeruginosa* colonization on lung function and anthropometric variables in children with cystic fibrosis. Pediatr. Pulmonol. 19, 10–15.

Peach, S.L., Borriello, S.P., Gaya, H., Barclay, F.E., Welch, A.R., September 1986. Asymptomatic carriage of *Clostridium difficile* in patients with cystic fibrosis. J. Clin. Pathol. 39 (9), 1013–1018.

Pencharz, P.B., Durie, P.R., 1993. Nutritional management of cystic fibrosis. Ann. Rev. Nutr. 13 (1), 111–136.

Pepin, J., Valiquette, L., Cossette, B., 2005. Mortality attributable to nosocomial *Clostridium difficile*-associated disease during an epidemic caused by a hypervirulent strain in Quebec. CMAJ 173, 1–6.

Perez-Cobas, A.E., et al., 2013. Differential effects of antibiotic therapy on the structure and function of human gut microbiota. PLoS One 8 (11), e80201.

Petrof, E.O., Gloor, G.B., Vanner, S.J., Weese, S.J., Carter, D., Daigneault, M.C., et al., 2013. Stool substitute transplant therapy for the eradication of *Clostridium difficile* infection: 'RePOOPulating' the gut. Microbiome 1 (1), 1–12.

Perron, G.G., Kryazhimskiy, S., Rice, D.P., Buckling, A., 2012. Multidrug therapy and evolution of antibiotic resistance: when order matters. Appl. Environ. Microbiol. 78 (17), 6137–6142.

Pitout, J.D., Chow, B.L., Gregson, D.B., Laupland, K.B., Elsayed, S., Church, D.L., 2007. Molecular epidemiology of metallo-β-lactamase-producing *Pseudomonas aeruginosa* in the Calgary Health Region: emergence of VIM-2-producing isolates. J. Clin. Microbiol. 45 (2), 294–298.

Pitout, J.D., Laupland, K.B., 2008. Extended-spectrum β-lactamase-producing Enterobacteriaceae: an emerging public-health concern. Lancet Infect. Dis. 8 (3), 159–166.

Plant, B.J., Goss, C.H., Plant, W.D., Bell, S.C., 2013. Management of comorbidities in older patients with cystic fibrosis. Lancet Respir. Med. 1 (2), 164–174.

Power, S.E., O'Toole, P.W., Stanton, C., Ross, R.P., Fitzgerald, G.F., 2014. Intestinal microbiota, diet and health. Br. J. Nutr. 111 (03), 387–402.

Pumbwe, L., et al., 2007. Bile salts enhance bacterial co-aggregation, bacterial-intestinal epithelial cell adhesion, biofilm formation and antimicrobial resistance of *Bacteroides fragilis*. Microb. Pathog. 43 (2), 78–87.

Queenan, A.M., Bush, K., 2007. Carbapenemases: the versatile β-lactamases. Clin. Microbiol. Rev. 20 (3), 440–458.

Quinton, P.M., 1990. Righting the wrong protein. Nature 347 (6290), 226.

Ramsey, B.W., Pepe, M.S., Quan, J.M., Otto, K.L., Montgomery, A.B., Williams-Warren, J., et al., 1999. Intermittent administration of inhaled tobramycin in patients with cystic fibrosis. New England J. Med. 340 (1), 23–30.

Ratjen, F., Döring, G., Nikolaizik, W.H., 2001. Effect of inhaled tobramycin on early *Pseudomonas aeruginosa* colonisation in patients with cystic fibrosis. Lancet 358 (9286), 983–984.

Rea, M.C., Sit, C.S., Clayton, E., O'Connor, P.M., Whittal, R.M., Zheng, J., et al., 2010. Thuricin CD, a posttranslationally modified bacteriocin with a narrow spectrum of activity against *Clostridium difficile*. Proc. Nat. Acad. Sci. 107 (20), 9352–9357.

Rea, M.C., Dobson, A., O'Sullivan, O., Crispie, F., Fouhy, F., Cotter, P.D., et al., 2011. Effect of broad-and narrow-spectrum antimicrobials on *Clostridium difficile* and microbial diversity in a model of the distal colon. Proc. Nat. Acad. Sci. 108 (Suppl. 1), 4639–4644.

Reynolds, P.E., November 1989. Structure, biochemistry and mechanism of action of glycopeptide antibiotics. Eur. J. Clin. Microbiol. Infect. Dis. 8 (11), 943–950. Endocarditis due to resistant organisms.

Reysset, G., 1996. Genetics of 5-Nitroimidazole resistance in *Bacteroides* species. Anaerobe 2 (2), 59–69.

Report EEJT, 2009. The bacterial challenge: time to react. A call to narrow the gap between multidrug-resistant bacteria in the EU and the development of new antibacterial agents. http://wwwemeaeuropaeu/docs/en_GB/document_library/Report/2009/11/WC500008770pdf.

Roca, I., Akova, M., Baquero, F., Carlet, J., Cavaleri, M., Coenen, S., Cohen, J., et al., 2015. The global threat of antimicrobial resistance: science for intervention. New Microbes New Infect. http://dx.doi.org/10.1016/j.nmni.2015.02.007.

Rolain, J.M., Parola, P., Cornaglia, G., 2010. New Delhi metallo-beta-lactamase (NDM-1): towards a new pandemia? Clin. Microbiol. Infect. 16 (12), 1699–1701.

Rodier, D.G., 2011. European Strategic Action Plan on Antibiotic Resistance. http://wwweurowhoint/__data/assets/pdf_file/0011/148988/RC61_Pres_Rodier_antibiotic_resistancepdf.

Rolfe, R.D., Helebian, S., Finegold, S.M., March 1981. Bacterial interference between *Clostridium difficile* and normal fecal flora. J. Infect. Dis. 143, 470–475.

Rousseau, C., et al., 2011. *Clostridium difficile* colonization in early infancy is accompanied by changes in intestinal microbiota composition. J. Clin. Microbiol. 49 (3), 858–865.

Russell, D.A., Ross, R.P., Fitzgerald, G.F., Stanton, C., 2011. Metabolic activities and probiotic potential of bifidobacteria. Int. J. Food Microbiol. 149 (1), 88–105.

Saiman, L., Marshall, B.C., Mayer-Hamblett, N., Burns, J.L., Quittner, A.L., Cibene, D.A., et al., 2003. Azithromycin in patients with cystic fibrosis chronically infected with *Pseudomonas aeruginosa*: a randomized controlled trial. JAMA 290 (13), 1749–1756.

Salyers, A.A., 1984. Bacteroides of the human lower intestinal tract. Ann. Rev. Microbiol. 38 (1), 293–313.

Salyers, A.A., et al., 2004. Human intestinal bacteria as reservoirs for antibiotic resistance genes. Trends Microbiol. 12 (9), 412–416.

Sawicki, G.S., Tiddens, H., 2012. Managing treatment complexity in cystic fibrosis: challenges and opportunities. Pediatr. Pulmonol. 47 (6), 523–533.

Scanlan, P.D., Buckling, A., Kong, W., Wild, Y., Lynch, S.V., Harrison, F., 2012. Gut dysbiosis in cystic fibrosis. J. Cystic Fibrosis 11 (5), 454–455.

Schippa, S., Iebba, V., Santangelo, F., Gagliardi, A., De Biase, R.V., Stamato, A., et al., 2013. Cystic fibrosis transmembrane conductance regulator (CFTR) allelic variants relate to shifts in faecal microbiota of cystic fibrosis patients. PloS One 8 (4), e61176.

Schloissnig, S., Arumugam, M., Sunagawa, S., Mitreva, M., Tap, J., Zhu, A., et al., 2013. Genomic variation landscape of the human gut microbiome. Nature 493 (7430), 45–50.

Schuster, A., Cynthia, H., Gerd, D., Martin, H.G., Freedom Study Group, 2013. Safety, efficacy and convenience of colistimethate sodium dry powder for inhalation (Colobreathe DPI) in patients with cystic fibrosis: a randomised study. Thorax 68 (4), 344–350.

Scott, K.P., Duncan, S.H., Flint, H.J., 2008. Dietary fibre and the gut microbiota. Nutr. Bull. 33 (3), 201–211.

Sharma, D., Singh Saharan, B., 2014. Simultaneous production of biosurfactants and bacteriocins by probiotic *Lactobacillus casei* MRTL3. Int. J. Microbiol. 2014.

Shipman, J.A., Berleman, J.E., Salyers, A.A., 2000. Characterization of four outer membrane proteins involved in binding starch to the cell surface of *Bacteroides thetaiotaomicron*. J. Bacteriol. 182 (19), 5365–5372.

Shoemaker, N.B., et al., 2001. Evidence for extensive resistance gene transfer among *Bacteroides* species and among Bacteroides and other genera in the human colon. Appl. Environ. Microbiol. 67 (2), 561–568.

Sjölund, M., et al., 2003. Long-term persistence of resistant Enterococcus species after antibiotics to eradicate *Helicobacter pylori*. Ann. Intern. Med. 139 (6), 483–487.

Smyth, A.R., Bell, S.C., Bojcin, S., Bryon, M., Duff, A., Flume, P., et al., 2014. European cystic fibrosis society standards of care: best practice guidelines. J. Cystic Fibrosis 13, S23–S42.

Somaraju, U.R., Solis-Moya, A., 2014. Pancreatic enzyme replacement therapy for people with cystic fibrosis. Cochrane Library. http://dx.doi.org/10.1002/14651858.

Sommer, M.O., et al., 2009. Functional characterization of the antibiotic resistance reservoir in the human microflora. Science 325 (5944), 1128–1131.

Stark, C., et al., 1993. Antimicrobial resistance in human oral and intestinal anaerobic microfloras. Antimicrob. Agents Chemother. 37 (8), 1665–1669.

Stecenko, A.A., Moran, A., 2010. Update on cystic fibrosis-related diabetes. Curr. Opin. Pulm. Med. 16 (6), 611–615.

Storm, D.R., et al., 1977. Polymyxin and related peptide antibiotics. Ann. Rev. Biochem. 46 (1), 723–763.

Strominger, J.L., Tipper, D.J., 1965. Bacterial cell wall synthesis and structure in relation to the mechanism of action of penicillins and other antibacterial agents. Am. J. Med. 39 (5), 708–721.

Sullivan, A., Edlund, C., Nord, C.E., 2001. Effect of antimicrobial agents on the ecological balance of human microflora. Lancet Infect. Dis. 1, 101–114.

Surawicz, C.M., Brandt, L.J., Binion, D.G., Ananthakrishnan, A.N., Curry, S.R., Gilligan, P.H., et al., 2013. Guidelines for diagnosis, treatment, and prevention of *Clostridium difficile* infections. Am. J. Gastroenterol. 108 (4), 478–498.

Szaff, M., Høiby, N., Flensborg, E.W., 1983. Frequent antibiotic therapy improves survival of cystic fibrosis patients with chronic *Pseudomonas aeruginosa* infection. Acta Paediatr. 72 (5), 651–657.

Taccetti, G., Campana, S., Festini, F., Mascherini, M., Döring, G., 2005. Early eradication therapy against *Pseudomonas aeruginosa* in cystic fibrosis patients. Eur. Respir. J. 26 (3), 458–461.

Taylor, S., et al., 1993. Glutathione peroxidase protects cultured mammalian cells from the toxicity of adriamycin and paraquat. Arch. Biochem. Biophys. 305 (2), 600–605.

Tipper, D., 1979. Mode of action of β-lactam antibiotics. Rev. Infect. Dis. 1 (1), 39–53.

Tenson, T., Lovmar, M., Ehrenberg, M., 2003. The mechanism of action of macrolides, lincosamides and streptogramin B reveals the nascent peptide exit path in the ribosome. J. Mol. Biol. 330 (5), 1005–1014.

Terhes, G., Maruyama, A., Latkóczy, K., Szikra, L., Konkoly-Thege, M., Princz, G., et al., 2014. In vitro antibiotic susceptibility profile of *Clostridium difficile* excluding PCR ribotype 027 outbreak strain in Hungary. Anaerobe 41–44.

Turnbaugh, P.J., Ley, R.E., Mahowald, M.A., Magrini, V., Mardis, E.R., Gordon, J.I., 2006. An obesity-associated gut microbiome with increased capacity for energy harvest. Nature 444 (7122), 1027–1131.

Turnbaugh, P.J., Ridaura, V.K., Faith, J.J., Rey, F.E., Knight, R., Gordon, J.I., 2009. The effect of diet on the human gut microbiome: a metagenomic analysis in humanized gnotobiotic mice. Sci. Transl. Med. 1 (6), 6ra14.

Turnbaugh, P.J., Gordon, J.I., 2009. The core gut microbiome, energy balance and obesity. J. Physiol. 587 (17), 4153–4158.

Tvede, M., Rask-Madsen, J., 1989. Bacteriotherapy for chronic relapsing *Clostridium difficile* diarrhoea in six patients. Lancet 333 (8648), 1156–1160.

Ubeda, C., et al., 2010. Vancomycin-resistant Enterococcus domination of intestinal microbiota is enabled by antibiotic treatment in mice and precedes bloodstream invasion in humans. J. Clin. Invest. 120 (12), 4332–4341.

Udekwu, K.I., Parrish, N., Ankomah, P., Baquero, F., Levin, B.R., 2009. Functional relationship between bacterial cell density and the efficacy of antibiotics. J. Antimicrob. Chemother. http://dx.doi.org/10.1093/jac/dkn554.

Uttley, L., Harnan, S., Cantrell, A., Taylor, C., Walshaw, M., Brownlee, K., Tappenden, P., 2013. Systematic review of the dry powder inhalers colistimethate sodium and tobramycin in cystic fibrosis. Eur. Respir. Rev. 22 (130), 476–486.

Valdez, J.C., Peral, M.C., Rachid, M., Santana, M., Perdigon, G., 2005. Interference of *Lactobacillus plantarum* with *Pseudomonas aeruginosa* in vitro and in infected burns: the potential use of probiotics in wound treatment. Clin. Microbiol. Infect. 11, 472–479.

Van Bambeke, F., Van Laethem, Y., Courvalin, P., Tulkens, P.M., 2004. Glycopeptide antibiotics. Drugs 64 (9), 913–936.

Videlock, E.J., Cremonini, F., 2012. Meta-analysis: probiotics in antibiotic-associated diarrhoea. Aliment. Pharmacol. Ther. 35 (12), 1355–1369.

Vighi, G., Marcucci, F., Sensi, L., Di Cara, G., Frati, F., 2008. Allergy and the gastrointestinal system. Clin. Exp. Immunol. 153 (s1), 3–6.

Villegas, M.V., Lolans, K., Correa, A., Kattan, J.N., Lopez, J.A., Quinn, J.P., 2007. First identification of *Pseudomonas aeruginosa* isolates producing a KPC-type carbapenem-hydrolyzing β-lactamase. Antimicrob. Agents Chemother. 51 (4), 1553–1555.

Viscidi, R., Willey, S., Bartlett, J.G., 1981. Isolation rates and toxigenic potential of *Clostridium difficile* isolates from various patient populations. Gastroenterology 81, 5–9.

Vonberg, R.P., et al., 2008. Infection control measures to limit the spread of *Clostridium difficile*. Clin. Microbiol. Infect. 14 (Suppl. 5), 2–20.

Waaij, V., 1989. The ecology of the human intestine and its consequences for overgrowth by pathogens such as *Clostridium difficile*. Ann. Rev. Microbiol. 43 (1), 69–87.

Wall, M.A., Terry, A.B., Eisenberg, J., McNamara, M., Cohen, R., 1983. Inhaled antibiotics in cystic fibrosis. Lancet 1, 1325.

Walsh, T.R., 2008. Clinically significant carbapenemases: an update. Curr. Opin. Infect. Dis. 21 (4), 367–371.

Warner, J.O., Taylor, B.W., Norman, A.P., Soothill, J.F., 1976. Association of cystic fibrosis with allergy. Arch. Dis. Child. 51 (7), 507–511.

Waters, V., Ratjen, F., 2006. Multidrug-resistant organisms in cystic fibrosis: management and infection-control issues. Expert Rev. Anti Infect. Ther. 4 (5).

Weiner, H.L., 2000. Oral tolerance, an active immunologic process mediated by multiple mechanisms. J. Clin. Invest. 106, 935–937.

Weiss, B., et al., 2010. Probiotic supplementation affects pulmonary exacerbations in patients with cystic fibrosis: a pilot study. Pediatr. Pulmonol. 45 (6), 536–540.

Welkon, C.J., Long, S.S., Thompson, C.M., Gilligan, P.H., 1985. *Clostridium difficile* in patients with cystic fibrosis. Am. J. Dis. Child. 139, 805–808.

Wells, J.M., Rossi, O., Meijerink, M., van Baarlen, P., 2011. Epithelial crosstalk at the microbiota–mucosal interface. Proc. Nat. Acad. Sci. 108 (Suppl. 1), 4607–4614.

Werlin, S.L., Benuri-Silbiger, I., Kerem, E., Adler, S.N., Goldin, E., Zimmerman, J., et al., 2010. Evidence of intestinal inflammation in patients with cystic fibrosis. J. Pediatr. Gastroenterol. Nutr. 51 (3), 304–308.

Wexler, H.M., 2007. Bacteroides: the good, the bad, and the nitty-gritty. Clin. Microbiol. Rev. 20 (4), 593–621.

White, H., Morton, A.M., Peckham, D.G., Conway, S.P., 2004. Dietary intakes in adult patients with cystic fibrosis–do they achieve guidelines? J. Cystic Fibrosis 3 (1), 1–7.

WHO, 2006. Toxicological Evaluation of Certain Veterinary Drug Residues in Food, vol. 57. World Health Organization.

Willing, B.P., Russell, S.L., Finlay, B.B., 2011. Shifting the balance: antibiotic effects on host–microbiota mutualism. Nat. Rev. Microbiol. 9 (4), 233–243.

Wills-Karp, M., Santeliz, J., Karp, C.L., 2001. The germless theory of allergic disease: revisiting the hygiene hypothesis. Nat. Rev. Immunol. 1 (1), 69–75.

Wolter, J., Seeney, S., Bell, S., Bowler, S., Masel, P., McCormack, J., 2002. Effect of long term treatment with azithromycin on disease parameters in cystic fibrosis: a randomised trial. Thorax 57 (3), 212–216.

Wright, E.A., et al., 2013. Sub-inhibitory concentrations of some antibiotics can drive diversification of *Pseudomonas aeruginosa* populations in artificial sputum medium. BMC Microbiol. 13, 170.

Wu, G.D., Chen, J., Hoffmann, C., Bittinger, K., Chen, Y.Y., Keilbaugh, S.A., et al., 2011. Linking long-term dietary patterns with gut microbial enterotypes. Science 334 (6052), 105–108.

Wybo, I., et al., 2007. Third Belgian multicentre survey of antibiotic susceptibility of anaerobic bacteria. J. Antimicrob. Chemother. 59 (1), 132–139.

Xu, J., et al., 2003. A genomic view of the human-*Bacteroides thetaiotaomicron* symbiosis. Science 299 (5615), 2074–2076.

Xu, D., Gao, J., Gillilland III, M., Wu, X., Song, I., Kao, J.Y., Owyang, C., 2014. Rifaximin alters intestinal bacteria and prevents stress-induced gut inflammation and visceral hyperalgesia in rats. Gastroenterology 146 (2), 484–496.

Yap, M.N., Yang, C.H., Charkowski, A.O., 2008. The response regulator HrpY of *Dickeya dadantii* 3937 regulates virulence genes not linked to the hrp cluster. Mol. Plant Microbe Inter. 21 (3), 304–314.

Zar, F.A., Bakkanagari, S.R., Moorthi, K.M., Davis, M.B., 2007. A comparison of vancomycin and metronidazole for the treatment of *Clostridium difficile*-associated diarrhea, stratified by disease severity. Clin. Infect. Dis. 45, 302–307.

Zebouh, M., Thomas, C., Honderlick, P., Lemee, L., Segonds, C., Wallet, F., Husson, M.O., 2008. Direct antimicrobial susceptibility testing method for analysis of sputum collected from patients with cystic fibrosis. J. Cystic Fibrosis 7 (3), 238–243.

Correlating the Gut Microbiome to Health and Disease

12

T.M. Marques, S. Holster, R. Wall, J. König, R.J. Brummer

Örebro University, Nutrition-Gut-Brain Interactions Research Centre, Faculty of Medicine and Health, Örebro, Sweden

W.M. de Vos

Wageningen University, Laboratory of Microbiology, Wageningen, The Netherlands; University of Helsinki, Haartman Institute, Department of Bacteriology and Immunology, Helsinki, Finland

INTRODUCTION

The human gut microbiota is a complex ecosystem that is estimated to be composed of approximately 10^{14} bacterial cells, which is 10 times more than the total number of human cells in the body (Zoetendal et al., 2008). Over 10 million microbial genes have been identified within the gut microbiota, illustrating the fact that the coding capacity of the microbes within it exceeds that of our own body cells (Li et al., 2014). Hence, this microbial community is commonly referred to as our hidden or forgotten "organ" as proposed 10 years ago (O'Hara and Shanahan, 2006).

The gut microbiota consists of a diverse population of mainly prokaryotes that are expected to have a symbiotic relationship with the human host. Most of these have an (facultative) anaerobic lifestyle and belong to a few abundant phyla, including the Firmicutes, Bacteroidetes, Actinobacteria, Proteobacteria, and Verrucomicrobia. The Firmicutes and Bacteroidetes phyla accommodate the most abundant species and constitute over 90% of the human gut microbiota (Bäckhed et al., 2005; Eckburg et al., 2005). The gut microbiota exerts a considerable influence on the host, being involved in food metabolism, immunomodulation, and pathogen exclusion. Thus the microbiome has a significant potential to affect our health by affecting our physiological, immunological, and nutritional status (Hooper et al., 1998; Neish, 2009).

From being almost sterile at birth, our gut is rapidly colonized in the first few days of life, being affected by such factors as mode of delivery (Grölund et al., 1999), type of feeding (Orrhage and Nord, 1999), and antibiotic therapy (Gibson et al., 2015). Although the gut microbiome develops rapidly in diversity and complexity in the first few years after birth, it becomes relatively stable in adulthood, and specific microbiota signatures have been detected in longitudinal analysis over 10 years (Rajilić-Stojanović et al., 2013). In addition, the composition of our microbiome is highly individual and similar in genetically related subjects (Turnbaugh et al., 2009).

The Gut-Brain Axis. http://dx.doi.org/10.1016/B978-0-12-802304-4.00012-8

Although our microbiome is relatively stable, it may be modified by various factors such as food components, major dietary changes, and pharmaceutical treatments that target the composition, stability, and activity of the microbiota.

After the discovery of microbial life, Antonie van Leeuwenhoek reported in 1681 the first observation relating a disturbed microbial composition to the diarrhea he was experiencing, possibly after drinking dirty Amsterdam canal water (Dobell, 1932). More than 2 centuries later, Metchnikoff hypothesized that replacing the "bad" bacteria in the gut with lactic acid bacteria could normalize bowel health and thus prolong life (Metchnikoff and Mitchell, 1907). Hence, it has long been speculated that the gut microbiota bears a significant functional role in maintaining gut health. Since these earlier observations numerous studies have been performed to elucidate what role the human gut microbiome plays in human health as a whole, and a total of more than 25 diseases and syndromes have been associated with the gut microbiota to date (de Vos and de Vos, 2012, Table 12.1). Most of our knowledge about this microbial organ and what role it plays in our physiology is becoming clearer thanks to recent advances in sequencing technology, which has helped us to reveal the complexity and composition of the gut microbiota. Dysbiosis is often used to designate an alteration of the composition of the gut microbiota, but this term is a misnomer because a healthy gut microbiota has not been well defined because it is also highly personalized, affected by diet, and extremely complex (Zoetendal et al., 2008; Zoetendal and de Vos, 2014). However, the presence of changes in gut microbiota composition has been described as being the major hallmark that is associated with, or contributes to, diseases that have been linked to the gut microbiome. Although, these are associations and not causalities in most cases, microbiota changes have been linked with diseases occurring within and outside of the gut, including inflammatory bowel disease (IBD; Sokol et al., 2008; Willing et al., 2010), irritable bowel syndrome (IBS; König and Brummer, 2014; Rajilić-Stojanović et al., 2011), obesity (Ley et al., 2006; Turnbaugh et al., 2006), type II diabetes (Qin et al., 2012; Karlsson et al., 2013), and colorectal cancer (CRC; Wang et al., 2012). Psychological disorders, such as anxiety and depression, are to some degree comorbidities in all of the above-mentioned diseases, and recent work has also suggested a potential role for the gut microbiota in behavior and mental health. Although the latter has only been reported in animal studies so far, the results have been striking (Heijtz et al., 2011; Bravo et al., 2011). One prominent example of this is a study by Collins et al. (2013), showing that the transplantation of a fecal microbiome from one mouse strain presenting a phenotypic set of behavior to another mouse strain resulted in the recipient strain displaying the behavioral phenotype of the donor. The aim of this chapter is to give an overview on the extensive role of our gut microbiome in health and disease.

GUT MICROBIOTA AND IMMUNE SYSTEM-RELATED DISEASES

Millions of years of coevolution have created a complex mutualistic relationship between the commensal microbiota and its host that begins at birth. The immune system shapes the microbiota composition and, in turn, the microbiota induces the maturation of the immune system and directs the development of immune responses

Table 12.1 Diseases (or Syndromes) That Are Found to be Associated With Deviations in the Intestinal Microbiota Composition

Level of Support	Diseases Associated With Fecal Microbiota	References
Considerable to high	C. difficile colitis	Khoruts et al. (2010), Petrof et al. (2013), and van Nood et al. (2013)
	Crohn's disease	Sokol et al. (2009) and Willing et al. (2010)
	Ulcerative colitis	Png et al. (2010), Lepage et al. (2011), Moayyedi et al. (2015), and Rossen et al. (2015)
	Irritable bowel syndrome	Saulnier et al. (2011), Rajilić-Stojanović et al. (2011), and Pozuelo et al. (2015)
	Colorectal cancer	Sobhani et al. (2011), Wang et al. (2012), and Keku et al. (2015)
	Celiac disease	Nistal et al. (2012), Di Cagno et al. (2011), Kalliomäki et al. (2012), and Giacomin et al. (2015)
	Atopic dermatitis	Bisgaard et al. (2011), Storrø et al. (2011), and Lynch et al. (2014)
	Asthma	Russel et al. (2012), Abrahamsson et al. (2014), and Arrieta et al. (2015)
	Rheumatoid arthritis	Scher and Abramson 2011, Scher et al. (2013), and Zhang et al. (2015)
	Type I diabetes	Giongo et al. (2011), Brown et al. (2011), Kostic et al. (2015), and Patterson et al. (2015)
	Type II diabetes	Larssen et al. (2010), Qin et al. (2012), and Karlsson et al. (2013)
	Obesity	Ley et al. (2006), Turnbaugh et al. (2009), Schwiertz et al. (2010), and Kasai et al. (2015)
	Nonalcoholic fatty liver disease	Spencer et al. (2011), Henao-Mejia et al. (2012), Zhu et al. (2013), and Jiang et al. (2015)

Continued

Table 12.1 Diseases (or Syndromes) That Are Found to be Associated With Deviations in the Intestinal Microbiota Composition—cont'd

Level of Support	Diseases Associated With Fecal Microbiota	References
Medium to uncertain	Alzheimer's disease	Qin et al. (2007), Lee et al. (2008), and Karri et al. (2010)
	Parkinson's disease	Forsyth et al. (2011) and Scheperjans et al. (2015)
	Autistic spectrum disorder	Wang et al. (2011a) and Williams et al. (2011, 2012)
	Chronic fatigue syndrome	Sheedy et al. (2009) and Frémont et al. (2013)
	Atherosclerosis	Koren et al. (2011), Koeth et al. (2013), and Yamashita et al. (2015)
	Cardiovascular disease	Wang et al. (2011b) and Lam et al. (2012)
	Depression and anxiety	Bravo et al. (2011) and Messaoudi et al. (2011)
	Frailty	van Tongeren et al. (2005) and Claesson et al. (2012)
	Graft vs. host disease	Murphy and Nguyen (2011), Vossen et al. (2014), and Eriguchi et al. (2015)
	Infant colic	de Weerth et al. (2013) and Roos et al. (2013)
	Multiple sclerosis	Berer et al. (2011) and Miyake et al. (2015)
	Retrovirus infection	Kane et al. (2011)
	Poliovirus infection	Kuss et al. (2011)

These are divided into different levels of support, varying from associations in multiple studies, microbiota targeting therapies, and specific model animal studies (considerable to high) to associations only or model animal studies only (medium to uncertain).
Adapted from de Vos, W.M., de Vos, E.A., 2012. Role of the intestinal microbiome in health and disease: from correlation to causation. Nutr. Rev. 70 (Suppl. 1), S45–S56.

(Kamada et al., 2013). The immune system has evolved, recognizing commensal bacteria and responding and adapting to foreign and self-molecules, hence protecting the host from pathogens while preserving the symbiotic relationship (Hooper et al., 2012). In turn, the gut bacterial community has developed to modulate structures and cells of the immune system, all of which have important roles in the process of tolerance and susceptibility to inflammation. Studies using germ-free (GF) animals have shown that the gut microbiota is required for the normal generation and maturation of gut-associated lymphoid tissues (Cebra et al., 1998) to regulate the development of specific immune cells in the gut, such as the T helper 17 (Th17) and Foxp3[+] regulatory T cells (Ivanov et al., 2008; Lathrop et al., 2011), and to induce the differentiation of immunoglobulin A–producing B cells (Strugnell and Wijburg, 2010). Therefore early-life exposure to microbial antigens is critical for a proper immune development. By recognizing self from nonself, presenting a broad range of antigens during the first days of life (critical window) will lower the risk for autoimmune diseases and exacerbated responsiveness to allergens later in life that may increase the susceptibility to allergies and asthma (Fujimura and Lynch, 2015; Hooper et al., 2012).

ALLERGIES AND ASTHMA

The prevalence of allergic diseases, such as atopic dermatitis (eczema), food allergies, and asthma has increased over the last decades, becoming a major health problem in developed countries. This increase has coincided with lifestyle-associated environmental changes that may affect the host microbiota, such as increased hygiene, smaller family sizes, dietary changes, and excessive antibiotic use (West et al., 2015). Indeed, the establishment of oral allergic sensitization in a murine model of food allergy has been associated with alterations in the intestinal microbiota (Rivas et al., 2013). Vancomycin treatment of newborn mice has been shown to reduce gut microbiota diversity, enhancing the susceptibility to experimental allergic asthma (Russel et al., 2012). The authors hypothesized that antibiotic exposure early in life selects for a community of microbes that disrupts the balance of proinflammatory and regulatory immune responses that may play key roles in disease onset. Moreover, several clinical studies have shown that a reduced diversity of intestinal microbiota at early life is associated with an increased risk of developing atopic diseases and asthma in infants (Abrahamsson et al., 2012, 2014; Bisgaard et al., 2011; Forno et al., 2008; Wang et al., 2008).

Epidemiological studies have shown an inverse relationship between rates of childhood allergies and exposure to microbial-rich environments, suggesting that exposure to high levels of certain allergens and bacteria early in life might be beneficial. In a study conducted by Ege et al. (2011), school children growing up in predominantly rural areas were shown to be protected from asthma and atopy whereas a study by Ownby et al. (2002) demonstrated that exposure to two or more dogs or cats in the first year of life reduced subsequent allergic sensitization. Of note, a birth cohort study in an inner-city environment conducted by Lynch et al. (2014) found the lowest rates of atopy and wheezing in children with higher bacterial diversity that had been exposed to high levels of cockroach, mouse, and cat allergen if compared with children with lower exposure to these allergens.

Substantial effort has been devoted to identifying specific bacterial species or taxa that correlate with the development of, or protection against, allergy-related disorders. However, the results are still conflicting and differ significantly depending on the study, probably because of differences in sample populations and the methods applied for microbiota analysis. Although Lynch et al. (2014) described the presence of allergy-protective bacteria, particularly from the *Prevotellaceae*, *Lachnospiraceae*, and *Ruminococcaceae* families, in the house dust of urban neighborhoods Ege et al. (2011) did not identify any protective microorganisms in the rural environment studied. Abrahamsson et al. (2012) reported a lower diversity of Bacteroidetes and Proteobacteria in infants with atopic eczema, but the same group did not find associations between asthma and the relative abundance of any phylum or genus in a second study (Abrahamsson et al., 2014). A recent study by Arrieta et al. (2015) found that babies that had low or undetectable levels of the bacterial genera *Lachnospira*, *Veillonella*, *Faecalibacterium*, and *Rothia* at 3 months of age had elevated risk to develop asthma-like symptoms by their first birthday, whereas infants at lower asthma risk had relatively robust levels of these bacteria in their intestine when they were 3 months old. It is interesting to note that the group confirmed the protective effect of these bacteria in a second experiment that showed an improvement in airway inflammation in GF mice inoculated with these four bacterial taxa. It is of interest to note that the absence of similar bacteria, including *Rothia* spp., were included in a classifier predicting later-life asthma in a large cohort of Finnish infants that had been exposed to unusually high levels of antibiotics earlier in life (Korpela et al., 2016).

RHEUMATOID ARTHRITIS

Gut microbiota aberrations may also play a role in rheumatoid arthritis (RA) onset and progression in genetically predisposed individuals (Scher and Abramson, 2011). RA is a chronic autoimmune disorder and its development is associated with the dysregulation of normal immune function with increased production of proinflammatory cytokines (eg, tumor necrosis factor [TNF]-α, interleukin [IL]-1, and IL-17) and activation of T and B lymphocytes (Abdollahi-Roodsaz et al., 2008). Animal models of inflammatory arthritis have demonstrated that bacterial colonization can be an environmental trigger for the development of the disease. Wu et al. (2010) showed that segmented filamentous bacteria (SFB) introduced into GF animals can induce Th17 cells to produce IL-17, a cytokine that stimulates the production of autoantibodies, provoking the onset of arthritis. However, it should be emphasized that SFB have only anecdotally been described to be present in humans. Hence, a recent study that further embarked on the molecular mechanism of SFB in inducing Th17 cell accumulation in mice also described the isolation of human bacteria that could mimic this signaling system (Atarashi et al., 2015).

In another animal study Abdollahi-Roodsaz et al. (2008) demonstrated that contamination of IL1rn−/− GF mice with a single species, *Lactobacillus bifidus*, results in the activation of toll-like receptor (TLR)-2 and TLR4 with rapid development of arthritis. Furthermore, clinical studies have been done to investigate if intestinal microbiota composition in patients with RA differs from healthy subjects. In a study conducted by Scher et al. (2013), the species *Prevotella copri* was found to be more abundant in patients suffering from untreated RA than in healthy subjects, but this discrepancy was not observed in chronic RA patients receiving treatment. Moreover, colonization of mice with *P. copri* exacerbated the severity of dextran sulfate sodium–induced colitis, suggesting that this organism has a potential proinflammatory function. Zhang et al. (2015) also reported alterations in the microbiota composition of RA patients when compared with healthy controls, which was partially resolved after RA treatment. Bacteria from the *Haemophilus* species were depleted, whereas *Lactobacillus salivarius* was overrepresented in individuals with RA, and this deviation was most marked in patients suffering with very active RA.

GUT MICROBIOTA AND INTESTINAL DISEASES
RECURRENT *CLOSTRIDIUM DIFFICILE* INFECTIONS

A large body of evidence has now accumulated indicating that, in addition to the presence of toxin-producing *Clostridium difficile*, this life-threatening disease is manifested in extreme colitis that cannot be cured with antibiotics, including the last-resort antibiotic vancomycin. Therapies that were already described in Chinese traditional medicine include changing the intestinal microbiota by inoculating new microbes via a process that is now known as fecal microbiota transplantation (FMT). In an observational study, FMT showed high efficacy in curing recurrent *Clostridium difficile* infection (CDI) patients using colonic transplantations (Mattila et al., 2012). In a comparative study in which recurrent CDI patients were treated with vancomycin, an intestinal lavage and vancomycin, or with duodenal FMT, only the latter was effective with a curing efficiency above 90% (van Nood et al., 2013). Molecular studies indicated that the intestinal microbiota of the recurrent CDI patients had a very low diversity coupled with overgrowth of inflammatory bacteria (Fuentes et al., 2014). This situation was immediately changed after FMT, and a healthy microbial community was established and sustained for long periods of time. This is the first and a unique example indicating that bugs are better than drugs and stimulated the use of FMT for a range of other diseases (Smits et al., 2013). Moreover, FMT has been used for other diseases, and its success is used to develop a range of products based on active intestinal microbes that can cure recurrent CDI and other diseases (de Vos, 2013).

INFLAMMATORY BOWEL DISEASE

IBD comprises several disorders that affect the gastrointestinal tract and are characterized by chronic inflammation. The most common and well-studied diseases are Crohn's disease and ulcerative colitis (UC). Microscopic colitis (MC), comprising lymphocytic colitis and collagenous colitis, is also regarded as IBD. The causes of IBD are still not understood. One hypothesis is that IBD is caused by an excessive immune response to the commensal gut microbiota in genetically susceptible subjects. In addition, a normal immune response to an altered microbiota is considered a putative pathophysiologic mechanism. Similar to IBS, several studies have been conducted to compare the intestinal microbiota in IBD in relation to healthy controls.

A common result is a reduced microbial diversity in IBD (Ott et al., 2004). With regard to the microbiota composition, results are more divergent. However, it seems that a lower abundance of butyrate- or propionate-producing bacteria, such as *Faecalibacterium prausnitzii* (Sokol et al., 2008) and *Akkermansia muciniphila* (Png et al., 2010; Rajilić-Stojanović et al., 2013), respectively, is a common feature. The localization of the disease and the different pathophysiologic mechanisms behind each case make interpretation of the intestinal microbiota composition difficult. For instance, Willing et al. (2010) reported that two different phenotypes in Crohn's disease, one localized in the ileum (ICD) and one localized in the colon (CCD), also resulted in a different microbiota composition. CCD patients had more Firmicutes compared with healthy subjects whereas ICD patients tended to have a lower abundance.

Fusobacterium nucleatum is one of the bacterial strains that is supposed to play a role in the pathogenesis of IBD. This bacterium is more abundant in colonic biopsies of IBD patients than in healthy controls and the strains isolated from inflamed tissue in IBD patients are more invasive in vivo (Strauss et al., 2011).

A critical question with regard to an altered microbiota composition in IBD is whether this microbial alteration either is secondary to the intestinal inflammation or an independent risk factor of IBD. Nevertheless, two recent clinical trials, applying FMT, have shown that exchanging the microbiota in UC patients may result in symptom improvement in at least a subset of the patients (Moayyedi et al., 2015; Rossen et al., 2015). It seems that success is dependent on repeated microbial transfers and is highly donor dependent.

MC is a chronic inflammatory disorder that is mainly characterized by its microscopic appearance. Two different types of MC have been described according to their histological aberrations. Collagenous colitis and lymphocytic colitis show an increased density of lymphocytes in the lamina propria of the colonic mucosa, but collagenous colitis also features a thickened subepithelial collagen layer. The pathophysiology of MC is not well understood, but the combination of an aberrant immune response and an altered microbiota composition seems to play a major role. Fischer et al. (2015) has described this altered microbiota composition in patients with MC. They found that the feces of patients with MC was significantly depleted in *Verrucomicrobia* (*Akkermansia* spp.) compared with feces of healthy subjects. In addition, other species such as *Bacteroides* and *Prevotella* differed in MC patients compared with healthy controls; however, no statistical significance was reached.

IRRITABLE BOWEL SYNDROME

IBS is one of the disorders known for the important role of the gut microbiome in its pathophysiology. This multifactorial disease affects 10–20% of the population. Patients are suffering from symptoms such as pain and cramps, diarrhea and/or constipation, bloating, flatulence, a feeling of incomplete defecation, and relief of pain or discomfort upon defecation. The etiology of IBS is still not well understood, and IBS is often diagnosed by excluding other intestinal diseases such as IBD. However, it is generally accepted that a dysregulation along the microbe-gut-brain axis is present in IBS, as shown by the high prevalence of psychological comorbidities and an increased visceral hypersensitivity in IBS patients (Kennedy et al., 2014). In addition, a low-grade intestinal inflammation is present in the intestinal mucosa of some patients, and there is evidence that the immune system reacts abnormally to the commensal microbiota, especially in the case of postinfectious IBS (Sundin et al., 2015a,b).

Many studies have investigated the intestinal microbiota of IBS patients and shown that it differs in composition and diversity compared with healthy controls (König and Brummer, 2014; Rajilić-Stojanović et al., 2011). However, results vary, probably because of differences in sampling and analysis techniques, various or missing classifications of patients into subgroups, and omitting the strong effect of dietary intake. In addition, it should be taken into account whether fecal or mucosal samples have been investigated because their composition differs substantially (Sundin et al., 2015a). Nevertheless, results so far provide evidence that the microbiota in IBS differs from healthy controls and that microbial metabolites also play an important role (Tana et al., 2010). A recently published study compared the fecal microbiota of 113 IBS patients with the microbiota in 66 healthy controls and showed that IBS patients have altered levels of butyrate- and methane-producing bacteria in their intestine and that those bacteria vary among different subtypes of IBS (Pozuelo et al., 2015). This study and others have shown correlations between the abundance of different types of bacterial strains and IBS symptoms (Malinen et al., 2010).

Additional evidence for the importance of the intestinal microbiota in IBS is the fact that treatment with probiotics and antibiotics have shown to improve IBS symptoms, even if this effect seems rather limited (~10% higher than placebo) (Hoveyda et al., 2009; Menees et al., 2012; Pimentel et al., 2011). Hence, optimization of probiotic strains and more effective ways of modifying the intestinal microbiota, such as by FMT, account for new promising therapeutic options for IBS.

COLORECTAL CANCER

An imbalance between the colonic microbiota and the intestinal epithelium might lead to an immune cell invasion and chronic inflammation, which in turn might result in colorectal carcinogenesis. Animal studies have shown that the presence of microbiota is necessary to develop CRC (Keku et al., 2015). Recently, a systematic review was published aiming to summarize the studies that have investigated the changes in microbiota and immune response in relation to colorectal carcinogenesis in human and animal studies (Borges, 2015). The authors report that some bacteria are more abundant (*Fusobacteria, Alistipes, Porphyromonadaceae, Coriobacteridae, Staphylococcaceae, Akkermansia* spp., and *Methanobacteriales*) whereas others are less abundant (*Bifidobacterium, Lactobacillus, Ruminococcus, Faecalibacterium* spp., *Roseburia*, and *Treponema*) in patients and laboratory animals with colorectal carcinomas. In addition, some butyrate-producing bacteria are reduced in the fecal material of CRC patients (Wang et al., 2012), which can be related to the hypothesis that butyrate plays a role in cancer prevention (Scharlau et al., 2009). However, two recent comprehensive metagenomic studies showed a strong correlation between the microbiota and CRC and even reported a microbiome-based classifier predicting the early CRC development (Zeller et al., 2014; Yu et al., 2015). It has been suggested that these microbiome-based markers are superior to fecal occult blood analysis, but this has to be further extensively tested. In addition, more research is needed to conclude whether microbiota aberrations are a cause or a consequence in CRC.

GUT MICROBIOTA AND DISEASES OF THE NERVOUS SYSTEM
ANXIETY AND DEPRESSION

Psychological disorders, such as anxiety and depression, are to some degree comorbidities in all of the diseases previously mentioned. The microbe-gut-brain axis is a well-accepted entity and is involved in these disorders. However, it remains uncertain whether mental and microbial factors are a cause or consequence.

A direct connection between the intestinal microbiota and mood disorders is well documented in animal models. GF mice show less anxiety-like behavior compared with conventionalized mice, suggesting that the development of this behavior can be affected by the intestinal microbiota (Neufeld et al., 2011). In addition, colonization of GF mice with microbiota of a different species resulted in behavioral changes (Bercik et al., 2011). In humans it is known that enteropathogens may affect mood, probably via the immune system. Reichenberg et al. (2001) showed in a placebo-controlled study that healthy volunteers experienced increased anxiety and depressive mood after intravenous infusion with *Salmonella abortus equi* endotoxins. The authors hypothesized that this effect on emotional perception was probably generated because of the host's immune system release of cytokines. Moreover, the common observation that many patients with chronic hepatitis C develop depression during interferon treatment led to the theory that depression is an inflammatory state (Udina et al., 2012).

Unfortunately, not many human studies on the effect of altered intestinal microbiota composition on brain function have been performed yet, but a few studies using probiotics showed an effect on mental factors. A milky drink containing the probiotic *Lactobacillus casei Shirota* improved the mood of volunteers with initially poor mood, but it had no effect on the general study populations (Benton et al., 2007). In addition, the administration of *Lactobacillus helveticus* R0052 and *Bifidobacterium longum* R0175 was studied in a double-blind, placebo-controlled, randomized trial (Messaoudi et al., 2011). Taking this mix of probiotics for 30 days improved psychological distress in healthy subjects.

AUTISTIC SPECTRUM DISORDER

Children with autistic spectrum disorder (ASD) are more likely to suffer from intestinal problems than children in the general population (Horvath et al., 1999). Several studies reported an altered microbiota composition in children with autism, indicating that microbiota possibly plays a role in this disorder. For instance, Wang et al. (2011a) used quantitative real-time polymerase chain reaction analysis to show that children with autism have lower relative abundance of *Bifidobacterium* species and mucolytic bacterium *A. muciniphila* in their feces compared with children without autism. It should be mentioned that the altered bowel habits per se could be the reason for an altered microbiota composition. In addition, altered microbiota composition in ileal and cecal mucosa has been reported (Williams et al., 2011, 2012). However, results are equivocal, probably because of different sampling and analysis methods as well as small patient numbers (König et al., 2015). This might be one of the reasons why no clinical trials have been published yet addressing potential therapeutic treatments to change the intestinal microbiota in ASD children. One small pilot study investigated the effect of vancomycin, an antibiotic that is poorly absorbed in the intestine, in children with autism and reported that autistic behavior was improved during the 8 weeks of intervention (Sandler et al., 2000). Although this result did not persist after treatment, it showed that the intestinal microbiota-brain connection might be of importance in ASD. In addition, the metabolites that are produced by gut microbiota, such as propionate, acetate, and valerate, were found in lower levels in patients with autism than in children from the general population, suggesting that in addition to the microbiota metabolites could also play an important role in ASD (Adams et al., 2011).

ALZHEIMER'S DISEASE

There is increasing evidence on impaired gastrointestinal function in Alzheimer's disease. Using an Alzheimer's disease male transgenic mouse model, Karri et al. (2010) showed that alterations in gastrointestinal tract morphology, a shift in microbiota composition, and an increase of amyloid protein expression in the gut play a key role in the pathophysiology of this disease. The amyloid precursor protein (APP) is found in many tissues in the body. Proteolysis of this protein results in generation of β-amyloid, which forms the amyloid plaques in the brain of Alzheimer's disease patients. In mice, APP expression increased after repeated injection of lipopolysaccharide (LPS; Lee et al., 2008), and systemic administration of LPS in mice leads to acute neurodegeneration (Qin et al., 2007). In addition, increased plasma levels of LPS were found in Alzheimer's disease patients (Zhang et al., 2009). The authors suggested that plasma LPS originates from translocation of commensal and pathogenic bacteria and may play an important role in the pathology of Alzheimer's disease, possibly through neuroinflammation. In a study recently published online it was reported that in the microbiota of a mouse model for Alzheimer's disease certain microbes were depleted, including *A. muciniphila* (Harach et al., 2015).

PARKINSON'S DISEASE

In addition to a dysfunctional motor system, up to 80% of Parkinson's disease patients suffer from constipation. It was long thought that the gastrointestinal problems in Parkinson's disease patients were a consequence of the disease (Abbott et al., 2001). However, half of all Parkinson's disease patients suffer from constipation before the onset of the actual disease, suggesting a relation between early gastrointestinal problems and later development of Parkinson's disease (König et al., 2015). It has been shown that Parkinson's disease patients have significantly increased gut permeability and an increased amount of *Escherichia coli* in sigmoid colon biopsies (Forsyth et al., 2011). Hypothetically, the *E. coli* could translocate to the epithelium and lamina propria because of this increased epithelial permeability. A study investigating the microbiota in Parkinson's disease patients showed that abundance of *Prevotellaceae* is reduced compared with healthy controls (Scheperjans et al., 2015). The abundance of *Enterobacteriacea* correlated with the severity of gait difficulty and postural instability, suggesting that the microbiota could be associated with the motor symptoms in Parkinson's disease.

GUT MICROBIOTA AND METABOLIC DISEASES
OBESITY

Obesity is a worldwide public health concern with multifactorial origins involving genetic, metabolic, and environmental factors. It is interesting to note that some individuals seem to be more susceptible to "obesogenic" environmental factors, such as sedentary lifestyles and high-calorie intake, than others (Tims et al., 2013). Although genome-wide association studies have identified several loci associated with obesity susceptibility, human genome variation itself cannot explain the observed variance in energy homeostasis and the apparent heritability of body mass index (BMI; Xia and Grant, 2013).

Numerous studies have revealed that the gut microbiota is strongly associated with host energy regulation and homeostasis and may play a critical role in the development of obesity. Bäckhed et al. (2004) were one of the first groups to suggest that the microbiota may be an environmental factor affecting the host predisposition toward adiposity. They showed that colonization of GF mice with microorganisms from conventionalized mice produces a rapid increase in total body fat content despite reduced food intake. The conventionalization of adult GF mice was shown to suppress *Fiaf* expression in their small intestines, stimulating hepatic triglyceride (TG) production and promoting lipoprotein lipase–directed incorporation of these TGs into adipocytes, thereby promoting storage of calories harvested from the diet. Furthermore, Turnbaugh et al. (2006) demonstrated that the gut microbiome in an ob/ob mouse model has an increased capacity to absorb energy from the diet and that this trait is transmissible. They showed that adult GF C57BL/6J mice colonized with a microbiota obtained from obese (ob/ob) donors exhibited a greater increase in body fat than mice colonized with a microbiota from lean donors. Other studies have focused on the short-chain fatty acid (SCFA) mechanisms thought to affect the host's energy metabolism and contribute to the pathogenesis of obesity. SCFAs produced by the gut microbiota were shown to interact with the G-protein–coupled receptor (GPR)-41 and GPR43, leading to the inhibition of lipolysis, affecting appetite, and increasing circulating levels of gut hormones (eg, peptide YY, leptin; Ge et al., 2008; Hong et al., 2005; Karaki et al., 2008;

Samuel et al., 2008). Kimura et al. (2013) described SCFAs as signaling molecules and GPR43 receptors as energy sensors, with their interaction suppressing the accumulation of fat in adipose tissue and stimulating the utilization of excess energy by other tissues to maintain metabolic homeostasis.

Investigations on the relationship between the gut microbiota ecology and obesity have yielded contradictory results. Previous studies by Ley et al. demonstrated a lower abundance of Bacteroidetes and a proportional increase in Firmicutes in genetically obese ob/ob mice (Ley et al., 2005) and in obese people (Ley et al., 2006) when compared with lean controls. Moreover, in the clinical study by Ley et al., the proportion of Bacteroidetes was shown to increase with weight loss when people followed low-calorie diets. These results led the group to hypothesize that the increased ratio of Firmicutes to Bacteroidetes could promote accumulation of adipose tissue and that manipulation of gut microbial communities could be an alternative approach in the treatment of obesity. Analogous to the results obtained by Ley et al. (2006), other clinical studies reported a significant reduction in the proportion of Bacteroidetes in obese patients compared with lean individuals (Armougom et al., 2009; Turnbaugh et al., 2009; Kasai et al., 2015). However, other studies have contradicted these findings (Table 12.2). Whereas Schwiertz et al. (2010) reported a lower ratio of Firmicutes to Bacteroidetes in obese adults compared with lean controls, other researchers have found no correlation between human obesity and the proportions of *Bacteroides* and Firmicutes (Duncan et al., 2008; Tims et al., 2013; Galley et al., 2014; Hu et al., 2015). In addition, studies looking into the association of obesity with gut microbiota diversity and changes in specific bacterial groups have also shown conflicting results, highlighting the importance of other factors such as age, geographical location, diet, and study methodology (sample size, microbiota-profiling methodologies, method sensitivity), which all would have to be taken into account when determining what role the human gut microbiota has in obesity. A recent study showed that Bacteroidetes were depleted in the intestinal samples of morbidly obese patients as compared with lean subjects (Verdam et al., 2013). Further analysis of this cohort using a metaproteomics approach showed that although their numbers were decreased, the activity of the Bacteroidetes was highly increased in morbidly obese patients, most likely as a consequence of their pH sensitivity (Kolmeder et al., 2015). This finding highlights the fact that it is the activity rather than the mere presence of intestinal microbes that determines their functionality.

TYPE II DIABETES

Type II diabetes (T2D) is a complex metabolic disorder influenced by genetic and environmental components and aggravated by several risk factors, including age, family history, diet, sedentary lifestyle, and obesity (Qin et al., 2012; Karlsson et al., 2013). Similar to obesity, T2D has become a major public health issue throughout the world. Both diseases are characterized by a state of chronic low-grade inflammation with abnormal expression and production of multiple inflammatory mediators accompanied by gut microbiota changes (Larsen et al., 2010).

Table 12.2 Reported Compositional Changes in the Human Gut Microbiome in Obese Subjects

References	Country	Subjects Age	Obese Subjects BMI (kg/m²)	Analytical Method	Microbiota in Obese Subjects		
					Diversity	Firmicutes/Bacteroidetes Ratio	Composition
Ley et al. (2006)	United States	21–65 years	30–43	16S rRNA sequencing	—	Higher	↑ Firmicutes ↓ Bacteroidetes
Duncan et al. (2008)	Scotland	—	≥30	16S rRNA-based quantitative FISH	—	No difference	—
Armougom et al. (2009)	France	17–72 years	≥30	RT-PCR	—	Higher	↑ Lactobacillus
Turnbaugh et al. (2009)	United States	21–32 years	≥30	16S rRNA sequencing/pyrosequencing	Lower	Higher	↑ Actinobacteria ↓ Bacteroidetes
Karlsson et al. (2013)	Sweden	4–5 years	17.6–25.8	qPCR and T-RFLP analysis	No difference	—	↑ Enterobacteriaceae ↓ Desulfovibrio and A. muciniphila-like bacteria
Schwiertz et al. (2010)	Germany	14–74 years	≥30	RT-PCR	—	Lower	↓ R. flavefaciens, C. leptum, and Bifidobacterium
Tims et al. (2013)	The Netherlands	19–43 years	Special classification for twins	HITChip	No difference	No difference	↑ E. ventriosum and R. intestinalis
Galley et al. (2014)	United States	18–27 months	≥30 (obese mothers)	Pyro-tag 16S sequencing	Higher	No difference	↑ Parabacteroides spp. and Oscillibacter spp. ↓ Blautia spp. and Eubacterium spp.
Hu et al. (2015)	Korea	13–16 years	≥30	Pyrosequencing	No difference	No difference	↑ Prevotella ↓ Bacteroides and Oscillibacter
Kasai et al. (2015)	Japan	<65 years	≥25	T-RFLP	Higher	Higher	↑ B. hydrogenotorophica, C. catus, E. ventriosum, R. bromii, and R. obeum ↓ B. faecichinchillae, B. thetaiotaomicron, B. wexlerae, C. bolteae, and F. plautii

BMI, body mass index; RT-PCR, reverse transcriptase polymerase chain reaction; FISH, fluorescence in situ hybridization; qPCR, quantitative polymerase chain reaction; T-RFLP, terminal restriction fragment length polymorphism; HITChip, human intestinal tract chip.

In a metagenomics study by Qin et al. (2012), Chinese patients with T2D were shown to have a moderate degree of gut microbial aberrations, with a decrease in the abundance of some universal butyrate-producing bacteria and an increase in various opportunistic pathogens, such as *Bacteroides caccae*, *Clostridium hathewayi*, *Clostridium ramosum*, *Clostridium symbiosum*, *Eggerthella lenta*, and *E. coli*. In addition, mucin-degrading species *A. muciniphila* and sulfate-reducing species *Desulfovibrio* sp. were also enriched in the samples of the T2D patients. In retrospect, the abundance of *A. muciniphila* could be attributed to the use of metformin in the T2D patients and the fact that metformin is stimulating the growth of this mucolytic bacterium (Lee and Ko, 2014). No significant difference in the within-sample diversity between T2D and control groups was observed, but this may be confounded by the drug use of the T2D patients. The functional changes in the T2D patients were characterized by an enrichment of markers of membrane transport of sugars; branched-chain amino acid, methane, and xenobiotic metabolism; and sulfate reduction. By contrast, a decreased level of bacterial chemotaxis, flagellar assembly, butyrate biosynthesis, and metabolism of cofactors and vitamins was observed in the T2D patients. Markers related to oxidative stress resistance and drug resistance were greatly enriched, suggesting that T2D patients may have a more hostile gut environment. Another large metagenomics study, conducted by Karlsson et al. (2013), also demonstrated compositional and functional alterations in the gut microbiome of European women with T2D. Increased numbers of *Lactobacillus* species and decreased numbers of *Clostridium* species were observed in the T2D group, and these changes were not correlated with BMI. The pathways that showed the highest scores for enrichment in T2D metagenomes were related to glycerol-lipid metabolism; fatty acid biosynthesis; and, as also observed by Qin et al., membrane transport and oxidative stress resistance. Both studies developed mathematical models based on the metagenomic profiles gathered and used that to identify individuals with T2D. However, when Karlsson et al. applied their European-cohort model to the Chinese cohort described by Qin et al., they discovered that the discriminant metagenomic markers for T2D found by them differed from the ones found by the Chinese group. This led the authors to suggest that, although both studies have found functional alterations of the gut microbiome directly linked to T2D development, metagenomic predictive tools for T2D should be specific for the age and geographical location of the populations studied. However, after correcting for the confounding use of metformin and other drugs, a series of robust signatures associated with T2D were found (Lee and Ko, 2014).

An altered microbiota in T2D may induce inflammatory processes and, in support of such a concept, several studies have demonstrated that patients with T2D exhibit a remarkable endotoxemia. In a study by Larsen et al. (2010), T2D was associated with a higher abundance of gram-negative bacteria, belonging to the phyla Bacteroidetes and Proteobacteria, and a lower abundance of Firmicutes. Higher levels of *Bacilli* and the *Lactobacillus* group were also observed in the diabetic subjects compared with controls. Of note, these compositional changes in the intestinal microbiota were not related with the individual's body mass. Although T2D is considered an attribute to obesity, in this study a higher *Bacteroidetes* to *Firmicutes* ratio correlated positively with higher blood glucose levels but negatively with higher body mass. These findings led the authors to suggest that overweight and diabetes are associated with different groups of intestinal microbiota and that levels of glucose tolerance should be considered when linking microbiota with obesity and other metabolic diseases. Correspondingly, Membrez et al. (2008) demonstrated that modulation of gut microbiota with antibiotics influences whole-body glucose homeostasis, independent of body weight/body fat mass. In antibiotic-treated mice, reduced liver TGs correlated with improved insulin resistance, suggesting that the influence of gut microbiota on glucose and liver metabolism may have similar mechanisms. Both groups hypothesized that higher amounts of gram-negative bacteria, as seen in cases of reduced glucose tolerance, increase the load of circulating LPS, which is known to cause acute whole-body insulin resistance and is a potent stimulator of inflammation (Cani et al., 2007). To further confirm this hypothesis, a clinical study by Jayashree et al. (2014) revealed increased levels of circulating LPS and LPS activity, associated with poor glycemic/lipid control and subclinical inflammation, in patients with T2D compared with control subjects. Moreover, Sato et al. (2014) also observed higher levels of LPS binding protein in plasma samples of Japanese T2D patients compared with control subjects. However, most of the gut bacteria detected in the higher rate in the blood of diabetic patients were gram positive, not gram negative. Similar to the data presented by others, counts of total *Lactobacillus* were significantly higher whereas fecal counts of the *Clostridium coccoides* group were significantly lower in T2D patients.

A relevant study was reported by Le Chatelier et al. (2013), who characterized a Danish cohort of subjects, many of whom were having metabolic-syndrome–like symptoms. Metagenomic analysis of the intestinal microbiota showed healthy subjects to have a highly diverse community with a high gene count whereas the subjects with signs of metabolic syndrome (MS) carried a microbial community with reduced diversity. This finding could be reproduced in a French obesity cohort, where it turned out that the high-diversity subjects responded better to a weight-loss diet than the low-diversity group (Cotillard et al., 2013).

NONALCOHOLIC FATTY LIVER DISEASE

Nonalcoholic fatty liver disease (NAFLD) is the hepatic manifestation of MS and the leading cause of chronic liver disease in the Western world. It is defined as the presence of fat accumulation in the hepatic cells in the absence of any secondary causes of liver injury, such as significant alcohol consumption, the use of steatogenic medications, or hereditary disorders (Aqel and DiBaise, 2015). NAFLD is characterized by a broad spectrum of hepatic pathology that ranges from simple steatosis to nonalcoholic steatohepatitis (NASH) and even cirrhosis, fibrosis, and hepatocellular carcinoma. Most individuals with NAFLD remain asymptomatic without any histological or biochemical injury, but 20% progress to develop

NASH, a chronic hepatic inflammation, characterized by steatosis, inflammation, and hepatocyte injury with or without cirrhosis (Henao-Mejia et al., 2012; Jiang et al., 2015).

Animal and human studies have demonstrated an important role for aberrations in gut microbiota composition in promoting liver diseases (Festi et al., 2014). Henao-Mejia et al. (2012) observed that inflammasome-deficient mice develop massive hepatic steatosis and liver inflammation accompanied by changes in the configuration of the gut microbiota. They found that *Porphyromonas*, a type of bacteria that has been associated with complications of chronic liver disease and with several components of the MS in mice and humans, was increased in the inflammasome-deficient mouse model. Inflammasome depletion was associated with a potentially pathogenic microbiota resulting in increased influx and accumulation of bacterial products, such as LPS, in the liver. This led to the stimulation of TLR4 and TLR9 and increased the expression of hepatic TNF-α expression, which drives NASH progression. Miele et al. (2009) also investigated the mechanisms underlying the transition from steatosis to NASH. They provided the first evidence that NAFLD in humans is associated with increased gut permeability and that this abnormality is related to the increased prevalence of small intestinal bacterial overgrowth (SIBO). In this study tight junction integrity disruption was shown, as evidenced by a lower expression of zona occludens-1 in the duodenal mucosa of patients with NAFLD compared with healthy subjects. The prevalence of SIBO in patients with NAFLD was more than twice as high compared with healthy subjects; however, the characteristics of the microbiota were not assessed in this study. Nevertheless, the composition of gut microbiota in patients with NAFLD was recently investigated in a comprehensive clinical study by Jiang et al. (2015). In this study gut microbiota changes were accompanied by increased intestinal permeability and inflammation in patients with NAFLD. Differences in the microbial population included increased levels of *Escherichia, Anaerobacter, Lactobacillus,* and *Streptococcus* and decreased levels of *Alistipes* and *Prevotella* in the feces of NAFLD patients compared with healthy subjects. Patients with NAFLD exhibited weakened mucosal barrier integrity within their intestinal mucosa with lower expression levels of occludin, widened tight junctions, and irregularly arranged microvilli. In addition, an impaired immune function was observed characterized by depleted numbers of CD4+ and CD8+ T lymphocytes in the lamina propria of the duodenal mucosa and higher levels of the proinflammatory cytokines in comparison to healthy controls.

In alignment with the results published by Jiang et al. (2015), Zhu et al. (2013) also reported increased levels of *Escherichia* in NASH patients when compared with controls. Moreover, NASH patients exhibited significantly elevated blood ethanol levels. These findings led the authors to suggest that a microbiota rich in alcohol-producing bacteria (such as *Escherichia*) stimulates the production of ethanol, leading to gut permeability disruption and generation of reactive oxygen species that cause inflammation of the liver already sensitized by the fat deposition.

The deficiency of an essential nutrient was also shown to contribute to the pathogenesis of NAFLD through microbiota disruption. Spencer et al. (2011) examined gut microbiomes of adult subjects who had fatty livers induced by a choline-deficient diet. Choline is an important component of cell membranes and is also important for lipid metabolism and synthesis of very-low–density lipoprotein in the liver. The group showed that choline deficiency may cause changes in gut microbiome composition, decreasing the levels of *Gammaproteobacteria* and increasing levels of *Erysipelotrichi*.

OVERVIEW OF SOME POTENTIAL THERAPIES THAT ARE CURRENTLY BEING USED TO RE-ESTABLISH A HEALTHY GUT MICROBIOTA

Given that a disturbed gut microbiota has been associated with numerous diseases, several therapeutic options are currently being used with an aim to re-establish a healthy, beneficial ecosystem within the gut. Such potential therapies include the use of probiotics and prebiotics, which act by increasing the numbers and/or activity of beneficial bacteria within the gut, and fecal transplantation, which introduces a healthy, diverse microbiota by replacing the existing microbiota. More than 1000 cultured bacterial isolates have been described in detail (Rajilić-Stojanović et al., 2012), a number that is ever increasing. This is of significant interest because culturing the intestinal microbiota has rather been neglected when the fast DNA-based approaches have been developed. A culturing renaissance is indeed taking place because it turns out that insight in cultures is needed when trying to develop new therapies.

To date, many examples of beneficial effects have been associated with the use of probiotic bacteria in health and various diseases, including IBS, obesity, and depression (Sanders et al., 2013). Beneficial effects of probiotics can be due to the direct effect of the bacterium itself, or the products it produces, as well as the effects that the probiotic bacterium has on the composition and/or activity of the resident microbiota. Indeed, probiotics can interact with the host's epithelial cells and other cells in the human body through physicochemical, enteroendocrine, and immune signals in the same way as the commensal gut microbiota, and although the use of a probiotic bacterium does not give rise to detectable changes in the composition of the fecal microbiota, its metabolic activity may be altered (McNulty et al., 2011). However, most of the data showing positive effects of different probiotic strains are obtained from animal models, and despite convincing and reproducible results from such studies, data from clinical trials are still uncertain. Reasons for this may partly include poor study design (dosage, time, etc.) and poor choice of strain. In addition, it should be pointed out that humans and mice have different microbiota. This is exemplified in the recent metagenomic comparison that revealed extensive functional similarity between mouse and man microbiota, but indicated that only 4% of the mouse microbial genes were found with high identity in the human microbiome (Xiao et al., 2015).

In comparison with probiotic studies, fewer well-designed clinical studies have been conducted using prebiotics. Prebiotics are growth substrates (eg, fructooligo-saccharides, galactooligosaccharides, inulin, resistant starch) that act as enhancers for bacteria that are already present in the human colon by stimulating their growth and/or activity. The most commonly used prebiotics specifically act as growth enhancers for lactobacilli and bifidobacteria; however, this concept of prebiotics has been expanded from solely focusing on the "bifidogenic effect" and nowadays it also includes other beneficial members of the gut microbiota. One example of this is the butyrate-producing bacterium *F. prausnitzii*, which currently is regarded as an important, functionally active bacterium within the human gut. For example, reduced numbers of *F. prausnitzii* have been detected in patients with Crohn's disease (Sokol et al., 2009), and given that this bacterium is also associated with antiinflammatory effects (Sokol et al., 2008), it makes it a strong target for disease therapy. *F. prausnitzii* has been shown to respond to inulin supplements and to pectins as growth substrates (Ramirez-Farias et al., 2009; Lopez-Silas et al., 2012). Thus, by increasing our knowledge about which bacterial species are present at lower abundance in a diseased state compared with a healthy state, this will enable us to selectively target these repressed bacteria by using a prebiotic substrate that we know can boost the growth and the activity of these bacteria. Prebiotic fibers, in addition to other nondigestible carbohydrates that we cannot break down with our own enzymes, can also give rise to SCFAs. SCFAs (acetate, propionate, and butyrate) are not only important for gut health, they also act as signaling molecules, for example by stimulating the production of gut and neuroactive peptides (Parnell and Relmer, 2009; Psichias et al., 2015). In addition, they can enter our circulatory system and thereby they may directly affect metabolism and the function of peripheral tissues (Smith et al., 2013; Gao et al., 2009).

An increasing number of diseases have been reported to be cured by using FMT (Smits et al., 2013; Rossen et al., 2015). As previously described, in this treatment the intestinal microbiota of a patient is removed via lavage and largely replaced by the fecal microbiota of a healthy donor. The success of FMT in recurrent CDI enormously stimulated the field, notably because it showed the power of microbes (van Nood et al., 2013). In more sophisticated comparative studies aimed to address the role of the intestinal microbiota, not only a transplantation with a healthy donor fecal microbiota was performed but also an autologous transplantation with the patient's own microbiota was performed in a blinded way. In this way it was shown that fecal microbiota is causing MS and only when a healthy donor microbiota was used was the hallmark of MS, insulin sensitivity, increased (Vrieze et al., 2012). Very recently, by using a similar approach, patients suffering from UC could be maintained in remission after transplantation with a healthy donor (Rossens et al., 2015). All of these FMT studies are highly relevant and demonstrate the impact of the intestinal microbiota. In some cases, such as in recurrent CDI, the transplantations are becoming mainstream. However, several issues associated with safety, delivery mode, and storage are limiting factors for large-scale treatments. Hence, considerable efforts are dedicated in designing so-called synthetic microbiomes (Petrof et al., 2013; de Vos, 2013). Other diseases are more complex and other avenues are taken, including reverse engineering, in which microbial taxa are identified based on careful analysis of the microbial changes in successful fecal transplantations (de Vos, 2013). These and other approaches of single intestinal strains that may improve health are currently under development. One is the intestinal mucosal inhabitant *A. muciniphila* (Belzer and de Vos, 2012). Mouse experiments have shown this unusual representative of the Verrucomicrobia to be capable of preventing diet-induced obesity and inflammation as well as regulatory T cell stimulation (Everard et al., 2013; Shin et al., 2014). The basis for this effect is an increased barrier function that recently was determined in human cell lines (Reunanen et al., 2015). These and other intestinal strains hold great promise to be developed into new therapeutic strains that can be used to improve human health and treat patients with deviations in the intestinal microbiota.

CONCLUSION

There is increasing evidence that changes in the gut microbiota are involved in common gut diseases such as IBS and IBD, that it is a partaker in systemic diseases such as allergies and metabolic diseases, and that it also may play a critical role in the development of stress-related disorders, such as anxiety and depression. However, understanding these microbiota changes and defining a healthy microbiome is challenging because of the tremendous complexity of the gut ecosystem and the huge variability between healthy individuals. Rapid advances in sequencing technology, made predominantly during the past decade, have expanded our knowledge about this second genome; nonetheless, further research is required to get new and deeper insights into what actual role the human gut microbiome plays in health and disease. A combination of classical microbiology (ie, culturing bacterial isolates of the gut microbiota), high-throughput sequencing techniques (including metatranscriptomics and metaproteomics), carefully designed animal experiments, and notably clinical trials are needed to establish cause-and-effect relationships and to establish interactions with key human cellular functions (ie, to understand microbiota-host relationships). On the basis of this, tailor-made treatment strategies, designed to target specific deviations in microbiome structure and functioning, may be developed.

ACKNOWLEDGMENTS

Research in the laboratories of the authors was supported by the Knowledge Foundation, Sweden, to R.J.B.; the Netherlands Organization for Scientific Research (Spinoza Award and SIAM Gravity Grant 024.002.002); the Finland Academy of Sciences (Grant 141130); and TEKES (Grant (329/31/2015) to W.M.dV.

REFERENCES

Abdollahi-Roodsaz, S., Joosten, L.A., Koenders, M.I., Devesa, I., Roelofs, M.F., Radstake, T.R., et al., 2008. Stimulation of TLR2 and TLR4 differentially skews the balance of T cells in a mouse model of arthritis. J. Clin. Investig. 118 (1), 205.

Abbott, R.D., Petrovitch, H., White, L.R., Masaki, K.H., Tanner, C.M., Curb, J.D., et al., 2001. Frequency of bowel movements and the future risk of Parkinson's disease. Neurology 57 (3), 456–462.

Abrahamsson, T.R., Jakobsson, H.E., Andersson, A.F., Björkstén, B., Engstrand, L., Jenmalm, M.C., 2012. Low diversity of the gut microbiota in infants with atopic eczema. J. Allergy Clin. Immunol. 129 (2), 434–440.

Abrahamsson, T.R., Jakobsson, H.E., Andersson, A.F., Björkstén, B., Engstrand, L., Jenmalm, M.C., 2014. Low gut microbiota diversity in early infancy precedes asthma at school age. Clin. Exp. Allergy 44 (6), 842–850.

Adams, J.B., Johansen, L.J., Powell, L.D., Quig, D., Rubin, R.A., 2011. Gastrointestinal flora and gastrointestinal status in children with autism–comparisons to typical children and correlation with autism severity. BMC Gastroenterology 11 (1), 22.

Aqel, B., DiBaise, J.K., 2015. Role of the gut microbiome in nonalcoholic fatty liver disease. Nutr. Clin. Pract. http://dx.doi.org/10.1177/0884533615605811.

Armougom, F., Henry, M., Vialettes, B., Raccah, D., Raoult, D., 2009. Monitoring bacterial community of human gut microbiota reveals an increase in *Lactobacillus* in obese patients and Methanogens in anorexic patients. PLoS One 4 (9), e7125.

Arrieta, M.C., Stiemsma, L.T., Dimitriu, P.A., Thorson, L., Russell, S., Yurist-Doutsch, S., et al., 2015. Early infancy microbial and metabolic alterations affect risk of childhood asthma. Sci. Transl. Med. 7 (307), 307ra152.

Atarashi, K., Tanoue, T., Ando, M., Kamada, N., Nagano, Y., Narushima, S., et al., 2015. Th17 cell induction by adhesion of microbes to intestinal epithelial cells. Cell 163 (2), 367–380.

Bäckhed, F., Ding, H., Wang, T., Hooper, L.V., Koh, G.Y., Nagy, A., et al., 2004. The gut microbiota as an environmental factor that regulates fat storage. Proc. Natl. Acad. Sci. U.S.A. 101 (44), 15718–15723.

Bäckhed, F., Ley, R.E., Sonnenburg, J.L., Peterson, D.A., Gordon, J.I., 2005. Host-bacterial mutualism in the human intestine. Science 307 (5717), 1915–1920.

Belzer, C., de Vos, W.M., 2012. Microbes inside—from diversity to function: the case of Akkermansia. ISME J. 6 (8), 1449–1458.

Benton, D., Williams, C., Brown, A., 2007. Impact of consuming a milk drink containing a probiotic on mood and cognition. Eur. J. Clin. Nutr. 61 (3), 355–361.

Bercik, P., Denou, E., Collins, J., Jackson, W., Lu, J., Jury, J., et al., 2011. The intestinal microbiota affect central levels of brain-derived neurotropic factor and behavior in mice. Gastroenterology 141 (2), 599–609.

Berer, K., Mues, M., Koutrolos, M., Al Rasbi, Z., Boziki, M., Johner, C., et al., 2011. Commensal microbiota and myelin autoantigen cooperate to trigger autoimmune demyelination. Nature 479 (7374), 538–541.

Bisgaard, H., Li, N., Bonnelykke, K., Chawes, B.L.K., Skov, T., Paludan-Müller, G., et al., 2011. Reduced diversity of the intestinal microbiota during infancy is associated with increased risk of allergic disease at school age. J. Allergy Clin. Immunol. 128 (3), 646–652.

Borges, C.M., 2015. Role of colonic microbiota in colorectal carcinogenesis: a systematic review. Rev. Esp. Enferm. Dig. 107.

Bravo, J.A., Forsythe, P., Chew, M.V., Escaravage, E., Savignac, H.M., Dinan, T.G., et al., 2011. Ingestion of *Lactobacillus* strain regulates emotional behavior and central GABA receptor expression in a mouse via the vagus nerve. Proc. Natl. Acad. Sci. U.S.A. 108 (38), 16050–16055.

Brown, C.T., Davis-Richardson, A.G., Giongo, A., Gano, K.A., Crabb, D.B., Mukherjee, N., et al., 2011. Gut microbiome metagenomics analysis suggests a functional model for the development of autoimmunity for type 1 diabetes. PLoS One 6 (10), e25792.

Cani, P.D., Amar, J., Iglesias, M.A., Poggi, M., Knauf, C., Bastelica, D., et al., 2007. Metabolic endotoxemia initiates obesity and insulin resistance. Diabetes 56 (7), 1761–1772.

Cebra, J.J., Periwal, S.B., Lee, G., Lee, F., Shroff, K.E., 1998. Development and maintenance of the gut-associated lymphoid tissue (GALT): the roles of enteric bacteria and viruses. J. Immunol. Res. 6 (1–2), 13–18.

Claesson, M.J., Jeffery, I.B., Conde, S., Power, S.E., O'Connor, E.M., Cusack, S., et al., 2012. Gut microbiota composition correlates with diet and health in the elderly. Nature 488 (7410), 178–184.

Collins, S.M., Kassam, Z., Bercik, P., 2013. The adoptive transfer of behavioral phenotype via the intestinal microbiota: experimental evidence and clinical implications. Curr. Opin. Microbiol. 16 (3), 240–245.

Cotillard, A., Kennedy, S.P., Kong, L.C., Prifti, P., Pons, F., et al., 2013. Dietary intervention impact on gut microbial gene richness. Nature 500, 585–588.

Di Cagno, R., De Angelis, M., De Pasquale, I., Ndagijimana, M., Vernocchi, P., Ricciuti, P., et al., 2011. Duodenal and faecal microbiota of celiac children: molecular, phenotype and metabolome characterization. BMC Microbiol. 11 (1), 219.

Dobell, C., 1932. Anthony Van Leeuwenhoek and His Little Animals. Harcourt Brace & Company, New York.

Duncan, S.H., Lobley, G.E., Holtrop, G., Ince, J., Johnstone, A.M., Louis, P., Flint, H.J., 2008. Human colonic microbiota associated with diet, obesity and weight loss. Int. J. Obes. 32 (11), 1720–1724.

Eckburg, P.B., Bik, E.M., Bernstein, C.N., Purdom, E., Dethlefsen, L., Sargent, M., et al., 2005. Diversity of the human intestinal microbial flora. Science 308 (5728), 1635–1638.

Ege, M.J., Mayer, M., Normand, A.C., Genuneit, J., Cookson, W.O., Braun-Fahrländer, C., et al., 2011. Exposure to environmental microorganisms and childhood asthma. N. Engl. J. Med. 364 (8), 701–709.

Everard, A., Belzer, C., Geurts, L., Ouwerkerk, J.P., Druart, C., Bindels, L.B., et al., 2013. Cross-talk between *Akkermansia muciniphila* and intestinal epithelium controls diet-induced obesity. Proc. Natl. Acad. Sci. U.S.A. 110 (22), 9066–9071.

Eriguchi, Y., Nakamura, K., Hashimoto, D., Shimoda, S., Shimono, N., Akashi, K., et al., 2015. Decreased secretion of Paneth cell α-defensins in graft-versus-host disease. Transpl. Infect. Dis. 17 (5), 702–706.

Festi, D., Schiumerini, R., Eusebi, L.H., Marasco, G., Taddia, M., Colecchia, A., 2014. Gut microbiota and metabolic syndrome. World J. Gastroenterol. 20 (43), 16079.

Fischer, H., Holst, E., Karlsson, F., Benoni, C., Toth, E., Olesen, M., et al., 2015. Altered microbiota in microscopic colitis. Gut. http://dx.doi.org/10.1136/gutjnl-2014-308956.

Forno, E., Onderdonk, A.B., McCracken, J., Litonjua, A.A., Laskey, D., Delaney, M.L., et al., 2008. Diversity of the gut microbiota and eczema in early life. Clin. Mol. Allergy 6 (11), 11.

Forsyth, C.B., Shannon, K.M., Kordower, J.H., Voigt, R.M., Shaikh, M., Jaglin, J.A., et al., 2011. Increased intestinal permeability correlates with sigmoid mucosa alpha-synuclein staining and endotoxin exposure markers in early Parkinson's disease. PLoS One 6 (12), e28032.

Frémont, M., Coomans, D., Massart, S., De Meirleir, K., 2013. High-throughput 16S rRNA gene sequencing reveals alterations of intestinal microbiota in myalgic encephalomyelitis/chronic fatigue syndrome patients. Anaerobe 22, 50–56.

Fuentes, S., van Nood, E., Tims, S., Heikamp-de Jong, I., Ter Braak, C.J., Keller, J.J., et al., 2014. Reset of a critically disturbed microbial ecosystem: faecal transplant in recurrent *Clostridium difficile* infection. ISME J. 8 (8), 1621–1633.

Fujimura, K.E., Lynch, S.V., 2015. Microbiota in allergy and asthma and the emerging relationship with the gut microbiome. Cell Host Microb. 17 (5), 592–602.

Galley, J.D., Bailey, M., Dush, C.K., Schoppe-Sullivan, S., Christian, L.M., 2014. Maternal obesity is associated with alterations in the gut microbiome in toddlers. PLoS One 9 (11), e113026.

Gao, Z., Yin, J., Zhang, J., Ward, R.E., Martin, R.J., Lefevre, M., Cefalu, W.T., Ye, J., 2009. Butyrate improves insulin sensitivity and increases energy expenditure in mice. Diabetes 58 (7), 1509–1517.

Ge, H., Li, X., Weiszmann, J., Wang, P., Baribault, H., Chen, J.L., et al., 2008. Activation of G protein-coupled receptor 43 in adipocytes leads to inhibition of lipolysis and suppression of plasma free fatty acids. Endocrinology 149 (9), 4519–4526.

Giacomin, P., Zakrzewski, M., Croese, J., Su, X., Sotillo, J., McCann, L., et al., 2015. Experimental hookworm infection and escalating gluten challenges are associated with increased microbial richness in celiac subjects. Sci. Rep. 5. http://dx.doi.org/10.1038/srep13797.

Gibson, M.K., Crofts, T.S., Dantas, G., 2015. Antibiotics and the developing infant gut microbiota and resistome. Curr. Opin. Microbiol. 27, 51–56.

Giongo, A., Gano, K.A., Crabb, D.B., Mukherjee, N., Novelo, L.L., Casella, G., et al., 2011. Toward defining the autoimmune microbiome for type 1 diabetes. ISME J. 5 (1), 82–91.

Grölund, M.M., Lehtonen, O.P., Eerola, E., Kero, P., 1999. Fecal microflora in healthy infants born by different methods of delivery: permanent changes in intestinal flora after cesarean delivery. J. Pediatr. Gastroenterol. Nutr. 28 (1), 19–25.

Harach, T., Marungruang, N., Dutilleul, N., Cheatham, V., Mc Coy, K.D., Neher, J.J., Jucker, M., Fåk, F., Lasser, T., Bolmont, T., 2015. Reduction of Alzheimer's Disease Beta-amyloid Pathology in the Absence of Gut Microbiota. http://arxiv.org/ftp/arxiv/papers/1509/1509.02273.pdf (access 31.10.15.).

Heijtz, R.D., Wang, S., Anuar, F., Qian, Y., Björkholm, B., Samuelsson, A., et al., 2011. Normal gut microbiota modulates brain development and behavior. Proc. Natl. Acad. Sci. U.S.A. 108 (7), 3047–3052.

Henao-Mejia, J., Elinav, E., Jin, C., Hao, L., Mehal, W.Z., Strowig, T., Flavell, R.A., 2012. Inflammasome-mediated dysbiosis regulates progression of NAFLD and obesity. Nature 482 (7384), 179–185.

Hong, Y.H., Nishimura, Y., Hishikawa, D., Tsuzuki, H., Miyahara, H., Gotoh, C., et al., 2005. Acetate and propionate short chain fatty acids stimulate adipogenesis via GPCR43. Endocrinology 146 (12), 5092–5099.

Hooper, L.V., Bry, L., Falk, P.G., Gordon, J.I., 1998. Host–microbial symbiosis in the mammalian intestine: exploring an internal ecosystem. Bioessays 20 (4), 336–343.

Hooper, L.V., Littman, D.R., Macpherson, A.J., 2012. Interactions between the microbiota and the immune system. Science 336 (6086), 1268–1273.

Horvath, K., Papadimitriou, J.C., Rabsztyn, A., Drachenberg, C., Tildon, J.T., 1999. Gastrointestinal abnormalities in children with autistic disorder. J. Pediatr. 135 (5), 559–563.

Hoveyda, N., Heneghan, C., Mahtani, K.R., Perera, R., Roberts, N., Glasziou, P., 2009. A systematic review and meta-analysis: probiotics in the treatment of irritable bowel syndrome. BMC Gastroenterol. 9 (1), 15.

Hu, H.J., Park, S.G., Jang, H.B., Choi, M.K., Park, K.H., Kang, J.H., et al., 2015. Obesity alters the microbial community profile in Korean adolescents. PLoS One 10 (7), e0134333.

Ivanov, I.I., de Llanos Frutos, R., Manel, N., Yoshinaga, K., Rifkin, D.B., Sartor, R.B., et al., 2008. Specific microbiota direct the differentiation of IL-17-producing T-helper cells in the mucosa of the small intestine. Cell Host Microb. 4 (4), 337–349.

Jayashree, B., Bibin, Y.S., Prabhu, D., Shanthirani, C.S., Gokulakrishnan, K., Lakshmi, B.S., et al., 2014. Increased circulatory levels of lipopolysaccharide (LPS) and zonulin signify novel biomarkers of proinflammation in patients with type 2 diabetes. Mol. Cell. Biochem. 388 (1–2), 203–210.

Jiang, W., Wu, N., Wang, X., Chi, Y., Zhang, Y., Qiu, X., et al., 2015. Dysbiosis gut microbiota associated with inflammation and impaired mucosal immune function in intestine of humans with non-alcoholic fatty liver disease. Sci. Rep. 5. http://dx.doi.org/10.1038/srep08096.

Kalliomäki, M., Satokari, R., Lähteenoja, H., Vähämiko, S., Grönlund, J., Routi, T., Salminen, S., 2012. Expression of microbiota, Toll-like receptors, and their regulators in the small intestinal mucosa in celiac disease. J. Pediatr. Gastroenterol. Nutr. 54 (6), 727–732.

Kamada, N., Seo, S.U., Chen, G.Y., Núñez, G., 2013. Role of the gut microbiota in immunity and inflammatory disease. Nat. Rev. Immunol. 13 (5), 321–335.

Kane, M., Case, L.K., Kopaskie, K., Kozlova, A., MacDearmid, C., Chervonsky, A.V., Golovkina, T.V., 2011. Successful transmission of a retrovirus depends on the commensal microbiota. Science 334 (6053), 245–249.

Karaki, S.I., Tazoe, H., Hayashi, H., Kashiwabara, H., Tooyama, K., Suzuki, Y., Kuwahara, A., 2008. Expression of the short-chain fatty acid receptor, GPR43, in the human colon. J. Mol. Histol. 39 (2), 135–142.

Karlsson, F.H., Tremaroli, V., Nookaew, I., Bergström, G., Behre, C.J., Fagerberg, B., et al., 2013. Gut metagenome in European women with normal, impaired and diabetic glucose control. Nature 498 (7452), 99–103.

Karri, S., Martinez, V.A., Coimbatore, G., 2010. Effect of dihydrotestosterone on gastrointestinal tract of male Alzheimer's disease transgenic mice. Indian J. Exp. Biol. 48 (5), 453–465.

Kasai, C., Sugimoto, K., Moritani, I., Tanaka, J., Oya, Y., Inoue, H., et al., 2015. Comparison of the gut microbiota composition between obese and non-obese individuals in a Japanese population, as analyzed by terminal restriction fragment length polymorphism and next-generation sequencing. BMC Gastroenterol. 15 (1), 100.

Keku, T.O., Dulal, S., Deveaux, A., Jovov, B., Han, X., 2015. The gastrointestinal microbiota and colorectal cancer. Am. J. Physiol. Gastrointest. Liver Physiol. 308 (5), G351–G363.

Kennedy, P.J., Cryan, J.F., Dinan, T.G., Clarke, G., 2014. Irritable bowel syndrome: a microbiome-gut-brain axis disorder? World J. Gastroenterol. 20 (39), 14105.

Khoruts, A., Dicksved, J., Jansson, J.K., Sadowsky, M.J., 2010. Changes in the composition of the human fecal microbiome after bacteriotherapy for recurrent *Clostridium* difficile-associated diarrhea. J. Clin. Gastroenterol. 44 (5), 354–360.

Kimura, I., Ozawa, K., Inoue, D., Imamura, T., Kimura, K., Maeda, T., Tsujimoto, G., 2013. The gut microbiota suppresses insulin-mediated fat accumulation via the short-chain fatty acid receptor GPR43. Nat. Commun. 4, 1829.

Koeth, R.A., Wang, Z., Levison, B.S., Buffa, J.A., Sheehy, B.T., Britt, E.B., et al., 2013. Intestinal microbiota metabolism of L-carnitine, a nutrient in red meat, promotes atherosclerosis. Nat. Med. 19 (5), 576–585.

Kolmeder, C.A., Ritari, J., Verdam, F.J., Muth, T., Keskitalo, S., Varjosalo, M., et al., 2015. Colonic metaproteomic signatures of active bacteria and the host in obesity. Proteomics 15 (20), 3544–3552.

König, J., Brummer, R.J., 2014. Alteration of the intestinal microbiota as a cause of and a potential therapeutic option in irritable bowel syndrome. Benefic. Microb. 5 (3), 247–261.

König, J., Ganda-Mall, J.P., Rangel, I., Edebol-Carlman, H., Brummer, R.J., 2015. The role of the gut microbiota in brain function. In: Venema, K., do Carmo, A.P. (Eds.), Probiotics and Prebiotics: Current Research and Future Trends. Caister Academic Press, Poole, UK.

Koren, O., Spor, A., Felin, J., Fåk, F., Stombaugh, J., Tremaroli, V., et al., 2011. Human oral, gut, and plaque microbiota in patients with atherosclerosis. Proc. Natl. Acad. Sci. U.S.A. 108 (Suppl. 1), 4592–4598.

Korpela, K., Salonen, A., Virta, L.J., Kekkonen, R.A., Forslund, K., Bork, P., de Vos, W.M., 2016. Intestinal microbiome is related to lifetime antibiotic use in Finnish pre-school children. Nat. Commun. 7, 10410. http://dx.doi.org/10.1038/ncomms10410.

Kostic, A.D., Gevers, D., Siljander, H., Vatanen, T., Hyötyläinen, T., Hämäläinen, A.M., et al., 2015. The dynamics of the human infant gut microbiome in development and in progression toward type 1 diabetes. Cell Host Microb. 17 (2), 260–273.

Kuss, S.K., Best, G.T., Etheredge, C.A., Pruijssers, A.J., Frierson, J.M., Hooper, L.V., et al., 2011. Intestinal microbiota promote enteric virus replication and systemic pathogenesis. Science 334 (6053), 249–252.

Lam, V., Su, J., Koprowski, S., Hsu, A., Tweddell, J.S., Rafiee, P., et al., 2012. Intestinal microbiota determine severity of myocardial infarction in rats. FASEB J. 26 (4), 1727–1735.

Larsen, N., Vogensen, F.K., Van Den Berg, F.W., Nielsen, D.S., Andreasen, A.S., Pedersen, B.K., et al., 2010. Gut microbiota in human adults with type 2 diabetes differs from non-diabetic adults. PLoS One 5 (2), e9085.

Lathrop, S.K., Bloom, S.M., Rao, S.M., Nutsch, K., Lio, C.W., Santacruz, N., et al., 2011. Peripheral education of the immune system by colonic commensal microbiota. Nature 478 (7368), 250–254.

Le Chatelier, E., Nielsen, T., Qin, J., Prifti, E., Hildebrand, F., Falony, G., et al., 2013. Richness of human gut microbiome correlates with metabolic markers. Nature 500 (7464), 541–546.

Lee, H., Ko, G., 2014. Effect of metformin on metabolic improvement and gut microbiota. Appl. Environ. Microbiol. 80 (19), 5935–5943.

Lee, J.W., Lee, Y.K., Yuk, D.Y., Choi, D.Y., Ban, S.B., Oh, K.W., Hong, J.T., 2008. Neuro-inflammation induced by lipopolysaccharide causes cognitive impairment through enhancement of beta-amyloid generation. J. Neuroinflammation 5 (1), 37.

Lepage, P., Häsler, R., Spehlmann, M.E., Rehman, A., Zvirbliene, A., Begun, A., et al., 2011. Twin study indicates loss of interaction between microbiota and mucosa of patients with ulcerative colitis. Gastroenterology 141 (1), 227–236.

Ley, R.E., Bäckhed, F., Turnbaugh, P., Lozupone, C.A., Knight, R.D., Gordon, J.I., 2005. Obesity alters gut microbial ecology. Proc. Natl. Acad. Sci. U.S.A. 102 (31), 11070–11075.

Ley, R.E., Turnbaugh, P.J., Klein, S., Gordon, J.I., 2006. Microbial ecology: human gut microbes associated with obesity. Nature 444 (7122), 1022–1023.

Li, J., Jia, H., Cai, X., Zhong, H., Feng, Q., Sunagawa, S., et al., 2014. An integrated catalog of reference genes in the human gut microbiome. Nat. Biotechnol. 32 (8), 834–841.

Lopez-Siles, M., Khan, T.M., Duncan, S.H., Harmsen, H.J., Garcia-Gil, L.J., Flint, H.J., 2012. Cultured representatives of two major phylogroups of human colonic *Faecalibacterium prausnitzii* can utilize pectin, uronic acids, and host-derived substrates for growth. Appl. Environ. Microbiol. 78 (2), 420–428.

Lynch, S.V., Wood, R.A., Boushey, H., Bacharier, L.B., Bloomberg, G.R., Kattan, M., et al., 2014. Effects of early-life exposure to allergens and bacteria on recurrent wheeze and atopy in urban children. J. Allergy Clin. Immunol. 134 (3), 593–601.

Malinen, E., Krogius-Kurikka, L., Lyra, A., Nikkilä, J., Jääskeläinen, A., Rinttilä, T., et al., 2010. Association of symptoms with gastrointestinal microbiota in irritable bowel syndrome. World J. Gastroenterol. 16 (36), 4532.

Mattila, E., Uusitalo–Seppälä, R., Wuorela, M., Lehtola, L., Nurmi, H., Ristikankare, M., et al., 2012. Fecal transplantation, through colonoscopy, is effective therapy for recurrent *Clostridium* difficile infection. Gastroenterology 142 (3), 490–496.

McNulty, N.P., Yatsunenko, T., Hsiao, A., Faith, J.J., Muegge, B.D., Goodman, A.L., et al., 2011. The impact of a consortium of fermented milk strains on the gut microbiome of gnotobiotic mice and monozygotic twins. Sci. Transl. Med. 3 (106), 106ra106.

Membrez, M., Blancher, F., Jaquet, M., et al., 2008. Gut microbiota modulation with norfloxacin and ampicillin enhances glucose tolerance in mice. FASEB J. 22, 2416–2426.

Menees, S.B., Maneerattannaporn, M., Kim, H.M., Chey, W.D., 2012. The efficacy and safety of rifaximin for the irritable bowel syndrome: a systematic review and meta-analysis. Am. J. Gastroenterol. 107 (1), 28–35.

Messaoudi, M., Lalonde, R., Violle, N., Javelot, H., Desor, D., Nejdi, A., et al., 2011. Assessment of psychotropic-like properties of a probiotic formulation (*Lactobacillus helveticus* R0052 and *Bifidobacterium longum* R0175) in rats and human subjects. Br. J. Nutr. 105 (05), 755–764.

Metchnikoff, E., Mitchell, P.C., 1907. The Prolongation of Life: Optimistic Studies. W. Heinemann, London (GP Putnam's Sons, New York).

Miele, L., Valenza, V., La Torre, G., Montalto, M., Cammarota, G., Ricci, R., et al., 2009. Increased intestinal permeability and tight junction alterations in nonalcoholic fatty liver disease. Hepatology 49 (6), 1877–1887.

Miyake, S., Kim, S., Suda, W., Oshima, K., Nakamura, M., Matsuoka, T., et al., 2015. Dysbiosis in the gut microbiota of patients with multiple sclerosis, with a striking depletion of species belonging to *Clostridia* XIVa and IV clusters. PLoS One 10 (9), e0137429.

Moayyedi, P., Surette, M.G., Kim, P.T., Libertucci, J., Wolfe, M., Onischi, C., et al., 2015. Fecal microbiota transplantation induces remission in patients with active ulcerative colitis in a randomized controlled trial. Gastroenterology 149 (1), 102–109.e6.

Murphy, S., Nguyen, V.H., 2011. Role of gut microbiota in graft-versus-host disease. Leuk. Lymphoma 52 (10), 1844–1856.

Neish, A.S., 2009. Microbes in gastrointestinal health and disease. Gastroenterology 136 (1), 65–80.

Neufeld, K.M., Kang, N., Bienenstock, J., Foster, J.A., 2011. Reduced anxiety-like behavior and central neurochemical change in germ-free mice. Neurogastroenterol. Motil. 23 (3), 255–264, e119.

Nistal, E., Caminero, A., Herrán, A.R., Arias, L., Vivas, S., de Morales, J.M.R., et al., 2012. Differences of small intestinal bacteria populations in adults and children with/without celiac disease: effect of age, gluten diet, and disease. Inflamm. Bowel Dis. 18 (4), 649–656.

van Nood, E., Vrieze, A., Nieuwdorp, M., Fuentes, S., Zoetendal, E.G., de Vos, W.M., et al., 2013. Duodenal infusion of donor feces for recurrent *Clostridium difficile*. N. Engl. J. Med. 368 (5), 407–415.

O'Hara, A.M., Shanahan, F., 2006. The gut flora as a forgotten organ. EMBO Rep. 7 (7), 688–693.

Orrhage, K., Nord, C.E., 1999. Factors controlling the bacterial colonization of the intestine in breastfed infants. Acta Paediatr. 88 (s430), 47–57.

Ott, S.J., Musfeldt, M., Wenderoth, D.F., Hampe, J., Brant, O., Fölsch, U.R., et al., 2004. Reduction in diversity of the colonic mucosa associated bacterial microflora in patients with active inflammatory bowel disease. Gut 53 (5), 685–693.

Ownby, D.R., Johnson, C.C., Peterson, E.L., 2002. Exposure to dogs and cats in the first year of life and risk of allergic sensitization at 6 to 7 years of age. Jama 288 (8), 963–972.

Patterson, E., Marques, T.M., O'Sullivan, O., Fitzgerald, P., Fitzgerald, G.F., Cotter, P.D., et al., 2015. Streptozotocin-induced type-1-diabetes disease onset in Sprague–Dawley rats is associated with an altered intestinal microbiota composition and decreased diversity. Microbiology 161 (Pt 1), 182–193.

Petrof, E.O., Gloor, G.B., Vanner, S.J., Weese, S.J., Carter, D., Daigneault, M.C., et al., 2013. Stool substitute transplant therapy for the eradication of *Clostridium difficile* infection: 'RePOOPulating' the gut. Microbiome 1 (1), 1–12.

Parnell, J.A., Relmer, R.A., 2009. Weight loss during oligofructose supplementation is associated with decreased ghrelin and increased peptide YY in overweight and obese adults. Am. J. Clin. Nutr. 89 (6), 1751–1759.

Psichias, A., Sleeth, M.L., Murphy, K.G., Brook, L., Bewick, G.A., Hanyaloglu, A.C., et al., 2015. The short chain fatty acid propionate stimulates GLP-1 and PYY secretion via free fatty acid receptor 2 in rodents. Intl. J. Obes. (London) 39 (3), 424–429.

Pimentel, M., Lembo, A., Chey, W.D., Zakko, S., Ringel, Y., Yu, J., et al., 2011. Rifaximin therapy for patients with irritable bowel syndrome without constipation. N. Engl. J. Med. 364 (1), 22–32.

Png, C.W., Lindén, S.K., Gilshenan, K.S., Zoetendal, E.G., McSweeney, C.S., Sly, L.I., et al., 2010. Mucolytic bacteria with increased prevalence in IBD mucosa augment in vitro utilization of mucin by other bacteria. Am. J. Gastroenterol. 105 (11), 2420–2428.

Pozuelo, M., Panda, S., Santiago, A., Mendez, S., Accarino, A., Santos, J., et al., 2015. Reduction of butyrate- and methane-producing microorganisms in patients with irritable bowel syndrome. Sci. Rep. 5.

Qin, J., Li, Y., Cai, Z., Li, S., Zhu, J., Zhang, F., et al., 2012. A metagenome-wide association study of gut microbiota in type 2 diabetes. Nature 490 (7418), 55–60.

Qin, L., Wu, X., Block, M.L., Liu, Y., Breese, G.R., Hong, J.S., et al., 2007. Systemic LPS causes chronic neuroinflammation and progressive neurodegeneration. Glia 55 (5), 453–462.

Rajilić-Stojanović, M., Biagi, E., Heilig, H.G., Kajander, K., Kekkonen, R.A., Tims, S., de Vos, W.M., 2011. Global and deep molecular analysis of microbiota signatures in fecal samples from patients with irritable bowel syndrome. Gastroenterology 141 (5), 1792–1801.

Rajilić-Stojanović, M., Heilig, H.G., Tims, S., Zoetendal, E.G., Vos, W.M., 2012. Long-term monitoring of the human intestinal microbiota composition. Environ. Microbiol. 15 (4), 1146–1159.

Rajilić-Stojanović, M., Shanahan, F., Guarner, F., de Vos, W.M., 2013. Phylogenetic analysis of dysbiosis in ulcerative colitis during remission. Inflamm. Bowel Dis. 19 (3), 481–488.

Ramirez-Farias, C., Slezak, K., Fuller, Z., Duncan, A., Holtrop, G., Louis, P., 2009. Effect of inulin on the human gut microbiota: stimulation of *Bifidobacterium adolescentis* and *Faecalibacterium prausnitzii*. Br. J. Nutr. 101 (4), 541–550.

Reichenberg, A., Yirmiya, R., Schuld, A., Kraus, T., Haack, M., Morag, A., Pollmächer, T., 2001. Cytokine-associated emotional and cognitive disturbances in humans. Arch. Gen. Psychiatry 58 (5), 445–452.

Reunanen, J., Kainulainen, V., Huuskonen, L., Ottman, N., Belzer, C., Huhtinen, H., et al., 2015. *Akkermansia muciniphila* adheres to enterocytes and strengthens the integrity of the epithelial cell layer. Appl. Environ. Microbiol. 81 (11), 3655–3662.

Rivas, M.N., Burton, O.T., Wise, P., Zhang, Y.Q., Hobson, S.A., Lloret, M.G., et al., 2013. A microbiota signature associated with experimental food allergy promotes allergic sensitization and anaphylaxis. J. Allergy Clin. Immunol. 131 (1), 201–212.

Roos, S., Dicksved, J., Tarasco, V., Locatelli, E., Ricceri, F., Grandin, U., Savino, F., 2013. 454 pyrosequencing analysis on faecal samples from a randomized DBPC trial of colicky infants treated with *Lactobacillus reuteri* DSM 17938. PLoS One 8 (2), e56710.

Rossen, N.G., Fuentes, S., van der Spek, M.J., Tijssen, J., Hartman, J.H., Duflou, A., et al., 2015. Findings from a randomized controlled trial of fecal transplantation for patients with ulcerative colitis. Gastroenterology 149 (1), 110–118.e4.

Russell, S.L., Gold, M.J., Hartmann, M., Willing, B.P., Thorson, L., Wlodarska, M., et al., 2012. Early life antibiotic-driven changes in microbiota enhance susceptibility to allergic asthma. EMBO Rep. 13 (5), 440–447.

Samuel, B.S., Shaito, A., Motoike, T., Rey, F.E., Backhed, F., Manchester, J.K., et al., 2008. Effects of the gut microbiota on host adiposity are modulated by the short-chain fatty-acid binding G protein-coupled receptor, Gpr41. Proc. Natl. Acad. Sci. U.S.A. 105 (43), 16767–16772.

Sanders, M.E., Guarner, F., Guerrant, R., Holt, P.R., Quigley, E.M., Sartor, R.B., et al., 2013. An update on the use and investigation of probiotics in health and disease. Gut 62 (5), 787–796.

Sandler, R.H., Finegold, S.M., Bolte, E.R., Buchanan, C.P., Maxwell, A.P., Väisänen, M.L., et al., 2000. Short-term benefit from oral vancomycin treatment of regressive-onset autism. J. Child Neurol. 15 (7), 429–435.

Saulnier, D.M., Riehle, K., Mistretta, T.A., Diaz, M.A., Mandal, D., Raza, S., et al., 2011. Gastrointestinal microbiome signatures of pediatric patients with irritable bowel syndrome. Gastroenterology 141 (5), 1782–1791.

Sato, J., Kanazawa, A., Ikeda, F., Yoshihara, T., Goto, H., Abe, H., et al., 2014. Gut dysbiosis and detection of "live gut bacteria" in blood of Japanese patients with type 2 diabetes. Diabet. Care 37 (8), 2343–2350.

Scharlau, D., Borowicki, A., Habermann, N., Hofmann, T., Klenow, S., Miene, C., et al., 2009. Mechanisms of primary cancer prevention by butyrate and other products formed during gut flora-mediated fermentation of dietary fibre. Mutat. Res. 682 (1), 39–53.

Scheperjans, F., Aho, V., Pereira, P.A., Koskinen, K., Paulin, L., Pekkonen, E., et al., 2015. Gut microbiota are related to Parkinson's disease and clinical phenotype. Mov. Disord. 30 (3), 350–358.

Scher, J.U., Abramson, S.B., 2011. The microbiome and rheumatoid arthritis. Nat. Rev. Rheumatol. 7 (10), 569–578.

Scher, J.U., Sczesnak, A., Longman, R.S., Segata, N., Ubeda, C., Bielski, C., et al., 2013. Expansion of intestinal *Prevotella copri* correlates with enhanced susceptibility to arthritis. eLife 2, e01202.

Schwiertz, A., Taras, D., Schäfer, K., Beijer, S., Bos, N.A., Donus, C., Hardt, P.D., 2010. Microbiota and SCFA in lean and overweight healthy subjects. Obesity 18 (1), 190–195.

Sheedy, J.R., Wettenhall, R.E., Scanlon, D., Gooley, P.R., Lewis, D.P., Mcgregor, N., et al., 2009. Increased D-lactic acid intestinal bacteria in patients with chronic fatigue syndrome. In Vivo 23 (4), 621–628.

Shin, N., Lee, J.W., Lee, B., Kim, M.S., Wong, T.B., et al., 2014. An increase in the *Akkermansia* spp. population induced by metformin treatment improves glucose homeostasis in diet-induced obese mice. Gut 63, 727–735.

Smith, P.M., Howitt, M.R., Panikov, N., Michaud, M., Gallini, C.A., Bohlooly-Y, M., et al., 2013. The microbial metabolites short-chain fatty acids, regulate colonic T_{reg} cell homeostasis. Science 341 (6145), 569–573.

Smits, L.P., Bouter, K.E., de Vos, W.M., Borody, T.J., Nieuwdorp, M., 2013. Therapeutic potential of fecal microbiota transplantation. Gastroenterology 145 (5), 946–953.

Sobhani, I., Tap, J., Roudot-Thoraval, F., Roperch, J.P., Letulle, S., Langella, P., et al., 2011. Microbial dysbiosis in colorectal cancer (CRC) patients. PLoS One 6 (1), e16393.

Sokol, H., Pigneur, B., Watterlot, L., Lakhdari, O., Bermúdez-Humarán, L.G., Gratadoux, J.J., et al., 2008. *Faecalibacterium prausnitzii* is an anti-inflammatory commensal bacterium identified by gut microbiota analysis of Crohn disease patients. Proc. Natl. Acad. Sci. U.S.A. 105 (43), 16731–16736.

Sokol, H., Seksik, P., Furet, J., Firmesse, O., Nion-Larmurier, I., Beaugerie, L., et al., 2009. Low counts of *Faecalibacterium prausnitzii* in colitis microbiota. Inflamm. Bowel Dis. 15 (8), 1183–1189.

Spencer, M.D., Hamp, T.J., Reid, R.W., Fischer, L.M., Zeisel, S.H., Fodor, A.A., 2011. Association between composition of the human gastrointestinal microbiome and development of fatty liver with choline deficiency. Gastroenterology 140 (3), 976–986.

Storrø, O., Øien, T., Langsrud, Ø., Rudi, K., Dotterud, C., Johnsen, R., 2011. Temporal variations in early gut microbial colonization are associated with allergen-specific immunoglobulin E but not atopic eczema at 2 years of age. Clin. Exp. Allergy 41 (11), 1545–1554.

Strauss, J., Kaplan, G.G., Beck, P.L., Rioux, K., Panaccione, R., DeVinney, R., et al., 2011. Invasive potential of gut mucosa-derived *Fusobacterium nucleatum* positively correlates with IBD status of the host. Inflamm. Bowel Dis. 17 (9), 1971–1978.

Strugnell, R.A., Wijburg, O.L., 2010. The role of secretory antibodies in infection immunity. Nat. Rev. Microbiol. 8 (9), 656–667.

Sundin, J., Rangel, I., Fuentes, S., Heikamp-de Jong, I., Hultgren-Hörnquist, E., Vos, W.M., Brummer, R.J., 2015a. Altered faecal and mucosal microbial composition in post-infectious irritable bowel syndrome patients correlates with mucosal lymphocyte phenotypes and psychological distress. Aliment. Pharmacol. Therap. 41 (4), 342–351.

Sundin, J., Rangel, I., Repsilber, D., Brummer, R.J., 2015b. Cytokine response after stimulation with key commensal bacteria differ in post–infectious irritable bowel syndrome (PI-IBS) patients compared to healthy subjects. PloS One 10 (9), e0134836.

Tana, C., Umesaki, Y., Imaoka, A., Handa, T., Kanazawa, M., Fukudo, S., 2010. Altered profiles of intestinal microbiota and organic acids may be the origin of symptoms in irritable bowel syndrome. Neurogastroenterol. Motil. 22 (5), 512–519, e115.

Tims, S., Derom, C., Jonkers, D.M., Vlietinck, R., Saris, W.H., Kleerebezem, M., et al., 2013. Microbiota conservation and BMI signatures in adult monozygotic twins. ISME J. 7 (4), 707–717.

Turnbaugh, P.J., Ley, R.E., Mahowald, M.A., Magrini, V., Mardis, E.R., Gordon, J.I., 2006. An obesity-associated gut microbiome with increased capacity for energy harvest. Nature 444 (7122), 1027–1131.

Turnbaugh, P.J., Hamady, M., Yatsunenko, T., Cantarel, B.L., Duncan, A., Ley, R.E., et al., 2009. A core gut microbiome in obese and lean twins. Nature 457 (7228), 480–484.

van Tongeren, S.P., Slaets, J.P., Harmsen, H.J.M., Welling, G.W., 2005. Fecal microbiota composition and frailty. Appl. Environ. Microbiol. 71 (10), 6438–6442.

Udina, M., Castellví, P., Moreno-España, J., Navinés, R., Valdés, M., Forns, X., et al., 2012. Interferon-induced depression in chronic hepatitis C: a systematic review and meta-analysis. J. Clin. Psychiatry 73 (8), 1128–1138.

de Vos, W.M., 2013. Fame and future of faecal transplantations–developing next-generation therapies with synthetic microbiomes. Microb. Biotechnol. 6 (4), 316–325.

de Vos, W.M., de Vos, E.A., 2012. Role of the intestinal microbiome in health and disease: from correlation to causation. Nutr. Rev. 70 (Suppl. 1), S45–S56.

Verdam, F.J., Fuentes, S., de Jonge, C., Zoetendal, E.G., Erbil, R., Greve, J.W., et al., 2013. Human intestinal microbiota composition is associated with local and systemic inflammation in obesity. Obesity 21 (12), E607–E615.

Vossen, J.M., Guiot, H.F., Lankester, A.C., Vossen, A.C., Bredius, R.G., Wolterbeek, R., et al., 2014. Complete suppression of the gut microbiome prevents acute graft-versus-host disease following allogeneic bone marrow transplantation. PLoS One 9 (9), e105706.

Vrieze, A., Van Nood, E., Holleman, F., Salojärvi, J., Kootte, R.S., Bartelsman, J.F., et al., 2012. Transfer of intestinal microbiota from lean donors increases insulin sensitivity in individuals with metabolic syndrome. Gastroenterology 143 (4), 913–916.

de Weerth, C., Fuentes, S., Puylaert, P., de Vos, W.M., 2013. Intestinal microbiota of infants with colic: development and specific signatures. Pediatrics 131 (2), e550–e558.

Wang, L., Christophersen, C.T., Sorich, M.J., Gerber, J.P., Angley, M.T., Conlon, M.A., 2011a. Low relative abundances of the mucolytic bacterium *Akkermansia muciniphila* and *Bifidobacterium* spp. in feces of children with autism. Appl. Environ. Microbiol. 77 (18), 6718–6721.

Wang, M., Karlsson, C., Olsson, C., Adlerberth, I., Wold, A.E., Strachan, D.P., et al., 2008. Reduced diversity in the early fecal microbiota of infants with atopic eczema. J. Allergy Clin. Immunol. 121 (1), 129–134.

Wang, T., Cai, G., Qiu, Y., Fei, N., Zhang, M., Pang, X., et al., 2012. Structural segregation of gut microbiota between colorectal cancer patients and healthy volunteers. ISME J. 6 (2), 320–329.

Wang, Z., Klipfell, E., Bennett, B.J., Koeth, R., Levison, B.S., DuGar, B., et al., 2011b. Gut flora metabolism of phosphatidylcholine promotes cardiovascular disease. Nature 472 (7341), 57–63.

West, C.E., Jenmalm, M.C., Prescott, S.L., 2015. The gut microbiota and its role in the development of allergic disease: a wider perspective. Clin. Exp. Allergy 45 (1), 43–53.

Williams, B.L., Hornig, M., Buie, T., Bauman, M.L., Cho Paik, M., Wick, I., et al., 2011. Impaired carbohydrate digestion and transport and mucosal dysbiosis in the intestines of children with autism and gastrointestinal disturbances. PLoS One 6 (9), e24585.

Williams, B.L., Hornig, M., Parekh, T., Lipkin, W.I., 2012. Application of novel PCR-based methods for detection, quantitation, and phylogenetic characterization of *Sutterella* species in intestinal biopsy samples from children with autism and gastrointestinal disturbances. MBio 3 (1), e00261–11.

Willing, B.P., Dicksved, J., Halfvarson, J., Andersson, A.F., Lucio, M., Zheng, Z., et al., 2010. A pyrosequencing study in twins shows that gastrointestinal microbial profiles vary with inflammatory bowel disease phenotypes. Gastroenterology 139 (6), 1844–1854.

Wu, H.J., Ivanov, I.I., Darce, J., Hattori, K., Shima, T., Umesaki, Y., et al., 2010. Gut-residing segmented filamentous bacteria drive autoimmune arthritis via T helper 17 cells. Immunity 32 (6), 815–827.

Xia, Q., Grant, S.F., 2013. The genetics of human obesity. Ann. N.Y. Acad. Sci. 1281 (1), 178–190.

Xiao, L., Feng, Q., Liang, S., Sonne, S.B., Xia, Z., Qiu, X., et al., 2015. A catalog of the mouse gut metagenome. Nat. Biotechnol. 33 (10), 1103–1108.

Yamashita, T., Kasahara, K., Emoto, T., Matsumoto, T., Mizoguchi, T., Kitano, N., et al., 2015. Intestinal immunity and gut microbiota as therapeutic targets for preventing atherosclerotic cardiovascular diseases. Circ. J. 79 (9), 1882–1890.

Yu, J., Feng, Q., Wong, S.H., Zhang, D., yi Liang, Q., Qin, Y., et al., 2015. Metagenomic analysis of faecal microbiome as a tool towards targeted non-invasive biomarkers for colorectal cancer. Gut. http://dx.doi.org/10.1136/gutjnl-2015-309800.

Zeller, G., Tap, J., Voigt, A.Y., Sunagawa, S., Kultima, J.R., Costea, P.I., et al., 2014. Potential of fecal microbiota for early-stage detection of colorectal cancer. Mol. Syst. Biol. 10 (11), 766.

Zhang, R., Miller, R.G., Gascon, R., Champion, S., Katz, J., Lancero, M., et al., 2009. Circulating endotoxin and systemic immune activation in sporadic amyotrophic lateral sclerosis (sALS). J. Neuroimmunol. 206 (1), 121–124.

Zhang, X., Zhang, D., Jia, H., Feng, Q., Wang, D., Liang, D., et al., 2015. The oral and gut microbiomes are perturbed in rheumatoid arthritis and partly normalized after treatment. Nat. Med. 21, 895–905.

Zhu, L., Baker, S.S., Gill, C., Liu, W., Alkhouri, R., Baker, R.D., Gill, S.R., 2013. Characterization of gut microbiomes in nonalcoholic steatohepatitis (NASH) patients: a connection between endogenous alcohol and NASH. Hepatology 57 (2), 601–609.

Zoetendal, E.G., Rajilić-Stojanović, M., De Vos, W.M., 2008. High-throughput diversity and functionality analysis of the gastrointestinal tract microbiota. Gut 57 (11), 1605–1615.

Zoetendal, E.G., de Vos, W.M., 2014. Effect of diet on the intestinal microbiota and its activity. Curr. Opin. Gastroenterol. 30 (2), 189–195.

The Hypothalamic-Pituitary-Adrenal Axis and Gut Microbiota: A Target for Dietary Intervention?

13

N. Sudo

Kyushu University, Department of Psychosomatic Medicine, Fukuoka, Japan

INTRODUCTION

The human intestine is inhabited by more than 1000 bacterial species and an estimated 10^{11}–10^{12} bacterial cells are present per gram of feces (Qin et al., 2010). These bacteria not only play a principal role in the postnatal maturation of the mammalian immune system (Sudo et al., 1997), but they also aid in the digestion and absorption of macromolecules and act as a barrier to gut pathogens by blocking attachment to gut binding sites, which is the first step of bacterial pathogenicity (Finlay, 1990). Moreover, it is rapidly becoming apparent that the gut microbiota plays a major role in the development and regulation of neuroendocrine systems such as the hypothalamic-pituitary-adrenal (HPA) axis. Our previous study on germ-free (GF) and gnotobiotic mice demonstrated that exposure to gut microbes is a critical environmental determinant that regulates the development of the HPA stress response and the setpoint for this axis (Sudo et al., 2004). Further progress in this field has since been achieved by several independent groups (Clarke et al., 2013; Gareau et al., 2011; Heijtza et al., 2011; Neufeld et al., 2011; Nishino et al., 2013; Crumeyrolle-Arias et al., 2014), and this concept is now integrated into an elaborate interaction among the microbiota, the gut, and the brain, which collectively are referred to as the microbiota-gut-brain axis (Collins and Bercik, 2009; Collins et al., 2012).

In this chapter we focus on bidirectional signaling between the gut microbiome and the host in terms of commensal microbiota affecting the HPA axis response, and we further discuss dietary factors, such as probiotics, as a possible therapeutic intervention for people with stress-related disorders.

THE HYPOTHALAMIC-PITUITARY-ADRENAL AXIS

The HPA axis is considered a central integrative system crucial for the successful physiological adaptation of an organism to stress. During stress corticotrophin-releasing hormone (CRH) and arginine vasopressin, the principal hypothalamic regulators of the

The Gut-Brain Axis. http://dx.doi.org/10.1016/B978-0-12-802304-4.00013-X

HPA axis, are released. CRH stimulates the secretion of adrenocorticotropin hormone (ACTH) from the anterior pituitary into the hypophyseal portal system via collateral fibers in the systemic circulation. ACTH leads to the secretion of glucocorticoids (GCs; cortisol in humans and corticosterone in rodents) from the adrenal cortex, the main target of ACTH. GCs are the final effectors of the HPA axis and regulate multiple bodily functions responsible for preparing the individual to cope with the demands of metabolic, physical, and psychological stressors (Chrousos and Gold, 1992).

The HPA axis is subjected to programming by early-life events. For example, as adults, neonatally handled animals exhibit dampened HPA responses to stress compared with nonhandled animals (Meaney et al., 1988). In contrast, adult animals exposed to repeated, prolonged maternal deprivation as neonates display increased HPA response to stress (Schmidt et al., 2002). These effects persist into adulthood, and the resulting hyperactivity of HPA responses is associated with the incidence of age-related neuropathology (Meaney et al., 1988), such as memory impairment in animals (Landfield et al., 1978, 1981) and humans (Lupien et al., 1998).

GUT MICROBIOTA: A CRITICAL FACTOR FOR DETERMINING THE HYPOTHALAMIC-PITUITARY-ADRENAL AXIS SETPOINT

Environmental factors, especially those which occur early in life, affect the development of the HPA axis. One such factor, the microbiota, is a major environmental force influencing host physiology and the development of the HPA response.

To explore the influence of the microbiota on the HPA axis, we investigated the HPA response to stress by comparing genetically identical mice that had no exposure to microorganisms (GF mice); mice raised with a normal functional microbiota, classified as specific pathogen free (SPF); and mice raised with a selected group of organisms (gnotobiotic; Sudo et al., 2004). We noted that the elevation in plasma ACTH and corticosterone responses to restraint stress were substantially higher in GF mice than in SPF mice (Table 13.1). To further elucidate the involvement of gut microbiota in the HPA stress response, gnotobiotic mice for which the gut flora was colonized with a single strain of bacterium in the neonatal period were tested for their susceptibility to restraint stress as adults. As summarized in Table 13.2, monoassociation with *Bifidobacterium infantis*, which is a representative inhabitant of the neonate's gut, but not *Bacteroides vulgatus* dampened the HPA stress response to the level observed in the SPF mice. The hormonal stress response in mice monocolonized with rabbit-derived enteropathogenic *Escherichia coli* (EPEC) was substantially higher than that in GF mice, although no such exaggerated response was found in the mice reconstituted with an EPEC mutant strain, ΔTir (Kenny et al., 1997). This particular strain is not internalized because of defects in the translocated intimin receptor. It is interesting to note that the enhanced HPA stress response of GF mice was partially corrected after reconstitution with SPF feces at an early stage of development whereas such a correction was not found when reconstitution was performed later in life. Therefore the microbe-induced reversal of the HPA axis setpoint

Table 13.1 Increased Plasma Adrenocorticotropin Hormone and Corticosterone Response to Restraint Stress in Germ-Free Mice[a]

	SPF		GF	
	ACTH (pg/mL)	Corticosterone (ng/mL)	ACTH (pg/mL)	Corticosterone (ng/mL)
Basal	46±13	19±5.6	49±12	23±4.2
1h RS	101±20	59±12	198±19***	129±20***
30min after RS	55±10	42±10	80±10*	83±16**

ACTH, adrenocorticotropin hormone; GF, germ-free; SPF, specific pathogen free; RS, restraint stress.
***$P<0.001$, **$P<0.01$, *$P<0.05$ significantly different from the corresponding SPF value.
[a]GF and SPF mice were subjected to a 1-h period of RS (n=6–11) per each time point, as previously described (Sudo et al., 2004).

Table 13.2 Effects of Restraint Stress on Plasma Adrenocorticotropin Hormone and Corticosterone Levels in the Gnotobiotic Mice[a]

	ACTH (pg/mL)		Corticosterone (ng/mL)	
	Basal	1h RS	Basal	1h RS
GF	66±12	188±16	19±3.9	131±12
SPF	54±6.1	106±20***	21±6.5	86±9.9***
Bifidobacterium infantis	60±9.8	113±15***	21±5.2	79±9.5***
Bacteroides vulgatus	63±9.9	166±14	17±6.8	140±14
EPEC	49±15	243±22*	19±6.6	172±20*
ΔTir	60±9.5	153±25	15±3.6	102±17

ACTH, adrenocorticotropin hormone; GF, germ-free; SPF, specific pathogen free; RS, restraint stress; EPEC, enteropathogenic Escherichia coli.
***$P<0.001$, *$P<0.05$ significantly different from the GF value.
[a]Plasma ACTH and corticosterone levels were measured at before or immediately after 1h RS in GF, SPF, and gnotobiotic mice reconstituted with a single strain with B. infantis, B. vulgatus, rabbit-derived EPEC, or EPEC mutant strain (ΔTir) at 9weeks of age as described previously (Sudo et al., 2004).

extended into adulthood, but only if bacterial colonization occurred early in life. Colonization as adults was ineffective, thus suggesting that there is a critical window of susceptibility to these effects with regard to the bacteria–host interaction.

ANTISTRESS EFFECTS OF PROBIOTICS

Barreau et al. (2004) have reported that probiotic treatment consisting of *Lactobacillus rhamnosus* and *Lactobacillus helveticus* can ameliorate enhanced basal HPA axis activity induced by maternal separation stress in rats, suggesting that probiotics normalize the activity of the HPA axis. The same treatment with probiotics also ameliorated water avoidance stress-induced elevations in serum corticosterone levels compared with placebo (Gareau et al., 2011). In line with these observations, Bravo et al. (2011) showed that the levels of stress-induced corticosterone are significantly lower in stressed mice fed *L. rhamnosus* compared with their control broth-fed counterparts. Thus these findings support the notion that probiotics exert a protective effect on stressed hosts.

PATHWAYS, MOLECULES, AND CELL TYPES INVOLVED IN MICROBIOTA-GUT-BRAIN SIGNALING

The exact mechanisms by which gut bacteria communicate with the brain and possibly alter its function and activity remain to be fully elucidated. The underlying pathways are most probably highly complex, and it is unlikely that any one single pathway or series of molecules are involved. However, some possible pathways and molecules, including recent topics, are reviewed here.

AFFERENT NEURAL SIGNALING

We demonstrated that administration of *B. infantis* to GF mice triggered a small, but significant, increase in plasma interleukin (IL)-6 levels without an associated elevation in plasma IL-1β. It is interesting to note that expression of the early gene product c-Fos in the hypothalamus was also noted 6h after the inoculation. However, pretreatment with anti-IL-6 antibody failed to affect the *B. infantis*-induced c-Fos response in the hypothalamus. In contrast, neonatal treatment with capsaicin partially suppressed this effect (Sudo, 2012). Moreover, inhibition of c-Fos responses were also sensitive to treatment with either granisetron, a serotonin (5-HT) type 3 receptor antagonist, or *p*-chlorophenylalanine, a 5-HT hydroxylase inhibitor (Fig. 13.1).

These results indicate that the brain responds to the presence of bacteria through a capsaicin-sensitive vagal or spinal afferent nerve pathway. The functional importance of this pathway in gut-brain signaling was further confirmed by an elegant study by Bravo and coworkers (Bravo et al., 2011), who demonstrated that surgical vagotomy inhibited anxiolytic and antidepressant effects of *L. rhamnosus*.

SHORT-CHAIN FATTY ACIDS

Short-chain fatty acids (SCFAs) are the end products of anaerobic bacterial fermentation in the gastrointestinal tract. Through their absorption and metabolism, the host is able to salvage energy from food not digested in the upper intestine. Under

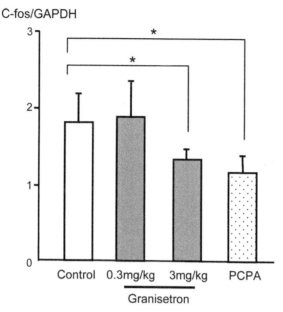

FIGURE 13.1 The effects of granisetron and PCPA on the hypothalamic c-Fos response upon exposure to *Bifidobacterium*.

GF mice were administered either 0.3 or 3 mg/kg granisetron or a corresponding vehicle (control) 30 min before intraperitoneal injection. A tryptophan hydroxylase inhibitor (PCPA) was administered intraperitoneally at a dose of 500 mg/kg for 2 consecutive days. These mice were given *Bifidobacterium infantis* and their hypothalamus c-Fos responses were examined as described previously (Sudo et al., 2004). The *bar graphs* show the relative band intensities from the densitometric analysis as the ratios of c-Fos to GAPDH mRNA after 30 cycles of amplification. All data are expressed as the mean ± SD ($n=5$). *Significant difference at $P<0.05$ compared with control values. *PCPA*, p-chlorophenylalanine; *GF*, germ-free; *GADPH*, glyceraldehyde-3-phosphate dehydrogenase.

physiological conditions, their production is entirely dependent on commensal microbes, and there are only negligible amounts of SCFA detectable in GF mice (Hoverstad and Midtvedt, 1986). As summarized in Table 13.3, association with fecal flora from SPF mice, which were formerly GF, resulted in a drastic elevation of cecal SCFA levels. Monoassociation with *B. infantis* or *B. vulgatus* also induced a small but significant elevation of cecal SCFA amounts in a strain specific-fashion.

SCFAs, such as acetate, butyrate, and propionate, also act as signal transduction molecules via G-protein coupled receptors (FFAR2, FFAR3, OLFR78, GPR109A) (Kasubuchi et al., 2015). Recent evidence suggests that gut microbiome-derived SCFAs not only exert multiple beneficial effects on the host's energy metabolism but also play a pivotal role in the regulation of the gut–brain signaling as described here.

Table 13.3 Short-Chain Fatty Acids in Cecal Content of Gnotobiotic Mice[a]

	(μmol/g Feces)			
	GF	EX-GF	*Bifidobacterium infantis*	*Bacteroides vulgatus*
Acetate	1.84±0.5	104.0±7.2**	4.28±0.55*	7.68±0.51**
Propionate	ND	3.0±0.16**	ND	2.30±0.24**
i-Butyrate	ND	2.0±0.08**	ND	0.29±0.03**
n-Butyrate	ND	3.4±0.32**	ND	ND
i-Valerate	ND	2.2±0.16**	ND	0.37±0.03**
n-Valerate	ND	3.0±0.14**	ND	ND
Total SCFA[b]	1.84±0.5	116.6±12.6**	4.28±0.55*	10.64±0.65**

GF, germ-free; SFCA, short chain fatty acid.
*$P<0.01$, **$P<0.001$ significantly different from the corresponding GF value, by Wilcoxon-Mann-Whitney test.
[a]GF mice were reconstituted with fecal flora from SPF mice (EX-GF), a single strain of B. infantis, or B. vulgatus. Cecal contents in the GF and reconstituted mice were immediately processed for SCFA analysis. The SCFA concentration was measured by gas chromatography, as described previously (Sudo et al., 2000).
[b]The total amounts of SCFAs are expressed as the sum of the amounts of acetate, propionate, i-butyrate, n-butylate, i-valerate, and n-valerate. All data are expressed as the means ±SD (n=6).

MOLECULAR AND CELLULAR TARGETS INFLUENCED BY THE MICROBIOTA, PROBIOTICS, AND SHORT-CHAIN FATTY ACIDS
LEAKY GUT AND BLOOD–BRAIN BARRIER PERMEABILITY

A potential mechanism by which probiotics may exhibit their beneficial activities is modulation of the epithelial barrier function (Dotan and Rachmilewitz, 2005; Sartor, 2004). This hypothesis is also supported by a study demonstrating that colonization of gnotobiotic mice with *Escherichia coli* Nissle 1917 resulted in an upregulation of the tight junction protein zonula occludens-1 in gut epithelial cells at the mRNA and protein levels (Ukena et al., 2007). Moreover, treatment with *Lactobacillus farciminis* and a specific myosin light-chain kinase inhibitor (ML-7) suppressed stress-induced increases in permeability and prevented the stress-induced HPA axis response through the inhibition of intestinal barrier impairment (Ait-Belgnaoui et al., 2012).

It is intriguing to note that GF mice have significantly increased permeability of the blood–brain barrier (BBB) during fetal development and in adulthood (Braniste et al., 2014). Interestingly, monocolonization with either *Clostridium tyrobutyricum* or *Bacteroides thetaiotaomicron* could restore BBB integrity and production of tight junction expression even in adult mice. Because these species produce SCFAs by fermentation of complex carbohydrates in the gut, it was subsequently observed that the SCFA butyrate was sufficient to restore BBB integrity.

MICROGLIA

Microglia cells are extremely sensitive not only to damage in the CNS but also to environmental challenges such as psychological stress (Chijiwa et al., 2015; Frank et al., 2013; Walker et al., 2013). A recent exciting study demonstrated that gut microbiota influence the CNS immune system by regulating microglial cell activation and homeostasis (Erny et al., 2015; Mosher and Wyss-Coray, 2015).

RNA sequencing showed striking differences in transcriptional profiles between microglia isolated from GF and SPF young adult mice. Of note, DNA damage-inducible transcript-4 (*Ddit4*), the product of which regulates cell growth, proliferation, and survival, was most elevated in microglia from GF mice compared with those from SPF mice. Other genes that were significantly upregulated in microglia from GF mice were *Sfp1* (encoding Pu.1) and *Csf1r*, which are highly expressed in developing microglia (Ginhoux et al., 2010; Kierdorf et al., 2013), whereas several genes involved in cell activation were downregulated. In addition, a greater percentage of microglia from GF mice expressed the surface proteins colony stimulating factor receptor-1 (CSFR1) F4/80, and CD31, which generally decline in abundance with cell maturation (Kierdorf et al., 2013). Overall, these findings are consistent with immature microglial characteristics in GF mice. It is interesting that increasing the microbiota complexity further, by co-housing partially recolonized animals with normal SPF animals, normalized microglial numbers and morphology as well as *Ddit4* levels. Moreover, when the GF mice were given a mixture of SCFAs in their drinking water, the microglial numbers, *Ddit4* mRNA levels, microglial morphology, and microglial expression of CSFR1 were normalized to those seen in SPF animals. Thus SCFAs appear to be important to the regulation of microglial maturation; however, the precise molecular mechanism by which SCFAs render microglia mature remains to be answered. Collectively, these findings clearly show that microglia are a critical link between microbiota and the brain.

EPIGENETICS

Epigenetic modulation of gene transcription, a recently proposed mechanism for regulating gene expression changes underlying neural plasticity, may be affected by early-life adversity, and, likewise, possibly by microbial colonization (Stilling et al., 2014). Early-life stress is considered to influence the epigenome on different levels, via distinct mechanisms (Klengel and Binder, 2015). For example, maternal separation stress affects the posttranslational modification of the epigenetic modifier methyl CpG binding protein-2 by phosphorylation, leading to a dissociation of the protein complex from the DNA strand (Chahrour et al., 2008). Alternatively, stress may directly influence the transcriptional regulation of epigenetic writers, readers, and erasers. Lee et al. (2011) demonstrated that in vitro exposure of a murine pituitary cell line, and in vivo exposure of mice, to the glucocorticoid analog dexamethasone caused a dose-dependent decrease in DNA (cytosine-5)-methyltransferase-1 expression and reduced DNA methylation at the murine *fkbp5* locus. An additional molecular mechanism leading to long-term epigenetic changes in response to stress is the activation of DNA binding proteins and specific transcription factors that lead to local changes in epigenetic profiles (Thomassin et al., 2001; Weaver et al., 2004). Another pathway that has been implicated in generating long-term epigenetic signatures of environmental exposure is the expression of small noncoding RNAs in the form of micro RNAs and their subsequent targeting of stress-relevant pathways (Haramati et al., 2011; Jung et al., 2015).

The possible molecules implicated as the link between epigenetics and gut microorganisms are still unclear. However, SCFAs may be key players, especially butyric acid, which is produced by obligate anaerobic bacteria such as *Clostridium* species. Butyric acid is also a prototype member of an emerging class of drugs, the histone deacetylase inhibitors (Tsankova et al., 2007). In fact, Schroeder et al. (2007) showed that systemic injection of butyrate induced histone hyperacetylation in the hippocampus and frontal cortex and exerted antidepressant-like effects in mice that were associated with increased brain-derived neurotrophic factor transcripts in the frontal cortex. Whether or not physiological levels of butyric acids can have the same effects on the brain is so far unknown. However, epigenetic modifications are undoubtedly important as a potential target of psychiatric treatments.

PROBIOTICS, PREBIOTICS, AND STRESS-RELATED DISORDERS

In the beginning of the 20th century, when the antidepressant drugs had not yet been developed, Phillips (1910) treated 18 melancholia patients with lactic acid bacillus. As a result, 11 patients fully recovered, 2 improved, the condition was unchanged in 4, and 1 died. All of the patients showed improvements in constipation and body weight gain. These findings had long been forgotten until probiotic intervention reemerged as a therapeutic potential in the 21st century. For example, in a clinical study healthy volunteers were given a combination of *L. helveticus* R0052 and *Bifidobacterium longum* R0175 or placebo in a double-blind, randomized, parallel-group study for 30 days and assessed using the Hopkins Symptom Checklist (HSCL-90), the Hospital Anxiety and Depression Scale (HADS), the Perceived Stress Scale, the Coping Checklist (CCL), and 24-h urinary-free cortisol (UFC; Messaoudi et al., 2011). Daily administration of probiotics alleviated psychological distress in volunteers such as global severity index, somatization, depression, and anger–hostility, as measured by the HSCL-90 scale, the HADS, and the CCL (problem solving) as well as by the UFC level. In the study examining the effects of prebiotics, 45 healthy volunteers received one of two prebiotics (fructooligosaccharides [FOS] or Bimuno-galactooligosaccharides [B-GOS]) or a placebo (maltodextrin) daily for 3 weeks (Schmidt et al., 2015). As a result, the salivary cortisol awakening response was significantly lower after B-GOS intake compared with placebo. Participants also showed decreased attentional vigilance to negative versus positive information in a dot-probe task after B-GOS compared with placebo intake. No effects were found after the administration of FOS. These results are consistent with previous findings of endocrine and anxiolytic effects of microbiota proliferation.

Thus accumulating high-quality evidence based on animal studies clearly shows a substantial crosstalk between gut microbes and brain functions; in contrast, clinical studies are still extremely limited. Well-controlled clinical trials with a large sample size are needed to demonstrate antistress effects of probiotics in humans.

CONCLUSION AND PERSPECTIVES

We are living in a bacterial world. Gut microbiota can have long-lasting and profound effects on the adult HPA axis and behaviors. Moreover, the recent findings provide strong evidence that SCFAs are a key player in the signaling from the gut to the brain. Probiotics or prebiotics would facilitate the design of new therapeutic approaches to stress-related disorders, such as anxiety and depression, by modulating gut microbiota-derived biochemical substances and influencing key pathways implicated in gut-brain communication.

REFERENCES

Ait-Belgnaoui, A., Durand, H., Cartier, C., Chaumaz, G., Eutamene, H., Ferrier, L., Houdeau, E., Fioramonti, J., Bueno, L., Theodorou, V., 2012. Prevention of gut leakiness by a probiotic treatment leads to attenuated HPA response to an acute psychological stress in rats. Psychoneuroendocrinology 37, 1885–1895.

Barreau, F., Ferrier, L., Fioramonti, J., Bueno, L., 2004. Neonatal maternal deprivation triggers long term alterations in colonic epithelial barrier and mucosal immunity in rats. Gut 53, 501–506.

Braniste, V., Al-Asmakh, M., Kowal, C., Anuar, F., Abbaspour, A., Toth, M., Korecka, A., Bakocevic, N., Ng, L.G., Kundu, P., Gulyas, B., Halldin, C., Hultenby, K., Nilsson, H., Hebert, H., Volpe, B.T., Diamond, B., Pettersson, S., 2014. The gut microbiota influences blood–brain barrier permeability in mice. Sci. Transl. Med. 6, 263ra158.

Bravo, J.A., Forsythe, P., Chew, M.V., Escaravage, E., Savignac, H.M., Dinan, T.G., Bienenstock, J., Cryan, J.F., 2011. Ingestion of *Lactobacillus* strain regulates emotional behavior and central GABA receptor expression in a mouse via the vagus nerve. Proc. Natl. Acad. Sci. U. S. A. 108, 16050–16055.

Chahrour, M., Sung, Y.J., Shaw, C., Zhou, X., Wong, S.T.C., Qin, J., Zoghbi, H.Y., 2008. MeCP2, a key contributor to neurological disease, activates and represses transcription. Science 320, 1224–1229.

Chijiwa, T., Oka, T., Lkhagvasuren, B., Yoshihara, K., Sudo, N., 2015. Prior chronic stress induces persistent polyI:C-induced allodynia and depressive-like behavior in rats: possible involvement of glucocorticoids and microglia. Physiol. Behav. 147, 264–273.

Chrousos, G., Gold, P., 1992. The concepts of stress and stress system disorders – overview of physical and behavioral homeostasis. J. Am. Med. Assoc. 267, 1244–1252.

Clarke, G., Grenham, S., Scully, P., Fitzgerald, P., Moloney, R.D., Shanahan, F., Dinan, T.G., Cryan, J.F., 2013. The microbiome-gut-brain axis during early life regulates the hippocampal serotonergic system in a sex-dependent manner. Mol. Psychiatry 18, 666–673.

Collins, S.M., Bercik, P., 2009. The relationship between intestinal microbiota and the central nervous system in normal gastrointestinal function and disease. Gastroenterology 136, 2003–2014.

Collins, S.M., Surette, M., Bercik, P., 2012. The interplay between the intestinal microbiota and the brain. Nat. Rev. Microbiol. 10, 735–742.

Crumeyrolle-Arias, M., Jaglin, M., Bruneau, A., Vancassel, S., Cardona, A., Dauge, V., Naudon, L., Rabot, S., 2014. Absence of the gut microbiota enhances anxiety-like behavior and neuroendocrine response to acute stress in rats. Psychoneuroendocrinology 42, 207–217.

Dotan, I., Rachmilewitz, D., 2005. Probiotics in inflammatory bowel disease: possible mechanisms of action. Curr. Opin. Gastroenterol. 21, 426–430.

Erny, D., Hrabě de Angelis, A.L., Jaitin, D., Wieghofer, P., Staszewski, O., David, E., Keren-Shaul, H., Mahlakoiv, T., Jakobshagen, K., Buch, T., Schwierzeck, V., Utermöhlen, O., Chun, E., Garrett, W.S., McCoy, K.D., Diefenbach, A., Staeheli, P., Stecher, B., Amit, I., Prinz, M., 2015. Host microbiota constantly control maturation and function of microglia in the CNS. Nat. Neurosci. 18, 965–977.

Finlay, B.B., 1990. Cell adhesion and invasion mechanisms in microbial pathogenesis. Curr. Opin. Cell Biol. 2, 815–820.

Frank, M.G., Watkins, L.R., Maier, S.F., 2013. Stress-induced glucocorticoids as a neuroendocrine alarm signal of danger. Brain Behav. Immun. 33, 1–6.

Gareau, M.G., Wine, E., Rodrigues, D.M., Cho, J.H., Whary, M.T., Philpott, D.J., MacQueen, G., Sherman, P.M., 2011. Bacterial infection causes stress-induced memory dysfunction in mice. Gut 60, 307–317.

Ginhoux, F., Greter, M., Leboeuf, M., Nandi, S., See, P., Gokhan, S., Mehler, M.F., Conway, S.J., Ng, L.G., Stanley, E.R., Samokhvalov, I.M., Merad, M., 2010. Fate mapping analysis reveals that adult microglia derive from primitive macrophages. Science 330, 841–845.

Haramati, S., Navon, I., Issler, O., Ezra-Nevo, G., Gil, S., Zwang, R., Hornstein, E., Chen, A., 2011. MicroRNA as repressors of stress-induced anxiety: the case of amygdalar miR-34. J. Neurosci. 31, 14191–14203.

Heijtza, R.D., Wang, S., Anuar, F., Qian, Y., Bjorkholm, B., Samuelsson, A., Hibberd, M.L., Forssberg, H., Pettersson, S., 2011. Normal gut microbiota modulates brain development and behavior. Proc. Natl. Acad. Sci. U. S. A. 108, 3047–3052.

Hoverstad, T., Midtvedt, T., 1986. Short-chain fatty acids in germfree mice and rats. J. Nutr. 116, 1772–1776.

Jung, S.H., Wang, Y., Kim, T., Tarr, A., Reader, B., Powell, N., Sheridan, J.F., 2015. Molecular mechanisms of repeated social defeat-induced glucocorticoid resistance: role of microRNA. Brain Behav. Immun. 44, 195–206.

Kasubuchi, M., Hasegawa, S., Hiramatsu, T., Ichimura, A., Kimura, I., 2015. Dietary gut microbial metabolites, short-chain fatty acids, and host metabolic regulation. Nutrients 7, 2839–2849.

Kenny, B., DeVinney, R., Stein, M., Reinscheid, D.J., Frey, E.A., Finlay, B.B., 1997. Enteropathogenic *E. coli* (EPEC) transfers its receptor for intimate adherence into mammalian cells. Cell 91, 511–520.

Kierdorf, K., Erny, D., Goldmann, T., Sander, V., Schulz, C., Perdiguero, E.G., Wieghofer, P., Heinrich, A., Riemke, P., Holscher, C., Muller, D.N., Luckow, B., Brocker, T., Debowski, K., Fritz, G., Opdenakker, G., Diefenbach, A., Biber, K., Heikenwalder, M., Geissmann, F., Rosenbauer, F., Prinz, M., 2013. Microglia emerge from erythromyeloid precursors via Pu.1- and Irf8-dependent pathways. Nat. Neurosci. 16, 273–280.

Klengel, T., Binder, E., 2015. Epigenetics of stress-related psychiatric disorders and gene × environment interactions. Neuron 86, 1343–1357.

Landfield, P.W., Baskin, R.K., Pitler, T.A., 1981. Brain aging correlates: retardation by hormonal-pharmacological treatments. Science 214, 581–584.

Landfield, P.W., Waymire, J.C., Lynch, G., 1978. Hippocampal aging and adrenocorticoids: quantitative correlations. Science 202, 1098–1102.

Lee, R.S., Tamashiro, K.L.K., Yang, X., Purcell, R.H., Huo, Y., Rongione, M., Potash, J.B., Wand, G.S., 2011. A measure of glucocorticoid load provided by DNA methylation of Fkbp5 in mice. Psychopharmacology 218, 303–312.

Lupien, S.J., de Leon, M., de Santi, S., Convit, A., Tarshish, C., Nair, N.P., Thakur, M., McEwen, B.S., Hauger, R.L., Meaney, M.J., 1998. Cortisol levels during human aging predict hippocampal atrophy and memory deficits. Nat. Neurosci. 1, 69–73.

Meaney, M.J., Aitken, D.H., van Berkel, C., Bhatnagar, S., Sapolsky, R.M., 1988. Effect of neonatal handling on age-related impairments associated with the hippocampus. Science 239, 766–768.

Messaoudi, M., Lalonde, R., Violle, N., Javelot, H., Desor, D., Nejdi, A., Bisson, J., Rougeot, C., Pichelin, M., Cazaubiel, M., Cazaubiel, J., 2011. Assessment of psychotropic-like properties of a probiotic formulation (*Lactobacillus helveticus* R0052 and *Bifidobacterium longum* R0175) in rats and human subjects. Br. J. Nutr. 105, 755–764.

Mosher, K.I., Wyss-Coray, T., 2015. Go with your gut: microbiota meet microglia. Nat. Neurosci. 18, 930–931.

Neufeld, K.M., Kang, N., Bienenstock, J., Foster, J.A., 2011. Reduced anxiety-like behavior and central neurochemical change in germ-free mice. Neurogastroenterol. Motil. 23, 255–264, e119.

Nishino, R., Mikami, K., Takahashi, H., Tomonaga, S., Furuse, M., Hiramoto, T., Aiba, Y., Koga, Y., Sudo, N., 2013. Commensal microbiota modulate murine behaviors in a strictly contamination-free environment confirmed by culture-based methods. Neurogastroenterol. Motil. 25, 521–528.

Phillips, J.G.P., 1910. The treatment of melancholia by the lactic acid bacillus. J. Mental Sci. 56, 422–431.

Qin, J., Li, R., Raes, J., Arumugam, M., Burgdorf, K.S., Manichanh, C., Nielsen, T., Pons, N., Levenez, F., Yamada, T., Mende, D.R., Li, J., Xu, J., Li, S., Li, D., Cao, J., Wang, B., Liang, H., Zheng, H., Xie, Y., Tap, J., Lepage, P., Bertalan, M., Batto, J.M., Hansen, T., Le Paslier, D., Linneberg, A., Nielsen, H.B., Pelletier, E., Renault, P., Sicheritz-Ponten, T., Turner, K., Zhu, H., Yu, C., Li, S., Jian, M., Zhou, Y., Li, Y., Zhang, X., Li, S., Qin, N., Yang, H., Wang, J., Brunak, S., Dore, J., Guarner, F., Kristiansen, K., Pedersen, O., Parkhill, J., Weissenbach, J., MetaHIT Consortium, Bork, P., Ehrlich, S.D., Wang, J., 2010. A human gut microbial gene catalogue established by metagenomic sequencing. Nature 464, 59–65.

Sartor, R.B., 2004. Therapeutic manipulation of the enteric microflora in inflammatory bowel diseases: antibiotics, probiotics, and prebiotics. Gastroenterology 126, 1620–1633.

Schmidt, K., Cowen, P.J., Harmer, C.J., Tzortzis, G., Errington, S., Burnet, P.W., 2015. Prebiotic intake reduces the waking cortisol response and alters emotional bias in healthy volunteers. Psychopharmacology 232, 1793–1801.

Schmidt, M., Oitzl, M.S., Levine, S., De Kloet, E.R., 2002. The HPA system during the postnatal development of CD1 mice and the effects of maternal deprivation. Dev. Brain Res. 139, 39–49.

Schroeder, F.A., Lin, C.L., Crusio, W.E., Akbarian, S., 2007. Antidepressant-like effects of the histone deacetylase inhibitor, sodium butyrate, in the mouse. Biol. Psychiatry 62, 55–64.

Stilling, R.M., Dinan, T.G., Cryan, J.F., 2014. Microbial genes, brain & behaviour – epigenetic regulation of the gut-brain axis. Genes Brain Behav. 13, 69–86.

Sudo, N., 2012. Role of microbiome in regulating the HPA axis and its relevance to allergy. Chem. Immunol. Allergy 98, 163–175.

Sudo, N., Chida, Y., Aiba, Y., Sonoda, J., Oyama, N., Yu, X., Kubo, C., Koga, Y., 2004. Postnatal microbial colonization programs the hypothalamic-pituitary-adrenal system for stress response in mice. J. Physiol. 558, 263–275.

Sudo, N., Aiba, Y., Takaki, A., Tanaka, K., Yu, X.N., Oyama, N., Koga, Y., Kubo, C., 2000. Dietary nucleic acids promote a shift in Th1/Th2 balance toward Th1-dominant immunity. Clin. Exp. Allergy 30, 979–987.

Sudo, N., Sawamura, S., Tanaka, K., Aiba, Y., Kubo, C., Koga, Y., 1997. The requirement of intestinal bacterial flora for the development of an IgE production system fully susceptible to oral tolerance induction. J. Immunol. 159, 1739–1745.

Thomassin, H., Flavin, M., Espinás, M., Grange, T., 2001. Glucocorticoid-induced DNA demethylation and gene memory during development. EMBO J. 20, 1974–1983.

Tsankova, N., Renthal, W., Kumar, A., Nestler, E.J., 2007. Epigenetic regulation in psychiatric disorders. Nat. Rev. Neurosci. 8, 355–367.

Ukena, S.N., Singh, A., Dringenberg, U., Engelhardt, R., Seidler, U., Hansen, W., Bleich, A., Bruder, D., Franzke, A., Rogler, G., Suerbaum, S., Buer, J., Gunzer, F., Westendorf, A.M., 2007. Probiotic *Escherichia coli* Nissle 1917 inhibits leaky gut by enhancing mucosal integrity. PloS One 2, e1308.

Walker, F.R., Nilsson, M., Jones, K., 2013. Acute and chronic stress-induced disturbances of microglial plasticity, phenotype and function. Curr. Drug Targets 14, 1262–1276.

Weaver, I.C.G., Cervoni, N., Champagne, F.A., D'Alessio, A.C., Sharma, S., Seckl, J.R., Dymov, S., Szyf, M., Meaney, M.J., 2004. Epigenetic programming by maternal behavior. Nat. Neurosci. 7, 847–854.

A Role for the Microbiota in Neurodevelopmental Disorders

14

J.M. Yano, E.Y. Hsiao

California Institute of Technology, Pasadena, CA, United States

INTRODUCTION

The interrelationship of the gastrointestinal (GI) system and the CNS has been recognized since the works of such notable 19th-century physiologists as Ivan Pavlov and Claude Bernard (Cryan and Dinan, 2012). However, only in recent decades has the scope and complexity of this gut–brain connection begun to be elucidated. Signaling between these systems can be mediated through multiple pathways (eg, neural, immune, and endocrine), all of which can be modulated by a wide range of genetic and environmental factors. Increasingly, an appreciation of the importance of commensal gut microbes to the health of the GI and nervous systems is apparent in the proliferation of scientific literature detailing the diverse array of physiological, psychological, and behavioral functions influenced by the gut microbiome (Collins et al., 2012; Cryan and Dinan, 2012). Although the microbial composition of the human gut is known to be affected by diet and other environmental factors, there is evidence for a "core microbiome" that remains stable in healthy individuals (Salonen et al., 2012). The microbial species composition of this core is commonly perturbed in disease.

Epidemiological studies highlight the connection among GI dysfunction, microbial dysbiosis, and psychiatric or neurological dysfunction. GI pathology, such as inflammatory bowel disease, is often co-morbid with psychiatric symptoms such as anxiety and depression (Graff et al., 2009). Furthermore, altered microbiota composition correlates with stress and depression with accompanying GI symptoms such as altered intestinal motility and decreased intestinal barrier integrity ("leaky gut"; Collins and Bercik, 2009). Because the evidence derived from human patient populations increasingly underlines the potential interactions among microbiota, gut, and brain, animal model studies have begun to probe the cause-and-effect relationship.

Multiple studies of germ-free (GF) animals (harboring no microbes) have revealed the importance of microbiota for normal brain function and behavior. For instance, GF mice exhibit an exaggerated stress response (in the form of elevated stress hormone release in response to restraint) when compared with mice with the normal complement of gut bacteria (Sudo et al., 2004). Interestingly, despite this heightened response to stress, GF mice also exhibit decreased levels of anxiety-like behaviors.

The Gut-Brain Axis. http://dx.doi.org/10.1016/B978-0-12-802304-4.00014-1

These behavioral changes are accompanied by alterations in neurotransmitter levels and gene expression profiles in the brain (Diaz Heijtz et al., 2011; Neufeld et al., 2011). Both the decreased baseline anxiety-like behaviors and the exaggerated stress response of GF animals are reversible through probiotic treatment (Diaz Heijtz et al., 2011; Sudo et al., 2004). GF mice also display deficits in sociability and social cognition, avoiding social contact that a normal mouse would pursue and fail to show the normal preference for familiar conspecifics versus novel ones. They also show increases in repetitive grooming behavior, which, along with social avoidance, is reversible through bacterial colonization (Desbonnet et al., 2014).

Such studies raise many questions regarding which microbes may be essential to normal brain development and behavior: Could a disrupted microbiome contribute to the pathogenesis of human neurodevelopmental disorders? Mechanistically how? Might such disorders be treatable via introduction of beneficial microbes, or by altering a disordered microbiome, toward a more favorable composition via diet or drugs?

AUTISM SPECTRUM DISORDER

Autism spectrum disorder (ASD) is a heterogeneous group of neurodevelopmental disorders, characterized by communication and language deficits, deficits in social interaction, restricted interests, and repetitive behavior. Symptoms and level of disability range from mild to severe, manifest in early childhood, and in most cases persist throughout adulthood. Although many studies have sought to identify reliable biomarkers for autism, and specific genetic, physiologic, metabolic, and neuroanatomical abnormalities have been correlated with ASD, the disorder is still diagnosed based on core behavioral symptoms (Walsh et al., 2011).

The global prevalence of autism diagnoses has increased dramatically (20- to 30-fold) since the late 1960s and early 1970s (~2 decades after autism was first defined in Leo Kanner's landmark case studies). Incidence rates as high as 1 in 68 children receiving a diagnosis of ASD have been reported. Although some of this prodigious increase may be attributed to increased awareness of autism, there has been much scientific interest in potential environmental causes.

Research into the etiology of ASD indicates that there are likely multiple pathways to pathogenesis. ASD has been recognized as a highly heritable disorder, and this has spurred many studies identifying genetic risk factors and their neurobiological consequences (Miles, 2011). However, several twin association and epidemiological studies reveal a previously underappreciated contribution of environmental risk factors to ASD (Hallmayer et al., 2011; Sandin et al., 2014). An increasing emphasis on environmental risk factors has led to new insights into how inflammation and other dysfunctional immune responses (Onore et al., 2012), environmental insults interacting with genetic susceptibility (Chaste and Leboyer, 2012), and disruption of the microbiome (Hsiao et al., 2013) may contribute to neurodevelopmental disorders.

Environmental factors that can lead to alterations in gut microbiota, such as high-carbohydrate diets, medication (eg, antibiotic use), and excessive hygiene practices, have been implicated in the rising incidence rate of ASD (Wang et al., 2011). Although a causal link between such factors and the pathogenesis of autism is currently still speculative, a growing body of literature linking ASD with GI dysfunction and altered gut microbiota, in addition to multiple animal studies in which probiotic treatments can correct behavioral deficits, indicates that a richer understanding of the gut-brain-microbiota axis may lead to effective new treatments of neurodevelopmental disorders.

GASTROINTESTINAL DYSFUNCTION IN AUTISM SPECTRUM DISORDER

Co-morbidity studies of ASD patient populations commonly report a significantly higher incidence of GI symptoms than that seen in the general population. Two such studies reported that the presence and severity of GI symptoms (commonly diarrhea, constipation, abdominal pain, and/or bloating) correlate with severity of ASD symptoms (Adams et al., 2011; Wang et al., 2011). Another found that the presence of GI symptoms is associated with higher degrees of social and language impairments in children with ASD (Gorrindo et al., 2012). Clinical reports indicate that the pain and discomfort of GI dysfunction exacerbates sleep disturbance, poor concentration, aggression, and self-injury in ASD individuals, making treatment of GI symptoms a significant target for improving quality of life (Buie et al., 2010).

It is difficult to pinpoint just how prevalent GI abnormalities are in the ASD patient population. Incidence rates range from 9% to 90% depending on the study, and there are wide variations in sample size, patient population selection, geographic location, and methods of assessing and defining GI dysfunction (Buie et al., 2010; Coury et al., 2012). Some studies report no higher incidence of GI disorder in ASD patients (Black et al., 2002). However, studies utilizing large patient populations (numbering in the thousands) do report a significant increase in chronic GI issues in ASD patients (Kohane et al., 2012; Mazurek et al., 2013). In addition, multiple independently conducted meta-analyses of the current literature have corroborated a genuinely higher prevalence of GI symptoms in ASD (Cao et al., 2013; McElhanon et al., 2014).

In addition to symptoms, GI pathology such as damage to intestinal mucosa and increased intestinal permeability (leaky gut) has been associated with ASD (D'Eufemia et al., 1996; de Magistris et al., 2010). One study reports that nonautistic first-degree relatives of individuals with ASD also show higher incidence rates of abnormal intestinal permeability, suggesting that hereditary factors may contribute (de Magistris et al., 2010). One genetic risk factor associated with the subset of ASD patients with co-morbid GI issues is a variant in the promoter of the gene for the MET receptor tyrosine kinase, a protein that functions in brain development and GI repair (Campbell et al., 2009). Likewise, variants of the serotonin transporter gene have been associated with autism (Prasad et al., 2009; Sutcliffe et al., 2005), and, in addition to its well-known importance as a neurotransmitter in the brain, serotonin is also crucial to maintaining normal GI function (Berger et al., 2009; Manocha and Khan, 2012).

Certain environmental risk factors for ASD are also associated with GI dysfunction, especially those known to trigger inflammation and other immune-related insults. Epidemiological studies have linked an increased risk of ASD in children to maternal infection during pregnancy (Atladottir et al., 2010) and familial history of autoimmune disease (Atladottir et al., 2009; Comi et al., 1999). Studies of proinflammatory factors in the gestational environment (eg, maternal blood, placenta, and amniotic fluid) find a correlation between elevated immune activity and increased risk for ASD (Abdallah et al., 2013; Brown et al., 2014; Croen et al., 2008). Intriguingly, a mouse model of ASD, induced by maternal immune activation (MIA) and initially developed to study the neurobehavioral effects of gestational exposure to inflammatory factors (Malkova et al., 2012; Shi et al., 2009), displays marked GI defects. In addition to deficits in sociability and communication, MIA offspring display decreased intestinal barrier integrity (mimicking the leaky gut seen in subsets of ASD patients). These deficits are detectable in juveniles and persist into adulthood (Hsiao et al., 2013).

MICROBIAL DYSBIOSIS IN AUTISM SPECTRUM DISORDER

Given the wide array of diseases and disorders in which disruption of the gut microbiome has been implicated (such as inflammatory bowel disease, obesity, and cardiovascular disease) and a growing appreciation of the impact that gut microbes have on host behavior, there has been much interest in the role of microbial dysbiosis in the pathogenesis of ASD (Blumberg and Powrie, 2012; Cryan and Dinan, 2012). An understanding of which gut microbes are under- or overrepresented in ASD, in addition to the physiological consequences resulting from such alterations to the microbial balance, may aid in the development of therapeutics aimed at restoring normal microbiota composition and function. As is the case with clinical studies linking ASD with GI dysfunction, the literature on microbial dysbiosis in ASD shows highly variable sample size, patient selection, and methodologies in addition to inconsistent reports on microbial composition (Cao et al., 2013). Which ASD-related differences regarding individual species or species clusters are identified varies depending on the study, and studies vary in their methods for collecting and identifying microbes. However, given the high heterogeneity of the disorder and the likelihood of multiple pathways to pathogenesis, the existence of a single characteristic "core" ASD microbiome profile seems unlikely.

The human gut microbiome contains trillions of individual microbes that contribute to digestion, GI motility, water and nutrient balance, and regulation of other microbes. Disruptions to the microbiome can lead to deficits in any of these functions. ASD patients tend to have a history of higher antibiotic use compared with the general population, and it has been speculated that this may induce alterations to the balance of the gut microbial ecosystem (Adams et al., 2011; Cryan and Dinan, 2012). In addition, many ASD individuals exhibit abnormal feeding behaviors such as a high aversion to novel or nonprocessed foods (Ibrahim et al., 2009; Kang et al., 2013). An abnormally restricted diet may contribute to an abnormal microbial balance, although it is possible that an existing microbial imbalance or other gut abnormality can be the cause of certain food aversions. Some ASD patients show a decreased ability to digest plant-based material, with lower serum levels of short-chain fatty acids (SCFAs), a by-product of the bacterial breakdown of dietary fiber (Adams et al., 2011). Others show deficiencies in production of certain enzymes and transporters utilized in the digestion of carbohydrates (Williams et al., 2011). An understanding of the cause-and-effect interactions among commensal microbes, pathogenic microbes, host genetics, behavior, and physiology is still in its early stages.

One of the commonly reported differences between ASD gut microbiota and that of non-ASD controls is that of an elevated relative abundance of Clostridia species (Finegold et al., 2002; Parracho et al., 2005; Song et al., 2004). Because Clostridia have previously been identified as toxin producers and the cause of human illness, one hypothesis is that an overgrowth of Clostridia (possibly induced by antibiotic treatment eliminating microbes that would have inhibited Clostridia proliferation) leads to toxin-induced neurobehavioral deficits in ASD (Parracho et al., 2005). Pathogenesis via altered levels of microbially derived molecules is a particular interest in microbial dysbiosis studies. In the MIA mouse model of autism, injection of a single metabolite (identified by comparative metabolomics as greatly elevated in MIA offspring exhibiting autistic-like behaviors) into normal mice was sufficient to induce increases in anxiety-like behavior (Hsiao et al., 2013). In addition, abnormal levels of SCFAs, common microbial products that are absorbed from the gut and circulated throughout the body, may contribute to disordered GI motility, immune activation, and neurotransmitter release (Nankova et al., 2014). One rodent model of ASD is induction of neurotoxicity via excessive amounts of the SCFA propionic acid (PPA) (El-Ansary and Al-Ayadhi, 2014; Shultz et al., 2014). These animals display social deficits and neurological abnormalities similar to those seen in ASD. The PPA model of ASD is particularly interesting because PPA and other fermentation products are known to be produced by Clostridia, *Bacteroidetes*, and *Desulfovibrio*, all of which have been associated with ASD (Macfabe, 2012).

A study of patients with a common subset of ASD (late-onset or regressive autism, in which behavioral development is normal until approximately 18 months then regresses to typical core symptoms of autism) revealed that bacteria of the genus *Desulfovibrio* was present in approximately half of the ASD patients but in none of the nonautistic controls (Finegold et al., 2010). Members of this genus can reduce sulfur and produce lipopolysaccharides. This lends particular interest to earlier reports that ASD children commonly present with low blood levels of sulfur and elevated blood levels of lipopolysaccharides, which correlate with reduced socialization (Emanuele et al., 2010).

Other microbiota alterations observed in ASD patients include decreased abundance of *Bifidobacterium* (Adams et al., 2011) and increased abundance of *Bacteroidetes* (Finegold et al., 2010), *Sutterella* (Williams et al., 2012), and *Lactobacillus* (Adams et al., 2011).

Animal models of environmentally induced ASD-like behaviors also mimic the reports of altered gut microbiota composition in humans. Valproic acid exposure in utero yields mouse offspring that exhibit the core behavioral abnormalities (social deficits, repetitive behavior, reduced communication) associated with ASD in addition to increased relative abundance of Clostridia species (de Theije et al., 2014). Mice in the MIA model of autism also display an increase in Clostridia (Hsiao et al., 2013).

PROBIOTICS IN THE TREATMENT OF NEURODEVELOPMENTAL DISORDERS

Animal models have been invaluable tools in research for potential therapeutics for GI disorders as well as neurobehavioral deficits. Factors affecting whether a particular species or combination of species of microbes may mitigate symptoms include mechanism of action and the developmental timing of treatment. Some probiotic studies identify vagal nerve signaling as an essential component of the mechanism of treatment (Bercik et al., 2011; Bravo et al., 2011). Others report that certain probiotic treatments only confer benefits when given to juveniles; treated adults show no improvement (Sudo et al., 2004).

Another factor is whether a particular treatment alters the profile of bacterial metabolites found in the host's circulation (Nicholson et al., 2012). This might be accomplished not only through the introduction of species that produce beneficial molecular products, but also by directly administrating isolated metabolites or reducing the overgrowth of species that produce toxic products.

In a mouse model of infection-induced colon inflammation, animals also exhibit increased anxiety-like behavior (Bercik et al., 2010). Oral treatment with the bacterial species *Bifidobacterium longum* relieved the anxiety effects of infection without affecting levels of inflammation, indicating that behavior and GI issues can be independently targeted (Bercik et al., 2011, 2010). Other probiotic studies, using another member of the *Bifidobacterium* genus, *Bifidobacterium infantis*, revealed that the exaggerated stress response of GF mice can be corrected through monocolonization (Sudo et al., 2004). Moreover, stress-induced GI inflammation and depressive-like behaviors in rats can be normalized by supplementation of the normal microbiota with *B. infantis* (Desbonnet et al., 2010).

Studies of lactic-acid producing bacteria of the genus *Lactobacillus* also demonstrate anxiolytic and antidepressive effects in probiotic treatments. *Lactobacillus rhamnosus* treatment can reduce stress-induced corticosterone production and the accompanying anxiety- and depressive-like behavior in rodents (Bravo et al., 2011). *L. rhamnosus* can also trigger changes in gamma-aminobutyric acid receptor expression profiles in the rodent brain, indicating the potential for certain microbes to enable behavioral changes by altering neural circuitry. Another species, *Lactobacillus helveticus*, also conveys protective effects against anxiety and memory deficits caused by a high-carbohydrate diet (Ohland et al., 2013).

One study combined two strains of bacteria in a single probiotic treatment and showed promising results regarding the ability to translate from rodent models to clinical studies (Messaoudi et al., 2011). The treatment combined bacterial strains that had demonstrated antiinflammatory properties in human intestinal cell cultures (genus *Lactobacillus*) and reduction of ulcerative colitis symptoms in human patients (genus *Bifidobacterium*). Oral administration of the probiotic mixture reduced anxiety-like behaviors in rats and self-reported symptoms of anxiety and depression in human subjects.

Aside from treatment with commensal species of gut microbes, one study fed mice *Mycobacterium vaccae*, an "ambient" aerobic microbe found in temperate environments, before a maze-learning task (Matthews and Jenks, 2013). Treated mice showed reduced anxiety-related behaviors when performing the task and improved maze completion time. The authors of this study highlight the potential for environmentally encountered microbes (which may have shared a long history of coevolution with humans before the relatively recent phenomena of urbanization and modern hygiene reduced the likelihood of exposure) to confer significant health benefits when used as probiotics.

A recent study of probiotic treatment relates more specifically to the panel of core symptoms seen in ASD (Hsiao et al., 2013). The MIA mouse model of ASD (mentioned earlier) is of particular interest as an animal model of neurodevelopmental disorder because of the many ways in which it mimics the human condition (Malkova et al., 2012; Shi et al., 2009). MIA offspring display a battery of behavioral abnormalities relevant to ASD, including increases in anxiety-like and repetitive behaviors, reduced sensorimotor gating, and deficits in vocal communication and social interaction. They also present with compromised intestinal barrier integrity, altered gut microbiome composition, and altered cytokine levels, also in common with a significant subset of ASD patients.

Bacteroides fragilis was selected as a candidate probiotic, based on its previously demonstrated ability to correct GI pathology in a mouse model of colitis (Mazmanian et al., 2008) and to protect against neuroinflammation in a mouse model of multiple sclerosis (Ochoa-Reparaz et al., 2010). *B. fragilis* corrects intestinal permeability and partially reverses the microbial dysbiosis and altered cytokine profile of MIA offspring (Hsiao et al., 2013). Most notably, *B. fragilis* treatment was able to correct many of the behavioral deficits seen in MIA offspring. Treatment corrected anxiety-like behavior and sensorimotor gating, decreased repetitive behavior, and increased communicative vocalization. Deficits in sociability and social preference remained, however, indicating that these deficits may arise through pathogenesis pathways independent of those regulating the other abnormalities seen in MIA offspring.

OTHER MICROBIOTA-RELATED TREATMENTS FOR AUTISM SPECTRUM DISORDER

Antibiotic treatment represents another means by which an unfavorable balance of gut microbes might be corrected to relieve symptoms. In a small clinical study of children with regressive-onset autism, oral administration of vancomycin led to an improvement in ASD-related behavioral symptoms (Sandler et al., 2000). However, the benefits were short lived and faded when antibiotic treatment was stopped. Such an observation is consistent with studies demonstrating the resilience of the microbiota in its ability to restore to pretreatment states relatively soon after antibiotic exposure (Lozupone et al., 2012).

It is interesting to note that several pharmacological therapies that show promise for treating core ASD symptoms exhibit antibiotic properties, raising the question of whether changes to the microbiome may contribute to their therapeutic effects. For example, D-cycloserine is a partial agonist of glutamatergic *N*-methyl-D-aspartic acid receptors and a broad-spectrum antibiotic used to treat tuberculosis. Preclinical studies reveal that D-cycloserine corrects core behavioral abnormalities in genetic and environmental animal models for ASD (Benson et al., 2013; Blundell et al., 2010; Deutsch et al., 2012; Modi and Young, 2011; Wellmann et al., 2014). Clinical trials further demonstrate beneficial effects of D-cycloserine in decreasing stereotypic behavior and improving social interaction in ASD individuals (Posey et al., 2004; Urbano et al., 2014). Rapamycin, a small-molecule inhibitor of the mechanistic target of rapamycin pathway, is another drug being explored for ASD with known antibiotic and immunosuppressant properties. Several studies demonstrate that rapamycin reverses neuropathological and behavioral abnormalities in animal models of ASD and tuberous sclerosis (Tsc) (Burket et al., 2014; Sato et al., 2012). Clinical trials of rapamycin in ASD and Tsc individuals are currently underway.

A therapeutic approach alternative to direct manipulation of the microbiota is dietary management. Several ASD children are placed on restricted diets, such as the gluten- and casein-free diet. Scientific evidence for the benefits of dietary therapy is lacking (Mari-Bauset et al., 2014) despite anecdotal evidence (from parental reports) that restricted diets improve physiological and behavioral abnormalities in ASD children (Harris and Card, 2012; Pennesi and Klein, 2012). It is interesting to note that dietary supplementation with the plant-derived phytochemical sulforaphane improved ASD behaviors in a placebo-controlled, randomized, double-blind clinical trial (Singh et al., 2014). Moreover, the high-fat, low-carbohydrate ketogenic diet improved ASD-related social deficits in two different mouse models of ASD (Ahn et al., 2014; Ruskin et al., 2013). One study demonstrated a protective effect of vitamin D against PPA-induced autistic-like behavior in rodents (Alfawaz et al., 2014), which is interesting in light of an increasing number of studies demonstrating a role for vitamin D in regulating the microbiome (Ly et al., 2011; Ooi et al., 2013). Future research along these lines may reveal other dietary supplements or regimens that may prove effective for treating symptoms of ASD.

FUTURE STUDIES

Exploring how the microbiome affects neurodevelopment and the manifestation of complex higher-order behaviors is an exciting frontier for investigation. Recent findings that indigenous gut microbes can modulate neural activity and various behaviors suggests that elucidating basic mechanisms by which the microbiota interacts with the nervous system will provide new insights into brain development and function and potentially uncover novel approaches for diagnosing, preventing, and/or treating symptoms of neurological disorders.

Animal and early clinical studies are beginning to suggest that targeting the microbiota may be a tractable strategy for treating behavioral and physiological symptoms of neurodevelopmental disorders. Although a preponderance of evidence points to a potential role for the microbiome in the etiopathogenesis and/or treatment of ASD, core behavioral abnormalities of ASD are similarly seen in various other neurodevelopmental disorders. Schizophrenia is interesting in this regard given its association with GI and immunological abnormalities (Severance et al., 2014). Particularly for ASD, additional research is needed to explore potential roles for the microbiome in animal models, especially those based on genetic risk factors for ASD. Although many preclinical studies reveal promising effects of probiotics in treating behavioral abnormalities, none have as yet been translated to clinical cohorts of neurodevelopmental disease. Issues with the clinical heterogeneity inherent to ASD and other behavioral disorders may pose significant challenges; appropriately powered studies that consider various well-defined subsets of ASD are needed to test the efficacy of microbe-based treatments. Furthermore, although fecal transplants are currently being explored for treatment of ASD, advancements in how live biotherapeutics are produced, administered, and designed may expand the therapeutic potential of probiotics for neurodevelopmental disorders.

REFERENCES

Abdallah, M.W., Larsen, N., Grove, J., Norgaard-Pedersen, B., Thorsen, P., Mortensen, E.L., Hougaard, D.M., 2013. Amniotic fluid inflammatory cytokines: potential markers of immunologic dysfunction in autism spectrum disorders. World J. Biol. Psychiatry 14, 528–538.

Adams, J.B., Johansen, L.J., Powell, L.D., Quig, D., Rubin, R.A., 2011. Gastrointestinal flora and gastrointestinal status in children with autism–comparisons to typical children and correlation with autism severity. BMC Gastroenterol. 11, 22.

Ahn, Y., Narous, M., Tobias, R., Rho, J.M., Mychasiuk, R., 2014. The ketogenic diet modifies social and metabolic alterations identified in the prenatal valproic acid model of autism spectrum disorder. Dev. Neurosci. 36, 371–380.

Alfawaz, H.A., Bhat, R.S., Al-Ayadhi, L., El-Ansary, A.K., 2014. Protective and restorative potency of vitamin D on persistent biochemical autistic features induced in propionic acid-intoxicated rat pups. BMC Complement. Altern. Med. 14, 416.

Atladottir, H.O., Pedersen, M.G., Thorsen, P., Mortensen, P.B., Deleuran, B., Eaton, W.W., Parner, E.T., 2009. Association of family history of autoimmune diseases and autism spectrum disorders. Pediatrics 124, 687–694.

Atladottir, H.O., Thorsen, P., Ostergaard, L., Schendel, D.E., Lemcke, S., Abdallah, M., Parner, E.T., 2010. Maternal infection requiring hospitalization during pregnancy and autism spectrum disorders. J. Autism Dev. Disord. 40, 1423–1430.

Benson, A.D., Burket, J.A., Deutsch, S.I., 2013. Balb/c mice treated with D-cycloserine arouse increased social interest in conspecifics. Brain. Res. Bull. 99, 95–99.

Bercik, P., Park, A.J., Sinclair, D., Khoshdel, A., Lu, J., Huang, X., Deng, Y., Blennerhassett, P.A., Fahnestock, M., Moine, D., et al., 2011. The anxiolytic effect of *Bifidobacterium longum* NCC3001 involves vagal pathways for gut-brain communication. Neurogastroenterol. Motil. 23, 1132–1139.

Bercik, P., Verdu, E.F., Foster, J.A., Macri, J., Potter, M., Huang, X., Malinowski, P., Jackson, W., Blennerhassett, P., Neufeld, K.A., et al., 2010. Chronic gastrointestinal inflammation induces anxiety-like behavior and alters central nervous system biochemistry in mice. Gastroenterology 139, 2102–2112. e2101.

Berger, M., Gray, J.A., Roth, B.L., 2009. The expanded biology of serotonin. Annu. Rev. Med. 60, 355–366.

Black, C., Kaye, J.A., Jick, H., 2002. Relation of childhood gastrointestinal disorders to autism: nested case-control study using data from the UK General Practice Research Database. BMJ 325, 419–421.

Blumberg, R., Powrie, F., 2012. Microbiota, disease, and back to health: a metastable journey. Sci. Transl. Med. 4, 137rv137.

Blundell, J., Blaiss, C.A., Etherton, M.R., Espinosa, F., Tabuchi, K., Walz, C., Bolliger, M.F., Sudhof, T.C., Powell, C.M., 2010. Neuroligin-1 deletion results in impaired spatial memory and increased repetitive behavior. J. Neurosci. 30, 2115–2129.

Bravo, J.A., Forsythe, P., Chew, M.V., Escaravage, E., Savignac, H.M., Dinan, T.G., Bienenstock, J., Cryan, J.F., 2011. Ingestion of *Lactobacillus* strain regulates emotional behavior and central GABA receptor expression in a mouse via the vagus nerve. Proc. Natl. Acad. Sci. U.S.A. 108, 16050–16055.

Brown, A.S., Sourander, A., Hinkka-Yli-Salomaki, S., McKeague, I.W., Sundvall, J., Surcel, H.M., 2014. Elevated maternal C-reactive protein and autism in a national birth cohort. Mol. Psychiatry 19, 259–264.

Buie, T., Campbell, D.B., Fuchs 3rd, G.J., Furuta, G.T., Levy, J., Vandewater, J., Whitaker, A.H., Atkins, D., Bauman, M.L., Beaudet, A.L., et al., 2010. Evaluation, diagnosis, and treatment of gastrointestinal disorders in individuals with ASDs: a consensus report. Pediatrics 125 (Suppl. 1), S1–S18.

Burket, J.A., Benson, A.D., Tang, A.H., Deutsch, S.I., 2014. Rapamycin improves sociability in the BTBR T(+)Itpr3(tf)/J mouse model of autism spectrum disorders. Brain Res. Bull. 100, 70–75.

Campbell, D.B., Buie, T.M., Winter, H., Bauman, M., Sutcliffe, J.S., Perrin, J.M., Levitt, P., 2009. Distinct genetic risk based on association of MET in families with co-occurring autism and gastrointestinal conditions. Pediatrics 123, 1018–1024.

Cao, X., Lin, P., Jiang, P., Li, C., 2013. Characteristics of the gastrointestinal microbiome in children with autism spectrum disorder: a systematic review. Shanghai Arch. Psychiatry 25, 342–353.

Chaste, P., Leboyer, M., 2012. Autism risk factors: genes, environment, and gene-environment interactions. Dialogues Clin. Neurosci. 14, 281–292.

Collins, S.M., Bercik, P., 2009. The relationship between intestinal microbiota and the central nervous system in normal gastrointestinal function and disease. Gastroenterology 136, 2003–2014.

Collins, S.M., Surette, M., Bercik, P., 2012. The interplay between the intestinal microbiota and the brain. Nat. Rev. Microbiol. 10, 735–742.

Comi, A.M., Zimmerman, A.W., Frye, V.H., Law, P.A., Peeden, J.N., 1999. Familial clustering of autoimmune disorders and evaluation of medical risk factors in autism. J. Child Neurol. 14, 388–394.

Coury, D.L., Ashwood, P., Fasano, A., Fuchs, G., Geraghty, M., Kaul, A., Mawe, G., Patterson, P., Jones, N.E., 2012. Gastrointestinal conditions in children with autism spectrum disorder: developing a research agenda. Pediatrics 130 (Suppl. 2), S160–S168.

Croen, L.A., Braunschweig, D., Haapanen, L., Yoshida, C.K., Fireman, B., Grether, J.K., Kharrazi, M., Hansen, R.L., Ashwood, P., Van de Water, J., 2008. Maternal mid-pregnancy autoantibodies to fetal brain protein: the early markers for autism study. Biol. Psychiatry 64, 583–588.

Cryan, J.F., Dinan, T.G., 2012. Mind-altering microorganisms: the impact of the gut microbiota on brain and behaviour. Nat. Rev. Neurosci. 13, 701–712.

D'Eufemia, P., Celli, M., Finocchiaro, R., Pacifico, L., Viozzi, L., Zaccagnini, M., Cardi, E., Giardini, O., 1996. Abnormal intestinal permeability in children with autism. Acta Paediatr. 85, 1076–1079.

Desbonnet, L., Clarke, G., Shanahan, F., Dinan, T.G., Cryan, J.F., 2014. Microbiota is essential for social development in the mouse. Mol. Psychiatry 19, 146–148.

Desbonnet, L., Garrett, L., Clarke, G., Kiely, B., Cryan, J.F., Dinan, T.G., 2010. Effects of the probiotic *Bifidobacterium infantis* in the maternal separation model of depression. Neuroscience 170, 1179–1188.

Deutsch, S.I., Pepe, G.J., Burket, J.A., Winebarger, E.E., Herndon, A.L., Benson, A.D., 2012. D-cycloserine improves sociability and spontaneous stereotypic behaviors in 4-week old mice. Brain Res. 1439, 96–107.

Diaz Heijtz, R., Wang, S., Anuar, F., Qian, Y., Bjorkholm, B., Samuelsson, A., Hibberd, M.L., Forssberg, H., Pettersson, S., 2011. Normal gut microbiota modulates brain development and behavior. Proc. Natl. Acad. Sci. U.S.A. 108, 3047–3052.

El-Ansary, A., Al-Ayadhi, L., 2014. Relative abundance of short chain and polyunsaturated fatty acids in propionic acid-induced autistic features in rat pups as potential markers in autism. Lipids Health Dis. 13, 140.

Emanuele, E., Orsi, P., Boso, M., Broglia, D., Brondino, N., Barale, F., di Nemi, S.U., Politi, P., 2010. Low-grade endotoxemia in patients with severe autism. Neurosci. Lett. 471, 162–165.

Finegold, S.M., Dowd, S.E., Gontcharova, V., Liu, C., Henley, K.E., Wolcott, R.D., Youn, E., Summanen, P.H., Granpeesheh, D., Dixon, D., et al., 2010. Pyrosequencing study of fecal microflora of autistic and control children. Anaerobe 16, 444–453.

Finegold, S.M., Molitoris, D., Song, Y., Liu, C., Vaisanen, M.L., Bolte, E., McTeague, M., Sandler, R., Wexler, H., Marlowe, E.M., et al., 2002. Gastrointestinal microflora studies in late-onset autism. Clin. Infect. Dis. 35, S6–S16.

Gorrindo, P., Williams, K.C., Lee, E.B., Walker, L.S., McGrew, S.G., Levitt, P., 2012. Gastrointestinal dysfunction in autism: parental report, clinical evaluation, and associated factors. Autism Res. 5, 101–108.

Graff, L.A., Walker, J.R., Bernstein, C.N., 2009. Depression and anxiety in inflammatory bowel disease: a review of comorbidity and management. Inflammatory Bowel Dis. 15, 1105–1118.

Hallmayer, J., Cleveland, S., Torres, A., Phillips, J., Cohen, B., Torigoe, T., Miller, J., Fedele, A., Collins, J., Smith, K., et al., 2011. Genetic heritability and shared environmental factors among twin pairs with autism. Arch. Gen. Psychiatry 68, 1095–1102.

Harris, C., Card, B., 2012. A pilot study to evaluate nutritional influences on gastrointestinal symptoms and behavior patterns in children with autism spectrum disorder. Complem. Ther. Med. 20, 437–440.

Hsiao, E.Y., McBride, S.W., Hsien, S., Sharon, G., Hyde, E.R., McCue, T., Codelli, J.A., Chow, J., Reisman, S.E., Petrosino, J.F., et al., 2013. Microbiota modulate behavioral and physiological abnormalities associated with neurodevelopmental disorders. Cell 155, 1451–1463.

Ibrahim, S.H., Voigt, R.G., Katusic, S.K., Weaver, A.L., Barbaresi, W.J., 2009. Incidence of gastrointestinal symptoms in children with autism: a population-based study. Pediatrics 124, 680–686.

Kang, D.W., Park, J.G., Ilhan, Z.E., Wallstrom, G., Labaer, J., Adams, J.B., Krajmalnik-Brown, R., 2013. Reduced incidence of Prevotella and other fermenters in intestinal microflora of autistic children. PloS One 8, e68322.

Kohane, I.S., McMurry, A., Weber, G., MacFadden, D., Rappaport, L., Kunkel, L., Bickel, J., Wattanasin, N., Spence, S., Murphy, S., et al., 2012. The co-morbidity burden of children and young adults with autism spectrum disorders. PloS One 7, e33224.

Lozupone, C.A., Stombaugh, J.I., Gordon, J.I., Jansson, J.K., Knight, R., 2012. Diversity, stability and resilience of the human gut microbiota. Nature 489, 220–230.

Ly, N.P., Litonjua, A., Gold, D.R., Celedon, J.C., 2011. Gut microbiota, probiotics, and vitamin D: interrelated exposures influencing allergy, asthma, and obesity? J. Allergy Clin. Immunol. 127, 1087–1094 quiz 1095–1086.

Macfabe, D.F., 2012. Short-chain fatty acid fermentation products of the gut microbiome: implications in autism spectrum disorders. Microb. Ecol. Health Dis. 23.

de Magistris, L., Familiari, V., Pascotto, A., Sapone, A., Frolli, A., Iardino, P., Carteni, M., De Rosa, M., Francavilla, R., Riegler, G., et al., 2010. Alterations of the intestinal barrier in patients with autism spectrum disorders and in their first-degree relatives. J. Pediatr. Gastroenterol. Nutr. 51, 418–424.

Malkova, N.V., Yu, C.Z., Hsiao, E.Y., Moore, M.J., Patterson, P.H., 2012. Maternal immune activation yields offspring displaying mouse versions of the three core symptoms of autism. Brain Behav. Immun. 26, 607–616.

Manocha, M., Khan, W.I., 2012. Serotonin and GI disorders: an update on clinical and experimental studies. Clin. Transl. Gastroenterol. 3, e13.

Mari-Bauset, S., Zazpe, I., Mari-Sanchis, A., Llopis-Gonzalez, A., Morales-Suarez-Varela, M., 2014. Evidence of the gluten-free and casein-free diet in autism spectrum disorders: a systematic review. J. Child Neurol. 29, 1718–1727.

Matthews, D.M., Jenks, S.M., 2013. Ingestion of *Mycobacterium vaccae* decreases anxiety-related behavior and improves learning in mice. Behav. Processes 96, 27–35.

Mazmanian, S.K., Round, J.L., Kasper, D.L., 2008. A microbial symbiosis factor prevents intestinal inflammatory disease. Nature 453, 620–625.

Mazurek, M.O., Vasa, R.A., Kalb, L.G., Kanne, S.M., Rosenberg, D., Keefer, A., Murray, D.S., Freedman, B., Lowery, L.A., 2013. Anxiety, sensory over-responsivity, and gastrointestinal problems in children with autism spectrum disorders. J. Abnorm. Child Psychol. 41, 165–176.

McElhanon, B.O., McCracken, C., Karpen, S., Sharp, W.G., 2014. Gastrointestinal symptoms in autism spectrum disorder: a meta-analysis. Pediatrics 133, 872–883.

Messaoudi, M., Lalonde, R., Violle, N., Javelot, H., Desor, D., Nejdi, A., Bisson, J.F., Rougeot, C., Pichelin, M., Cazaubiel, M., et al., 2011. Assessment of psychotropic-like properties of a probiotic formulation (*Lactobacillus helveticus* R0052 and *Bifidobacterium longum* R0175) in rats and human subjects. Br. J. Nutr. 105, 755–764.

Miles, J.H., 2011. Autism spectrum disorders–a genetics review. Gen. Med. 13, 278–294.

Modi, M.E., Young, L.J., 2011. D-cycloserine facilitates socially reinforced learning in an animal model relevant to autism spectrum disorders. Biol. Psychiatry 70, 298–304.

Nankova, B.B., Agarwal, R., MacFabe, D.F., La Gamma, E.F., 2014. Enteric bacterial metabolites propionic and butyric acid modulate gene expression, including CREB-dependent catecholaminergic neurotransmission, in PC12 cells–possible relevance to autism spectrum disorders. PloS One 9, e103740.

Neufeld, K.M., Kang, N., Bienenstock, J., Foster, J.A., 2011. Reduced anxiety-like behavior and central neurochemical change in germ-free mice. Neurogastroenterol. Motil. 23, 255–264. e119.

Nicholson, J.K., Holmes, E., Kinross, J., Burcelin, R., Gibson, G., Jia, W., Pettersson, S., 2012. Host-gut microbiota metabolic interactions. Science 336, 1262–1267.

Ochoa-Reparaz, J., Mielcarz, D.W., Ditrio, L.E., Burroughs, A.R., Begum-Haque, S., Dasgupta, S., Kasper, D.L., Kasper, L.H., 2010. Central nervous system demyelinating disease protection by the human commensal *Bacteroides fragilis* depends on polysaccharide A expression. J. Immunol. 185, 4101–4108.

Ohland, C.L., Kish, L., Bell, H., Thiesen, A., Hotte, N., Pankiv, E., Madsen, K.L., 2013. Effects of *Lactobacillus helveticus* on murine behavior are dependent on diet and genotype and correlate with alterations in the gut microbiome. Psychoneuroendocrinology 38, 1738–1747.

Onore, C., Careaga, M., Ashwood, P., 2012. The role of immune dysfunction in the pathophysiology of autism. Brain Behav. Immun. 26, 383–392.

Ooi, J.H., Li, Y., Rogers, C.J., Cantorna, M.T., 2013. Vitamin D regulates the gut microbiome and protects mice from dextran sodium sulfate-induced colitis. J. Nutr. 143, 1679–1686.

Parracho, H.M., Bingham, M.O., Gibson, G.R., McCartney, A.L., 2005. Differences between the gut microflora of children with autistic spectrum disorders and that of healthy children. J. Med. Microbiol. 54, 987–991.

Pennesi, C.M., Klein, L.C., 2012. Effectiveness of the gluten-free, casein-free diet for children diagnosed with autism spectrum disorder: based on parental report. Nutr. Neurosci. 15, 85–91.

Posey, D.J., Kem, D.L., Swiezy, N.B., Sweeten, T.L., Wiegand, R.E., McDougle, C.J., 2004. A pilot study of D-cycloserine in subjects with autistic disorder. Am. J. Psychiatry 161, 2115–2117.

Prasad, H.C., Steiner, J.A., Sutcliffe, J.S., Blakely, R.D., 2009. Enhanced activity of human serotonin transporter variants associated with autism. Philos. Trans. R. Soc. Lond. B Biol. Sci. 364, 163–173.

Ruskin, D.N., Svedova, J., Cote, J.L., Sandau, U., Rho, J.M., Kawamura Jr., M., Boison, D., Masino, S.A., 2013. Ketogenic diet improves core symptoms of autism in BTBR mice. PloS One 8, e65021.

Salonen, A., Salojarvi, J., Lahti, L., de Vos, W.M., 2012. The adult intestinal core microbiota is determined by analysis depth and health status. Clin. Microbiol. Infect. 18 (Suppl. 4), 16–20.

Sandin, S., Lichtenstein, P., Kuja-Halkola, R., Larsson, H., Hultman, C.M., Reichenberg, A., 2014. The familial risk of autism. JAMA 311, 1770–1777.

Sandler, R.H., Finegold, S.M., Bolte, E.R., Buchanan, C.P., Maxwell, A.P., Väisänen, M.L., Nelson, M.N., Wexler, H.M., 2000. Short-term benefit from oral vancomycin treatment of regressive-onset autism. J. Child Neurol. 15, 429–435.

Sato, A., Kasai, S., Kobayashi, T., Takamatsu, Y., Hino, O., Ikeda, K., Mizuguchi, M., 2012. Rapamycin reverses impaired social interaction in mouse models of tuberous sclerosis complex. Nat. Commun. 3, 1292.

Severance, E.G., Yolken, R.H., Eaton, W.W., 2014. Autoimmune diseases, gastrointestinal disorders and the microbiome in schizophrenia: more than a gut feeling. Schizophr. Res. 14, 319–313. http://dx.doi.org/10.1016/j.schres.2014.06.027.

Shi, L., Smith, S.E., Malkova, N., Tse, D., Su, Y., Patterson, P.H., 2009. Activation of the maternal immune system alters cerebellar development in the offspring. Brain Behav. Immun. 23, 116–123.

Shultz, S.R., Aziz, N.A., Yang, L., Sun, M., MacFabe, D.F., O'Brien, T.J., 2014. Intracerebroventricular injection of propionic acid, an enteric metabolite implicated in autism, induces social abnormalities that do not differ between seizure-prone (FAST) and seizure-resistant (SLOW) rats. Behav. Brain Res. 278C, 542–548.

Singh, K., Connors, S.L., Macklin, E.A., Smith, K.D., Fahey, J.W., Talalay, P., Zimmerman, A.W., 2014. Sulforaphane treatment of autism spectrum disorder (ASD). Proc. Natl. Acad. Sci. U.S.A. 111, 15550–15555.

Song, Y., Liu, C., Finegold, S.M., 2004. Real-time PCR quantitation of clostridia in feces of autistic children. Appl. Environ. Microbiol. 70, 6459–6465.

Sudo, N., Chida, Y., Aiba, Y., Sonoda, J., Oyama, N., Yu, X.N., Kubo, C., Koga, Y., 2004. Postnatal microbial colonization programs the hypothalamic-pituitary-adrenal system for stress response in mice. J. Physiol. 558, 263–275.

Sutcliffe, J.S., Delahanty, R.J., Prasad, H.C., McCauley, J.L., Han, Q., Jiang, L., Li, C., Folstein, S.E., Blakely, R.D., 2005. Allelic heterogeneity at the serotonin transporter locus (SLC6A4) confers susceptibility to autism and rigid-compulsive behaviors. Am. J. Hum. Genet. 77, 265–279.

de Theije, C.G., Wopereis, H., Ramadan, M., van Eijndthoven, T., Lambert, J., Knol, J., Garssen, J., Kraneveld, A.D., Oozeer, R., 2014. Altered gut microbiota and activity in a murine model of autism spectrum disorders. Brain Behav. Immun. 37, 197–206.

Urbano, M., Okwara, L., Manser, P., Hartmann, K., Herndon, A., Deutsch, S.I., 2014. A trial of D-cycloserine to treat stereotypies in older adolescents and young adults with autism spectrum disorder. Clin. Neuropharmacol. 37, 69–72.

Walsh, P., Elsabbagh, M., Bolton, P., Singh, I., 2011. In search of biomarkers for autism: scientific, social and ethical challenges. Nat. Rev. Neurosci. 12, 603–612.

Wang, L.W., Tancredi, D.J., Thomas, D.W., 2011. The prevalence of gastrointestinal problems in children across the United States with autism spectrum disorders from families with multiple affected members. J. Dev. Behav. Pediatr. 32, 351–360.

Wellmann, K.A., Varlinskaya, E.I., Mooney, S.M., 2014. D-Cycloserine ameliorates social alterations that result from prenatal exposure to valproic acid. Brain Res. Bull. 108, 1–9.

Williams, B.L., Hornig, M., Buie, T., Bauman, M.L., Cho Paik, M., Wick, I., Bennett, A., Jabado, O., Hirschberg, D.L., Lipkin, W.I., 2011. Impaired carbohydrate digestion and transport and mucosal dysbiosis in the intestines of children with autism and gastrointestinal disturbances. PloS One 6, e24585.

Williams, B.L., Hornig, M., Parekh, T., Lipkin, W.I., 2012. Application of novel PCR-based methods for detection, quantitation, and phylogenetic characterization of Sutterella species in intestinal biopsy samples from children with autism and gastrointestinal disturbances. mBio 3.

Altering the Gut Microbiome for Cognitive Benefit?

15

K. Huynh[a], M. Schneider[a]

University of California San Diego, Department of Medicine, La Jolla, CA, United States

M.G. Gareau

University of California Davis, Department of Anatomy, Davis, CA, United States

INTRODUCTION

The complex connection between the commensal intestinal microbiota and behavior, including cognitive function, has received increasing attention in recent years. Because altered cognitive function is an important component of numerous clinical pathologies, including, but not limited to, metabolic diseases, intestinal diseases, and mood disorders, a role for the microbiota in modulating these diseases could have important clinical implications. Colloquially known as "the forgotten organ," the intestinal microbiota has been well established as an important intermediary in the context of anxiety and depression (Borre et al., 2014; Mayer et al., 2014; Tillisch, 2014). However, the influence of these gut bacterial populations is likely to extend further, to include cognition, via the proposed microbiota-gut-brain axis. Research investigating the exciting interplay between factors modulating the gut microbiota and their subsequent influence on cognitive function is in its infancy, although the field is rapidly growing (Gareau et al., 2010). To study the effect of the intestinal microbiota on memory and cognition, investigators have turned to studying, if, and how, factors that modify the gut microbiota could lead to changes in overall cognitive function (Gareau, 2014). Although a precise mechanism underlying the effects of the microbiota in cognition remains to be confirmed, the current hypotheses focus on the interplay among neural, endocrine, and immune pathways (Cryan and Dinan, 2012). This chapter serves to survey the existing literature and summarize how altering the microbiota via dietary manipulation and probiotic or prebiotic administration may be of cognitive benefit, while also discussing potential mechanisms by which the gut microbiota communicates with the brain.

---

[a]These authors contributed equally.

FACTORS INFLUENCING COGNITION
DIETARY FACTORS

Among the most important factors that contribute to the development and maintenance of the intestinal microbiota is not surprisingly diet. Short- and long-term changes in dietary intake significantly influence the gut microbiome (Wu et al., 2011). Short-term changes in the microbiota after dietary intervention were found to occur rapidly and modestly whereas long-term changes in healthy volunteers correlated with enterotype clustering in a cross-sectional analysis (Wu et al., 2011). A growing body of evidence exists linking these diet-induced changes in the composition of the gut microbiota to altered cognitive capacities, including learning and memory.

One of the early studies designed to assess the effect of dietary changes on the composition of the microbiota, and subsequent behavioral impact, examined the effects of a 50% lean ground-beef–enriched chow diet on behavioral outcomes in mice. These mice not only had a significantly more diverse microbiota, but they performed better in behavioral cognition tests (hole-board open-field test) compared with control animals (Li et al., 2009). Although no single intestinal microbiota profile exists that is deemed a gold standard of health, certain ratios of bacterial phyla implicate a more healthy state of the gut microbiome; increased diversity is generally associated with overall health. Recent findings in the literature suggest that dietary modifications may prevent or treat various psychiatric syndromes, often with co-morbidities in the gastrointestinal tract and neuropsychological function.

Breastfeeding and Bacterial Colonization

Longitudinal studies, beginning in infancy, have provided important insights into the development of the gut microbiota and how early composition affects cognition later in life. It has been demonstrated that nutritional sources are one of the most influential factors in infantile gut colonization—second only to mode of birth (vaginal or cesarean; Koenig et al., 2011). Whether a baby is initially breast-fed or formula-fed is key to the ratio and quantity of intestinal bacterial communities, which also likely influences lifelong cognitive functioning (Mulle et al., 2013). Breast milk is important in establishing the foundational microbial communities of a healthy intestinal tract (Rogier et al., 2014). Because breast milk is a source of lactic acid bacteria (*Lactobacillus* and *Bifidobacteria*), which have beneficial functions, these bacterial populations often serve as biomarkers of a healthy infant gut (Mulle et al., 2013). Breast-fed and formula-fed babies have largely different trajectories of gut microbiome development, with breast-fed babies ultimately establishing a microbiome associated with healthier cognitive functioning. In fact, studies by Horwood et al. showed that breast-fed babies subsequently demonstrate enhanced academic performance later in life as compared with their formula-fed peers (Horwood and Fergusson, 1998); later studies suggest that the microbiota may influence this improved cognition, but without causal evidence (Mulle et al., 2013).

Studies on autism spectrum disorder (ASD), a disorder that is highly co-morbid with heightened social anxiety and characterized by delayed cognitive development and impaired motor function and learning (Allsop et al., 2014; Chukoskie et al., 2013), have further established the correlation between breastfeeding and healthy cognitive function. Babies with a delayed start to breastfeeding or those who feed for a shorter period of time were found to have an elevated risk for ASD (Mulle et al., 2013) whereas others have demonstrated a dose-response pattern in which continuous breastfeeding in the first 6 months through 2 years of age correlated with decreased risk of autism (Tanoue and Oda, 1989). Although this correlation is likely multifactorial and the lack of breastfeeding is certainly not necessarily causal of ASD, feeding patterns do lead to atypical gut populations and dysbiosis, which are also correlated with ASD development (Tomova et al., 2015). It is interesting to note that 90% of children with ASD typically exhibit picky eating behaviors and generally prefer starches and processed foods while refusing fruits and vegetables. A key function of the healthy gut microbiome (especially *Bacteriodetes*) is to assist in the breakdown of complex plant polysaccharides and nondigestible material. A diet high in plant material—exactly the foods ASD children reject—supports this beneficial microbial community (Mulle et al., 2013). The directionality, or possible bidirectionality, between dysbiosis and ASD behavior remains unresolved, although anecdotal reports of improved behavior in children with ASD after dietary manipulations, such as gluten-free and casein-free diets, suggest that dysbiosis may in part contribute to ASD behavior (Mulle et al., 2013). This area in ASD research requires further study.

High-Fat Diet and Obesity

Not only does the microbiota reflect early-life diet and shape early cognitive function, but it may also reflect long-term dietary habits and mediate the cognitive risks associated with obesity or an unhealthy diet. A diet high in fat and sugar is associated with altered cognitive function in the form of deficiencies in learning, memory, and executive function as well as depression, anxiety, and dementia (Pyndt Jorgensen et al., 2014). Studies have shown that a high-fat diet (HFD) can induce a shift in the ratios of *Bacteriodetes* to *Firmicutes* populations by reducing the former and increasing the latter as well as decreasing the overall diversity of the microbial population (Khan et al., 2014; Turnbaugh et al., 2006). In a groundbreaking preclinical study, Bruce–Keller et al. transferred the cecal and colonic contents of donor mice fed an HFD to nonobese recipient mice (C57BL/6). This resulted in the synchronized transfer of the cognitive deficits associated with the donor HFD fed and obese mice to the recipient mice (Bruce-Keller et al., 2014). This study sought to identify the effect on cognitive deficits, including memory, executive function, and stereotypical behavior (marble burying), of HFD-induced dysbiosis in the absence of obesity and nutritional deficits. Upon confirming, through ribosomal DNA phylogenetics, that the protocol successfully transfers the bacterial communities among mice and produces a distinct microbiota footprint, behavioral tests were performed to evaluate the cognitive function of these mice. Mice colonized with a microbiota from an unhealthy-diet donor showed elevated anxiety-like behavior and decreased memory as compared with mice colonized with microbiota from nonobese donors. Moreover, specific synapse-associated proteins, including phosphorylated synapsin-1, were significantly reduced in the HFD-shaped microbiota mice, suggesting decreased synapse density and plasticity. It was also noted that recipient mice show evidence of increased intestinal permeability (Bruce-Keller et al., 2014). A concomitant elevation in serum endotoxin and lymphocyte expression of toll-like receptor-4, reflecting proinflammatory and immune responses, were also observed (Bruce-Keller et al., 2014). This study provided the first definitive findings that the microbiota-induced changes after HFD are sufficient to disrupt brain physiology and function in mice, even in the absence of altered diet, obesity, or metabolic syndrome.

The complicated relationship between diet and the brain is further substantiated by studies that have demonstrated that HFD-induced changes to the microbiota can result in anxiety-like and depressive behaviors in mice subjected to chronic social stress (Finger et al., 2011). Although the mechanisms by which gut microbes affect behavior and mediate stress, anxiety, and depression are not well understood, physiological changes suggest that multiple possible mechanisms could be involved, including immune activation (Bruce-Keller et al., 2014) or direct interactions with neural activities. Activation of the immune system and altered neural activity are associated with neurological or psychiatric disorders. Maintaining a healthy diet, and in the future, therapeutic manipulation of the microbiota to achieve that of a healthy nonobese person, could be effective in mitigating prevalence and severity of neuropsychiatric disorders (Bruce-Keller et al., 2014).

Exercise is a common way to combat obesity and was once thought to prevent the health detriments of an HFD. Many studies have demonstrated, using insulin readouts and glucose monitoring, that exercise modulates changes in cognitive function associated with HFD (Jung and Kang, 2010). A recent mouse behavioral and microbiota study demonstrated that exercise improved cognitive-learning abilities of mice fed an HFD; however, the prominent anxiety-like behavior was not ameliorated with exercise (Kang et al., 2014). Upon further investigation into the composition of the intestinal microbiota, using 16S rRNA hypervariable sequencing to identify the fingerprint regions of different bacterial taxa, results showed unique bacterial communities among mice fed an HFD with and without exercise as compared with mice raised on a normal chow diet. The HFD and the exercise groups showed shifts in the composition of the microbiota from normal chow-fed and conventionally housed mice but in orthogonal directions. This led the group to conclude that exercise and diet affect the gut microbiota in unrelated ways, and that exercise likely does not mitigate the cognitive disruption of an HFD via the microbiota-gut-brain axis (Kang et al., 2014). Further studies are necessary to better understand the interplay between diet and exercise in shaping a healthy intestinal microbiome.

Depression

Depression is currently one of the leading causes of global disease burden, and the need for effective prevention and treatment is significant. Major depressive disorders

(MDDs) are frequently associated with cognitive disturbances and elevated anxiety; mouse models display decreased spatial and associative learning and loss of cognitive flexibility (Darcet et al., 2014). The intestinal microbiota is a clear health factor that regulates the risk of developing depressive disorders (Dash et al., 2015). The correlation between diet-induced microbiota changes and risk of depression is now under investigation. A recent systematic review and meta-analysis, including results from 13 observational studies, concluded that a healthy diet may be associated with reduced onset of depression. Similarly, diets high in sugar and fat yield an increased propensity toward psychological symptoms, suggesting a role for the microbiota-gut-brain axis (Lai et al., 2014). It has even been suggested that the microbiota may elicit cravings for foods that fuel bacterial fitness, rather than host health, and that increased microbial diversity may limit bacterial control over dietary choices (Alcock et al., 2014).

Carbohydrate consumption, especially fiber, is important in determining the overall intestinal microbial composition and leads to the increased production of antiinflammatory short-chain fatty acids (SCFAs). These SCFAs promote a shift toward colonization of beneficial bacterial species while competitively excluding detrimental, pathogenic bacteria (Havenaar, 2011). Fiber provides the building blocks for bacterial fermentation to SCFAs such as acetate, propionate, and butyrate—all of which subdue the colonic inflammatory response typically associated with depressive disorders (Kaczmarczyk et al., 2012). The success of using SCFAs as a means to increase beneficial bacteria and improve cognitive function remains to be studied.

Serotonin

The gut microbiota can also influence serotonin (5-HT) locally in the gut and centrally in the brain. Germ-free mice were demonstrated to have increased plasma tryptophan levels and a decrease in the kyneurine:tryptophan ratio, largely regulated by tryptophan-2,3-dioxygenase (TDO) and indoleamine-2,3-dioxygenase (IDO) (Clarke et al., 2013). Interferon (IFN)-γ is a potent inducer of TDO, responsible for kyneurine production from tryphophan and resulting in decreased tryptophan availability for production of 5-HT. This reduced circulation of tryptophan is documented to functionally affect mood and even reinstate depressive symptoms in patients who previously responded positively to selective 5-HT reuptake inhibitors (Young, 2013). A decrease in 5-HT synthesis by TDO/IDO is observed in many disorders, including in patients with irritable bowel syndrome (O'Mahony et al., 2015). 5-HT levels are intrinsically related to depression, thus providing a possible explanation that connects the immune response to depressive behavior. Clinical and experimental evidence document that increased peripheral cytokine levels and inflammation are also associated with depression-like symptoms and neuropsychological disturbances in humans (Grigoleit et al., 2011). However, it remains to be determined whether modulating the microbiota to affect 5-HT biosynthesis will be clinically relevant for cognitive benefit.

Inflammation and Infection

The induction of colonic inflammatory pathways associated with unhealthy diets has been causally related to depression after psychological and pathological stressors and may, in part, occur as a consequence of the immunological host response (Lawson et al., 2013). Lipopolysaccharide (LPS) from the outer membrane of gram-negative bacteria can elicit a major inflammatory response when sensed by the host immune system. In fact, when LPS was given systemically to mice it enhanced their sickness response and depression-like behaviors (Lawson et al., 2013). Researchers discovered that increased translocation of LPS from the gut can induce depression and detected elevated antibodies against LPS in mouse models of chronic depression (Maes et al., 2008). The authors also found accompanying stress-sensitive inflammation and noted increased production of proinflammatory cytokines, including interleukin (IL)-1β, IL-6, tumor necrosis factor (TNF)-α, and IFNγ (Maes, 2008). These data suggest that an immune response related to dysbiosis may contribute to depressive behaviors.

Given the association among the microbiota-gut-brain axis, the inflammatory state of the gut, and depression, researchers are now exploring potential clinical applications. In fact, modifying a diet to be less inflammatory and healthier has recently been shown to prevent depression (Dash et al., 2015). Altering the diet may prove to be the first line of defense against delaying or preventing depressive disorders and be a readily accessible mode of modifying the gut microbial composition for treatment of common mood disorders, especially depression. Furthermore, depression is an important psychiatric comorbidity in cognitive disorders of later life (Nihonmatsu-Kikuchi et al., 2013), eliciting further interest in the study of the gut-microbiota-brain axis's role in cognitive decline associated with aging.

Aging

The diet-microbiota effect has become the object of intense research in relation to cognitive aging and neurodegenerative disease, including clinical dementia and Alzheimer's disease. Epidemiological evidence provides support that diet may be a key player in preventing cognitive decline. Cognitive decline includes decreased sensory, motor, and higher cognitive functions that occur as a result of age-related changes and diseases in elderly populations (Caracciolo et al., 2014). The microbiota of older people is significantly less diverse than younger people and displays greater variation between individuals (Guigoz et al., 2008; Jumpertz et al., 2011; Woodmansey, 2007). This reduced diversity of the intestinal microbiota is the current suspected cause of cognitive decline via the microbiota-gut-brain axis because reduced diversity may lead to colonization with opportunistic pathogenic bacteria at the expense of the symbiotic healthy bacteria. The hypothesized mechanism of microbiota-gut-brain interactions resulting in cognitive decline is similar to that of depression; age-related changes in the intestinal microbiota may lead to low-grade inflammation in the gut causing a systemic release of inflammatory mediators that in turn activate glial cells and cause neuroinflammation. This inflammation of the brain, as discussed previously, is characteristic of most cognition-related diseases (Caracciolo et al., 2014).

A clinical study evaluated the overall health and cognitive function of 160 elderly people with varying diets, microbiota profiles, and residence location; clustering subjects by diet differentiated the cohort by the same residence location and microbiota groupings whereas clustering by microbiota composition most significantly correlated with measures of fragility, co-morbidity, nutritional status, and inflammation. In addition, those who lived in long-term care facilities had a characteristically less diverse microbiota than those living integrated in the community as well as higher levels of proinflammatory markers (TNF-α, IL-6, IL-8, and C-reactive protein; Claesson et al., 2012). This study supports the role of diet-driven microbiota alterations in elderly health decline. Although these results are promising of a potential correlation, further research is needed to establish the roles of each bacterial family in the gut and to derive specific mechanisms of communication within the microbiota-gut-brain axis.

PROBIOTIC INTERVENTIONS AND COGNITIVE FUNCTION

The beneficial role of probiotics in supporting the composition of the host microbiota in healthy and diseased states is frequently debated in clinical research. However, recent studies have reported that probiotics can ameliorate defects in intestinal physiology, dysbiosis, behavior, and cognition (Gareau, 2014).

PROBIOTIC INTERVENTION IN A HEALTHY CONTEXT

Although probiotics have been shown to treat various diseases, many people take probiotics on a daily basis to promote general health and well-being. Recently, the possibilities of probiotics having a positive cognitive effect in health have emerged. Healthy adult BALB/c mice treated with *L. rhamnosus* JB-1 were shown to display reduced anxiety-like activity and induction in transcriptional changes in three subtypes of gamma-aminobutyric acid (GABA) receptors in the hippocampus, amygdala, and cingulate cortex (Bravo et al., 2011). The changes observed correlate with previous studies that implicate the GABA-ergic pathways that directly influence cognitive processes (Cryan and Slattery, 2010; Jacobson et al., 2007; Rudolph and Mohler, 2014). Overall, it suggests that administration of *L. rhamnosus* to healthy mice can improve GABA-ergic pathways leading to improved memory, reduced fear conditioning, and antidepressive effects (Bravo et al., 2011). It is interesting to note that the GABA changes that correlated with *L. rhamnosus* administration were not observed in vagotomized mice, suggesting that the vagus nerve plays a major role in this process (Bravo et al., 2011). More recently it was demonstrated that similar beneficial effects on baseline behavior could also be observed after administration of bifidobacteria species, including *B. longum* 1714 and *B. breve* 1205 to an inherently anxious mouse strain (Savignac et al., 2014).

Probiotics have also been shown to influence brain activity in healthy human subjects. In a recent clinical study, healthy women were given fermented milk products for 4 weeks, which was followed by functional magnetic resonance imaging of the brain. Researchers found that probiotic treatment altered activity in areas of the brain that process sensation and emotion (Tillisch et al., 2013). Likewise, in a double-blind, randomized, parallel, placebo-controlled clinical study, 55 subjects (both men and women) were subjected to either a probiotic cocktail containing *L. helveticus* R0052 and *B. longum* R0175 or placebo. After 30 days of administration, subjects were assessed through established psychoanalytical tests. Hopkins Symptom Checklist-90 (HSCL-90) and Coping Checklist (CCL) were used to evaluate numerous possible psychopathologies and cognitive functions. Relative to baseline levels recorded before the beginning of treatment, the HSCL-90 results showed significant improvement in depression and somatization ratings in individuals taking probiotics, whereas CCL showed that this same group displayed an improved problem-solving score and lowered self-blame scores (Messaoudi et al., 2011). These studies indicate that probiotics can modulate brain activity in healthy subjects.

PROBIOTICS AND COGNITION IN THE CONTEXT OF DISEASE

Despite a wealth of preclinical and experimental data supporting their beneficial effects, clinical studies involving probiotics in patients have shown inconsistent findings. Recent meta-analyses evaluating the effectiveness of probiotics in clinical settings have concluded that probiotics are effective in treating functional gastrointestinal disorders such as irritable bowel syndrome (Ford et al., 2014; Ortiz-Lucas et al., 2013). However, the data are less convincing for inflammatory bowel diseases (IBDs), which suggest that probiotics may be of benefit in ulcerative colitis but not in Crohn's disease (Bernstein, 2014). Nonetheless, numerous clinical studies have demonstrated that probiotics have significant health benefits in the context of *H. pylori* eradication as well as conferring protection against *C. difficile* infection (Dang et al., 2014; Hickson, 2011). Current work investigating the role of probiotics on the microbiota-gut-brain axis shows that the benefits of probiotics are limited to specific strains and that each strain or combination of strains can confer cognitive benefits in different disease states.

INFLAMMATION AND INFECTION

The immune system regulates key processes after infection and inflammation in the gut, and as such it is postulated to play a role in modulating the communication between the gut and the brain. Mice without an adaptive immune system are significantly impaired in cognitive processes such as learning and memory (Brynskikh et al., 2008; Kipnis et al., 2008). Studies of the microbiota-gut-brain axis using mouse models lacking an adaptive immune system, such as Rag1(−/−), show that these mice are innately anxious and exhibit cognitive defects accompanied by alterations in colonic physiology (Smith et al., 2014). However, treatment of Rag1 (−/−) mice with *L. rhamnosus* and *L. helveticus*, starting at weaning, was able to correct the defects in memory, anxiety, and colonic physiology (Smith et al., 2014), suggesting that probiotics could overcome behavioral defects in an immune-deficient host in the absence of adaptive immune cells. In female Wistar rats, administration of *L. farciminis* before exposure to an acute physical stress was shown to protect the animals from stress-induced changes in blood LPS levels as well as IL-6 and TNF-α expression (Ait-Belgnaoui et al., 2012). These studies indicate that the microbiota could be modulating behavior and cognition in part via the immune system.

The interrelationship among diet, behavior, and inflammation was studied in a mouse model of IBD in IL10-deficient (−/−) mice, which spontaneously develop intestinal inflammation resembling human IBD (Kole and Maloy, 2014). IL10−/− mice were placed on a Western diet, itself associated with colonic inflammation (Thorburn et al., 2014), supplemented with or without probiotic. Administration of a Western diet modulated the microbiota in wild-type and IL10−/− mice (Ohland et al., 2013). Administration of *L. helveticus* R0052 improved memory, decreased anxiety-like behavior relative to controls, and ameliorated colonic damage (Ohland et al., 2013). This study highlights the connection among diet, the microbiota, intestinal inflammation, and behavior or cognitive function and illustrates the complexity of these interactions.

Dysbiosis in patients with IBD has been identified suggesting that the microbiota may play a role in disease development (Frank et al., 2007). IBD is characterized by acute inflammation as well as increased barrier permeability, colloquially known as "leaky gut" (Antoni et al., 2014). A leaky gut is believed to allow passage of LPS and other endotoxins across the intestinal barrier, contributing to the strong inflammatory response seen in patients with IBD. In the chronic dextran sodium sulfate (DSS) mouse model of IBD, which causes distal colonic disease resembling colitis, the probiotic *B. longum* was shown to normalize anxiety-like behavior relative to controls (Bercik et al., 2011). Amelioration of anxiety-like behavior was not observed in vagotomized mice, implicating the vagus nerve as a major pathway in the microbiota-gut-brain axis. In a separate study that utilized the same DSS model, *B. longum* was found to reduce colonic lesions, neutrophil infiltration, and edema (Elian et al., 2014).

Mechanistic studies have identified the aryl hydrocarbon receptor (AhR) as playing a major role in modulating inflammation (Esser et al., 2009; Stevens et al., 2009). AhRs detect the presence of bacterial aromatic compounds, such as bacterial pigments, and initiate the transcription of defensive processes in epithelial cells (Moura-Alves et al., 2014). AhR is downregulated in colonic tissues of patients with IBD (Monteleone et al., 2011), suggesting that it may be involved in mitigating pathogenesis. AhRs may also play a role in neurodevelopmental pathways that regulate cognitive processes. Adult AhR−/− mice display deficits in hippocampal-dependent processes and decreased cell survival and differentiation in the dentate gyrus (Latchney et al., 2013). Persistent AhR activation was also found to display similar defects in memory and neurological changes observed in AhR−/− mice. It has been shown that heat-killed probiotics, such as *L. bulgaricus* OLL1181, can inhibit DSS-induced colitis through activation of the AhR pathway (Takamura et al., 2011). In a groundbreaking study, researchers were able to identify a specific AhR activator derived from the probiotic *P. freudenreichii* ET-3 (Fukumoto et al., 2014). The AhR activator, 1,4-dihydroxy-2-naphtoic acid, a precursor of vitamin K2, was found to inhibit DSS-induced colitis as well as LPS-induced IL-6 production (Fukumoto et al., 2014). Therefore probiotics may help to improve barrier function and mitigate cognitive consequences associated with persistent AhR activation. Further work is still needed to fully evaluate the effects of AhR activation on cognitive processes. It is likely that multiple routes of communication may govern this process. These studies suggest that changes in behavior, including anxiety-like behavior and cognitive deficits, induced after induction of inflammation, can be modulated by administration of probiotics.

In the context of infection, gastrointestinal inflammation after *T. muris* nematode infection can induce anxiety-like behavior in mice as well as decreased expression of brain-derived neurotrophic factor (BDNF) in the hippocampal region (Bercik et al., 2010). Administration of the probiotic *B. longum* during infection normalized behavior and levels of BDNF expression in CNS neurons (Bercik et al., 2010). In mice challenged with *C. rodentium*, a murine pathogen used to model bacterial diarrheal disease, stress-induced cognitive deficits and dysbiosis were observed. However, pretreatment with a probiotic cocktail containing *L. helveticus* and *L. rhamnosus*, starting 7 days before infection, normalized the microbiota, prevented cognitive dysfunction, and normalized hippocampal BDNF (Gareau et al., 2011). The exact mechanism by which probiotics could modulate changes in the brain and behavior remain to be elucidated.

METABOLIC DISORDERS

Metabolic disorders are characterized by the inability to properly utilize and/or store energy, with the most prominent metabolic disorder being diabetes. Metabolic disorders have been associated with cognitive decline including decreased mental flexibility and memory deficits (Panza et al., 2010). Elderly patients with impaired glucose tolerance have greater impaired cognitive functions including verbal and visual-spatial memory relative to healthy groups (Vanhanen et al., 1998). Current research suggests that probiotics may be able to ameliorate cognitive decline associated with metabolic disorders. In the streptozocin-induced rat model of type I diabetes, diabetic male Wistar rats exhibited spatial memory impairments relative to control rats. However, *L. acidophilus* ATCC 4356, *B. lactis* DSM 10,140, and *L. fermentum* ATCC 9338 restored cognitive function in diabetic rats (Davari et al., 2013). Moreover, diabetic rats showed impaired long-term potentiation (LTP) and excitatory postsynaptic potentials (EPSPs) in the CA1 region at baseline (Davari et al., 2013). LTP and the measured EPSPs in the CA1 region are implicated in learning and memory (Davari et al., 2013). However, LTP and EPSPs were restored in diabetic animals administered probiotics (Davari et al., 2013). In rats with hyperammonemia (HA), 5-HT metabolism was found to be increased in the cerebellum, hippocampus, and prefrontal cortex; however, rats that were given *L. helveticus* NS8 showed a reduced metabolism of 5-HT (Luo et al., 2014). High levels of 5-HT are associated with increased anxiety-like behavior in rat models (Laugeray et al., 2011). Mice with HA were observed to display cognitive defects and anxiety-like behavior; administration of *L. helveticus* NS8 effectively prevented these behavioral deficits

(Luo et al., 2014). In addition, levels of 5-HT and 5-hydroxyindoleacetic acid were also found to be reduced in HA rats administered probiotics. The results of both of these recent studies demonstrate that probiotic administration causes changes in brain activity and cognition in rodents with metabolic syndromes.

SCHIZOPHRENIA

There is growing evidence suggesting that a connection exists between neurological disorders and the gut microbiota. Schizophrenia is a severe and devastating mental disorder that is characterized by abnormal social behavior and altered perception of reality. Genetic risk factors are estimated to play a causal role in schizophrenia development in 30% of cases; despite an astonishing 80% heritability rate of implicated genes (Singh et al., 2014). Thus it is currently hypothesized that the development of schizophrenic symptoms involves interplay between the gut microbiota and genetic factors. Schizophrenia studies using an inducible mouse model demonstrate altered baseline microbiota and memory deficits (Pyndt Jorgensen et al., 2014). Although there is great potential for probiotics as a possible alternative, or adjunct, treatment option for schizophrenia further investigation is still needed.

PREBIOTIC INTERVENTION AND COGNITIVE FUNCTION

Prebiotics can modulate the growth and distribution of beneficial microorganisms in the gut; commonly studied prebiotics include, but are not limited to, fructooligosaccharides (FOS), galactooligosaccharides (GOS), and inulin, and more recently human milk oligosaccharides (HMOs). Studies have demonstrated that prebiotics can modulate brain activity and biochemistry. Adult male rats that were fed FOS and GOS for 5 weeks showed increased hippocampal expression of BDNF and N-methyl-D-aspartic acid (NMDA) receptors, both important in hippocampal-dependent learning and memory (Savignac et al., 2013). NMDA receptors and their association with the gut microbiota have not been investigated, but there are speculations that NMDA receptor agonists such as D-alanine, which is found in bacterial cell walls, may influence serum levels (Savignac et al., 2013).

In a clinical study, 45 volunteers were given GOS, FOS, or placebo. Patients who received GOS demonstrated decreased salivary cortisol levels, suggesting that prebiotics can influence the hypothalamic-pituitary-adrenal (HPA) axis (Schmidt et al., 2014). Vigilance reaction times were also measured; high vigilance reaction times are typical of highly anxious individuals (Koster et al., 2005). Patients in the GOS-supplemented arm of the study demonstrated decreased vigilance toward negative signals compared with placebo, indicating that GOS administration was associated with decreased anxiety (Schmidt et al., 2014).

HMOs are increasingly being recognized as being capable of modulating the microbiota in infants (Bode, 2012), and they promote the growth of *B. longum infantis* in breast-fed infants (Sela et al., 2012). They are thought to function in a prebiotic manner to shape the microbiota in the first few weeks of life (De Leoz et al., 2014). It has also been well established that HMOs are capable of ameliorating disease, specifically necrotizing enterocolitis in very low birth–weight infants (Underwood et al., 2014). The ability for HMOs to provide a beneficial effect on behavior and cognitive function has not yet been addressed; however, given the role for the microbiota in modulating the gut-brain axis, it seems plausible that they could provide a beneficial effect. Administration of sialic acid, a key component of HMOs, to formula-fed piglets improved learning (Wang et al., 2007), supporting the hypothesis that HMOs may modulate the microbiota to benefit cognitive function.

CONCLUSIONS

A role for the modulation of the microbiota by dietary factors, probiotics, or prebiotics for the improvement of cognitive function is under increased investigation. Although much progress has been made in the field, including identification of possible neuronal and humoral factors involved in the regulation of the microbiota-gut-brain axis, research in this emerging field is complex (Table 15.1). Dietary factors are variable among study participants. Furthermore, the multifactorial biological interactions of dietary factors, probiotics, and prebiotics may lead to confounding or synergistic effects that are similarly difficult to control for appropriately.

Immunological factors, cytokines, the vagus nerve, and sensory signaling, as well as the HPA axis, have all been shown to influence communication between the gut and the brain. Many mechanisms are likely to be enlisted by the diet and microbiota to affect cognition, making the identification of the role of one variable in one pathway challenging (Fig. 15.1). In both diseased and healthy states these microbiota-gut-brain axis factors may synergistically influence brain function, cognition, and behavior. Altering the gut-microbiota in several systemic GI and CNS disorders leads to cognitive improvements. Future studies that decipher mechanistic underpinnings of the microbiota-gut-brain axis will expand clinical applications and lead to the identification of specific targets for improved cognitive treatment outcomes.

Table 15.1 Complicating Factors Affecting the Study of the Modulation of the Microbiota for Cognitive Function in Humans

1. Reliably assessing dietary intake qualitatively and quantitatively
2. Time of exposure to a dietary intervention or probiotic supplementation
3. Multifactorial nature of potential biological interactions that could lead to synergistic or counteracting effects
4. Large variability among dietary consumption, uptake, availability to tissues
5. Different probiotic strains confer health benefits through different mechanisms

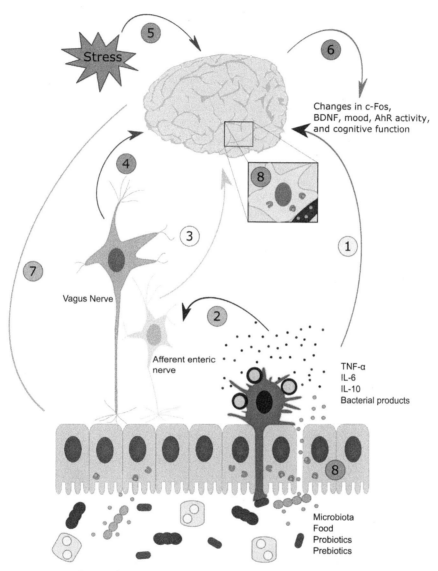

FIGURE 15.1 Proposed mechanisms of communication in the microbiota-gut-brain axis.

Although the pathway of communication among the microbiota, gut, and brain remains to be fully elucidated, numerous pathways have been proposed based on preclinical studies in rodent models. (1) Humoral factors including cytokines (TNF-α, IL-6, and IL-10) and bacteria-associated molecules (short-chain fatty acids) and lipopolysaccharides. (2) Cytokines modulate afferent enteric neurons involved in nociception. (3) Communication between afferent enteric neurons and the brain. (4) Vagus nerve intestinal innervation. (5) Stress-induced activation of the HPA axis resulting in cognitive decline. (6) Gene activation and behavioral changes associated with cognitive deficits. (7) HPA axis effects on regulating intestinal barrier function and motility. (8) AhR can modulate intestinal barrier and cognitive function. *TNF*, tumor necrosis factor; *IL*, interleukin; *HPA*, hypothalamic-pituitary-adrenal; *AhR*, aryl hydrocarbon receptor; *BDNF*, brain-derived neurotrophic factor.

REFERENCES

Ait-Belgnaoui, A., Durand, H., Cartier, C., Chaumaz, G., Eutamene, H., Ferrier, L., Houdeau, E., Fioramonti, J., Bueno, L., Theodorou, V., 2012. Prevention of gut leakiness by a probiotic treatment leads to attenuated HPA response to an acute psychological stress in rats. Psychoneuroendocrinology 37, 1885–1895.

Alcock, J., Maley, C.C., Aktipis, C.A., 2014. Is eating behavior manipulated by the gastrointestinal microbiota? Evolutionary pressures and potential mechanisms. BioEssays 36, 940–949.

Allsop, S.A., Vander Weele, C.M., Wichmann, R., Tye, K.M., 2014. Optogenetic insights on the relationship between anxiety-related behaviors and social deficits. Front Behav. Neurosci. 8, 241.

Antoni, L., Nuding, S., Wehkamp, J., Stange, E.F., 2014. Intestinal barrier in inflammatory bowel disease. World J. Gastroenterol. 20, 1165–1179.

Bercik, P., Park, A.J., Sinclair, D., Khoshdel, A., Lu, J., Huang, X., Deng, Y., Blennerhassett, P.A., Fahnestock, M., Moine, D., Berger, B., Huizinga, J.D., Kunze, W., McLean, P.G., Bergonzelli, G.E., Collins, S.M., Verdu, E.F., 2011. The anxiolytic effect of *Bifidobacterium longum* NCC3001 involves vagal pathways for gut-brain communication. Neurogastroenterol. Motil. 23, 1132–1139.

Bercik, P., Verdu, E.F., Foster, J.A., Macri, J., Potter, M., Huang, X., Malinowski, P., Jackson, W., Blennerhassett, P., Neufeld, K.A., Lu, J., Khan, W.I., Corthesy-Theulaz, I., Cherbut, C., Bergonzelli, G.E., Collins, S.M., 2010. Chronic gastrointestinal inflammation induces anxiety-like behavior and alters central nervous system biochemistry in mice. Gastroenterology 139, 2102–2112.e1.

Bernstein, C.N., 2014. Antibiotics, probiotics and prebiotics in IBD. Nestle Nutr. Inst. Workshop Ser. 79, 83–100.

Bode, L., 2012. Human milk oligosaccharides: every baby needs a sugar mama. Glycobiology 22, 1147–1162.

Borre, Y.E., Moloney, R.D., Clarke, G., Dinan, T.G., Cryan, J.F., 2014. The impact of microbiota on brain and behavior: mechanisms & therapeutic potential. Adv. Exp. Med. Biol. 817, 373–403.

Bravo, J.A., Forsythe, P., Chew, M.V., Escaravage, E., Savignac, H.M., Dinan, T.G., Bienenstock, J., Cryan, J.F., 2011. Ingestion of *Lactobacillus* strain regulates emotional behavior and central GABA receptor expression in a mouse via the vagus nerve. Proc. Natl. Acad. Sci. U.S.A. 108, 16050–16055.

Bruce-Keller, A.J., Salbaum, J.M., Luo, M., Blanchard, E.t., Taylor, C.M., Welsh, D.A., Berthoud, H.R., 2014. Obese-type gut microbiota induce neurobehavioral changes in the absence of obesity. Biol. Psychiatry 77 (7), 607–615.

Brynskikh, A., Warren, T., Zhu, J., Kipnis, J., 2008. Adaptive immunity affects learning behavior in mice. Brain Behav. Immun. 22, 861–869.

Caracciolo, B., Xu, W., Collins, S., Fratiglioni, L., 2014. Cognitive decline, dietary factors and gut-brain interactions. Mech. Ageing Dev. 136–137, 59–69.

Chukoskie, L., Townsend, J., Westerfield, M., 2013. Motor skill in autism spectrum disorders: a subcortical view. Int. Rev. Neurobiol. 113, 207–249.

Claesson, M.J., Jeffery, I.B., Conde, S., Power, S.E., O'Connor, E.M., Cusack, S., Harris, H.M., Coakley, M., Lakshminarayanan, B., O'Sullivan, O., Fitzgerald, G.F., Deane, J., O'Connor, M., Harnedy, N., O'Connor, K., O'Mahony, D., van Sinderen, D., Wallace, M., Brennan, L., Stanton, C., Marchesi, J.R., Fitzgerald, A.P., Shanahan, F., Hill, C., Ross, R.P., O'Toole, P.W., 2012. Gut microbiota composition correlates with diet and health in the elderly. Nature 488, 178–184.

Clarke, G., Grenham, S., Scully, P., Fitzgerald, P., Moloney, R.D., Shanahan, F., Dinan, T.G., Cryan, J.F., 2013. The microbiome-gut-brain axis during early life regulates the hippocampal serotonergic system in a sex-dependent manner. Mol. Psychiatry 18, 666–673.

Cryan, J.F., Dinan, T.G., 2012. Mind-altering microorganisms: the impact of the gut microbiota on brain and behaviour. Nat. Rev. Neurosci. 13, 701–712.

Cryan, J.F., Slattery, D.A., 2010. GABAB receptors and depression. Current status. Adv. Pharmacol. 58, 427–451.

Dang, Y., Reinhardt, J.D., Zhou, X., Zhang, G., 2014. The effect of probiotics supplementation on *Helicobacter pylori* eradication rates and side effects during eradication therapy: a meta-analysis. PLoS One 9, e111030.

Darcet, F., Mendez-David, I., Tritschler, L., Gardier, A.M., Guilloux, J.P., David, D.J., 2014. Learning and memory impairments in a neuroendocrine mouse model of anxiety/depression. Front Behav. Neurosci. 8, 136.

Dash, S., Clarke, G., Berk, M., Jacka, F.N., 2015. The gut microbiome and diet in psychiatry: focus on depression. Curr. Opin. Psychiatry 28, 1–6.

Davari, S., Talaei, S.A., Alaei, H., Salami, M., 2013. Probiotics treatment improves diabetes-induced impairment of synaptic activity and cognitive function: behavioral and electrophysiological proofs for microbiome-gut-brain axis. Neuroscience 240, 287–296.

De Leoz, M.L., Kalanetra, K.M., Bokulich, N.A., Strum, J.S., Underwood, M.A., German, J.B., Mills, D.A., Lebrilla, C.B., 2014. Human milk glycomics and gut microbial genomics in infant feces show a correlation between human milk oligosaccharides and gut microbiota: a proof-of-concept study. J. Proteome Res. 14 (1), 491–502.

Elian, S.D., Souza, E.L., Vieira, A.T., Teixeira, M.M., Arantes, R.M., Nicoli, J.R., Martins, F.S., 2014. *Bifidobacterium longum* subsp. infantis BB-02 attenuates acute murine experimental model of inflammatory bowel disease. Benef. Microbe. 1–10.

Esser, C., Rannug, A., Stockinger, B., 2009. The aryl hydrocarbon receptor in immunity. Trends Immunol. 30, 447–454.

Finger, B.C., Dinan, T.G., Cryan, J.F., 2011. High-fat diet selectively protects against the effects of chronic social stress in the mouse. Neuroscience 192, 351–360.

Ford, A.C., Quigley, E.M., Lacy, B.E., Lembo, A.J., Saito, Y.A., Schiller, L.R., Soffer, E.E., Spiegel, B.M., Moayyedi, P., 2014. Efficacy of prebiotics, probiotics, and synbiotics in irritable bowel syndrome and chronic idiopathic constipation: systematic review and meta-analysis. Am. J. Gastroenterol. 109, 1547–1561 quiz 1546, 1562.

Frank, D.N., St Amand, A.L., Feldman, R.A., Boedeker, E.C., Harpaz, N., Pace, N.R., 2007. Molecular-phylogenetic characterization of microbial community imbalances in human inflammatory bowel diseases. Proc. Natl. Acad. Sci. U.S.A. 104, 13780–13785.

Fukumoto, S., Toshimitsu, T., Matsuoka, S., Maruyama, A., Oh-Oka, K., Takamura, T., Nakamura, Y., Ishimaru, K., Fujii-Kuriyama, Y., Ikegami, S., Itou, H., Nakao, A., 2014. Identification of a probiotic bacteria-derived activator of the aryl hydrocarbon receptor that inhibits colitis. Immunol. Cell Biol. 92, 460–465.

Gareau, M.G., 2014. Microbiota-gut-brain axis and cognitive function. Adv. Exp. Med. Biol. 817, 357–371.

Gareau, M.G., Sherman, P.M., Walker, W.A., 2010. Probiotics and the gut microbiota in intestinal health and disease. Nat. Rev. Gastroenterol. Hepatol. 7, 503–514.

Gareau, M.G., Wine, E., Rodrigues, D.M., Cho, J.H., Whary, M.T., Philpott, D.J., Macqueen, G., Sherman, P.M., 2011. Bacterial infection causes stress-induced memory dysfunction in mice. Gut 60, 307–317.

Grigoleit, J.S., Kullmann, J.S., Wolf, O.T., Hammes, F., Wegner, A., Jablonowski, S., Engler, H., Gizewski, E., Oberbeck, R., Schedlowski, M., 2011. Dose-dependent effects of endotoxin on neurobehavioral functions in humans. PLoS One 6, e28330.

Guigoz, Y., Dore, J., Schiffrin, E.J., 2008. The inflammatory status of old age can be nurtured from the intestinal environment. Curr. Opin. Clin. Nutr. Metab. Care 11, 13–20.

Havenaar, R., 2011. Intestinal health functions of colonic microbial metabolites: a review. Benef. Microbe. 2, 103–114.

Hickson, M., 2011. Probiotics in the prevention of antibiotic-associated diarrhoea and *Clostridium difficile* infection. Therap. Adv. Gastroenterol. 4, 185–197.

Horwood, L.J., Fergusson, D.M., 1998. Breastfeeding and later cognitive and academic outcomes. Pediatrics 101, E9.

Jacobson, L.H., Kelly, P.H., Bettler, B., Kaupmann, K., Cryan, J.F., 2007. Specific roles of GABA(B(1)) receptor isoforms in cognition. Behav. Brain Res. 181, 158–162.

Jumpertz, R., Le, D.S., Turnbaugh, P.J., Trinidad, C., Bogardus, C., Gordon, J.I., Krakoff, J., 2011. Energy-balance studies reveal associations between gut microbes, caloric load, and nutrient absorption in humans. Am. J. Clin. Nutr. 94, 58–65.

Jung, H.L., Kang, H.Y., 2010. Effects of endurance exercise and high-fat diet on insulin resistance and ceramide contents of skeletal muscle in Sprague-Dawley rats. Korean Diabetes J. 34, 244–252.

Kaczmarczyk, M.M., Miller, M.J., Freund, G.G., 2012. The health benefits of dietary fiber: beyond the usual suspects of type 2 diabetes mellitus, cardiovascular disease and colon cancer. Metabolism 61, 1058–1066.

Kang, S.S., Jeraldo, P.R., Kurti, A., Miller, M.E., Cook, M.D., Whitlock, K., Goldenfeld, N., Woods, J.A., White, B.A., Chia, N., Fryer, J.D., 2014. Diet and exercise orthogonally alter the gut microbiome and reveal independent associations with anxiety and cognition. Mol. Neurodegener. 9, 36.

Khan, N.A., Raine, L.B., Donovan, S.M., Hillman, C.H., 2014. IV. The cognitive implications of obesity and nutrition in childhood. Monogr. Soc. Res. Child Dev. 79, 51–71.

Kipnis, J., Derecki, N.C., Yang, C., Scrable, H., 2008. Immunity and cognition: what do age-related dementia, HIV-dementia and 'chemo-brain' have in common? Trends Immunol. 29, 455–463.

Koenig, J.E., Spor, A., Scalfone, N., Fricker, A.D., Stombaugh, J., Knight, R., Angenent, L.T., Ley, R.E., 2011. Succession of microbial consortia in the developing infant gut microbiome. Proc. Natl. Acad. Sci. U.S.A. 108 (Suppl. 1), 4578–4585.

Kole, A., Maloy, K.J., 2014. Control of intestinal inflammation by interleukin-10. Curr. Top Microbiol. Immunol. 380, 19–38.

Koster, E.H., Verschuere, B., Crombez, G., Van Damme, S., 2005. Time-course of attention for threatening pictures in high and low trait anxiety. Behav. Res. Ther. 43, 1087–1098.

Lai, J.S., Hiles, S., Bisquera, A., Hure, A.J., McEvoy, M., Attia, J., 2014. A systematic review and meta-analysis of dietary patterns and depression in community-dwelling adults. Am. J. Clin. Nutr. 99, 181–197.

Latchney, S.E., Hein, A.M., O'Banion, M.K., DiCicco-Bloom, E., Opanashuk, L.A., 2013. Deletion or activation of the aryl hydrocarbon receptor alters adult hippocampal neurogenesis and contextual fear memory. J. Neurochem. 125, 430–445.

Laugeray, A., Launay, J.M., Callebert, J., Surget, A., Belzung, C., Barone, P.R., 2011. Evidence for a key role of the peripheral kynurenine pathway in the modulation of anxiety- and depression-like behaviours in mice: focus on individual differences. Pharmacol. Biochem. Behav. 98, 161–168.

Lawson, M.A., Parrott, J.M., McCusker, R.H., Dantzer, R., Kelley, K.W., O'Connor, J.C., 2013. Intracerebroventricular administration of lipopolysaccharide induces indoleamine-2,3-dioxygenase-dependent depression-like behaviors. J. Neuroinflammation 10, 87.

Li, W., Dowd, S.E., Scurlock, B., Acosta-Martinez, V., Lyte, M., 2009. Memory and learning behavior in mice is temporally associated with diet-induced alterations in gut bacteria. Physiol. Behav. 96, 557–567.

Luo, J., Wang, T., Liang, S., Hu, X., Li, W., Jin, F., 2014. Ingestion of *Lactobacillus* strain reduces anxiety and improves cognitive function in the hyperammonemia rat. Sci. China Life Sci. 57, 327–335.

Maes, M., 2008. The cytokine hypothesis of depression: inflammation, oxidative & nitrosative stress (IO&NS) and leaky gut as new targets for adjunctive treatments in depression. Neuro Endocrinol. Lett. 29, 287–291.

Maes, M., Kubera, M., Leunis, J.C., 2008. The gut-brain barrier in major depression: intestinal mucosal dysfunction with an increased translocation of LPS from gram negative enterobacteria (leaky gut) plays a role in the inflammatory pathophysiology of depression. Neuro.Endocrinol. Lett. 29, 117–124.

Mayer, E.A., Knight, R., Mazmanian, S.K., Cryan, J.F., Tillisch, K., 2014. Gut microbes and the brain: paradigm shift in neuroscience. J. Neurosci. 34, 15490–15496.

Messaoudi, M., Lalonde, R., Violle, N., Javelot, H., Desor, D., Nejdi, A., Bisson, J.F., Rougeot, C., Pichelin, M., Cazaubiel, M., Cazaubiel, J.M., 2011. Assessment of psychotropic-like properties of a probiotic formulation (*Lactobacillus helveticus* R0052 and *Bifidobacterium longum* R0175) in rats and human subjects. Br. J. Nutr. 105, 755–764.

Monteleone, I., Rizzo, A., Sarra, M., Sica, G., Sileri, P., Biancone, L., MacDonald, T.T., Pallone, F., Monteleone, G., 2011. Aryl hydrocarbon receptor-induced signals up-regulate IL-22 production and inhibit inflammation in the gastrointestinal tract. Gastroenterology 141, 237–248 248.e1.

Moura-Alves, P., Fae, K., Houthuys, E., Dorhoi, A., Kreuchwig, A., Furkert, J., Barison, N., Diehl, A., Munder, A., Constant, P., Skrahina, T., Guhlich-Bornhof, U., Klemm, M., Koehler, A.B., Bandermann, S., Goosmann, C., Mollenkopf, H.J., Hurwitz, R., Brinkmann, V., Fillatreau, S., Daffe, M., Tummler, B., Kolbe, M., Oschkinat, H., Krause, G., Kaufmann, S.H., 2014. AhR sensing of bacterial pigments regulates antibacterial defence. Nature 512, 387–392.

Mulle, J.G., Sharp, W.G., Cubells, J.F., 2013. The gut microbiome: a new frontier in autism research. Curr. Psychiatry Rep. 15, 337.

Nihonmatsu-Kikuchi, N., Hayashi, Y., Yu, X.J., Tatebayashi, Y., 2013. Depression and Alzheimer's disease: novel postmortem brain studies reveal a possible common mechanism. J. Alzheimers Dis. 37, 611–621.

O'Mahony, S.M., Clarke, G., Borre, Y.E., Dinan, T.G., Cryan, J.F., 2015. Serotonin, tryptophan metabolism and the brain-gut-microbiome axis. Behav. Brain Res. 277, 32–48.

Ohland, C.L., Kish, L., Bell, H., Thiesen, A., Hotte, N., Pankiv, E., Madsen, K.L., 2013. Effects of *Lactobacillus helveticus* on murine behavior are dependent on diet and genotype and correlate with alterations in the gut microbiome. Psychoneuroendocrinology 38 (9), 1738–1747.

Ortiz-Lucas, M., Tobias, A., Saz, P., Sebastian, J.J., 2013. Effect of probiotic species on irritable bowel syndrome symptoms: a bring up to date meta-analysis. Rev. Esp. Enferm. Dig. 105, 19–36.

Panza, F., Frisardi, V., Capurso, C., Imbimbo, B.P., Vendemiale, G., Santamato, A., D'Onofrio, G., Seripa, D., Sancarlo, D., Pilotto, A., Solfrizzi, V., 2010. Metabolic syndrome and cognitive impairment: current epidemiology and possible underlying mechanisms. J. Alzheimers Dis. 21, 691–724.

Pyndt Jorgensen, B., Hansen, J.T., Krych, L., Larsen, C., Klein, A.B., Nielsen, D.S., Josefsen, K., Hansen, A.K., Sorensen, D.B., 2014. A possible link between food and mood: dietary impact on gut microbiota and behavior in BALB/c mice. PLoS One 9, e103398.

Rogier, E.W., Frantz, A.L., Bruno, M.E., Wedlund, L., Cohen, D.A., Stromberg, A.J., Kaetzel, C.S., 2014. Secretory antibodies in breast milk promote long-term intestinal homeostasis by regulating the gut microbiota and host gene expression. Proc. Natl. Acad. Sci. U.S.A. 111, 3074–3079.

Rudolph, U., Mohler, H., 2014. GABAA receptor subtypes: therapeutic potential in Down syndrome, affective disorders, schizophrenia, and autism. Annu. Rev. Pharmacol. Toxicol. 54, 483–507.

Savignac, H.M., Corona, G., Mills, H., Chen, L., Spencer, J.P., Tzortzis, G., Burnet, P.W., 2013. Prebiotic feeding elevates central brain derived neurotrophic factor, N-methyl-D-aspartate receptor subunits and D-serine. Neurochem. Int. 63, 756–764.

Savignac, H.M., Kiely, B., Dinan, T.G., Cryan, J.F., 2014. Bifidobacteria exert strain-specific effects on stress-related behavior and physiology in BALB/c mice. Neurogastroenterol. Motil. 26, 1615–1627.

Schmidt, K., Cowen, P.J., Harmer, C.J., Tzortzis, G., Errington, S., Burnet, P.W., 2014. Prebiotic intake reduces the waking cortisol response and alters emotional bias in healthy volunteers. Psychopharmacology (Berl) 232 (10), 1793–1801.

Sela, D.A., Garrido, D., Lerno, L., Wu, S., Tan, K., Eom, H.J., Joachimiak, A., Lebrilla, C.B., Mills, D.A., 2012. *Bifidobacterium longum* subsp. infantis ATCC 15697 alpha-fucosidases are active on fucosylated human milk oligosaccharides. Appl. Environ. Microbiol. 78, 795–803.

Singh, S., Kumar, A., Agarwal, S., Phadke, S.R., Jaiswal, Y., 2014. Genetic insight of schizophrenia: past and future perspectives. Gene 535, 97–100.

Smith, C.J., Emge, J.R., Berzins, K., Lung, L., Khamishon, R., Shah, P., Rodrigues, D.M., Sousa, A.J., Reardon, C., Sherman, P.M., Barrett, K.E., Gareau, M.G., 2014. Probiotics normalize the gut-brain-microbiota axis in immunodeficient mice. Am. J. Physiol. Gastrointest. Liver Physiol. 307, G793–G802.

Stevens, E.A., Mezrich, J.D., Bradfield, C.A., 2009. The aryl hydrocarbon receptor: a perspective on potential roles in the immune system. Immunology 127, 299–311.

Takamura, T., Harama, D., Fukumoto, S., Nakamura, Y., Shimokawa, N., Ishimaru, K., Ikegami, S., Makino, S., Kitamura, M., Nakao, A., 2011. *Lactobacillus bulgaricus* OLL1181 activates the aryl hydrocarbon receptor pathway and inhibits colitis. Immunol. Cell Biol. 89, 817–822.

Tanoue, Y., Oda, S., 1989. Weaning time of children with infantile autism. J. Autism Dev. Disord. 19, 425–434.

Thorburn, A.N., Macia, L., Mackay, C.R., 2014. Diet, metabolites, and "western-lifestyle" inflammatory diseases. Immunity 40, 833–842.

Tillisch, K., 2014. The effects of gut microbiota on CNS function in humans. Gut Microbe. 5, 404–410.

Tillisch, K., Labus, J., Kilpatrick, L., Jiang, Z., Stains, J., Ebrat, B., Guyonnet, D., Legrain-Raspaud, S., Trotin, B., Naliboff, B., Mayer, E.A., 2013. Consumption of fermented milk product with probiotic modulates brain activity. Gastroenterology 144, 1394–1401.e1-4.

Tomova, A., Husarova, V., Lakatosova, S., Bakos, J., Vlkova, B., Babinska, K., Ostatnikova, D., 2015. Gastrointestinal microbiota in children with autism in Slovakia. Physiol. Behav. 138, 179–187.

Turnbaugh, P.J., Ley, R.E., Mahowald, M.A., Magrini, V., Mardis, E.R., Gordon, J.I., 2006. An obesity-associated gut microbiome with increased capacity for energy harvest. Nature 444, 1027–1031.

Underwood, M.A., Arriola, J., Gerber, C.W., Kaveti, A., Kalanetra, K.M., Kananurak, A., Bevins, C.L., Mills, D.A., Dvorak, B., 2014. *Bifidobacterium longum* subsp. infantis in experimental necrotizing enterocolitis: alterations in inflammation, innate immune response, and the microbiota. Pediatr. Res. 76, 326–333.

Vanhanen, M., Koivisto, K., Kuusisto, J., Mykkanen, L., Helkala, E.L., Hanninen, T., Riekkinen Sr., P., Soininen, H., Laakso, M., 1998. Cognitive function in an elderly population with persistent impaired glucose tolerance. Diabetes Care 21, 398–402.

Wang, B., Yu, B., Karim, M., Hu, H., Sun, Y., McGreevy, P., Petocz, P., Held, S., Brand-Miller, J., 2007. Dietary sialic acid supplementation improves learning and memory in piglets. Am. J. Clin. Nutr. 85, 561–569.

Woodmansey, E.J., 2007. Intestinal bacteria and ageing. J. Appl. Microbiol. 102, 1178–1186.

Wu, G.D., Chen, J., Hoffmann, C., Bittinger, K., Chen, Y.Y., Keilbaugh, S.A., Bewtra, M., Knights, D., Walters, W.A., Knight, R., Sinha, R., Gilroy, E., Gupta, K., Baldassano, R., Nessel, L., Li, H., Bushman, F.D., Lewis, J.D., 2011. Linking long-term dietary patterns with gut microbial enterotypes. Science 334, 105–108.

Young, S.N., 2013. Acute tryptophan depletion in humans: a review of theoretical, practical and ethical aspects. J. Psychiatry Neurosci. 38, 294–305.

The Influence of Diet and the Gut Microbiota in Schizophrenia

16

R.H. Ghomi
University of Washington, Seattle, WA, United States

K. Nemani
New York University School of Medicine, New York, NY, United States

INTRODUCTION

The *Diagnostic and Statistical Manual of Mental Disorders*, 5th edition, defines and characterizes schizophrenia as the presence of delusions, hallucinations, disorganized speech and behavior, and other symptoms that cause social or occupational dysfunction that persist for at least 6 months (American Psychiatric Association and DSM-5 Task Force, 2013). The World Health Organization's International Classification of Diseases, 10th revision, similarly defines schizophrenia ("WHO | International Classification of Diseases (ICD)," 2010), except requiring only 1 month of symptom duration, emphasizing their recommendation to avoid delaying diagnosis and noting 1 month of symptoms as a sufficient threshold for diagnosis. Both systems of classification attempt to describe and unify a complex syndrome with no single cause but rather resulting from the interplay of countless variables including social, genetic, epigenetic, biological, dietary, and many other factors. Both systems also attempt to simplify a complex syndrome unique to each individual into discrete signs and symptoms, which in turn are targets for research and therapy. This simplification may explain to some degree why pharmacotherapy has inevitably failed to show great treatment promise—each drug is aimed at mechanisms shared by many functions to treat specific symptoms rather than any unique syndrome. Lifetime prevalence rates, which are likely conservative because of limited identification of affected individuals, are consistently estimated to be approximately 1% or 10/1000 persons (Saha et al., 2005). The relatively significant prevalence has driven robust research efforts to understand this syndrome with the hopes of finding new pathways for treatment. Gut-brain research is a promising field for not only understanding a major aspect of the pathophysiology of schizophrenia but also for creating possibilities for novel interventions, potentially without the significant treatment limiting side effects of current antipsychotics.

Perhaps the most significant lesson to be drawn from this chapter is the contribution of all of the above factors to each patient's unique presentation of signs and

The Gut-Brain Axis. http://dx.doi.org/10.1016/B978-0-12-802304-4.00016-5

symptoms, which the syndrome of schizophrenia intends to capture. In other words, it could be stated that a certain genotype or environment predisposes to schizophrenia and, at the same time, schizophrenia predisposes to a certain genotype or environment. This new perspective is a shift from biological reductionism, which has dominated modern medicine and was only made possible by continued scientific research revealing the complexity and challenge of reducing this syndrome to any one specific pathway. Schizophrenia has been a historically difficult disease process to describe with only weak effects found in much of the literature when looking at single causes in isolation. The data that follow arose from investigations precipitated by the observations gleaned from many such studies, including genome-wide association studies investigating thousands of small single nucleotide polymorphisms (SNPs) carrying weak-effect associations that cumulatively could explain approximately 30% of the underlying genetic risk for schizophrenia (Singh et al., 2014).

Accordingly, we now know that genetics can predispose a patient to certain environmental stressors that can lead to epigenetic changes (Babenko et al., 2014), further predisposing to the same stressors, thereby propagating the risk of the illness across generations. By conferring protection and resilience, these epigenetic changes can increase exposure to further environmental stressors. Knowing the bidirectional nature of disease, we aim to explore one pathway in schizophrenia that both contributes to and is reinforced by the disease state—namely, the gut-brain axis—all the while noting that without behavior and context there would be no diagnosis of schizophrenia.

The goal of this chapter is to focus on the gut-brain axis and the bidirectional mechanisms by which diet affects the gut environment, which in turn affects the brain and behavior of those with schizophrenia. Other chapters in this text focus on specific areas of gut-brain signaling and should be referred to for further details pertinent to our discussion. The opportunities for intervention and disease modification, specifically in the form of dietary changes including the addition of prebiotics and probiotics, will also be discussed. Finally, the perspective of schizophrenia as a multifaceted and complex interplay of many factors in a behavioral context will allow for the most comprehensive understanding of the disease process and investigation of effective interventions in the future.

GUT-BRAIN PATHWAYS IN SCHIZOPHRENIA

To study schizophrenia, many validated methods have been used; however, most of the following discussion cites use of several validated symptom tracking tools in humans, such as a the Positive and Negative Syndrome Scale (PANSS), to capture and monitor the symptoms of schizophrenia treatment targets. Much of the gut-brain research in schizophrenia has been elucidated through the use of animal models, which creates a different set of challenges in creating a valid model of schizophrenia based on observable behaviors in mice that may be correlated to human behaviors. Many such models have emerged, including the maternal immune activation mouse model (Ibi et al., 2011), which is established by treating neonatal mice with a toll-like receptor ligand (polyriboinosinic-polyribocytidylic acid) to induce a strong innate immune response leading to schizophrenia-like behaviors in adulthood. Germ-free (GF) mice have also been used in the context of studying schizophrenia to create a model in which manipulation of bacterial colonization is possible and controlled. There are preclinical counterparts to the human symptom scales, such as a three-chamber sociability test, which is able to demonstrate changes in socially driven behavior in mice, which are then extrapolated to the social behavior changes seen in schizophrenia. Likewise, memory can be tested in mice using a maze, and neuroanatomic and physiologic correlates can be drawn by observing the hippocampus in these mice. These behaviors are then observed when one or more variables are manipulated (eg, observing social behavior in mice colonized with specific bacteria at different points in their development). These methods serve to elucidate not only the pathophysiology of gut-brain pathways but also possibilities for therapeutic interventions. Several established pathways of how such alterations may play a role in schizophrenia are discussed in this first section.

NEURODEVELOPMENT

After birth, a newborn's gastrointestinal (GI) tract is populated with microbes from the environment that are now known to play a critical role in the development of the brain (Douglas-Escobar et al., 2013). The gestational age, mode of delivery, and the newborn's type of diet may have significant and lasting effects on the composition of the microbiome (Dominguez-Bello et al., 2010; Mshvildadze et al., 2008; Penders et al., 2006). In fact, term infants (not premature) born vaginally (not by C-section) and exclusively fed breast milk (no formula) were found to have the most bifidobacteria and least *Clostridium difficile* and *Escherichia coli*. The microbiota modulate a range of neurotrophins and proteins such as brain-derived neurotrophic factor (BDNF), serotonin, and N-methyl-D-aspartate (NMDA), all previously shown to be involved in brain development and plasticity (Diaz Heijtz et al., 2011; Douglas-Escobar et al., 2013). Both genetics and environment together guide pre- and postnatal brain development.

BRAIN-DERIVED NEUROTROPHIC FACTOR

BDNF has been shown to be a key modulator of brain development and is affected by genetics and environmental factors, including the gut microbiota, establishing a link between the gut microbiome and the pathophysiology of schizophrenia (Nieto et al., 2013). Lower BDNF expression has been found in patients with schizophrenia in multiple brain regions including the hippocampus and prefrontal cortex (Thompson Ray et al., 2011; Weickert et al., 2003). This correlates with the executive and memory dysfunction seen in schizophrenia (Bilder et al., 2000). Prenatal stress in mice was found to downregulate expression of BDNF through DNA methylation (Dong et al., 2014), a mechanism by which environmental modulation may contribute to a schizophrenia phenotype through epigenetic changes. Gut microbiota has been shown to be a mediator of brain development through modulation of neurotrophins, including synaptophysin, postsynaptic density protein-95, and BNDF in mouse models (Diaz Heijtz et al., 2011; Douglas-Escobar et al., 2013). Both GF and specific pathogen free mice have been compared to normal controls in various tests of behavior measuring activity levels, correlating to anxiety-like behaviors. There is evidence of a critical window during early development during which the absence of the microbiome appears to have behavioral effects that persist into adulthood and are perhaps modulated in part by BDNF. GF mice when inoculated with normal gut flora within a 6-week window were found to display anxiety-like behaviors similar to those observed in control animals whereas when GF mice were inoculated at 14 weeks anxiety-like behavior persisted (Neufeld et al., 2011a,b; Sudo et al., 2004). Clinically translating the findings is challenging given the difficulty in identifying and distinguishing anxiety symptoms within the disease course of schizophrenia as a possible separate disorder or in the context of positive and negative symptoms of schizophrenia with relative decreases and increases in anxiety, respectively.

SEROTONIN

Serotonin is a primary signaling neurotransmitter in the CNS and a key target for much pharmacologic therapeutics in psychiatric conditions, including schizophrenia. The role of serotonin in schizophrenia has been studied for decades and is central to the development of second-generation antipsychotics, the antipsychotic effects of which in schizophrenia are attributed, to some degree, to their effect at serotonin receptors in the CNS. The role of serotonin in the pathogenesis of symptoms seen in schizophrenia has been elucidated through extensive multimodality studies (Bleich et al., 1988). Serotonin system alterations have been correlated with specific symptoms of schizophrenia, and the newer atypical antipsychotics, differing mainly by their activity at serotonin receptors, appear to have greater efficacy in treating negative symptoms and schizophrenia resistant to typical antipsychotics. Quantitative differences in serotonin have also been observed in patients with schizophrenia, further strengthening the link between serotonin and schizophrenia. More recently, work demonstrating the role of the gut-brain axis in regulating serotonin, specifically in the hippocampus of GF mice, demonstrated increased levels of hippocampal serotonin compared with control mice (Clarke et al., 2013). Of note, even after colonizing the mice with a normal microbiota, the increased hippocampal serotonin levels were maintained. However, plasma tryptophan (the main precursor to serotonin synthesis) was found to be significantly elevated in male GF mice. Although tryptophan levels were restored to control levels after colonization with normal microflora in the gut, hippocampal serotonin was unchanged, again indicating the importance of early-life brain development and the difficulty in reversing changes in the CNS later in life. This work demonstrated the modulation of the deficit in anxiety-like behavior in GF mice, which normalized after colonization later in life. Reduced anxiety is a commonly utilized component of schizophrenia measured in mouse models.

N-METHYL-D-ASPARTATE

NMDA is another neurotransmitter in the CNS that plays a major role in the pathophysiology of schizophrenia. NMDA receptors are a type of glutamate receptor involved in the control of synaptic plasticity in memory function. Data have shown that NMDA receptor antagonists produce schizophrenia-like symptoms. On the other hand, agents that enhance NMDA receptor function reduce negative symptoms and improve cognition (Coyle, 2012), leading to the conclusion that NMDA and its receptors play an important role in schizophrenia. Studies in GF mice have established a link between NMDA signaling and the gut microbiota. Such abnormalities in NMDA system functioning observed in GF mice parallel, to some degree, decreased NMDA receptor expression seen in individuals with schizophrenia (Coyle, 2012; Sudo et al., 2004). A decrease in the expression of the NMDA receptor subunit 2A was found in the cortex and hippocampus of GF animals compared with controls (Sudo et al., 2004). Separately, a downregulation of the NMDA receptor subunit 2B in the central amygdala of GF mice has also been reported (Neufeld et al., 2011a,b). Given the important role that the NMDA 2B receptor subunit plays in amygdala-dependent fear learning (Rodrigues et al., 2001), this finding may explain the decreased anxiety-like behavior seen in GF mice. Given that normal development of the microbiome is necessary to stimulate brain plasticity through the appropriate expression of NMDA receptors, it is possible that an altered microbiome may contribute to the NMDA receptor dysfunction seen in schizophrenia.

INFLAMMATION AND IMMUNITY IN SCHIZOPHRENIA

Inflammatory responses contribute to the symptomatology of schizophrenia through several known mechanisms to which the gut-brain axis may contribute and that we will discuss here. These mechanisms include alterations in gut permeability, which closely link to the stress response and provide an opportunity by which pathogenic, food, and antigens can communicate with the brain, directly affecting the course of schizophrenia. The impact of psychological stress on intestinal barrier dysfunction and schizophrenia will be discussed further in the context of the hypothalamic-pituitary-adrenal (HPA) axis.

GUT BARRIER DYSFUNCTION

It is well established that inflammatory processes are accompanied by disruption of the epithelial barrier. Moreover, several pathogens have been demonstrated to affect the permeability of the GI tract (John et al., 2011). One of the initial studies to point to an association between inflammation of the GI tract and schizophrenia came from an autopsy study of 82 patients that found that 92% had colitis, 88% had enteritis, and 50% had gastritis (Buscaino, 1953; Hemmings, 2004). Many early studies also linked circulating antibodies to dietary antigens with schizophrenia. One such study attracting attention to this area demonstrated abnormal intestinal permeability as a feature of hospitalized schizophrenia patients with Celiac disease (Wood et al., 1987). Abnormalities of the epithelial barrier in schizophrenia may occur as a consequence of changes in tight junction proteins or function. Tight junctions create a paracellular barrier to the diffusion of water and solutes in the gut as well as the blood–brain barrier. This barrier plays a role in blocking exogenous pathogenic substances from entering the body and the brain (Wei and Huang, 2013). Structural proteins identified within tight junctions include occludins, claudins, and zona occludens (Fanning et al., 1999). Of note, an SNP within *CLDN5*, the gene coding for the tight junction protein claudin-5, was found to be associated with schizophrenia in a Chinese population (Sun et al., 2004; Wu et al., 2010). A defect in this gene may contribute to increased intestinal permeability in individuals with schizophrenia and increase their vulnerability to harmful environmental exposures.

INFECTION

Infections and the consequent immune response have been investigated for their potential role in the pathogenesis of schizophrenia. Maternal infections during pregnancy have been associated with increased risk of schizophrenia in offspring (Fineberg and Ellman, 2013). A pathogen of particular interest in this context is *Toxoplasma gondii*, a coccidian protozoon of the apicomplexa family. Infection with *T. gondii* has been used to create models of colitis and ileitis (Bereswill et al., 2010; Craven et al., 2012; Erridge et al., 2010; Hand et al., 2012; Muñoz et al., 2009; Schreiner and Liesenfeld, 2009). Significant correlations between antibodies to food antigens and those to *T. gondii* have also been reported (Severance et al., 2012). Several meta-analyses have consistently shown odds ratios favoring *T. gondii* as a risk factor for schizophrenia ranging from 1.68 to 2.73 (Monroe et al., 2014; Torrey et al., 2012). Although *T. gondii* may modify host behavior through a direct effect on the CNS (Gatkowska et al., 2012; Torrey et al., 2007, 2012; Webster, 2001; Xiao et al., 2012), a role for the gut in this regard cannot be fully discounted. *Saccharomyces cerevisiae*, a commensal fungus, serves as another marker of intestinal inflammation and bacterial translocation. In a study measuring antibodies to *S. cerevisiae*, elevated antibody levels were found in recent onset and chronic schizophrenia patients (Severance et al., 2012). Soluble CD14 (sCD14), another marker of bacterial translocation, was found to be significantly elevated and to confer a 3.1-fold increase in odds of association with schizophrenia when compared with controls in studies in antipsychotic-naïve and treated patients (Severance et al., 2013). It is interesting to note that the same study also uncovered an association between sCD14 and gluten antibodies in antipsychotic-naïve schizophrenia patients.

Memory dysfunction has been well established as a symptom or sign of schizophrenia, with significant effect sizes found in several areas of cognition, the largest being in verbal learning and memory (Ranganath et al., 2008). Some of the memory dysfunction seen in schizophrenia may be mediated through the gut microbiota. To explore this relationship, mice were exposed to *Citrobacter rodentium*, a known effacing and immune-activating pathogen. It is interesting to note that behavioral abnormalities were not observed when nonstressed mice, with an intact gut microflora, were infected. However, when control mice were exposed to stress, memory dysfunction was observed and persisted after the bacteria were cleared from the gut, and intestinal injury had resolved (Gareau et al., 2011). Furthermore, pretreatment with probiotics, including *Lactobacillus*, before infection prevented stress-induced memory deficits, increases in serum corticosterone levels, and colonic epithelial cell crypt depth. Infection-induced reductions in BDNF expression were also restored by probiotic pretreatment. GF mice were also observed to have memory impairment with or without stress exposure.

AUTOIMMUNITY

A greater incidence of autoimmune disorders has consistently been shown in schizophrenia patients and their relatives compared with controls (Benros et al., 2012; Eaton et al., 2006). Antibodies against specific brain areas, dubbed "antibrain antibodies," have been found in several regions including the hippocampus, amygdala, and frontal cortex (Strous and Shoenfeld, 2006). A great deal of progress has been made to elucidate the role of autoimmune processes in schizophrenia as a cause and a consequence. The intestinal microbiota has been shown to play a critical role in fostering immunological tolerance by interacting with gut mucosal cells to regulate production of chemokines and cytokines (Neish, 2009). Changes in microbiota composition affect the functioning of the immune system through lymphocyte accumulation and differentiation in the GI tract (Artis, 2008; Nemani et al., 2015). Molecular mimicry is a prevailing theory as a driver of the increasing autoimmunity seen in the general population (Kohm et al., 2003). Foreign antigens may share enough similarity in peptide structural sequence with self-peptides to induce autoreactivity of T or B cells against one's own tissue and cells. Molecular mimicry may be one of several pathways explaining the mechanism of heightened immune responses observed consistently in schizophrenia patients. The plethora of evidence linking schizophrenia to autoimmune processes allows for investigation of more direct linkages to the microbiome.

DIET AND SCHIZOPHRENIA

The effect of diet on the microbiome is well established (David et al., 2014). Dietary changes as a risk factor for schizophrenia have been studied in immigrants; emigration from sub-Saharan African and Caribbean nations to the United Kingdom has been shown to be a risk factor for developing schizophrenia (Cantor-Graae and Selten, 2005). One hypothesis rooted in the microbiome asserts that the dramatic change in diet with such geographical movement could explain to some degree the variable incidence in schizophrenia in these migrants. The significantly lower consumption of wheat products in these populations as compared with those in developed countries is an example used to support this hypothesis. Multiple studies have documented immune dysregulation in individuals with schizophrenia, suggesting a heightened and prolonged immune response to certain antigens (Benros et al., 2014; Dimitrov et al., 2013; McAllister, 2014). The mechanisms of allergic responses to food antigens has been shown to be affected by changes to the gut flora (Kim and Sampson, 2012). Antigens from the diet, including bovine casein and gluten, are discussed here.

GLUTEN SENSITIVITY

Increased immune sensitivity to gluten has been described in schizophrenia since the 1950s (Cascella et al., 2011; Dickerson et al., 2010; Dohan, 1966; Dohan et al., 1984; Karlsson et al., 2012; Reichelt and Landmark, 1995; Singh and Kay, 1976), and the co-occurrence of schizophrenia with Celiac disease has been established. Celiac disease is an immune-mediated enteropathy triggered by gluten-containing grains including wheat, rye, and barley in genetically predisposed individuals (Briani et al., 2008). Epidemiologic data have shown a higher prevalence of Celiac disease among patients with schizophrenia in some studies (Cascella et al., 2011; Eaton et al., 2006); however, this is not universal (Ludvigsson et al., 2007; Peleg et al., 2004; West et al., 2006). In particular, Dohan spent his career investigating the epidemiology of schizophrenia, specifically the link with Celiac disease and wheat consumption. He discovered a direct correlation in the incidence of schizophrenia with wheat consumption across populations. Health registers show a relative risk of 3.2 for schizophrenia in individuals with an earlier diagnosis of Celiac disease whereas the relative risk for schizophrenia in individuals with a diagnosis of Crohn's disease and ulcerative colitis was 1.4 (Eaton et al., 2004).

Anti-tissue transglutaminase (anti-tTG), anti-endomysial antibodies, and anti-gliadin antibodies (AGA) are characteristic of Celiac disease. As we previously reported, several studies have shown increased sensitivity to gluten in schizophrenia patients based on AGA (Cascella et al., 2011; Dickerson et al., 2010; Jin et al., 2012; Okusaga et al., 2013). However, the immune response of patients with schizophrenia differs from that of patients with Celiac disease when specific classes of antibodies are evaluated. Using blood samples from the Clinical Antipsychotic Trials of Intervention Effectiveness (CATIE), it was found that 23.1% of the sample with schizophrenia had AGA but not anti-tTG antibodies compared with 3.1% of the comparison sample (Cascella et al., 2011). The difference in antigenic specificity has been replicated when immune responses to gluten have been studied in schizophrenia as compared with Celiac disease, shedding light on the consistently elevated AGA response in both diseases but the different response in transglutaminase antibodies pointing to both a shared and separate pathophysiology (Samaroo et al., 2010). Non-Celiac gluten sensitivity (NCGS) is recognized as a gluten-mediated disorder that is distinct from Celiac disease and a relationship between NCGS and neuropsychiatric disorders, including autism and schizophrenia, has also been demonstrated (Catassi et al., 2013).

BOVINE CASEIN SENSITIVITY

Bovine casein derived from milk products is another antigen capable of inducing a prolonged immune response. Increased levels of casein antibodies have been found in individuals with schizophrenia before and after diagnosis (Niebuhr et al., 2011; Severance et al., 2010). A study of 855 members of the US military discharged with a schizophrenia diagnosis and 1165 healthy controls demonstrated increased casein immunoglobulin G (IgG) antibody levels. Among those with a high initial level, casein IgG was predictive of an 18% increase in hazard ratio of schizophrenia (Niebuhr et al., 2011).

Increased intestinal permeability is one means by which gluten and casein antigens could gain entry into the systemic circulation and generate a humoral immune response (Severance et al., 2012). This may trigger an inflammatory cascade with the potential to affect brain structure and function (Carter, 2009). Given the evidence of a heightened immune reaction to gluten and bovine casein in schizophrenia patients, it is possible that these antigens are inducing an immune reaction that is detrimental to the brain. It is also possible that pathogenic antigens gain entry into the brain through defects in tight junctions that are present in the blood–brain barrier as well as the gut (Sun et al., 2004; Wu et al., 2010).

METABOLIC DYSFUNCTION AND SCHIZOPHRENIA

When comparing healthy subjects to those with diabetes and obesity, the microbiome appears to be significantly different in composition, and these changes correlate with blood glucose (Larsen et al., 2010; Turnbaugh et al., 2009). Animal studies have demonstrated that the gut flora can control how energy is extracted from the diet and how it is stored in the body (Turnbaugh et al., 2006). Changing the composition of gut flora can lead to disturbances in fat and sugar metabolism, driving metabolic syndrome, specifically obesity and insulin resistance (Bäckhed et al., 2007, 2004; Turnbaugh et al., 2006). Bacterial endotoxins, such as lipopolysaccharides, have long been known to be a primary driver of systemic inflammatory responses during infection. This inflammatory response also contributes to obesity and insulin resistance. More recently, the composition of the gut flora has been observed to modulate systemic exposure to bacterial endotoxins, and may, through associated inflammatory responses, represent a common link between metabolic syndrome and neurobehavioral syndromes, such as schizophrenia (Cani et al., 2008, 2007; Creely et al., 2007). Schizophrenia patients are at an increased risk for the development of metabolic syndrome due to intrinsic metabolic abnormalities (Ryan et al., 2003) and as a consequence of their antipsychotic treatment (Fan et al., 2013).

Elevations in serum proinflammatory cytokines have been found in schizophrenia patients when compared with controls (Francesconi et al., 2011; Kunz et al., 2011; Pedrini et al., 2012; Song et al., 2013), and the severity of clinical symptoms correlates with the level of inflammatory markers (Fan et al., 2007, 2010; Hope et al., 2013). Increasing evidence suggests the metabolic syndrome observed in many individuals with schizophrenia is associated with an upregulated inflammatory and immune process (Fan et al., 2010; Leonard et al., 2012; Miller et al., 2013). It is likely that changes in the microbiome influence the inflammatory status of these individuals, which puts them at risk for metabolic dysfunction. In GF animal models, normally protected from obesity, changes in gut flora alter risk of diet-induced obesity through changes in fatty acid metabolism (Bäckhed et al., 2007).

Although increased rates of metabolic dysfunction are present in antipsychotic-naïve individuals with schizophrenia, antipsychotic medication has been shown to further increase metabolic dysfunction. The weight gain induced by antipsychotics appears to be partially mediated by changes in the microbiome. For instance, when female rats were given olanzapine, an atypical antipsychotic known to cause metabolic dysfunction, significant changes in the bacterial composition of the gut microbiome were observed, including an increase in *Firmicutes* and decrease in *Bacteriodetes* (Davey et al., 2012). An associated increase in systemic inflammatory cytokines was also observed. Progress in dissecting the effects of disease pathology from those of antipsychotic treatment have been hindered by evidence showing that metabolic dysfunction occurs in schizophrenia patients who are not being treated with antipsychotic medications but who subsequently respond to treatment. Therefore the reputation of second-generation antipsychotics for causing metabolic syndrome is not as clearly demarcated as previously believed. Certain inflammatory markers, such as interleukin (IL)-1β, IL-6, and transforming growth factor-β, have been established to increase during acute exacerbations of psychotic symptoms and normalize in response to antipsychotic treatment, making them better state-related markers. Other inflammatory markers, such as IL-12, interferon-γ, tumor necrosis factor-α, and soluble IL receptor-2, appear to be better trait markers as their levels remain elevated even after antipsychotic treatment (Miller et al., 2011). A recent study reported variable cytokine levels in antipsychotic-naïve, first-episode schizophrenia patients, with only IL-10 significantly correlated with improvements in symptom scores (de Witte et al., 2014). These results indicate a deeper level of complexity involving the inflammatory response, the microbiota, and antipsychotic treatment in the development of the metabolic dysfunction seen in schizophrenia.

HYPOTHALAMIC-PITUITARY-ADRENAL AXIS

It is well known that stress disrupts the integrity of the GI tract (Collins and Bercik, 2009; Lambert, 2009; Söderholm and Perdue, 2001). High levels of stress in childhood and adulthood have also been well documented in patients with psychosis (Fisher et al., 2009; Laursen et al., 2007). One of the mechanisms by which physical and psychological stress increases intestinal permeability is through the increased secretion of corticotrophin-releasing hormone (CRH). The HPA axis is a vital part of normal functioning, controlling physiological responses to a wide range of stresses. CRH modulates gut neuroimmune responses via mucosal immune cells and inflammatory mediators, which contribute to disruption of the intestinal barrier (Al-Sadi and Ma, 2007; Keita et al., 2010; Saunders et al., 2002; Turner, 2009). A recent meta-analysis reviewed studies using models of social stress to investigate HPA axis response. Whereas individuals with schizophrenia had a normal cortisol production rate, their cortisol levels were lower than controls in anticipation of and after exposure to social stress (Ciufolini et al., 2014). Another recent meta-analysis showed a small but consistent finding of increased morning cortisol levels in schizophrenia patients, more so in those with an established diagnosis (Girshkin et al., 2014). An enhanced HPA axis response to stress may contribute to the biological vulnerability to psychosis through direct effects on the CNS and indirect effects on the intestinal tract.

MICROBIOTA-GUT-BRAIN INTERVENTIONS IN SCHIZOPHRENIA
DIET

Seven clinical trials have been published examining the effects of a gluten-free diet on schizophrenia symptoms (Kalaydjian et al., 2006). These early studies included schizophrenia patients who had not been tested for antibodies, and they had variable outcomes. Nonetheless, resolution of schizophrenia symptoms after initiation of a gluten-free diet has been described in case reports (De Santis et al., 1997; Jackson et al., 2012; Jansson et al., 1984; Kraft and Westman, 2009). There are also at least two current trials underway investigating the effects of gluten removal on schizophrenia symptoms in AGA-positive individuals. Data from these trials and future studies are needed to determine the effect of a gluten-free diet on the subpopulation of people with schizophrenia who are sensitive to gluten. An investigation in 1973 identified earlier hospital discharge rates for relapsed schizophrenia patients fed a cereal-free, milk-free diet (Dohan and Grasberger, 1973); however, the effect of a casein-free diet in isolation on schizophrenia has yet to be investigated.

The bacterial metabolite butyrate, a short-chain fatty acid and known histone deacetylase inhibitor, is produced by gut bacteria and has been shown to be effective in reversing phencyclidine (PCP)-induced behavioral abnormalities in animal models of schizophrenia (Aoyama et al., 2014). Butyrate was shown to attenuate decreases in histone acetylation and in expression of gamma-aminobutyric acid-related genes induced by PCP treatment in the prefrontal cortex.

ANTIMICROBIALS

Alteration of the gut commensal microbiota with antibiotics has been shown to modify the susceptibility to autoimmune demyelinating processes of the CNS, such as those seen in multiple sclerosis (Ochoa-Repáraz et al., 2009). The protection afforded by antimicrobials is associated with a shift in the immune response from T helper (Th)-1/Th17 toward antiinflammatory Th2-type responses (Ochoa-Repáraz et al., 2010). Minocycline, a second-generation tetracycline, is currently under investigation as an adjunct treatment in schizophrenia. To date there has been some early evidence of its efficacy in treating negative symptoms (Jhamnani et al., 2013; Khodaie-Ardakani et al., 2014; Liu et al., 2014) and treatment-resistant schizophrenia (Qurashi et al., 2014). Although tetracycline is believed to have a neuroprotective effect due to its antiinflammatory action and ability to enhance glutamate neuro-transmission (Liu et al., 2014), its immunomodulatory properties as mediated by gut microbiota have yet to be investigated and may play a role.

PREBIOTICS

Prebiotics have also been explored as an avenue for modulating BDNF and NMDA receptors, previously shown to be modulated with probiotics and known to play a role in the pathophysiology of schizophrenia. Fructo-oligosaccharide and galacto-oligosaccharides are known soluble fibers and prebiotics, that when digested by gut bacteria, are associated with proliferation of specific species. Prebiotics have been associated with increased hippocampal BDNF and NMDA receptor subunits, which correlated with anxiolytic and improved cognitive function effects (Savignac et al., 2013). A recent study showed that *Bifidobacterium breve* raises fatty acid concentrations in the brain (Wall et al., 2012). Arachadonic acid and docohexaenoic acid play important roles in neurodevelopmental processes and are of particular significance to individuals with schizophrenia, as relatively low levels have been reported in this population (McNamara, 2011). There is some evidence that supplementation with omega-3 fatty acids improves symptoms in schizophrenia (Stafford et al., 2013).

PROBIOTICS

There is promising clinical evidence to support a role of probiotic interventions in reducing anxiety, decreasing the stress response, and improving mood in animal (Arseneault-Bréard et al., 2012; Bravo et al., 2011; Messaoudi et al., 2011) and human studies (Logan and Katzman, 2005; Messaoudi et al., 2011; Rao et al., 2009). The mechanisms underlying these effects are not known, but it has been hypothesized that reductions in the effects of proinflammatory cytokines and modification of nutritional status through direct effects of B vitamins, omega-3 fatty acids, and minerals may play a role (Cryan and O'Mahony, 2011; Logan and Katzman, 2005). Probiotics have also been found to improve lactose digestion, which may reduce the interference that high intestinal lactose concentrations have on serotonin availability through effects on L-tryptophan metabolism (Ledochowski et al., 1998). Because patients with schizophrenia often suffer from an increased stress response, compromised nutritional status, increased inflammatory status, and lactose sensitivity, probiotic interventions have promising therapeutic potential.

One probiotic that has shown to positively affect neuronal function in an animal model is VSL#3. This is thought to occur through its effects on long-term potentiation (LTP), the mechanism underlying neural plasticity. Neural plasticity is a vital quality of the human brain, allowing neurons in the brain to change functionally in response to a stimulus or stress. LTP describes the ability for neural synapses to change chemically in response to activity, either strengthening or weakening connections with other neurons. This mechanism is altered in schizophrenia through several pathways, including dysfunction of NMDA receptors, abnormalities in activity-dependent genes, and disturbances in cortical excitability (Hasan et al., 2011). LTP has successfully been modulated through the use of the probiotic mixture,

VSL#3. Middle-aged rats with deficits in hippocampal LTP treated with VSL#3 displayed changes in their intestinal microbiota and gene expression in brain tissue and improvements in LTP (Distrutti et al., 2014). However, whether VSL#3 could be of benefit in schizophrenia-related LTP dysfunction has yet to be studied.

Probiotic interventions have been shown to improve obesity-associated dyslipidemia and insulin resistance in animal models (Yu et al., 2013) and reduce weight gain and fat mass (Ji et al., 2012). Oral administration of *Lactobacillus gasseri* SBT2055 in healthy overweight humans has been found to reduce abdominal visceral and subcutaneous fat (Kadooka et al., 2010). The antiobesity effects of probiotics may have therapeutic potential for patients with schizophrenia given their higher risk metabolic profile. A recent study in rats reported that co-administration of antibiotics attenuated olanzapine-induced alterations in the microbiota and olanzapine-induced metabolic disturbances including weight gain, visceral fat deposition, elevated plasma free fatty acids, and macrophage infiltration of adipose tissue (Davey et al., 2013). These findings suggest that the microbiota might be a novel treatment target for metabolic co-morbidity in patients with schizophrenia.

To date there has been one randomized control trial exploring the effects of probiotic supplementation on schizophrenia symptoms (Dickerson et al., 2014). In this trial 65 outpatients with schizophrenia were assigned to 14 weeks of adjunctive probiotic (combined *Lactobacillus rhamnosus* strain GG and *Bifidobacterium animalis* subsp. lactis strain Bb12) or placebo therapy. No difference was found in the PANSS between the two groups, although patients in the probiotic group were less likely to develop severe bowel difficulty over the course of the trial. The patients in this trial were chronically ill with a mean duration of illness of over 25 years. It is possible that trials focusing on patients presenting earlier in their course of illness may yield different results, as might trials that provide longer probiotic supplementation.

FECAL MICROBIAL TRANSPLANTATION

Although probiotics and antibiotics may be the best known and commercially available options to treat GI dysbiosis, fecal microbiota transplantation is an old procedure that has been rediscovered as a cutting-edge option for the restoration of gut microbiota. There has been growing interest in the use of fecal microbiota transplantation for the treatment of patients with chronic GI infections and inflammatory bowel diseases. There has also been interest of late in its therapeutic potential for extraintestinal conditions including cardiometabolic disease and autoimmune disorders (Smits et al., 2013). A better understanding of the microbiome in schizophrenia needs to be gained before the therapeutic potential of fecal transplantation can be explored.

SUMMARY

This chapter summarizes several pathways in which the gut-brain axis functions to affect the symptoms and course of schizophrenia. These pathways represent a subset of known pathways and likely an even smaller subset of those that have yet to be uncovered. Those of significance include gut permeability, infection and autoimmunity, diet and food antigens, metabolic dysfunction, and HPA axis activity. We also explored current and future areas of intervention including changes to diet; micro- and macronutrients; the role of antibiotics, pre-, and probiotics; and the expanding application of fecal transplantation. All of these topics serve to illustrate the diverse manifestation of the gut-brain axis and its specific effect on a complex syndrome. Although studies continue to reveal an altered microbiome in patients with schizophrenia as compared with controls (Yolken and Dickerson, 2014), the conclusion should be clear: the role of the gut-brain axis in schizophrenia is real and deserves continued attention. Further integration into practice is warranted to improve the care offered to patients who suffer from this illness.

REFERENCES

Al-Sadi, R.M., Ma, T.Y., 2007. IL-1beta causes an increase in intestinal epithelial tight junction permeability. J. Immunol. Baltim. Md. 1950 (178), 4641–4649.

American Psychiatric Association, DSM-5 Task Force, 2013. Diagnostic and Statistical Manual of Mental Disorders: DSM-5.

Aoyama, Y., Mouri, A., Toriumi, K., Koseki, T., Narusawa, S., Ikawa, N., Mamiya, T., Nagai, T., Yamada, K., Nabeshima, T., 2014. Clozapine ameliorates epigenetic and behavioral abnormalities induced by phencyclidine through activation of dopamine D1 receptor. Int. J. Neuropsychopharmacol. Off. Sci. J. Coll. Int. Neuropsychopharmacol. CINP 17, 723–737. http://dx.doi.org/10.1017/S1461145713001466.

Arseneault-Bréard, J., Rondeau, I., Gilbert, K., Girard, S.-A., Tompkins, T.A., Godbout, R., Rousseau, G., 2012. Combination of *Lactobacillus helveticus* R0052 and *Bifidobacterium longum* R0175 reduces post-myocardial infarction depression symptoms and restores intestinal permeability in a rat model. Br. J. Nutr. 107, 1793–1799. http://dx.doi.org/10.1017/S0007114511005137.

Artis, D., 2008. Epithelial-cell recognition of commensal bacteria and maintenance of immune homeostasis in the gut. Nat. Rev. Immunol. 8, 411–420. http://dx.doi.org/10.1038/nri2316.

Babenko, O., Kovalchuk, I., Metz, G.A.S., 2014. Stress-induced perinatal and transgenerational epigenetic programming of brain development and mental health. Neurosci. Biobehav. Rev. 48C, 70–91. http://dx.doi.org/10.1016/j.neubiorev.2014.11.013.

Bäckhed, F., Ding, H., Wang, T., Hooper, L.V., Koh, G.Y., Nagy, A., Semenkovich, C.F., Gordon, J.I., 2004. The gut microbiota as an environmental factor that regulates fat storage. Proc. Natl. Acad. Sci. U. S. A. 101, 15718–15723. http://dx.doi.org/10.1073/pnas.0407076101.

Bäckhed, F., Manchester, J.K., Semenkovich, C.F., Gordon, J.I., 2007. Mechanisms underlying the resistance to diet-induced obesity in germ-free mice. Proc. Natl. Acad. Sci. U. S. A. 104, 979–984. http://dx.doi.org/10.1073/pnas.0605374104.

Benros, M.E., Eaton, W.W., Mortensen, P.B., 2014. The epidemiologic evidence linking autoimmune diseases and psychosis. Biol. Psychiatry 75, 300–306. http://dx.doi.org/10.1016/j.biopsych.2013.09.023.

Benros, M.E., Mortensen, P.B., Eaton, W.W., 2012. Autoimmune diseases and infections as risk factors for schizophrenia. Ann. N. Y. Acad. Sci. 1262, 56–66. http://dx.doi.org/10.1111/j.1749-6632.2012.06638.x.

Bereswill, S., Muñoz, M., Fischer, A., Plickert, R., Haag, L.-M., Otto, B., Kühl, A.A., Loddenkemper, C., Göbel, U.B., Heimesaat, M.M., 2010. Anti-inflammatory effects of resveratrol, curcumin and simvastatin in acute small intestinal inflammation. PLoS One 5, e15099. http://dx.doi.org/10.1371/journal.pone.0015099.

Bilder, R.M., Goldman, R.S., Robinson, D., Reiter, G., Bell, L., Bates, J.A., Pappadopulos, E., Willson, D.F., Alvir, J.M., Woerner, M.G., Geisler, S., Kane, J.M., Lieberman, J.A., 2000. Neuropsychology of first-episode schizophrenia: initial characterization and clinical correlates. Am. J. Psychiatry 157, 549–559.

Bleich, A., Brown, S.L., Kahn, R., van Praag, H.M., 1988. The role of serotonin in schizophrenia. Schizophr. Bull. 14, 297–315.

Bravo, J.A., Forsythe, P., Chew, M.V., Escaravage, E., Savignac, H.M., Dinan, T.G., Bienenstock, J., Cryan, J.F., 2011. Ingestion of *Lactobacillus* strain regulates emotional behavior and central GABA receptor expression in a mouse via the vagus nerve. Proc. Natl. Acad. Sci. U. S. A. 108, 16050–16055. http://dx.doi.org/10.1073/pnas.1102999108.

Briani, C., Samaroo, D., Alaedini, A., 2008. Celiac disease: from gluten to autoimmunity. Autoimmun. Rev. 7, 644–650. http://dx.doi.org/10.1016/j.autrev.2008.05.006.

Buscaino, V., 1953. Patologia extraneurale della schizofrenia. Fegato, tubo digerente, sistema reticolo-endoteliale. Acta Neurol. (Napoli) VIII 1–60.

Cani, P.D., Amar, J., Iglesias, M.A., Poggi, M., Knauf, C., Bastelica, D., Neyrinck, A.M., Fava, F., Tuohy, K.M., Chabo, C., Waget, A., Delmée, E., Cousin, B., Sulpice, T., Chamontin, B., Ferrières, J., Tanti, J.-F., Gibson, G.R., Casteilla, L., Delzenne, N.M., Alessi, M.C., Burcelin, R., 2007. Metabolic endotoxemia initiates obesity and insulin resistance. Diabetes 56, 1761–1772. http://dx.doi.org/10.2337/db06-1491.

Cani, P.D., Bibiloni, R., Knauf, C., Waget, A., Neyrinck, A.M., Delzenne, N.M., Burcelin, R., 2008. Changes in gut microbiota control metabolic endotoxemia-induced inflammation in high-fat diet-induced obesity and diabetes in mice. Diabetes 57, 1470–1481. http://dx.doi.org/10.2337/db07-1403.

Cantor-Graae, E., Selten, J.-P., 2005. Schizophrenia and migration: a meta-analysis and review. Am. J. Psychiatry 162, 12–24. http://dx.doi.org/10.1176/appi.ajp.162.1.12.

Carter, C.J., 2009. Schizophrenia susceptibility genes directly implicated in the life cycles of pathogens: cytomegalovirus, influenza, herpes simplex, rubella, and *Toxoplasma gondii*. Schizophr. Bull. 35, 1163–1182. http://dx.doi.org/10.1093/schbul/sbn054.

Cascella, N.G., Kryszak, D., Bhatti, B., Gregory, P., Kelly, D.L., Mc Evoy, J.P., Fasano, A., Eaton, W.W., 2011. Prevalence of celiac disease and gluten sensitivity in the United States clinical antipsychotic trials of intervention effectiveness study population. Schizophr. Bull. 37, 94–100. http://dx.doi.org/10.1093/schbul/sbp055.

Catassi, C., Bai, J.C., Bonaz, B., Bouma, G., Calabrò, A., Carroccio, A., Castillejo, G., Ciacci, C., Cristofori, F., Dolinsek, J., Francavilla, R., Elli, L., Green, P., Holtmeier, W., Koehler, P., Koletzko, S., Meinhold, C., Sanders, D., Schumann, M., Schuppan, D., Ullrich, R., Vécsei, A., Volta, U., Zevallos, V., Sapone, A., Fasano, A., 2013. Non-celiac gluten sensitivity: the new frontier of gluten related disorders. Nutrients 5, 3839–3853. http://dx.doi.org/10.3390/nu5103839.

Ciufolini, S., Dazzan, P., Kempton, M.J., Pariante, C., Mondelli, V., 2014. HPA axis response to social stress is attenuated in schizophrenia but normal in depression: evidence from a meta-analysis of existing studies. Neurosci. Biobehav. Rev. 47, 359–368. http://dx.doi.org/10.1016/j.neubiorev.2014.09.004.

Clarke, G., Grenham, S., Scully, P., Fitzgerald, P., Moloney, R.D., Shanahan, F., Dinan, T.G., Cryan, J.F., 2013. The microbiome-gut-brain axis during early life regulates the hippocampal serotonergic system in a sex-dependent manner. Mol. Psychiatry 18, 666–673. http://dx.doi.org/10.1038/mp.2012.77.

Collins, S.M., Bercik, P., 2009. The relationship between intestinal microbiota and the central nervous system in normal gastrointestinal function and disease. Gastroenterology 136, 2003–2014. http://dx.doi.org/10.1053/j.gastro.2009.01.075.

Coyle, J.T., 2012. NMDA receptor and schizophrenia: a brief history. Schizophr. Bull. 38, 920–926. http://dx.doi.org/10.1093/schbul/sbs076.

Craven, M., Egan, C.E., Dowd, S.E., McDonough, S.P., Dogan, B., Denkers, E.Y., Bowman, D., Scherl, E.J., Simpson, K.W., 2012. Inflammation drives dysbiosis and bacterial invasion in murine models of ileal Crohn's disease. PLoS One 7, e41594. http://dx.doi.org/10.1371/journal.pone.0041594.

Creely, S.J., McTernan, P.G., Kusminski, C.M., Fisher, ff M., Da Silva, N.F., Khanolkar, M., Evans, M., Harte, A.L., Kumar, S., 2007. Lipopolysaccharide activates an innate immune system response in human adipose tissue in obesity and type 2 diabetes. Am. J. Physiol. Endocrinol. Metab. 292, E740–E747. http://dx.doi.org/10.1152/ajpendo.00302.2006.

Cryan, J.F., O'Mahony, S.M., 2011. The microbiome-gut-brain axis: from bowel to behavior. Neurogastroenterol. Motil. Off. J. Eur. Gastrointest. Motil. Soc. 23, 187–192. http://dx.doi.org/10.1111/j.1365-2982.2010.01664.x.

Davey, K.J., Cotter, P.D., O'Sullivan, O., Crispie, F., Dinan, T.G., Cryan, J.F., O'Mahony, S.M., 2013. Antipsychotics and the gut microbiome: olanzapine-induced metabolic dysfunction is attenuated by antibiotic administration in the rat. Transl. Psychiatry 3, e309. http://dx.doi.org/10.1038/tp.2013.83.

Davey, K.J., O'Mahony, S.M., Schellekens, H., O'Sullivan, O., Bienenstock, J., Cotter, P.D., Dinan, T.G., Cryan, J.F., 2012. Gender-dependent consequences of chronic olanzapine in the rat: effects on body weight, inflammatory, metabolic and microbiota parameters. Psychopharmacology (Berl.) 221, 155–169. http://dx.doi.org/10.1007/s00213-011-2555-2.

David, L.A., Maurice, C.F., Carmody, R.N., Gootenberg, D.B., Button, J.E., Wolfe, B.E., Ling, A.V., Devlin, A.S., Varma, Y., Fischbach, M.A., Biddinger, S.B., Dutton, R.J., Turnbaugh, P.J., 2014. Diet rapidly and reproducibly alters the human gut microbiome. Nature 505, 559–563. http://dx.doi.org/10.1038/nature12820.

De Santis, A., Addolorato, G., Romito, A., Caputo, S., Giordano, A., Gambassi, G., Taranto, C., Manna, R., Gasbarrini, G., 1997. Schizophrenic symptoms and SPECT abnormalities in a coeliac patient: regression after a gluten-free diet. J. Intern. Med. 242, 421–423.

Diaz Heijtz, R., Wang, S., Anuar, F., Qian, Y., Björkholm, B., Samuelsson, A., Hibberd, M.L., Forssberg, H., Pettersson, S., 2011. Normal gut microbiota modulates brain development and behavior. Proc. Natl. Acad. Sci. U. S. A. 108, 3047–3052. http://dx.doi.org/10.1073/pnas.1010529108.

Dickerson, F., Stallings, C., Origoni, A., Vaughan, C., Khushalani, S., Leister, F., Yang, S., Krivogorsky, B., Alaedini, A., Yolken, R., 2010. Markers of gluten sensitivity and celiac disease in recent-onset psychosis and multi-episode schizophrenia. Biol. Psychiatry 68, 100–104. http://dx.doi.org/10.1016/j.biopsych.2010.03.021.

Dickerson, F.B., Stallings, C., Origoni, A., Katsafanas, E., Savage, C., Schweinfurth, L., Goga, J., Khushalani, S., Yolken, R.H., 2014. Effect of probiotic supplementation on schizophrenia symptoms and association with gastrointestinal functioning: a randomized, placebo-controlled trial. Prim Care Companion CNS Disord. 16 (1). http://dx.doi.org/10.4088/PCC.13m01579.

Dimitrov, D.H., Lee, S., Yantis, J., Valdez, C., Paredes, R.M., Braida, N., Velligan, D., Walss-Bass, C., 2013. Differential correlations between inflammatory cytokines and psychopathology in veterans with schizophrenia: potential role for IL-17 pathway. Schizophr. Res. 151, 29–35. http://dx.doi.org/10.1016/j.schres.2013.10.019.

Distrutti, E., O'Reilly, J.-A., McDonald, C., Cipriani, S., Renga, B., Lynch, M.A., Fiorucci, S., 2014. Modulation of intestinal microbiota by the probiotic VSL#3 resets brain gene expression and ameliorates the age-related deficit in LTP. PLoS One 9, e106503. http://dx.doi.org/10.1371/journal.pone.0106503.

Dohan, F.C., 1966. Wheat "consumption" and hospital admissions for schizophrenia during World War II. A preliminary report. Am. J. Clin. Nutr. 18, 7–10.

Dohan, F.C., Grasberger, J.C., 1973. Relapsed schizophrenics: earlier discharge from the hospital after cereal-free, milk-free diet. Am. J. Psychiatry 130, 685–688.

Dohan, F.C., Harper, E.H., Clark, M.H., Rodrigue, R.B., Zigas, V., 1984. Is schizophrenia rare if grain is rare? Biol. Psychiatry 19, 385–399.

Dominguez-Bello, M.G., Costello, E.K., Contreras, M., Magris, M., Hidalgo, G., Fierer, N., Knight, R., 2010. Delivery mode shapes the acquisition and structure of the initial microbiota across multiple body habitats in newborns. Proc. Natl. Acad. Sci. U. S. A. 107, 11971–11975. http://dx.doi.org/10.1073/pnas.1002601107.

Dong, E., Dzitoyeva, S.G., Matrisciano, F., Tueting, P., Grayson, D.R., Guidotti, A., 2014. Brain-derived neurotrophic factor epigenetic modifications associated with schizophrenia-like phenotype induced by prenatal stress in mice. Biol. Psychiatry 77 (6), 589–596. http://dx.doi.org/10.1016/j.biopsych.2014.08.012.

Douglas-Escobar, M., Elliott, E., Neu, J., 2013. Effect of intestinal microbial ecology on the developing brain. JAMA Pediatr. 167, 374–379. http://dx.doi.org/10.1001/jamapediatrics.2013.497.

Eaton, W., Mortensen, P.B., Agerbo, E., Byrne, M., Mors, O., Ewald, H., 2004. Coeliac disease and schizophrenia: population based case control study with linkage of Danish national registers. BMJ 328, 438–439.

Eaton, W.W., Byrne, M., Ewald, H., Mors, O., Chen, C.-Y., Agerbo, E., Mortensen, P.B., 2006. Association of schizophrenia and autoimmune diseases: linkage of Danish national registers. Am. J. Psychiatry 163, 521–528. http://dx.doi.org/10.1176/appi.ajp.163.3.521.

Erridge, C., Duncan, S.H., Bereswill, S., Heimesaat, M.M., 2010. The induction of colitis and ileitis in mice is associated with marked increases in intestinal concentrations of stimulants of TLRs 2, 4, and 5. PLoS One 5, e9125. http://dx.doi.org/10.1371/journal.pone.0009125.

Fanning, A.S., Mitic, L.L., Anderson, J.M., 1999. Transmembrane proteins in the tight junction barrier. J. Am. Soc. Nephrol. JASN 10, 1337–1345.

Fan, X., Borba, C.P.C., Copeland, P., Hayden, D., Freudenreich, O., Goff, D.C., Henderson, D.C., 2013. Metabolic effects of adjunctive aripiprazole in clozapine-treated patients with schizophrenia. Acta Psychiatr. Scand. 127, 217–226. http://dx.doi.org/10.1111/acps.12009.

Fan, X., Liu, E.Y., Freudenreich, O., Park, J.H., Liu, D., Wang, J., Yi, Z., Goff, D., Henderson, D.C., 2010. Higher white blood cell counts are associated with an increased risk for metabolic syndrome and more severe psychopathology in non-diabetic patients with schizophrenia. Schizophr. Res. 118, 211–217. http://dx.doi.org/10.1016/j.schres.2010.02.1028.

Fan, X., Pristach, C., Liu, E.Y., Freudenreich, O., Henderson, D.C., Goff, D.C., 2007. Elevated serum levels of C-reactive protein are associated with more severe psychopathology in a subgroup of patients with schizophrenia. Psychiatry Res. 149, 267–271. http://dx.doi.org/10.1016/j.psychres.2006.07.011.

Fineberg, A.M., Ellman, L.M., 2013. Inflammatory cytokines and neurological and neurocognitive alterations in the course of schizophrenia. Biol. Psychiatry 73, 951–966. http://dx.doi.org/10.1016/j.biopsych.2013.01.001.

Fisher, H., Morgan, C., Dazzan, P., Craig, T.K., Morgan, K., Hutchinson, G., Jones, P.B., Doody, G.A., Pariante, C., McGuffin, P., Murray, R.M., Leff, J., Fearon, P., 2009. Gender differences in the association between childhood abuse and psychosis. Br. J. Psychiatry J. Ment. Sci. 194, 319–325. http://dx.doi.org/10.1192/bjp.bp.107.047985.

Francesconi, L.P., Ceresér, K.M., Mascarenhas, R., Stertz, L., Gama, C.S., Belmonte-de-Abreu, P., 2011. Increased annexin-V and decreased TNF-α serum levels in chronic-medicated patients with schizophrenia. Neurosci. Lett. 502, 143–146. http://dx.doi.org/10.1016/j.neulet.2011.06.042.

Gareau, M.G., Wine, E., Rodrigues, D.M., Cho, J.H., Whary, M.T., Philpott, D.J., Macqueen, G., Sherman, P.M., 2011. Bacterial infection causes stress-induced memory dysfunction in mice. Gut 60, 307–317. http://dx.doi.org/10.1136/gut.2009.202515.

Gatkowska, J., Wieczorek, M., Dziadek, B., Dzitko, K., Dlugonska, H., 2012. Behavioral changes in mice caused by *Toxoplasma gondii* invasion of brain. Parasitol. Res. 111, 53–58. http://dx.doi.org/10.1007/s00436-011-2800-y.

Girshkin, L., Matheson, S.L., Shepherd, A.M., Green, M.J., 2014. Morning cortisol levels in schizophrenia and bipolar disorder: a meta-analysis. Psychoneuroendocrinology 49, 187–206. http://dx.doi.org/10.1016/j.psyneuen.2014.07.013.

Hand, T.W., Dos Santos, L.M., Bouladoux, N., Molloy, M.J., Pagán, A.J., Pepper, M., Maynard, C.L., Elson 3rd, C.O., Belkaid, Y., 2012. Acute gastrointestinal infection induces long-lived microbiota-specific T cell responses. Science 337, 1553–1556. http://dx.doi.org/10.1126/science.1220961.

Hasan, A., Nitsche, M.A., Rein, B., Schneider-Axmann, T., Guse, B., Gruber, O., Falkai, P., Wobrock, T., 2011. Dysfunctional long-term potentiation-like plasticity in schizophrenia revealed by transcranial direct current stimulation. Behav. Brain Res. 224, 15–22. http://dx.doi.org/10.1016/j.bbr.2011.05.017.

Hemmings, G., 2004. Schizophrenia. Lancet 364, 1312–1313. http://dx.doi.org/10.1016/S0140-6736(04)17181-X.

Hope, S., Ueland, T., Steen, N.E., Dieset, I., Lorentzen, S., Berg, A.O., Agartz, I., Aukrust, P., Andreassen, O.A., 2013. Interleukin 1 receptor antagonist and soluble tumor necrosis factor receptor 1 are associated with general severity and psychotic symptoms in schizophrenia and bipolar disorder. Schizophr. Res. 145, 36–42. http://dx.doi.org/10.1016/j.schres.2012.12.023.

Ibi, D., Nagai, T., Nabeshima, T., Yamada, K., 2011. [PolyI: C-induced neurodevelopmental animal model for schizophrenia]. Nihon Shinkei Seishin Yakurigaku Zasshi 31, 201–207.

Jackson, J., Eaton, W., Cascella, N., Fasano, A., Warfel, D., Feldman, S., Richardson, C., Vyas, G., Linthicum, J., Santora, D., Warren, K.R., Carpenter Jr., W.T., Kelly, D.L., 2012. A gluten-free diet in people with schizophrenia and anti-tissue transglutaminase or anti-gliadin antibodies. Schizophr. Res. 140, 262–263. http://dx.doi.org/10.1016/j.schres.2012.06.011.

Jansson, B., Kristjánsson, E., Nilsson, L., 1984. [Schizophrenic psychosis disappearing after patient is given gluten-free diet]. Läkartidningen 81, 448–449.

Jhamnani, K., Shivakumar, V., Kalmady, S., Rao, N.P., Venkatasubramanian, G., 2013. Successful use of add-on minocycline for treatment of persistent negative symptoms in schizophrenia. J. Neuropsychiatry Clin. Neurosci. 25 (1), E06–E07. http://dx.doi.org/10.1176/appi.neuropsych.11120376.

Jin, S.-Z., Wu, N., Xu, Q., Zhang, X., Ju, G.-Z., Law, M.H., Wei, J., 2012. A study of circulating gliadin antibodies in schizophrenia among a Chinese population. Schizophr. Bull. 38, 514–518. http://dx.doi.org/10.1093/schbul/sbq111.

Ji, Y.S., Kim, H.N., Park, H.J., Lee, J.E., Yeo, S.Y., Yang, J.S., Park, S.Y., Yoon, H.S., Cho, G.S., Franz, C.M.A.P., Bomba, A., Shin, H.K., Holzapfel, W.H., 2012. Modulation of the murine microbiome with a concomitant anti-obesity effect by *Lactobacillus rhamnosus* GG and *Lactobacillus sakei* NR28. Benef. Microbe. 3, 13–22. http://dx.doi.org/10.3920/BM2011.0046.

John, L.J., Fromm, M., Schulzke, J.-D., 2011. Epithelial barriers in intestinal inflammation. Antioxid. Redox Signal. 15, 1255–1270. http://dx.doi.org/10.1089/ars.2011.3892.

Kadooka, Y., Sato, M., Imaizumi, K., Ogawa, A., Ikuyama, K., Akai, Y., Okano, M., Kagoshima, M., Tsuchida, T., 2010. Regulation of abdominal adiposity by probiotics (*Lactobacillus gasseri* SBT2055) in adults with obese tendencies in a randomized controlled trial. Eur. J. Clin. Nutr. 64, 636–643. http://dx.doi.org/10.1038/ejcn.2010.19.

Kalaydjian, A.E., Eaton, W., Cascella, N., Fasano, A., 2006. The gluten connection: the association between schizophrenia and celiac disease. Acta Psychiatr. Scand. 113, 82–90. http://dx.doi.org/10.1111/j.1600-0447.2005.00687.x.

Karlsson, H., Blomström, Å., Wicks, S., Yang, S., Yolken, R.H., Dalman, C., 2012. Maternal antibodies to dietary antigens and risk for nonaffective psychosis in offspring. Am. J. Psychiatry 169, 625–632. http://dx.doi.org/10.1176/appi.ajp.2012.11081197.

Keita, A.V., Söderholm, J.D., Ericson, A.-C., 2010. Stress-induced barrier disruption of rat follicle-associated epithelium involves corticotropin-releasing hormone, acetylcholine, substance P, and mast cells. Neurogastroenterol. Motil. Off. J. Eur. Gastrointest. Motil. Soc. 22, 770–778, e221–e222. http://dx.doi.org/10.1111/j.1365-2982.2010.01471.x.

Khodaie-Ardakani, M.-R., Mirshafiee, O., Farokhnia, M., Tajdini, M., Hosseini, S.-M.-R., Modabbernia, A., Rezaei, A., Salehi, B., Yekehtaz, H., Ashrafi, M., Tabrizi, M., Akhondzadeh, S., 2014. Minocycline add-on to risperidone for treatment of negative symptoms in patients with stable schizophrenia: randomized double-blind placebo-controlled study. Psychiatry Res. 215 (3), 540–546. http://dx.doi.org/10.1016/j.psychres.2013.12.051.

Kim, J.S., Sampson, H.A., 2012. Food allergy: a glimpse into the inner workings of gut immunology. Curr. Opin. Gastroenterol. 28, 99–103. http://dx.doi.org/10.1097/MOG.0b013e32834e7b60.

Kohm, A.P., Fuller, K.G., Miller, S.D., 2003. Mimicking the way to autoimmunity: an evolving theory of sequence and structural homology. Trends Microbiol. 11, 101–105.

Kraft, B.D., Westman, E.C., 2009. Schizophrenia, gluten, and low-carbohydrate, ketogenic diets: a case report and review of the literature. Nutr. Metab. 6, 10. http://dx.doi.org/10.1186/1743-7075-6-10.

Kunz, M., Ceresér, K.M., Goi, P.D., Fries, G.R., Teixeira, A.L., Fernandes, B.S., Belmonte-de-Abreu, P.S., Kauer-Sant'Anna, M., Kapczinski, F., Gama, C.S., 2011. Serum levels of IL-6, IL-10 and TNF-α in patients with bipolar disorder and schizophrenia: differences in pro- and anti-inflammatory balance. Rev. Bras. Psiquiatr. 33, 268–274.

Lambert, G.P., 2009. Stress-induced gastrointestinal barrier dysfunction and its inflammatory effects. J. Anim. Sci. 87, E101–E108. http://dx.doi.org/10.2527/jas.2008-1339.

Larsen, N., Vogensen, F.K., van den Berg, F.W.J., Nielsen, D.S., Andreasen, A.S., Pedersen, B.K., Al-Soud, W.A., Sørensen, S.J., Hansen, L.H., Jakobsen, M., 2010. Gut microbiota in human adults with type 2 diabetes differs from non-diabetic adults. PLoS One 5, e9085. http://dx.doi.org/10.1371/journal.pone.0009085.

Laursen, T.M., Munk-Olsen, T., Nordentoft, M., Bo Mortensen, P., 2007. A comparison of selected risk factors for unipolar depressive disorder, bipolar affective disorder, schizoaffective disorder, and schizophrenia from a Danish population-based cohort. J. Clin. Psychiatry 68, 1673–1681.

Ledochowski, M., Sperner-Unterweger, B., Fuchs, D., 1998. Lactose malabsorption is associated with early signs of mental depression in females: a preliminary report. Dig. Dis. Sci. 43, 2513–2517.

Leonard, B.E., Schwarz, M., Myint, A.M., 2012. The metabolic syndrome in schizophrenia: is inflammation a contributing cause? J. Psychopharmacol. Oxf. Engl. 26, 33–41. http://dx.doi.org/10.1177/0269881111431622.

Liu, F., Guo, X., Wu, R., Ou, J., Zheng, Y., Zhang, B., Xie, L., Zhang, L., Yang, L., Yang, S., Yang, J., Ruan, Y., Zeng, Y., Xu, X., Zhao, J., 2014. Minocycline supplementation for treatment of negative symptoms in early-phase schizophrenia: a double blind, randomized, controlled trial. Schizophr. Res. 153 (1), 169–176.

Logan, A.C., Katzman, M., 2005. Major depressive disorder: probiotics may be an adjuvant therapy. Med. Hypotheses 64, 533–538. http://dx.doi.org/10.1016/j.mehy.2004.08.019.

Ludvigsson, J.F., Osby, U., Ekbom, A., Montgomery, S.M., 2007. Coeliac disease and risk of schizophrenia and other psychosis: a general population cohort study. Scand. J. Gastroenterol. 42, 179–185. http://dx.doi.org/10.1080/00365520600863472.

McAllister, A.K., 2014. Major histocompatibility complex I in brain development and schizophrenia. Biol. Psychiatry 75, 262–268. http://dx.doi.org/10.1016/j.biopsych.2013.10.003.

McNamara, R.K., 2011. Omega-3 fatty acid deficiency: a preventable risk factor for schizophrenia? Schizophr. Res. 129, 215–216. http://dx.doi.org/10.1016/j.schres.2010.12.017.

Messaoudi, M., Lalonde, R., Violle, N., Javelot, H., Desor, D., Nejdi, A., Bisson, J.-F., Rougeot, C., Pichelin, M., Cazaubiel, M., Cazaubiel, J.-M., 2011. Assessment of psychotropic-like properties of a probiotic formulation (*Lactobacillus helveticus* R0052 and *Bifidobacterium longum* R0175) in rats and human subjects. Br. J. Nutr. 105, 755–764. http://dx.doi.org/10.1017/S0007114510004319.

Miller, B.J., Buckley, P., Seabolt, W., Mellor, A., Kirkpatrick, B., 2011. Meta-analysis of cytokine alterations in schizophrenia: clinical status and antipsychotic effects. Biol. Psychiatry 70, 663–671. http://dx.doi.org/10.1016/j.biopsych.2011.04.013.

Miller, B.J., Mellor, A., Buckley, P., 2013. Total and differential white blood cell counts, high-sensitivity C-reactive protein, and the metabolic syndrome in non-affective psychoses. Brain Behav. Immun. 31, 82–89. http://dx.doi.org/10.1016/j.bbi.2012.08.016.

Monroe, J.M., Buckley, P.F., Miller, B.J., 2014. Meta-analysis of anti-*Toxoplasma gondii* IgM antibodies in acute psychosis. Schizophr. Bull. 41 (4), 989–998. http://dx.doi.org/10.1093/schbul/sbu159.

Mshvildadze, M., Neu, J., Mai, V., 2008. Intestinal microbiota development in the premature neonate: establishment of a lasting commensal relationship? Nutr. Rev. 66, 658–663. http://dx.doi.org/10.1111/j.1753-4887.2008.00119.x.

Muñoz, M., Heimesaat, M.M., Danker, K., Struck, D., Lohmann, U., Plickert, R., Bereswill, S., Fischer, A., Dunay, I.R., Wolk, K., Loddenkemper, C., Krell, H.-W., Libert, C., Lund, L.R., Frey, O., Hölscher, C., Iwakura, Y., Ghilardi, N., Ouyang, W., Kamradt, T., Sabat, R., Liesenfeld, O., 2009. Interleukin (IL)-23 mediates *Toxoplasma gondii*-induced immunopathology in the gut via matrixmetalloproteinase-2 and IL-22 but independent of IL-17. J. Exp. Med. 206, 3047–3059. http://dx.doi.org/10.1084/jem.20090900.

Neish, A.S., 2009. Microbes in gastrointestinal health and disease. Gastroenterology 136, 65–80. http://dx.doi.org/10.1053/j.gastro.2008.10.080.

Nemani, K., Hosseini Ghomi, R., McCormick, B., Fan, X., 2015. Schizophrenia and the gut-brain axis. Prog. Neuropsychopharmacol. Biol. Psychiatry 56, 155–160. http://dx.doi.org/10.1016/j.pnpbp.2014.08.018.

Neufeld, K.-A.M., Kang, N., Bienenstock, J., Foster, J.A., 2011a. Effects of intestinal microbiota on anxiety-like behavior. Commun. Integr. Biol. 4, 492–494. http://dx.doi.org/10.4161/cib.4.4.15702.

Neufeld, K.M., Kang, N., Bienenstock, J., Foster, J.A., 2011b. Reduced anxiety-like behavior and central neurochemical change in germ-free mice. Neurogastroenterol. Motil. Off. J. Eur. Gastrointest. Motil. Soc. 23, 255–264, e119. http://dx.doi.org/10.1111/j.1365-2982.2010.01620.x.

Niebuhr, D.W., Li, Y., Cowan, D.N., Weber, N.S., Fisher, J.A., Ford, G.M., Yolken, R., 2011. Association between bovine casein antibody and new onset schizophrenia among US military personnel. Schizophr. Res. 128, 51–55. http://dx.doi.org/10.1016/j.schres.2011.02.005.

Nieto, R., Kukuljan, M., Silva, H., 2013. BDNF and schizophrenia: from neurodevelopment to neuronal plasticity, learning, and memory. Front. Psychiatry 4, 45. http://dx.doi.org/10.3389/fpsyt.2013.00045.

Ochoa-Repáraz, J., Mielcarz, D.W., Ditrio, L.E., Burroughs, A.R., Foureau, D.M., Haque-Begum, S., Kasper, L.H., 2009. Role of gut commensal microflora in the development of experimental autoimmune encephalomyelitis. J. Immunol. 183 (10), 6041–6050. http://dx.doi.org/10.4049/jimmunol.0900747.

Ochoa-Repáraz, J., Mielcarz, D.W., Haque-Begum, S., Kasper, L.H., 2010. Induction of a regulatory B cell population in experimental allergic encephalomyelitis by alteration of the gut commensal microflora. Gut Microbes. 1 (2), 103–108. http://dx.doi.org/10.4161/gmic.1.2.11515.

Okusaga, O., Yolken, R.H., Langenberg, P., Sleemi, A., Kelly, D.L., Vaswani, D., Giegling, I., Hartmann, A.M., Konte, B., Friedl, M., Mohyuddin, F., Groer, M.W., Rujescu, D., Postolache, T.T., 2013. Elevated gliadin antibody levels in individuals with schizophrenia. World J. Biol. Psychiatry Off. J. World Fed. Soc. Biol. Psychiatry 14, 509–515. http://dx.doi.org/10.3109/15622975.2012.747699.

Pedrini, M., Massuda, R., Fries, G.R., de Bittencourt Pasquali, M.A., Schnorr, C.E., Moreira, J.C.F., Teixeira, A.L., Lobato, M.I.R., Walz, J.C., Belmonte-de-Abreu, P.S., Kauer-Sant'Anna, M., Kapczinski, F., Gama, C.S., 2012. Similarities in serum oxidative stress markers and inflammatory cytokines in patients with overt schizophrenia at early and late stages of chronicity. J. Psychiatr. Res. 46, 819–824. http://dx.doi.org/10.1016/j.jpsychires.2012.03.019.

Peleg, R., Ben-Zion, Z.I., Peleg, A., Gheber, L., Kotler, M., Weizman, Z., Shiber, A., Fich, A., Horowitz, Y., Shvartzman, P., 2004. "Bread madness" revisited: screening for specific celiac antibodies among schizophrenia patients. Eur. Psychiatry J. Assoc. Eur. Psychiatr. 19, 311–314. http://dx.doi.org/10.1016/j.eurpsy.2004.06.003.

Penders, J., Thijs, C., Vink, C., Stelma, F.F., Snijders, B., Kummeling, I., van den Brandt, P.A., Stobberingh, E.E., 2006. Factors influencing the composition of the intestinal microbiota in early infancy. Pediatrics 118, 511–521. http://dx.doi.org/10.1542/peds.2005-2824.

Qurashi, I., Collins, J., Chaudhry, I., Husain, N., 2014. Promising use of minocycline augmentation with clozapine in treatment-resistant schizophrenia. J. Psychopharmacol. 28 (7), 707–708. http://dx.doi.org/10.1177/0269881114527358.

Ranganath, C., Minzenberg, M., Ragland, J.D., 2008. The cognitive neuroscience of memory function and dysfunction in schizophrenia. Biol. Psychiatry 64, 18–25. http://dx.doi.org/10.1016/j.biopsych.2008.04.011.

Rao, S., Srinivasjois, R., Patole, S., 2009. Prebiotic supplementation in full-term neonates: a systematic review of randomized controlled trials. Arch. Pediatr. Adolesc. Med. 163, 755–764. http://dx.doi.org/10.1001/archpediatrics.2009.94.

Reichelt, K.L., Landmark, J., 1995. Specific IgA antibody increases in schizophrenia. Biol. Psychiatry 37, 410–413. http://dx.doi.org/10.1016/0006-3223(94)00176-4.

Rodrigues, S.M., Schafe, G.E., LeDoux, J.E., 2001. Intra-amygdala blockade of the NR2B subunit of the NMDA receptor disrupts the acquisition but not the expression of fear conditioning. J. Neurosci. Off. J. Soc. Neurosci. 21, 6889–6896.

Ryan, M.C.M., Collins, P., Thakore, J.H., 2003. Impaired fasting glucose tolerance in first-episode, drug-naive patients with schizophrenia. Am. J. Psychiatry 160, 284–289.

Saha, S., Chant, D., Welham, J., McGrath, J., 2005. A systematic review of the prevalence of schizophrenia. PLoS Med. 2, e141. http://dx.doi.org/10.1371/journal.pmed.0020141.

Samaroo, D., Dickerson, F., Kasarda, D.D., Green, P.H.R., Briani, C., Yolken, R.H., Alaedini, A., 2010. Novel immune response to gluten in individuals with schizophrenia. Schizophr. Res. 118, 248–255. http://dx.doi.org/10.1016/j.schres.2009.08.009.

Saunders, P.R., Santos, J., Hanssen, N.P.M., Yates, D., Groot, J.A., Perdue, M.H., 2002. Physical and psychological stress in rats enhances colonic epithelial permeability via peripheral CRH. Dig. Dis. Sci. 47, 208–215.

Savignac, H.M., Corona, G., Mills, H., Chen, L., Spencer, J.P.E., Tzortzis, G., Burnet, P.W.J., 2013. Prebiotic feeding elevates central brain derived neurotrophic factor, N-methyl-D-aspartate receptor subunits and D-serine. Neurochem. Int. 63, 756–764. http://dx.doi.org/10.1016/j.neuint.2013.10.006.

Schreiner, M., Liesenfeld, O., 2009. Small intestinal inflammation following oral infection with *Toxoplasma gondii* does not occur exclusively in C57BL/6 mice: review of 70 reports from the literature. Mem. Inst. Oswaldo Cruz 104, 221–233.

Severance, E.G., Alaedini, A., Yang, S., Halling, M., Gressitt, K.L., Stallings, C.R., Origoni, A.E., Vaughan, C., Khushalani, S., Leweke, F.M., Dickerson, F.B., Yolken, R.H., 2012. Gastrointestinal inflammation and associated immune activation in schizophrenia. Schizophr. Res. 138, 48–53. http://dx.doi.org/10.1016/j.schres.2012.02.025.

Severance, E.G., Dickerson, F.B., Halling, M., Krivogorsky, B., Haile, L., Yang, S., Stallings, C.R., Origoni, A.E., Bossis, I., Xiao, J., Dupont, D., Haasnoot, W., Yolken, R.H., 2010. Subunit and whole molecule specificity of the anti-bovine casein immune response in recent onset psychosis and schizophrenia. Schizophr. Res. 118, 240–247. http://dx.doi.org/10.1016/j.schres.2009.12.030.

Severance, E.G., Gressitt, K.L., Stallings, C.R., Origoni, A.E., Khushalani, S., Leweke, F.M., Dickerson, F.B., Yolken, R.H., 2013. Discordant patterns of bacterial translocation markers and implications for innate immune imbalances in schizophrenia. Schizophr. Res. 148, 130–137. http://dx.doi.org/10.1016/j.schres.2013.05.018.

Singh, M.M., Kay, S.R., 1976. Wheat gluten as a pathogenic factor in schizophrenia. Science 191, 401–402.

Singh, S., Kumar, A., Agarwal, S., Phadke, S.R., Jaiswal, Y., 2014. Genetic insight of schizophrenia: past and future perspectives. Gene 535, 97–100. http://dx.doi.org/10.1016/j.gene.2013.09.110.

Smits, L.P., Bouter, K.E., de Vos, W.M., Borody, T.J., Nieuwdorp, M., 2013. Therapeutic potential of fecal microbiota transplantation. Gastroenterology. 145 (5), 946–953. http://dx.doi.org/10.1053/j.gastro.2013.08.058.

Söderholm, J.D., Perdue, M.H., 2001. Stress and gastrointestinal tract. II. Stress and intestinal barrier function. Am. J. Physiol. Gastrointest. Liver Physiol. 280, G7–G13.

Song, X., Fan, X., Song, X., Zhang, J., Zhang, W., Li, X., Gao, J., Harrington, A., Ziedonis, D., Lv, L., 2013. Elevated levels of adiponectin and other cytokines in drug naïve, first episode schizophrenia patients with normal weight. Schizophr. Res. 150, 269–273. http://dx.doi.org/10.1016/j.schres.2013.07.044.

Stafford, M.R., Jackson, H., Mayo-Wilson, E., Morrison, A.P., Kendall, T., 2013. Early interventions to prevent psychosis: systematic review and meta-analysis. BMJ 346, f185.

Strous, R.D., Shoenfeld, Y., 2006. Schizophrenia, autoimmunity and immune system dysregulation: a comprehensive model updated and revisited. J. Autoimmun. 27, 71–80. http://dx.doi.org/10.1016/j.jaut.2006.07.006.

Sudo, N., Chida, Y., Aiba, Y., Sonoda, J., Oyama, N., Yu, X.-N., Kubo, C., Koga, Y., 2004. Postnatal microbial colonization programs the hypothalamic-pituitary-adrenal system for stress response in mice. J. Physiol. 558, 263–275. http://dx.doi.org/10.1113/jphysiol.2004.063388.

Sun, Z.-Y., Wei, J., Xie, L., Shen, Y., Liu, S.-Z., Ju, G.-Z., Shi, J.-P., Yu, Y.-Q., Zhang, X., Xu, Q., Hemmings, G.P., 2004. The CLDN5 locus may be involved in the vulnerability to schizophrenia. Eur. Psychiatry J. Assoc. Eur. Psychiatr. 19, 354–357. http://dx.doi.org/10.1016/j.eurpsy.2004.06.007.

Thompson Ray, M., Weickert, C.S., Wyatt, E., Webster, M.J., 2011. Decreased BDNF, trkB-TK$^+$ and GAD67 mRNA expression in the hippocampus of individuals with schizophrenia and mood disorders. J. Psychiatry Neurosci. JPN. 36, 195–203. http://dx.doi.org/10.1503/jpn.100048.

Torrey, E.F., Bartko, J.J., Lun, Z.-R., Yolken, R.H., 2007. Antibodies to *Toxoplasma gondii* in patients with schizophrenia: a meta-analysis. Schizophr. Bull. 33, 729–736. http://dx.doi.org/10.1093/schbul/sbl050.

Torrey, E.F., Bartko, J.J., Yolken, R.H., 2012. *Toxoplasma gondii* and other risk factors for schizophrenia: an update. Schizophr. Bull. 38, 642–647. http://dx.doi.org/10.1093/schbul/sbs043.

Turnbaugh, P.J., Hamady, M., Yatsunenko, T., Cantarel, B.L., Duncan, A., Ley, R.E., Sogin, M.L., Jones, W.J., Roe, B.A., Affourtit, J.P., Egholm, M., Henrissat, B., Heath, A.C., Knight, R., Gordon, J.I., 2009. A core gut microbiome in obese and lean twins. Nature 457, 480–484. http://dx.doi.org/10.1038/nature07540.

Turnbaugh, P.J., Ley, R.E., Mahowald, M.A., Magrini, V., Mardis, E.R., Gordon, J.I., 2006. An obesity-associated gut microbiome with increased capacity for energy harvest. Nature 444, 1027–1031. http://dx.doi.org/10.1038/nature05414.

Turner, J.R., 2009. Intestinal mucosal barrier function in health and disease. Nat. Rev. Immunol. 9, 799–809. http://dx.doi.org/10.1038/nri2653.

Wall, R., Marques, T.M., O'Sullivan, O., Ross, R.P., Shanahan, F., Quigley, E.M., Dinan, T.G., Kiely, B., Fitzgerald, G.F., Cotter, P.D., Fouhy, F., Stanton, C., 2012. Contrasting effects of *Bifidobacterium breve* NCIMB 702258 and *Bifidobacterium breve* DPC 6330 on the composition of murine brain fatty acids and gut microbiota. Am. J. Clin. Nutr. 95, 1278–1287. http://dx.doi.org/10.3945/ajcn.111.026435.

Webster, J.P., 2001. Rats, cats, people and parasites: the impact of latent toxoplasmosis on behaviour. Microbe. Infect. Inst. Pasteur 3, 1037–1045.

Weickert, C.S., Hyde, T.M., Lipska, B.K., Herman, M.M., Weinberger, D.R., Kleinman, J.E., 2003. Reduced brain-derived neurotrophic factor in prefrontal cortex of patients with schizophrenia. Mol. Psychiatry 8, 592–610. http://dx.doi.org/10.1038/sj.mp.4001308.

Wei, Q., Huang, H., 2013. Insights into the role of cell-cell junctions in physiology and disease. Int. Rev. Cell Mol. Biol. 306, 187–221. http://dx.doi.org/10.1016/B978-0-12-407694-5.00005-5.

West, J., Logan, R.F., Hubbard, R.B., Card, T.R., 2006. Risk of schizophrenia in people with coeliac disease, ulcerative colitis and Crohn's disease: a general population-based study. Aliment. Pharmacol. Ther. 23, 71–74. http://dx.doi.org/10.1111/j.1365-2036.2006.02720.x.

WHO | International Classification of Diseases (ICD) [WWW Document], 2010. WHO. URL http://www.who.int/classifications/icd/en/ (accessed 11.23.14.).

de Witte, L., Tomasik, J., Schwarz, E., Guest, P.C., Rahmoune, H., Kahn, R.S., Bahn, S., 2014. Cytokine alterations in first-episode schizophrenia patients before and after antipsychotic treatment. Schizophr. Res. 154, 23–29. http://dx.doi.org/10.1016/j.schres.2014.02.005.

Wood, N.C., Hamilton, I., Axon, A.T., Khan, S.A., Quirke, P., Mindham, R.H., McGuigan, K., Prison, H.M., 1987. Abnormal intestinal permeability. An aetiological factor in chronic psychiatric disorders? Br. J. Psychiatry J. Ment. Sci. 150, 853–856.

Wu, N., Zhang, X., Jin, S., Liu, S., Ju, G., Wang, Z., Liu, L., Ye, L., Wei, J., 2010. A weak association of the CLDN5 locus with schizophrenia in Chinese case-control samples. Psychiatry Res. 178, 223. http://dx.doi.org/10.1016/j.psychres.2009.11.019.

Xiao, J., Kannan, G., Jones-Brando, L., Brannock, C., Krasnova, I.N., Cadet, J.L., Pletnikov, M., Yolken, R.H., 2012. Sex-specific changes in gene expression and behavior induced by chronic *Toxoplasma* infection in mice. Neuroscience 206, 39–48. http://dx.doi.org/10.1016/j.neuroscience.2011.12.051.

Yolken, R., Dickerson, F., 2014. The microbiome: the missing link in the pathogenesis of schizophrenia. Neurol. Psychiatry Brain Res. 20, 26–27. http://dx.doi.org/10.1016/S0920-9964(14)70050-7.

Yu, R.-Q., Yuan, J.-L., Ma, L.-Y., Qin, Q.-X., Wu, X.-Y., 2013. [Probiotics improve obesity-associated dyslipidemia and insulin resistance in high-fat diet-fed rats]. Zhongguo Dang Dai Er Ke Za Zhi Chin. J. Contemp. Pediatr. 15, 1123–1127.

Alcohol-Dependence and the Microbiota-Gut-Brain Axis

17

P. Stärkel
*Saint Luc University Hospital, Department of Hepato-Gastroenterology, Brussels, Belgium;
Catholic University of Louvain, Laboratory of Hepato-Gastroenterology, Institute of
Experimental and Clinical Research (IREC), Brussels, Belgium*

S. Leclercq
*Catholic University of Louvain, Institute of Neuroscience and Department of Adult
Psychiatry, Brussels, Belgium*

N.M. Delzenne
*Catholic University of Louvain, Louvain Drug Research Institute, Metabolism and Nutrition
Research Group, Brussels, Belgium*

P. de Timary
*Catholic University of Louvain, Institute of Neuroscience and Department of Adult
Psychiatry, Brussels, Belgium; Saint Luc University Hospital, Department of Adult
Psychiatry, Brussels, Belgium*

ALCOHOL AND GUT BARRIER FUNCTION: WHAT HAVE ANIMAL AND HUMAN STUDIES TAUGHT US?

Alcohol abuse is one of the leading causes of chronic liver disease and liver-related deaths worldwide. The gastrointestinal tract is undoubtedly the first interface of the body that is confronted with the toxic effects of orally administered alcohol. However, the gut could also be a target for developing new strategies to limit the systemic toxic effects of alcohol and to reduce alcohol-induced organ damage beyond the gastrointestinal tract itself. Therefore it is of utmost importance to better understand how alcohol alters the function of the gut and to determine how these alterations influence cellular processes in distant organs, including the brain and the liver.

ALCOHOL, TIGHT JUNCTION FUNCTION, AND GUT PERMEABILITY

It has been known for decades that acute and chronic alcohol consumption can disrupt the intestinal epithelial barrier resulting in increased gut permeability. In the 1980s animal and human studies suggested that increased intestinal leakage occurred after alcohol administration and that this effect is possibly related to destabilization

The Gut-Brain Axis. http://dx.doi.org/10.1016/B978-0-12-802304-4.00017-7

of the intercellular junctions of the epithelium (Worthington et al., 1978; Bjarnason et al., 1984; Draper et al., 1983; Lavö et al., 1992; Bode et al., 1991; Bode and Bode, 2003). Although perhaps forgotten, the gut has once again gained much interest in the context of alcohol abuse disorders in recent years. The suspicion that alcohol-induced alterations in intestinal permeability has been confirmed in preclinical animal models as well as in patients with alcohol abuse disorders (Keshavarzian et al., 1994, 2009; Leclercq et al., 2012). Alcohol and its main oxidative metabolite, acetaldehyde, likely alter the intestinal ultrastructure by disrupting epithelial tight junction integrity, in particular the tight junction proteins occludin and zonula occludens-1 (ZO-1; Wang et al., 2014a,b; Elamin et al., 2012; Dunagan et al., 2012; Rao, 2008; Zhong et al., 2010). As a consequence, microbial products such as lipopolysaccharide (LPS) and peptidoglycans can translocate from the intestinal lumen and subsequently reach the bloodstream, liver, or brain, which are particularly sensitive to alcohol-induced damage (Rao, 2009; Leclercq et al., 2012, 2014b). Recent data confirm that chronic alcohol administration in animal models (Pascual et al., 2015; Szabo and Lippai, 2014; Maraslioglu et al., 2014), as well as acute and chronic alcohol abuse in humans (Bala et al., 2014; Leclercq et al., 2014b), can lead to an increase in acute phase protein levels and an increase in proinflammatory cytokines such as tumor necrosis factor (TNF)-α, interleukin (IL)-6, and IL-1β in the systemic circulation, thereby establishing a chronic inflammatory state. These observations have incited researchers to propose new concepts based on the existence of a gut-liver, gut-brain, or even a gut-liver-brain axis, which might not only play a role in organ damage but also in alcohol dependence.

MOLECULAR MECHANISMS UNDERLYING ALCOHOL-INDUCED DISRUPTION OF THE GUT BARRIER

To date the exact molecular mechanisms underlying increased intestinal permeability remain largely unknown. Most studies use cell culture–based systems; in vivo studies investigating the pathways that induce intestinal barrier disruption after chronic alcohol administration are scarce. However, oxidative stress appears to play a role because acetaldehyde induces epithelial cell monolayer disruption as a consequence of tight-junction protein redistribution (Rao, 2008). Moreover, Cyp2e1 protein and activity, the principal cytochrome P450 enzyme that metabolizes alcohol, is expressed in the intestine and is upregulated by chronic alcohol use. Cyp2e1 contributes to oxidative stress in the intestine, and Cyp2e1 knock-out mice are resistant to alcohol-induced gut "leakiness." Moreover, small interfering (si)RNA knockdown of Cyp2e1 in an epithelial cell line prevented alcohol-induced increases in permeability, and emerging data suggest that Cyp2e1-mediated effects may involve upregulation of the circadian clock proteins, CLOCK (circadian locomotor output cycles kaput) and PER2 (period circadian clock-2; Forsyth et al., 2013, 2014).

Recent animal studies point to the potential involvement of a TNF-α/nuclear factor-κB (NFkB) pathway in alcohol-induced intestinal barrier dysfunction. For example, in animal models of chronic alcohol administration it has been demonstrated that increased TNF-α production by inflammatory cells of the intestinal lamina propria occurs concomitantly with increased expression of NFkB (Chen et al., 2015a; Chang et al., 2013). Moreover, TNF-α is released by intestinal epithelial cells upon stimulation with increasing concentrations of alcohol (Amin et al., 2009). Of note, TNF-receptor I partially influences tight-junction disruption through activation of the myosin light-chain kinase (MLCK); MLCK expression correlates with barrier disruption in vitro (Zolotarevsky et al., 2002; Elamin et al., 2014a). TNF-α can also induce phosphorylation of the Forkhead transcription factor (FoxO4), leading to its inactivation and consequent stimulation of NFkB (Chang et al., 2013). Activation of inducible nitric oxide synthases (iNOS) in vitro and in vivo could also play a role in alcohol-induced intestinal barrier disruption (Banan et al., 2000; Tang et al., 2009). iNOS and ethanol-induced intracellular release of Ca^{2+}, and subsequent activation of RhoA (Ras homolog gene family, member A), is one mechanism by which alcohol could influence intestinal barrier function (Tong et al., 2013a,b; Elamin et al., 2014b). Although data in humans are scarce, studies tend to confirm that increased expression of TNF-α is a characteristic feature of duodenal biopsies from alcohol-dependent (AD) patients (Chen et al., 2015a); MLCK upregulation has also been reported in healthy volunteers in response to alcohol exposure (Elamin et al., 2014a). Taken together, the available evidence supports the involvement of TNF-α as an important tight-junction regulator in the intestine in response to chronic alcohol exposure (Fig. 17.1).

However, TNF-α is not likely to be the only factor controlling intestinal barrier function. It is part of a complex network involving several potential mediators, such as Snail, protein phosphatase 2A, extracellular signal-regulated kinase, protein kinase C, protein tyrosine phosphatase, and hepatocyte nuclear factor 4α, all of which have been implicated in alcohol-related intestinal barrier dysfunction (Elamin et al., 2014a,c; Forsyth et al., 2011; Dunagan et al., 2012; Samak et al., 2011; Suzuki et al., 2008; Atkinson et al., 2001; Zhong et al., 2010).

EFFECTS OF ALCOHOL ON THE GUT MUCUS LAYER

The intestinal mucus layer forms a physical barrier between the underlying epithelium and the lumen of the gastrointestinal tract and protects the epithelium against noxious agents, viruses, and pathogenic bacteria. It consists of two separate sublayers: the inner layer is attached to the epithelial cell layer and is devoid of bacteria and the outer layer, which can be washed off easily, is colonized by bacteria (Matsuo et al., 1997; Johanssen et al., 2008). The intestinal mucus layer is composed of mucins (Muc), which are synthesized and secreted by intestinal goblet cells (van Klinken et al., 1999). There are three gastrointestinal-secreted mucins—Muc2, Muc5AC, and Muc6—which are characteristically large, heavily O-glycosylated glycoproteins assembled into oligomers that contribute to the viscous properties of the intestinal mucus layer (McGuckin et al., 2011). The intestinal membrane-bound mucins Muc1, Muc3-4, Muc12-13, and Muc17 protect against pathogens that have the capacity to penetrate the inner mucus layer (Linden et al., 2008). Rodent studies and human studies in alcoholics demonstrate that

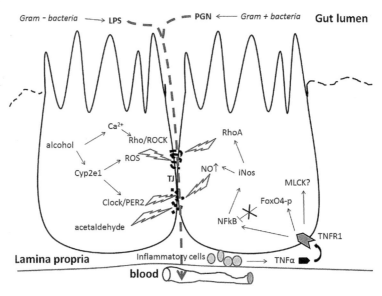

FIGURE 17.1

Cellular mechanisms possibly contributing to disruption of TJs. Alterations, in particular of occludin and ZO, and increased gut permeability in response to alcohol abuse allow translocation of bacterial products (eg, LPS and PGN) from the gut lumen into the blood stream. *TJ*, Tight junction; *LPS*, lipopolysaccharide; *PGN*, peptidoglycans; *ROS*, reactive oxygen species; *TNFα*, tumor necrosis factor-α; *TNFR1*, tumor necrosis factor receptor-1; *iNOS*, inducible nitric oxide synthase; *NO*, nitric oxide; *MLCK*, myosin light chain kinase; *FoxO*, forkhead box "other"; *NFkB*, nuclear factor-κB; *Cyp2e1*, cytochrome P450 2e1; *CLOCK*, circadian locomotor output cycles kaput; *PER2*, period circadian clock-2.

the mucus layer thickens in response to alcohol (Hartmann et al., 2013; Grewal and Mahmood, 2009); this could be interpreted as a protective response to alcohol intake. A downside of this seemingly protective response is impairment of the vigorous immune-defense system that enterocytes can mount against bacteria.

Chronic alcohol exposure also suppresses the gene and protein expression of regenerating islet-derived genes (Reg)—Reg3b and Reg3g—in rodents and humans (Hartmann et al., 2013). Both molecules are secreted into the mucus layer where they have been implicated in intestinal homeostasis and exhibit antimicrobial activity (Dessein et al., 2009). Probiotic-mediated restoration of Reg3g levels, or knockdown of Muc2, results in a reduced thickness of the mucus layer in rodents exposed to alcohol and a decrease in bacterial translocation (Hartmann et al., 2013; Chen et al., 2015b). These data indicate that alcohol-induced changes in the composition of the mucus layer might contribute to the dysfunction of the intestinal barrier. This concept is further supported by the observation that alcohol both dissolves and extracts lipids from the mucus, resulting in a decrease in mucosal surface hydrophobicity, which is also an important element of the gut barrier (Qin and Deitch, 2015).

In conclusion, alcohol-induced epithelial cell damage impairs the mucosal innate immune system and results in a failure of intestinal homeostasis. In addition to the potential mechanisms outlined here, alcohol also influences the gut-associated immune system (Choudhry et al., 2002; Maier et al., 1999). However, there is currently still much speculation about how alcohol triggers intestinal changes and/or inflammation.

ALCOHOL-INDUCED CHANGES ON THE GUT MICROBIOTA

Evidence now supports that certain aspects of health and disease may depend on the status of the microbiota (Nicholson et al., 2012). Intestinal bacteria have been shown to shape and modulate the immune system (Hooper et al., 2012), to participate in the maintenance of a healthy intestinal barrier (Guarner et al., 2003), and to influence brain function and behavior. Therefore disruption of the gut microbiota, known as dysbiosis, can lead to various diseases, including inflammatory bowel diseases, colon cancer, irritable bowel syndrome, obesity and metabolic syndrome, nonalcoholic fatty liver diseases, autoimmune diseases, and changes in mood and behavior (Flint et al., 2014). One important consequence of gut dysbiosis is disruption of gut barrier function. Such disruption might subsequently promote the unchecked passage or translocation of bacterial elements such as LPS or peptidoglycans across the gut wall, which may, in turn, bind to host receptors and promote systemic inflammation. Such processes have already been described in the context of obesity and related metabolic diseases (Cani et al., 2009).

GUT MICROBIOTA-DERIVED METABOLITES

Colonic bacteria can ferment nutrients, endogenous host-derived substrates (eg, mucus and pancreatic enzymes), and dietary components that escape digestion in the upper part of the gastrointestinal tract. Two types of bacterial fermentation occur in the colon (Hamer et al., 2012): carbohydrate fermentation and protein fermentation.

Carbohydrate fermentation occurs mainly in the proximal part of the colon, the metabolic endpoint of which is the generation of short-chain fatty acids (SCFAs). Acetate, propionate, and butyrate represent the main SCFAs found in fecal samples. SCFAs, particularly butyrate, have been shown to have beneficial impacts on health and well-being. These include provision of energy for colonocytes, inhibition of pathogen growth (by pH modulation), and improved mineral and ion absorption. SCFAs also reinforce various components of the colonic defense barrier, have anti-inflammatory properties, improve insulin sensitivity, and have been demonstrated to promote satiety (Hamer et al., 2008; Arora et al., 2011). After carbohydrate fermentation, particular intestinal bacteria can catalyze the reduction of acetate to acetaldehyde and then to ethanol (Macfarlane et al., 2003). These bacteria are termed ethanol-producing bacteria. Therefore ethanol found in the gut can have two origins: exogenous (alcohol consumption) and endogenous (produced by bacterial enzymes).

On the other hand, protein fermentation involves the fermentation of dietary peptides as well as mucus and pancreatic enzymes and takes place in the distal colon. This process generates potentially toxic substances. The fermentation of branched-chain amino acids (BCAAs—valine, isoleucine, and leucine) leads to the production of branched-chain fatty acids (BCFAs) such as 2-methyl propanoic acid, 2-methyl butanoic acid, and 3-methyl butanoic acid. The bacterial degradation of aromatic amino acids tyrosine and tryptophan results in the production of phenolic and indole compounds, respectively. The end products of tyrosine metabolism include mainly phenol and 4-methyl phenol whereas tryptophan degradation generates indole and 3-methyl indole (also called skatole). Fermentation of sulfur amino acids by sulfate-reducing bacteria results in the production of hydrogen sulfide (H_2S). Of note, SCFAs can also arise from protein fermentation, but in small amounts. Phenolic and sulfur-containing compounds are potentially toxic. For instance, phenols are believed to act as co-carcinogens (Bone et al., 1976). Moreover, two independent studies have shown that phenol exposure decreases transepithelial electric resistance in a concentration-dependent manner in parallel with an increase in the paracellular flux of mannitol or dextran fluorescein isothiocyanate in intestinal epithelial cell culture (Hughes et al., 2008; McCall et al., 2009). The change in paracellular permeability observed after phenol treatment correlates with mislocalization of the tight junction proteins claudin-1 and ZO-1 to the cytosol (McCall et al., 2009). In contrast, indole has been shown to reinforce the epithelial intestinal cell barrier in vitro (Bansal et al., 2010). H_2S produced by sulfate-reducing bacteria is an extremely toxic agent that has been shown to induce genomic DNA damage in colonocytes (Attene-Ramos et al., 2006). It is important to note that BCFAs, phenolic, and indolic compounds are not produced by human enzymes; therefore they are unique colonic bacterial metabolites.

EFFECT OF ETHANOL ON GUT MICROBIOTA COMPOSITION

The idea that the gut microbiota could be altered by ethanol consumption came from experimental and clinical data demonstrating that the bacterial endotoxin LPS is an important factor in the development of alcoholic liver disease. Indeed, elevated endotoxin levels and liver injury are observed in rats administered ethanol (Nanji et al., 1993) and in alcoholics (Parlesak et al., 2000; Fukui et al., 1991; Bode et al., 1987). Lowering serum endotoxin levels by antibiotics (Adachi et al., 1995), dietary oats (Keshavarzian et al., 2001), or probiotics (Forsyth et al., 2009; Nanji et al., 1994) attenuates ethanol-induced liver damage in rats. Thus endotoxin, and possibly other gut-derived bacterial products, may be involved in the development of liver disease in alcoholics. Three possible mechanisms have been proposed to explain elevated blood endotoxin levels in alcoholics: an increased production of endotoxins by an abnormal gut microbiota composition or bacterial overgrowth (Yan et al., 2011; Bode et al., 1984; Casafont et al., 1996); an increased permeation of endotoxins through the gut wall due to gut leakiness; or decreased function of liver Kupffer cells, which are responsible for endotoxin clearance.

The first experimental study investigating whether chronic ethanol consumption affects gut bacterial composition was conducted in 2009 (Mutlu et al., 2009). This study showed that chronic ethanol treatment induced alterations of the mucosa-associated colonic bacterial microbiota in rats. The authors hypothesized that dysbiosis could contribute to endotoxemia and liver disease by increasing endotoxin production and by disruption of gut barrier function. Subsequent studies investigated in more detail the changes in the microbiome using pyrosequencing technology, described a reduced abundance of Firmicutes and *Lactobacillus*, and increased Bacteroidetes in mice continuously fed ethanol (Yan et al., 2011). Others demonstrated that chronic alcohol consumption by mice induced a reduction in Firmicutes (unclassified Lachnospiraceae and Ruminococcaceae) and Bacteroidetes and an increase in Proteobacteria, Actinobacteria, and *Lactobacillus* (Bull-Otterson et al., 2013). The authors suggest that alcohol-induced microbial shifts could potentially be driven by a change in luminal pH. The discrepancies observed across different animal studies could be due to the different periods of alcohol feeding and methodological differences. However, in animals, at least an improvement of alcohol-induced dysbiosis has been reported after supplementation with prebiotics (Yan et al., 2011; Mutlu et al., 2009) and probiotics (Mutlu et al., 2009; Bull-Otterson et al., 2013).

However, in humans few studies have tried to correlate changes in the gut microbiota with alcohol consumption. Kirpich et al. found decreased numbers of *Bifidobacterium*, *Lactobacillus*, and *Enterococcus* in alcoholics compared with healthy controls (Kirpich et al., 2008). After 5 days of probiotic supplementation and alcohol abstinence these bacteria returned to numbers seen in control subjects. In 2012, Mutlu et al. characterized the gut microbiota composition in alcoholics using next-generation sequencing technologies and showed that only a subgroup of alcoholics had an altered colonic microbiota composition (Mutlu et al., 2012): 31% of subjects were defined as dysbiotic. The study included alcoholic subjects with and without liver disease as well as those actively drinking and sober alcoholics. The mucosa-associated dysbiosis was represented by lower abundances of Bacteroidetes and a higher abundance of Proteobacteria. These results suggest that chronic alcohol consumption, rather than liver disease, is the most important event in terms of determining changes in the gut microbiota. Moreover, the effects of alcohol abuse were not temporary because sober (>1 month) alcoholics were also considered dysbiotic. The authors suggest that dysbiosis could contribute to gut leakiness, but this remains speculative because intestinal permeability was not measured.

Metabolomics analysis of fecal samples has been applied in the context of numerous digestive tract disorders, including colorectal cancers, irritable bowel syndrome, and inflammatory bowel diseases. In 2013 Xie et al. characterized the metabolic alterations of the whole gastrointestinal tract contents in rats after 8 weeks of chronic ethanol consumption. Elevated acetic acid levels were observed in the upper part of the intestine in ethanol-fed rats, presumably because of the oxidation of ethanol to acetaldehyde and subsequent oxidation by mucosal or bacterial aldehyde dehydrogenase to acetic acid. However, ethanol consumption induced a significant decrease in colonic SCFAs, BCAAs, and BCFAs (Xie et al., 2013).

MICROBIOTA-DERIVED METABOLITES, GUT PERMEABILITY, AND ALCOHOL DEPENDENCE

We performed a study in AD patients to investigate the potential link among gut permeability, gut microbiota, and behavioral markers of addiction severity (Leclercq et al., 2014b). The observation that some, but not all, AD subjects develop gut leakiness indicates that chronic alcohol dependence is necessary, but is not sufficient alone, to cause gut dysfunction. Thus other factors in addition to direct toxicity of alcohol may be involved. We showed that AD subjects presenting with increased intestinal permeability also had altered gut microbial composition and activity. It is interesting to note that we observed that *Lactobacillus* spp. and *Bifidobacterium* spp., as well as bacteria from the family Ruminococcaceae, were increased during alcohol abstinence and inversely correlated with intestinal permeability. These bacteria are known to have a beneficial effect on gut barrier function (Madesen et al., 2001). Among Ruminococcaceae bacteria, *Faecalibacterium prausnitzii* is particularly interesting. This species is also depleted in Crohn's disease (Sokol et al., 2008) and ulcerative colitis (Machiels et al., 2013) and has been shown to have in vitro and in vivo antiinflammatory properties (Sokol et al., 2008). Indeed, supernatants from *F. prausnitzii* cultures inhibit IL-8 secretion and NFκB activation in intestinal epithelial cells stimulated with IL-1β (Sokol et al., 2008). In our study, AD patients who presented with low levels of *F. prausnitzii* had higher plasma levels of IL-8, and these variables were significantly and negatively correlated (Leclercq et al., 2014b). Taken together, our results show that alterations in microbial composition are associated with increased intestinal permeability and increased plasma levels of proinflammatory cytokines.

Our results also suggest that bacterial-derived metabolites may be involved in the regulation of gut barrier function; therefore they could indirectly contribute to alcohol-induced toxicity. The metabolite differences observed were as a consequence of protein fermentation and the formation of BCFAs, indolic compounds, and other potentially toxic metabolites such as phenolic and sulfur-containing compounds. However, it is important to note that the main beneficial products of carbohydrate fermentation (eg, the SCFAs) were not different between AD and control subjects (Nicholson et al., 2012). Production of phenolic compounds in the gut also depends on microbial composition (Bures et al., 1990) or the metabolic activity of the microbiota (Lord et al., 2008). Phenol is increased in AD subjects who also display increased intestinal permeability. The toxic effect of phenol on intestinal epithelial cells has been demonstrated in two independent in vitro studies (Hughes et al., 2008; McCall et al., 2009), both of which confirm that phenol is a potential driver of gut barrier dysfunction. Another phenolic compound, 4-methyl phenol (also called *p*-cresol), is decreased in AD subjects, who also display deficits in intestinal permeability, during alcohol withdrawal and is associated with an increase in *Lactobacillus* spp., *Bifidobacterium* spp., and *Ruminococcaceae*, which are associated with the production of *p*-cresol (Ward et al., 1987; Yokoyama et al., 1979). Moreover, bacterial metabolism of tryptophan results in various indolic compounds (Yokoyama et al., 1979; Zheng

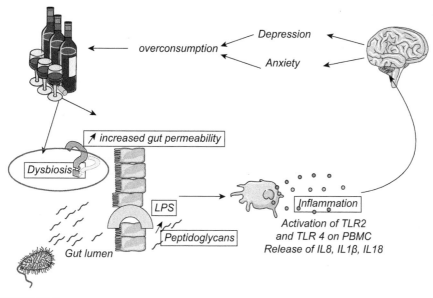

FIGURE 17.2

The vicious circle of alcohol dependence. Alcohol-induced dysbiosis and bacterial overgrowth contribute to intestinal tight-junction disruption, increased gut permeability, and translocation of bacterial products into the blood. PBMCs are activated and produce inflammatory cytokines. This systemic inflammatory response influences brain mechanisms and behavioral patterns perpetuating alcohol seeking. *PBMCs*, Peripheral blood mononuclear cells; *TLR*, toll-like receptor; *IL*, interleukin; *LPS*, lipopolysaccharide.

et al., 2011). In vitro studies have shown these to improve intestinal cell barrier function and to decrease proinflammatory cytokine expression (Bansal et al., 2010; Venkatesh et al., 2014). It is interesting to note that the level of 3-methyl indole was diminished in AD subjects with high intestinal permeability and who also presented with increased plasma IL-8 levels. Taken together, these observations support a protective role of indolic-producing gut microbes on gut barrier function and inflammation and a detrimental role for phenol-producing bacteria. Supporting the concept of a microbiota-gut-brain axis, we showed that AD subjects with gut dysfunction also had higher scores for depression, anxiety, and alcohol craving at the end of a detoxification program (Leclercq et al., 2014b; Fig. 17.2).

CONTRIBUTION OF GENETIC AND ENVIRONMENTAL FACTORS TO ALCOHOL-ASSOCIATED DYSBIOSIS

The underlying cause of alcohol-induced dysbiosis and gut barrier dysfunction are likely multiple, especially given that nutritional disorders, genetics, lifestyle, and mental and biological stress are all associated with alcohol dependence. Nutritional intakes, in particular, are strongly altered in alcohol dependence. Therefore dietary changes could, to some degree, be responsible for the development of dysbiosis observed in a subset of AD patients. Dysbiosis may also occur independent of alcohol consumption. However, this hypothesis has yet to be completely tested. An independent study conducted on a population of AD subjects (de Timary et al., 2012) demonstrated that on average alcohol accounted for almost 40% of caloric intake; intake of proteins, lipids, and carbohydrates were all significantly reduced compared with healthy controls. No differences in fat or fiber intake between nondysbiotic and dysbiotic AD subjects have been reported (Mutlu et al., 2012). However, nutritional assessments were performed on a very limited number of subjects in this particular study. In another study from our own group, plasma prealbumin levels, used as a marker of the nutritional status (Shenkin et al., 2006), did not differ between low and high intestinal permeability grouped AD subjects. Therefore these observations do not support the influence of diet as a distinguishing factor between dysbiotic and nondysbiotic AD subjects. Of course other factors may explain the dysbiosis observed in AD subjects, including genetics, lifestyle, and stress. It is plausible that genetic variation exists between subjects with dysbiosis and subjects with a normal gut microbiota. Evidence from adoption and twin studies support the conclusion that a proportion of the risk for development of alcohol dependence relates to genetics (Mayfield et al., 2008).

Disrupted circadian rhythms may also contribute to the differential susceptibility to alcohol-induced gut leakiness in a subset of alcoholics (Swanson et al., 2011; Summa et al., 2013; Forsyth et al., 2013). Circadian rhythms control various biological processes including sleep/wake cycles, body temperature, hormone secretion, glucose homeostasis, immune function, and intestinal function. In this regard circadian genes have been shown to control the expression of tight-junction genes involved in the regulation of intestinal permeability (Kyoto et al., 2014). Disruption of circadian rhythms has deleterious consequences for health and has been associated with metabolic syndrome, cardiovascular disease, cancer, and intestinal disorders. Lifestyle factors such as shift work, late-night activity, jet lag, and timing of food intake and alcohol consumption are all disrupters of circadian rhythmicity (Voigt et al., 2013). An in vitro study has demonstrated that alcohol disrupts intestinal epithelial cell permeability in parallel with an upregulation of the circadian clock genes *CLOCK* and *PER2*. Moreover, knockdown of these genes prevented alcohol-induced increases in epithelial permeability in vitro (Swanson et al., 2011). Further studies are now warranted to determine whether the expression of intestinal circadian genes is altered in alcoholic patients and whether such changes can differentiate alcoholics with and without a leaky gut.

The question of stress also deserves comment because changes in microbial composition have been reported in the context of stress in animal (Bailey et al., 2011; Galley et al., 2014) and human studies (Holdeman et al., 1976; Knowles et al., 2008). In some individuals, alcohol consumption is considered as an attempt to cope with stress (Zimmermann et al., 2007). Moreover, stress is known to alter the activity of the hypothalamic-pituitary-adrenal (HPA) axis; stress triggers the release of corticotropin-releasing factor (CRF) in the hypothalamus, causing adrenocorticotrophic hormone secretion from the pituitary gland and subsequently glucocorticoids (corticosterone in rodents and cortisol in humans) from the adrenal glands. In an animal model of early-life stress, the maternal separation (MS) model, enhanced activity of the HPA axis, increased hypothalamic CRH (Arborelius et al., 1999), and elevated levels of serum corticosterone (Gareau et al., 2007) are characteristic features of MS. CRF has also been implicated in stress-induced intestinal abnormalities (Söderholm et al., 2002), including increased colonic permeability (Saunders et al., 2002) and mucin release (Castagliuolo et al., 1996). Probiotic treatment (*Lactobacillus rhamnosus* and *Lactobacillus helveticus*) of MS rat pups normalizes corticosterone levels and ameliorates colonic dysfunction (Gareau et al., 2007). In adult rats, chronic peripheral administration of CRF, mimicking chronic stress, also caused an increase in serum corticosterone levels and colonic barrier dysfunction (Teitelbaum et al., 2008). In human studies, elevated plasma cortisol concentrations and enhanced cerebrospinal fluid levels of CRH have been observed in patients suffering from depression and anxiety (Arborelius et al., 1999; Van Eck et al., 1996). Therefore we assessed salivary cortisol levels in AD and control subjects. Our preliminary data revealed that patients with high intestinal permeability had higher cortisol levels than subjects with low intestinal permeability.

However, to date we still do not exactly know what causes the dysbiosis observed in AD subjects; whether it is a consequence of chronic alcohol abuse or whether preexiting dysbiosis contributes to the development of a more severe form of alcohol dependence in susceptible individuals is unknown. In practice it is almost impossible to evaluate the gut microbiota of subjects before the diagnosis of alcohol dependence. To overcome this limitation, patients who have completed their withdrawal programs and who relapse after several months or several years of abstinence may prove to be a useful cohort in which to study changes in the gut microbiota in the context of alcohol dependence.

DO CHANGES IN THE GUT INFLUENCE BRAIN AND BEHAVIOR IN ALCOHOL USE DISORDERS?

PSYCHOLOGICAL AND BEHAVIORAL CHANGES IN ALCOHOL DEPENDENCE

Alcohol dependence is one of the most frequent psychiatric disorders and currently represents the second cause of death and morbidity worldwide (Hall, 2012). The societal burden of alcohol dependence is great and is largely due to its consequences on health (Rehm et al., 2013) and criminality. Moreover, alcohol dependence is considered as a hazard to self and to others (Nutt et al., 2010). Alcohol addiction results from a complex interaction among a score of biological, psychological, and social dimensions (Volkow et al., 2004). Several factors contribute to the development of alcohol dependence. These are not only genetic (Schuckit, 2000) and personality related (Finn, 2002) but also include the interaction between ethanol consumption and brain reward circuits (Koob and Le Moal, 2008). The positive reinforcement that drinking exerts on further ethanol intake is at least partially associated with the production of dopamine or neuropeptides belonging to the opioid family. Furthermore, as with other addictions, alcohol use disorders also occur as a consequence of a decrease in executive functions (Noël et al., 2001). More precisely, alcohol use disorders result from an imbalance between automatic affective processes, likely generated in the limbic system, and reflexive control processes arising from the frontocortical areas (Friese, 2011). Another important dimension of alcohol use disorders is the relationship between compulsive drinking and emotional processes, in which drinking is often triggered by affective situations—most often negative emotions. In particular, a strong correlation has repeatedly been observed between alcohol craving and depression or anxiety (Andersohn and Kiefer, 2004; Cordovil de Sousa Uva et al., 2010; de Timary et al., 2013). This negative reinforcement process has been described as the "dark side" of the addiction by some (Koob and Le Moal, 2005) and may explain a large proportion of relapses in abstinent AD subjects (Zywiak et al., 2003). Concerning the social difficulties encountered by subjects presenting with alcohol use disorders, several processes may participate, including difficulties in social cognition, manifested by a difficulty to correctly interpret the emotions of others (Kornreich et al., 2003; Maurage et al., 2009; Uekerman et al., 2008), and deficits in theory of mind (Uekermann et al., 2007; Maurage et al., 2015). In addition to these aspects, the shame and the stigma associated with alcohol use disorders (Saunders et al., 2006) also contributes to the social isolation experienced by sufferers. These are likely reinforced by the stigmatization of those suffering from alcohol use disorders within society (Schomerus et al., 2011) and the heightened sensitivity of these individuals to social rejection (Maurage et al., 2012).

The possibility that the gut, or the gut microbiota, participate in the development of alcohol use disorders certainly deserves greater attention. Such a concept is supported by several lines of evidence in animal studies. However, to correctly evaluate the role of the gut in the development of the disease, behavioral studies, taking into account the biopsychosocial complexity of the disease described earlier, will need to be developed.

Recent interest on the possible role of the gut and the microbiota in the development of psychiatric disorders mainly arises from animal studies that have clearly established a relationship among the microbiota, gut, and the brain (Cryan and Dinan, 2012). Studies examining the effect of gut dysbiosis in psychiatric disorders have mainly focused on the development of mood symptoms (eg, depression and anxiety; for review see in Foster and McVey Neufeld, 2013; Luna and Foster, 2014; Dash et al., 2015; Jiang et al., 2015; Naseribafrouei et al., 2014) and the development of profound social impairments such as those observed in autism spectrum disorders (Adams et al., 2011; Finegold et al., 2012; Hsiao et al., 2013). Gut-brain interactions are bidirectional by nature, and stress has been shown to induce an increase in intestinal permeability (Gareau et al., 2007) and to alter the gut microbiota (Bailey et al., 2011). Three aspects will be developed further in this section of our chapter exploring the possible relationship among the gut, the brain, and behavior in alcohol use disorder. These are the sickness behavior theory, brain inflammation, and dysbiosis.

THE SICKNESS BEHAVIOR THEORY AND SYMPTOMS ASSOCIATED WITH ALCOHOL DEPENDENCE

Anyone who has experienced a bacterial or viral infection knows what it means to "feel sick" (Konzman et al., 2002; Dantzer et al., 2008). Sickness behaviors are characterized by lassitude, fatigue, inability to concentrate, loss of appetite, irritability, altered sleep pattern, and withdrawal from normal social activities. These banal symptoms contribute to a highly organized strategy of the organism to fight infection and facilitate recovery after pathogen exposure. This strategy is called sickness behavior and comprises three components: fever, neuroendocrine changes (ie, increased HPA axis activity), and alterations in behavior. It is important to emphasize that such changes in behavior are not only restricted to situations of infection but have also been described in various psychopathological situations, in particular in depression (Konzman et al., 2002; Dantzer et al., 2008). However, it is less common to associate alcohol dependence or alcohol use disorders with sickness behavior. Indeed, comparison can be drawn between the behavioral changes described here associated with an infection and the symptoms experienced during a hangover (Lund, 2007). Furthermore, at the beginning of a detoxification, AD subjects also present with important symptoms of depression, anxiety, and fatigue (Cordovil de Sousa Uva et al., 2010). These symptoms largely improve during the course of a detoxification (Andersohn and Kiefer, 2004; de Timary et al., 2008).

Sickness behavior, which occurs subsequent to infection, is known to be triggered by proinflammatory cytokines. Indeed, infectious pathogens encounter dendritic cells, blood monocytes, and tissue macrophages, which express pattern-recognition receptors such as toll-like receptors (TLRs). In humans, 10 TLRs have been identified which, for the most part, recognize mainly viral and bacterial structures (Akira et al., 2006; Sandor et al., 2005). For instance, LPS, a component of the cell wall of gram-negative bacteria, is recognized by TLR4 whereas peptidoglycan originating mainly from gram-positive bacteria is recognized by TLR2 (Takeuchi et al., 1999; Silhavy et al., 2010). Upon TLR activation, a signal transduction cascade leads to transcription factor activation and, in the end, cytokine production, including TNF-α, IL-1β, and IL-6 (Kawaiand Akira, 2007). These peripherally produced inflammatory cytokines can subsequently reach the brain, where they in turn can stimulate further cytokine production that manifests in the development of sickness behavior (Fig. 17.3).

However, when inflammation is prolonged, as occurs in chronic inflammatory diseases, sickness behaviors may transform into depressive symptoms. Several studies have suggested a role for proinflammatory cytokines in the development of depression (Yirmiya, 1996; Yirmiya et al., 1999; Smith, 1991). Depressed individuals have increased circulating levels of proinflammatory cytokines (Maes, 1999). Furthermore, the prevalence of depressive disorders in patients afflicted with chronic inflammatory diseases is higher than normal. Clinical evidence implicating a role for inflammation in

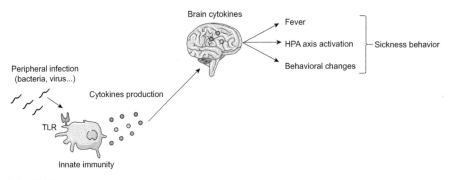

FIGURE 17.3

Cytokine-induced sickness behavior after peripheral infection. TLRs on cells of the innate immune system become activated by infectious particles leading to proinflammatory cytokine production participating in sickness behavior. *TLR*, Toll-like receptor; *HPA*, hypothalamic-pituitary-adrenal.

the development of depression can be gleaned from studies in patients receiving immunotherapy treatments. For example, 45% of cancer or hepatitis C patients treated with IFN-α and IL-2 developed symptoms of depression (Capuron et al., 2000, 2001; Musselman et al., 2001). Furthermore, preclinical behavioral studies further implicate a role for cytokines as causative factors in depression (Dantzer et al., 1999). More recently, a study examining the effect of endotoxin in healthy humans established causality between the immune response to endotoxin and altered behavior (Schedlowski et al., 2014). For instance, injection of *Salmonella abortus* endotoxin induced an increase in serum TNF-α, IL-6, and cortisol as well as the development of a depressed mood, increased anxiety, and a decrease in memory performance (Reichenberg et al., 2001). Similar results were obtained after vaccination of healthy volunteers with *Salmonella typhi*, who reported negative changes in mood (Wright et al., 2005). Taken together, such animal and human studies demonstrate that a proinflammatory state greatly increases the incidence of mood disturbance.

It has been shown that heavy drinkers may present with increased LPS and cytokine levels after a binge drinking episode (Bala et al., 2014). We have also shown an increase in intestinal permeability and LPS levels in AD subjects at the beginning of a detoxification period (Leclercq et al., 2012); these markers regressed to the levels observed in control subjects after 18 days of abstinence. Moreover, depression and anxiety-related symptoms and craving also decreased in the same patients during abstinence. Proinflammatory cytokine levels partially regressed after detoxification. Positive correlations were observed between plasma cytokine levels and alcohol craving, depression, and anxiety. In another study, in which we measured inflammation in mononuclear cells extracted from the blood of AD subjects at the beginning of alcohol withdrawal, inflammation correlated with alcohol intake (Leclercq et al., 2014a). We again observed a correlation between alcohol craving, in particular with the obsessive dimension of craving and inflammation. More specifically, IL-8 regressed during alcohol withdrawal and explained a large fraction of the variation in craving—49% of the variance. These observations collectively suggest an association between inflammation and alcohol consumption in which the amount of alcohol consumed induces an increase in inflammation that may in turn induce craving, likely through negative reinforcement processes. A similar vicious cycle has also been described between drinking and inflammation measured at the level of the brain.

Leclercq et al. (2014a) propositioned that the systemic inflammation observed in AD subjects originates, at least in part, in the gut, in particular, because of the translocation of bacterial components, such as LPS and peptidoglycans across the gut barrier. On the other hand, the same study also supports that inflammation, and in particular the increase in plasma TNF-α and IL-6, may not arise because of direct activation of gut immune components by bacterial products, but they may be generated indirectly by other target organs, such as the liver. Several mechanisms have been proposed to explain how inflammation may induce sickness behavior and depression. These include neural transmission by afferent projections of the vagus nerve to the brain (Schedlowski et al., 2014), a humoral route involving the blood–brain barrier, and tryptophan metabolism.

NEUROINFLAMMATION AND ALCOHOL DEPENDENCE

In addition to the known role for inflammation in the development of alcoholic liver diseases (Szabo et al., 2011), several lines of evidence suggest that excessive alcohol consumption also induces inflammation at the level of the brain. Evidence for an effect of ethanol on CNS inflammation arises from various studies that have described increases in inflammatory markers in cultures of rat brain slices (Zhou and Crews, 2010), murine macrophages (Fernandez-Lizarbe et al., 2008), primary microglia (Fernandez-Lizarbe et al., 2009), and astrocytes (Alfonso-Loeches et al., 2010). An inflammatory response has also been observed in rodents (Crews et al., 2006, 2013; Kane et al., 2014) that consume ethanol in a binge manner and in mice chronically exposed to ethanol consumption (Whitman et al., 2013; Lippai et al., 2013). Evidence of neuroinflammation has also been observed in human brains of AD subjects collected postmortem (Crews et al., 2013; Vetreno et al., 2013; He and Crews, 2008). A detailed review of the different inflammatory pathways activated in these models is provided in an excellent review and perspective by Robinson et al. (2014). Animal models support a relationship between alcohol consumption and the immune response (Wu et al., 2012; Harris and Blednov, 2013; Harris, 2014). For example, injection of TLR4 siRNA into the central amygdala of alcohol-preferring rats reduced ethanol self-administration (Liu et al., 2011). However, studies in TLR4 knock-out mice did not support this finding (Pascual et al., 2011). Nonetheless, injection of LPS has been shown to produce a prolonged increase in ethanol self-administration in mice (Blednov et al., 2011). Overlap in genes activated by ethanol and LPS has also been observed in mouse brain (Osterndorff-Kahanek et al., 2013, 2015). These authors demonstrated important changes in the expression of immune-related genes in microglia, astrocytes, and neuronal cells in various regions of the brain, including the amygdala, the nucleus accumbens, and the prefrontal cortex of mice in response to ethanol vapor exposure, further supporting an immunomodulatory role for ethanol in CNS inflammation. Some of the genes induced by ethanol are also regulated by LPS via a TLR4-dependent pathway (Gupta et al., 2013; Lee et al., 2013). In the context of alcohol dependence, approximately 10% of all of the genes in the human brain, particularly in the frontal cortex, for which expression was altered, were associated with inflammatory processes (Liu et al., 2006). Moreover, alterations in inflammatory signaling pathways have been observed after examination of human brains of chronic alcoholics (Okvist et al., 2007; Edenberg et al., 2008). However, other pathways, for instance those involving peptido-glycan and TLR2, have not yet been studied in detail in alcohol dependence. However, based on our own findings, it is likely that such pathways could also play a role in the pathophysiology of alcohol dependence (Leclercq et al., 2014a). However, the question remains as to whether inflammation associated with alcohol dependence is associated with neurodegeneration (El Khoury, 2010).

DYSBIOSIS AND THE COMPLEXITY OF SYMPTOMS IN ALCOHOL USE DISORDERS

The origins of inflammation associated with alcohol dependence are far from being clearly understood. This inflammation may arise from various sources; however, reported evidence confirms the existence of a disrupted gut barrier and gut microbi-ota in a subpopulation of AD patients (Leclercq et al., 2014b). These findings support the possibility that inflammation arises directly from the gut or may be associated with gut-derived bacterial products (Leclercq et al., 2014a). The fact that these altera-tions also correlate with more severe patterns of alcohol dependence, characterized by increased expression of craving, depression, and anxiety after a period of alcohol withdrawal, further supports the role of gut dysbiosis in the disorder (Leclercq et al., 2014b). Earlier reports implicating the gut in the development of AD also highlight a role for gut hormones in this regard (Leggio et al., 2011; Engel and Jerlhag, 2014).

The gut microbiota secretes more than 100 different metabolites (Clarke et al., 2014), suggesting that it could also act as an endocrine organ. Given the evidence that the microbiota can interact with the vagus nerve (Forsythe et al., 2014) and host stress systems (Moloney et al., 2014), it is of utmost importance to assess, at a behavioral level, these communication pathways in the context of alcohol use disorders. Beyond the negative reinforcement/sickness behavior hypothesis already discussed, dysbiosis could also have an influence on other aspects of the disease. Positive reinforcement processes as well as impulsivity factors, which are generally associated with the dis-order, are also likely to play an important role. Whether gut dysbiosis itself, or in con-junction with alcohol drinking, is related to alterations in impulsivity or in positive reinforcement processes deserves further exploration. Social isolation and deficits in social cognition also play a very important role in episodes of relapse (Zywiak et al., 2003). Deficits in theory of mind, defined as the difficulty in correctly interpreting the intentions or goals of other people, have been established in at least a subpopulation of AD subjects (Maurage et al., 2015). Whether these difficulties are related to gut-derived metabolites or to an effect of prolonged inflammation have yet to be determined.

CONCLUSION

In conclusion, exciting new evidence links the gut and its microbiota to a large spectrum of diseases, including alcohol dependence. Investigating novel concepts such as a gut-brain axis, or even a gut-liver-brain axis, as initiating or modulating the psychological symptoms and behavioral changes associated with AD will pave the way for further translational research in this area and the development of novel therapeutic approaches directed toward the gut and microbiota in managing this disorder.

REFERENCES

Adachi, Y., Moore, L.E., Bradford, B.U., Gao, W., Thurman, R.G., 1995. Antibiotics prevent liver injury in rats following long-term exposure to ethanol. Gastroenterology 108, 218–224.

Adams, J.B., Johansen, L.J., Powell, L.D., Quig, D., Rubin, R.A., 2011. Gastrointestinal flora and gastrointestinal status in children with autism–comparisons to typical children and correlation with autism severity. BMC Gastroenterol. 11, 22.

Akira, S., Uematsu, S., Takeuchi, O., 2006. Pathogen recognition and innate immunity. Cell 124 (4), 783–801.

Alfonso-Loeches, S., Pascual-Lucas, M., Blanco, A.M., Sanchez-Vera, I., Guerri, C., 2010. Pivotal role of TLR4 receptors in alcohol-induced neuroinflammation and brain damage. J. Neurosci. 30 (24), 8285–8295.

Amin, P.B., Diebel, L.N., Liberati, D.M., 2009. Dose-dependent effects of ethanol and E. coli on gut permeability and cytokine production. J. Surg. Res. 157 (2), 187–192.

Andersohn, F., Kiefer, F., 2004. Depressive mood and craving during alcohol withdrawal: association and interaction. Ger. J. Psychiatry 7, 6–11.

Arborelius, L., Owens, M.J., Plotsky, P.M., Nemeroff, C.B., 1999. The role of corticotropin-releasing factor in depression and anxiety disorders. J. Endocrinol. 160, 1–12.

Arora, T., Sharma, R., Frost, G., 2011. Propionate. Anti-obesity and satiety enhancing factor? Appetite 56, 511–515.

Atkinson, K.J., Rao, R.K., 2001. Role of protein tyrosine phosphorylation in acetaldehyde-induced disruption of epithelial tight junctions. Am. J. Physiol. Gastrointest. Liver Physiol. 280, G1280–G1288.

Attene-Ramos, M.S., Wagner, E.D., Plewa, M.J., Gaskins, H.R., 2006. Evidence that hydrogen sulfide is a genotoxic agent. Mol. Cancer Res. 4, 9–14.

Bailey, M.T., Dowd, S.E., Galley, J.D., Hufnagle, A.R., Allen, R.G., Lyte, M., 2011. Exposure to a social stressor alters the structure of the intestinal microbiota: implications for stressor-induced immunomodulation. Brain Behav. Immun. 25 (3), 397–407.

Bala, S., Marcos, M., Gattu, A., Catalano, D., Szabo, G., 2014. Acute binge drinking increases serum endotoxin and bacterial DNA levels in healthy individuals. PLoS One 9 (5), e96864.

Banan, A., Fields, J.Z., Decker, H., Zhang, Y., Keshavarzian, A., 2000. Nitric oxide and its metabolites mediate ethanol-induced microtubule disruption and intestinal barrier dysfunction. J. Pharmacol. Exp. Ther. 294 (3), 997–1008.

Bansal, T., Alaniz, R.C., Wood, T.K., Jayaraman, A., 2010. The bacterial signal indole increases epithelial-cell tight-junction resistance and attenuates indicators of inflammation. Proc. Natl. Acad. Sci. U.S.A. 107, 228–233.

Bjarnason, I., Peters, T.J., Wise, R.J., 1984. The leaky gut of alcoholism: possible route of entry for toxic compounds. Lancet 1 (8370), 179–182.

Blednov, Y.A., Benavidez, J.M., Geil, C., Perra, S., Morikawa, H., Harris, R.A., 2011. Activation of inflammatory signaling by lipopolysaccharide produces a prolonged increase of voluntary alcohol intake in mice. Brain Behav. Immun. 25 (Suppl. 1), S92–S105.

Bode, C., Vollmer, E., Hug, J., Bode, J.C., 1991. Increased permeability of the gut to polyethylene glycol and dextran in rats fed alcohol. Ann. N.Y. Acad. Sci. 625, 837–840.

Bode, C., Bode, J.C., 2003. Effect of alcohol consumption on the gut. Best Pract. Res. Clin. Gastroenterol. 17 (4), 575–592.

Bode, C., Kugler, V., Bode, J.C., 1987. Endotoxemia in patients with alcoholic and non-alcoholic cirrhosis and in subjects with no evidence of chronic liver disease following acute alcohol excess. J. Hepatol. 4, 8–14.

Bode, J.C., Bode, C., Heidelbach, R., Dürr, H.K., Martini, G.A., 1984. Jejunal microflora in patients with chronic alcohol abuse. Hepatogastroenterology 31, 30–34.

Bone, E., Tamm, A., Hill, M., 1976. The production of urinary phenols by gut bacteria and their possible role in the causation of large bowel cancer. Am. J. Clin. Nutr. 29, 1448–1454.

Bull-Otterson, L., Feng, W., Kirpich, I., et al., 2013. Metagenomic analyses of alcohol induced pathogenic alterations in the intestinal microbiome and the effect of *Lactobacillus rhamnosus* GG treatment. PLoS One 8, e53028.

Bures, J., et al., 1990. Excretion of phenol and p-cresol in the urine in fasting obese individuals and in persons treated with total enteral nutrition. Cas. Lek. Cesk. 129, 1166–1171.

Cani, P.D., Possemiers, S., Van de Wiele, T., Guiot, Y., Everard, A., Rottier, O., Geurts, L., Naslain, D., Neyrinck, A., Lambert, D.M., Muccioli, G.G., Delzenne, N.M., 2009. Changes in gut microbiota control inflammation in obese mice through a mechanism involving GLP-2-driven improvement of gut permeability. Gut 58, 1091–1103.

Capuron, L., Ravaud, A., Dantzer, R., 2000. Early depressive symptoms in cancer patients receiving interleukin 2 and/or interferon alfa-2b therapy. J. Clin. Oncol. 18 (10), 2143–2151.

Capuron, L., Ravaud, A., Gualde, N., Bosmans, E., Dantzer, R., Maes, M., Neveu, P.J., 2001. Association between immune activation and early depressive symptoms in cancer patients treated with interleukin-2-based therapy. Psychoneuroendocrinology 26 (8), 797–808.

Casafont Morencos, F., de las Heras Castaño, G., Martín Ramos, L., López Arias, M.J., Ledesma, F., Pons Romero, F., 1996. Small bowel bacterial overgrowth in patients with alcoholic cirrhosis. Dig. Dis. Sci. 41, 552–556.

Castagliuolo, I., Lamont, J.T., Qiu, B., Fleming, S.M., Bhaskar, K.R., Nikulasson, S.T., Kornetsky, C., Pothoulakis, C., 1996. Acute stress causes mucin release from rat colon: role of corticotropin releasing factor and mast cells. Am. J. Physiol. 271, G884–G892.

Chang, B., Sang, L., Wang, Y., Tong, J., Wang, B., 2013. The role of FoxO4 in the relationship between alcohol-induced intestinal barrier dysfunction and liver injury. Int. J. Mol. Med. 31 (3), 569–576.

Chen, P., Stärkel, P., Turner, J.R., Ho, S.B., Schnabl, B., 2015a. Dysbiosis-induced intestinal inflammation activates tumor necrosis factor receptor I and mediates alcoholic liver disease in mice. Hepatology 61 (3), 883–894.

Chen, P., Torralba, M., Tan, J., Embree, M., Zengler, K., Stärkel, P., van Pijkeren, J.P., DePew, J., Loomba, R., Ho, S.B., Bajaj, J.S., Mutlu, E.A., Keshavarzian, A., Tsukamoto, H., Nelson, K.E., Fouts, D.E., Schnabl, B., 2015b. Supplementation of saturated long-chain fatty acids maintains intestinal eubiosis and reduces ethanol-induced liver injury in mice. Gastroenterology 148 (1), 203–214.

Choudhry, M.A., Fazal, N., Goto, M., Gamelli, R.L., Sayeed, M.M., 2002. Gut-associated lymphoid T cell suppression enhances bacterial translocation in alcohol and burn injury. Am. J. Physiol. Gastrointest. Liver Physiol. 282, G937–G947.

Clarke, G., Stilling, R.M., Kennedy, P.J., Stanton, C., Cryan, J.F., Dinan, T.G., 2014. Minireview: gut microbiota: the neglected endocrine organ. Mol. Endocrinol 28 (8), 1221–1238.

Cordovil De Sousa Uva, M., Luminet, O., Cortesi, M., Constant, E., Derely, M., De Timary, P., 2010. Distinct effects of protracted withdrawal on affect, craving, selective attention and executive functions among alcohol-dependent patients. Alcohol Alcohol. 45, 241–246.

Crews, F., Nixon, K., Kim, D., Joseph, J., Shukitt-Hale, B., Qin, L., Zou, J., 2006. BHT blocks NF-kappaB activation and ethanol-induced brain damage. Alcohol. Clin. Exp. Res. 30 (11), 1938–1949.

Crews, F.T., Qin, L., Sheedy, D., Vetreno, R.P., Zou, J., 2013. High mobility group box 1/ Toll-like receptor danger signaling increases brain neuroimmune activation in alcohol dependence. Biol. Psychiatry 73 (7), 602–612.

Cryan, J.F., Dinan, T.G., 2012. Mind-altering microorganisms: the impact of the gut microbiota on brain and behaviour. Nat. Rev. Neurosci. 13 (10), 701–712.

Dantzer, R., O'Connor, J.C., Freund, G.G., Johnson, R.W., Kelley, K.W., 2008. From inflammation to sickness and depression: when the immune system subjugates the brain. Nat. Rev. Neurosci. 9, 46–56.

Dantzer, R., Wollman, E., Vitkovic, L., Yirmiya, R., 1999. Cytokines and depression: fortuitous or causative association? Mol. Psychiatry 4 (4), 328–332.

Dash, S., Clarke, G., Berk, M., Jacka, F.N., 2015. The gut microbiome and diet in psychiatry: focus on depression. Curr. Opin. Psychiatry 28, 1–6.

Dessein, R., Gironella, M., Vignal, C., Peyrin-Biroulet, L., Sokol, H., Secher, T., Lacas-Gervais, S., Gratadoux, J.J., Lafont, F., Dagorn, J.C., Ryffel, B., Akira, S., Langella, P., Nunez, G., Sirard, J.C., Iovanna, J., Simonet, M., Chamaillard, M., 2009. Toll-like receptor 2 is critical for induction of Reg3 beta expression and intestinal clearance of Yersinia pseudotuberculosis. Gut 58, 771–776.

Draper, L.R., Gyure, L.A., Hall, J.G., Robertson, D., 1983. Effect of alcohol on the integrity of the intestinal epithelium. Gut 24 (5), 399–404.

Dunagan, M., Chaudhry, K., Samak, G., Rao, R.K., 2012. Acetaldehyde disrupts tight junctions in caco-2 cell monolayers by a protein phosphatase 2A-dependent mechanism. Am. J. Physiol. Gastrointest. Liver Physiol. 303, G1356–G1364.

Edenberg, H.J., Xuei, X., Wetherill, L.F., Bierut, L., Bucholz, K., Dick, D.M., Hesselbrock, V., Kuperman, S., Porjesz, B., Schuckit, M.A., Tischfield, J.A., Almasy, L.A., Nurnberger Jr., J.I., Foroud, T., 2008. Association of NFKB1, which encodes a subunit of the transcription factor NF-kappaB, with alcohol dependence. Hum. Mol. Genet. 17 (7), 963–970.

Elamin, E., Jonkers, D., Juuti-Uusitalo, K., van Ijzendoorn, S., Troost, F., Duimel, H., Broers, J., Verheyen, F., Dekker, J., Masclee, A., 2012. Effects of ethanol and acetaldehyde on tight junction integrity: in vitro study in a three dimensional intestinal epithelial cell culture model. PLoS One 7 (4), e35008.

Elamin, E., Masclee, A., Troost, F., Pieters, H.J., Keszthelyi, D., Aleksa, K., Dekker, J., Jonkers, D., 2014a. Ethanol impairs intestinal barrier function in humans through mitogen activated protein kinase signaling: a combined in vivo and in vitro approach. PLoS One 9 (9), e107421.

Elamin, E., Masclee, A., Dekker, J., Jonkers, D., 2014b. Ethanol disrupts intestinal epithelial tight junction integrity through intracellular calcium-mediated Rho/ROCK activation. Am. J. Physiol. Gastrointest. Liver Physiol. 306 (8), G677–G685.

Elamin, E., Masclee, A., Troost, F., Dekker, J., Jonkers, D., 2014c. Activation of the epithelial-to-mesenchymal transition factor snail mediates acetaldehyde-induced intestinal epithelial barrier disruption. Alcohol. Clin. Exp. Res. 38, 344–353.

El Khoury, J., 2010. Neurodegeneration and the neuroimmune system. Nat. Med. 16, 1369–1370.

Engel, J.A., Jerlhag, E., 2014. Role of appetite-regulating peptides in the pathophysiology of addiction: implications for pharmacotherapy. CNS Drugs 28, 875–886.

Fernandez-Lizarbe, S., Pascual, M., Gascon, M.S., Blanco, A., Guerri, C., 2008. Lipid rafts regulate ethanol-induced activation of TLR4 signaling in murine macrophages. Mol. Immunol. 45 (7), 2007–2016.

Fernandez-Lizarbe, S., Pascual, M., Guerri, C., 2009. Critical role of TLR4 response in the activation of microglia induced by ethanol. J. Immunol. 183 (7), 4733–4744.

Finegold, S.M., Downes, J., Summanen, P.H., 2012. Microbiology of regressive autism. Anaerobe 18, 260–262.

Finn, P.R., 2002. Motivation, working memory, and decision making: a cognitive-motivational theory of personality vulnerability to alcoholism. Behav. Cogn. Neurosci. Rev. 1 (3), 183–205.

Flint, H.J., Duncan, S.H., Louis, P., 2014. Gut microbiome and obesity. In: Kushner, R.F., Bessesen, D.H. (Eds.), Treat. Obese Patient. Springer New York, New York, NY, pp. 73–82.

Forsyth, C.B., Farhadi, A., Jakate, S.M., Tang, Y., Shaikh, M., Keshavarzian, A., 2009. Lactobacillus GG treatment ameliorates alcohol-induced intestinal oxidative stress, gut leakiness, and liver injury in a rat model of alcoholic steatohepatitis. Alcohol 43, 163–172.

Forsyth, C.B., Tang, Y., Shaikh, M., Zhang, L., Keshavarzian, A., 2011. Role of snail activation in alcohol-induced iNOS-mediated disruption of intestinal epithelial cell permeability. Alcohol. Clin. Exp. Res. 35 (9), 1635–1643.

Forsyth, C.B., Voigt, R.M., Shaikh, M., Tang, Y., Cederbaum, A.I., Turek, F.W., Keshavarzian, A., 2013. Role for intestinal CYP2E1 in alcohol-induced circadian gene-mediated intestinal hyperpermeability. Am. J. Physiol. Gastrointest. Liver Physiol. 305 (2), G185–G195.

Forsyth, C.B., Voigt, R.M., Keshavarzian, A., 2014. Intestinal CYP2E1: a mediator of alcohol-induced gut leakiness. Redox Biol. 3, 40–46.

Forsythe, P., Bienenstock, J., Kunze, W.A., 2014. Vagal pathways for microbiome-brain-gut axis communication. Adv. Exp. Med. Biol. 817, 115–133.

Foster, J.A., McVey Neufeld, K.A., 2013. Gut-brain axis: how the microbiome influences anxiety and depression. Trends Neurosci. 36 (5), 305–312.

Friese, M., Hofmann, W., Wiers, R.W., 2011. On taming horses and strengthening riders: recent developments in research on interventions to improve self-control in health behaviors. Self Identity 10, 336–351.

Fukui, H., Brauner, B., Bode, J.C., Bode, C., 1991. Plasma endotoxin concentrations in patients with alcoholic and non-alcoholic liver disease: reevaluation with an improved chromogenic assay. J. Hepatol. 12, 162–169.

Galley, J.D., Nelson, M.C., Yu, Z., Dowd, S.E., Walter, J., Kumar, P.S., Lyte, M., Bailey, M.T., 2014. Exposure to a social stressor disrupts the community structure of the colonic mucosa-associated microbiota. BMC Microbiol. 14, 189.

Gareau, M.G., Jury, J., MacQueen, G., Sherman, P.M., Perdue, M.H., 2007. Probiotic treatment of rat pups normalises corticosterone release and ameliorates colonic dysfunction induced by maternal separation. Gut 56, 1522–1528.

Grewal, R.K., Mahmood, A., 2009. Ethanol effects on mucin glycosylation of mucins in rat intestine. Ann. Gastroenterol. 22, 178–183.

Guarner, F., Malagelada, J.-R., 2003. Gut flora in health and disease. Lancet 361, 512–519.

Gupta, A., Cooper, Z.A., Tulapurkar, M.E., Potla, R., Maity, T., Hasday, J.D., Singh, I.S., 2013. Toll-like receptor agonists and febrile range hyperthermia synergize to induce heat shock protein 70 expression and extracellular release. J. Biol. Chem. 288 (4), 2756–2766.

Hall, M.D., 2012. Alcoholism and depression. Home Healthc. Nurse 30, 543–550.

Hamer, H.M., De, P., Windey, K., Verbeke, K., 2012. Functional analysis of colonic bacterial metabolism: relevant to health? Am. J. Physiol. Gastrointest. Liver Physiol. 302, G1–G9.

Hamer, H.M., Jonkers, D., Venema, K., Vanhoutvin, S., Troost, F.J., Brummer, R.J., 2008. The role of butyrate on colonic function. Aliment. Pharmacol. Ther. 27, 104–119.

Harris, A., 2014. Endotoxins, alcohol consumption and neuroimmune signaling: a vicious cycle. In: Presentation at the 53rd Meeting of the American College of Neuropsychopharmacology.

Harris, R.A., Blednov, Y.A., 2013. Neuroimmune genes and alcohol drinking behavior. In: Cui, C., Grandison, L., Noronha, A. (Eds.), Neural-Immune Interactions in Brain Function and Alcohol Related Disorders. Springer, New York, pp. 425–440.

Hartmann, P., Chen, P., Wang, H.J., Wang, L., McCole, D.F., Brandl, K., Stärkel, P., Belzer, C., Hellerbrand, C., Tsukamoto, H., Ho, S.B., Schnabl, B., 2013. Deficiency of intestinal mucin-2 ameliorates experimental alcoholic liver disease in mice. Hepatology 58 (1), 108–119.

He, J., Crews, F.T., 2008. Increased MCP-1 and microglia in various regions of the human alcoholic brain. Exp. Neurol. 210 (2), 349–358.

Holdeman, L.V., Good, I.J., Moore, W.E., 1976. Human fecal flora: variation in bacterial composition within individuals and a possible effect of emotional stress. Appl. Environ. Microbiol. 31, 359–375.

Hooper, L.V., Littman, D.R., Macpherson, A.J., 2012. Interactions between the Microbiota.

Hsiao, E.Y., McBride, S.W., Hsien, S., Sharon, G., Hyde, E.R., McCue, T., Codelli, J.A., Chow, J., Reisman, S.E., Petrosino, J.F., et al., 2013. Microbiota modulate behavioral and physiological abnormalities associated with neurodevelopmental disorders. Cell 155, 1451–1463.

Hughes, R., Kurth, M.J., McGilligan, V., McGlynn, H., Rowland, I., 2008. Effect of colonic bacterial metabolites on caco-2 cell paracellular permeability in vitro. Nutr. Cancer 60, 259–266.

Jiang, H., Ling, Z., Zhang, Y., Mao, H., Ma, Z., Yin, Y., Wang, W., Tang, W., Tan, Z., Shi, J., Li, L., Ruan, B., April 13, 2015. Altered fecal microbiota composition in patients with major depressive disorder. Brain Behav. Immun. 48, 186–194. http://dx.doi.org/10.1016/j.bbi.2015.03.016. pii:S0889–1591(15)00110-5 (Epub ahead of print).

Johansson, M.E., Phillipson, M., Petersson, J., Velcich, A., Holm, L., Hansson, G.C., 2008. The inner of the two Muc2 mucin-dependent mucus layers in colon is devoid of bacteria. Proc. Natl. Acad. Sci. U.S.A. 105, 15064–15069.

Kane, C.J., Phelan, K.D., Douglas, J.C., Wagoner, G., Johnson, J.W., Xu, J., Phelan, P.S., Drew, P.D., 2014. Effects of ethanol on immune response in the brain: region-specific changes in adolescent versus adult mice. Alcohol. Clin. Exp. Res. 38 (2), 384–391.

Kawai, T., Akira, S., 2007. Signaling to NF-kappaB by toll-like receptors. Trends Mol. Med. 13, 460–469.

Keshavarzian, A., Fields, J.Z., Vaeth, J., Holmes, E.W., 1994. The differing effects of acute and chronic alcohol on gastric and intestinal permeability. Am. J. Gastroenterol. 89, 2205–2211.

Keshavarzian, A., Farhadi, A., Forsyth, C.B., Rangan, J., Jakate, S., Shaikh, M., Banan, A., Fields, J.Z., 2009. Evidence that chronic alcohol exposure promotes intestinal oxidative stress, intestinal hyperpermeability and endotoxemia prior to development of alcoholic steatohepatitis in rats. J. Hepatol. 50 (3), 538–547.

Keshavarzian, A., Choudhary, S., Holmes, E.W., Yong, S., Banan, A., Jakate, S., Fields, J.Z., 2001. Preventing gut leakiness by oats supplementation ameliorates alcohol-induced liver damage in rats. J. Pharmacol. Exp. Ther. 299, 442–448.

Kirpich, I.A., Solovieva, N.V., Leikhter, S.N., Shidakova, N.A., Lebedeva, O.V., Sidorov, P.I., Bazhukova, T.A., Soloviev, A.G., Barve, S.S., McClain, C.J., Cave, M., 2008. Probiotics restore bowel flora and improve liver enzymes in human alcohol-induced liver injury: a pilot study. Alcohol 42, 675–682.

van Klinken, B.J., Einerhand, A.W., Duits, L.A., Makkink, M.K., Tytgat, K.M., Renes, I.B., Verburg, M., et al., 1999. Gastrointestinal expression and partial cDNA cloning of murine Muc2. Am. J. Physiol. 276, G115–G124.

Knowles, S.R., Nelson, E.A., Palombo, E.A., 2008. Investigating the role of perceived stress on bacterial flora activity and salivary cortisol secretion: a possible mechanism underlying susceptibility to illness. Biol. Psychol. 77, 132–137.

Konsman, J.P., Parnet, P., Dantzer, R., 2002. Cytokine-induced sickness behaviour: mechanisms and implications. Trends Neurosci. 25, 154–159.

Koob, G.F., Le Moal, M., 2008. Neurobiological mechanisms for opponent motivational processes in addiction. Philos. Trans. R. Soc. B. Biol. Sci. 363 (1507), 3113.

Koob, G.F., Le Moal, M., 2005. Plasticity of reward neurocircuitry and the 'dark side' of drug addiction. Nat. Neurosci. 8, 1442–1444.

Kornreich, C., Foisy, M.-L., Philippot, P., Dan, B., Tecco, J., Noel, X., Hess, U., Pelc, I., Verbanck, P., 2003. Impaired emotional facial expression recognition in alcoholics, opiate dependence subjects, methadone maintained subjects and mixed alcohol-opiate antecedents subjects compared with normal controls. Psychiatry Res. 119, 251–260.

Kyoko, O., Kono, H., Ishimaru, K., Miyake, K., Kubota, T., Ogawa, H., Okumura, K., Shibata, S., Nakao, A., 2014. Expressions of tight junction proteins occludin and claudin-1 are under the circadian control in the mouse large intestine: implications in intestinal permeability and susceptibility to colitis. PLoS One 9, e98016.

Lavö, B.1, Colombel, J.F., Knutsson, L., Hällgren, R., 1992. Acute exposure of small intestine to ethanol induces mucosal leakage and prostaglandin E2 synthesis. Gastroenterology 102 (2), 468–473.

Leclercq, S., Cani, P.D., Neyrinck, A.M., Stärkel, P., Jamar, F., Mikolajczak, M., Delzenne, N.M., de Timary, P., 2012. Role of intestinal permeability and inflammation in the biological and behavioral control of alcohol-dependent subjects. Brain Behav. Immun. 26 (6), 911–918.

Leclercq, S., Matamoros, S., Cani, P.D., Neyrinck, A.M., Jamar, F., Stärkel, P., Windey, K., Tremaroli, V., Bäckhed, F., Verbeke, K., de Timary, P., Delzenne, N.M., 2014a. Intestinal permeability, gut-bacterial dysbiosis, and behavioral markers of alcohol-dependence severity. Proc. Natl. Acad. Sci. U.S.A. 111 (42), E4485–E4493.

Leclercq, S., De Saeger, C., Delzenne, N., de Timary, P., Stärkel, P., 2014b. Role of inflammatory pathways, blood mononuclear cells, and gut-derived bacterial products in alcohol dependence. Biol. Psychiatry 76 (9), 725–733.

Lee, K.H., Jeong, J., Yoo, C.G., 2013. Positive feedback regulation of heat shock protein 70 (Hsp70) is mediated through toll-like receptor 4-PI3K/Akt-glycogen synthase kinase-3beta pathway. Exp. Cell Res. 319 (1), 88–95.

Leggio, L., Addolorato, G., Cippitelli, A., Jerlhag, E., Kampov-Polevoy, A.B., Swift, R.M., 2011. Role of feeding-related pathways in alcohol dependence: a focus on sweet preference, NPY, and ghrelin. Alcohol. Clin. Exp. Res. 35, 194–202.

Linden, S.K., Florin, T.H., McGuckin, M.A., 2008. Mucin dynamics in intestinal bacterial infection. PLoS One 3, e3952.

Lippai, D., Bala, S., Petrasek, J., Csak, T., Levin, I., Kurt-Jones, E.A., Szabo, G., 2013. Alcohol-induced IL-1beta in the brain is mediated by NLRP3/ASC inflammasome activation that amplifies neuroinflammation. J. Leukoc. Biol. 94 (1), 171–182.

Liu, J., Lewohl, J.M., Harris, R.A., Iyer, V.R., Dodd, P.R., Randall, P.K., Mayfield, R.D., 2006. Patterns of gene expression in the frontal cortex discriminate alcoholic from nonalcoholic individuals. Neuropsychopharmacology 31 (7), 1574–1582.

Liu, J., Yang, A.R., Kelly, T., Puche, A., Esoga, C., June Jr., H.L., Elnabawi, A., Merchenthaler, I., Sieghart, W., June Sr., H.L., Aurelian, L., 2011. Binge alcohol drinking is associated with GABA$_A$ alpha2-regulated toll-like receptor 4 (TLR4) expression in the central amygdala. Proc. Natl. Acad. Sci. U.S.A. 108 (11), 4465–4470.

Lord, R.S., Bralley, J.A., 2008. Clinical applications of urinary organic acids. Part 2. Dysbiosis markers. Altern. Med. Rev. 13, 292–306.

Luna, R.A., Foster, J.A., 2014. Gut brain axis: diet microbiota interactions and implications for modulation of anxiety and depression. Curr. Opin. Biotechnol. 32C, 35–41.

Lund, I., 2007. Drinking on the premises in Norway: young adults' use of public drinking places. Addict. Behav. 32 (12), 2737–2746.

Macfarlane, S., Macfarlane, G.T., 2003. Regulation of short-chain fatty acid production. Proc. Nutr. Soc. 62, 67–72.

Machiels, K., Joossens, M., Sabino, J., De Preter, V., Arijs, I., Eeckhaut, V., Ballet, V., Claes, K., Van Immerseel, F., Verbeke, K., Ferrante, M., Verhaegen, J., Rutgeerts, P., Vermeire, S., 2013. A decrease of the butyrate-producing species *Roseburia hominis* and *Faecalibacterium prausnitzii* defines dysbiosis in patients with ulcerative colitis. Gut 63 (8), 1275–1283.

Madsen, K., Cornish, A., Soper, P., McKaigney, C., Jijon, H., Yachimec, C., Doyle, J., Jewell, L., De Simone, C., 2001. Probiotic bacteria enhance murine and human intestinal epithelial barrier function. Gastroenterology 121, 580–591.

Maier, A., Bode, C., Fritz, P., Bode, J.C., 1999. Effects of chronic alcohol abuse on duodenal mononuclear cells in man. Dig. Dis. Sci. 44 (4), 691–696.

Maraslioglu, M., Oppermann, E., Blattner, C., Weber, R., Henrich, D., Jobin, C., Schleucher, E., Marzi, I., Lehnert, M., 2014. Chronic ethanol feeding modulates inflammatory mediators, activation of nuclear factor-κB, and responsiveness to endotoxin in murine Kupffer cells and circulating leukocytes. Mediators Inflamm. 2014, 808695.

Maes, M., 1999. Major depression and activation of the inflammatory response system. In: Dantzer, R., Wollman, E.E., Yirmiya, R. (Eds.), Cytokines, Stress, and Depression. Springer, US, pp. 25–46. Available from: http://link.springer.com/chapter/10.1007/978-0-585-37970-8_2.

Matsuo, K., Ota, H., Akamatsu, T., Sugiyama, A., Katsuyama, T., 1997. Histochemistry of the surface mucous gel layer of the human colon. Gut 40, 782–789.

Maurage, P., Campanella, S., Philippot, P., Charest, I., Martin, S., de Timary, P., 2009. Impaired emotional facial expression decoding in alcoholism is also present for emotional prosody and body postures. Alcohol Alcohol. 44, 476–485.

Maurage, P., Joassin, F., Philippot, P., Heeren, A., Vermeulen, N., Mahau, P., Delperdange, C., Corneille, O., Luminet, O., de Timary, P., 2012. Disrupted regulation of social exclusion in alcohol dependence: an fMRI study. Neuropsychopharmacology 37 (9), 2067–2075.

Maurage, F., de Timary, P., Tecco, J.M., Lechantre, S., Samson, D., 2015. Theory of mind difficulties in patients with alcohol dependence: beyond the prefrontal cortex dysfunction hypothesis. Alcohol. Clin. Exp. Res. 39 (6), 980–988.

Mayfield, R.D., Harris, R.A., Schuckit, M.A., 2008. Genetic factors influencing alcohol dependence. Br. J. Pharmacol. 154, 275–287.

McCall, I.C., Betanzos, A., Weber, D.A., Nava, P., Miller, G.W., Parkos, C.A., 2009. Effects of phenol on barrier function of a human intestinal epithelial cell line correlate with altered tight junction protein localization. Toxicol. Appl. Pharmacol. 241, 61–70.

McGuckin, M.A., Linden, S.K., Sutton, P., Florin, T.H., 2011. Mucin dynamics and enteric pathogens. Nat. Rev. Microbiol. 9, 265–278.

Moloney, R.D., Desbonnet, L., Clarke, G., Dinan, T.G., Cryan, J.F., 2014. The microbiome: stress, health and disease. Mamm. Genome J. Int. Mamm. Genome Soc. 25, 49–74.

Musselman, D.L., Lawson, D.H., Gumnick, J.F., Manatunga, A.K., Penna, S., Goodkin, R.S., Greiner, K., Nemeroff, C.B., Miller, A.H., 2001. Paroxetine for the prevention of depression induced by high-dose interferon alfa. N. Engl. J. Med. 344 (13), 961–966.

Mutlu, E., Keshavarzian, A., Engen, P., Forsyth, C.B., Sikaroodi, M., Gillevet, P., 2009. Intestinal dysbiosis: a possible mechanism of alcohol-induced endotoxemia and alcoholic steatohepatitis in rats. Alcohol. Clin. Exp. Res. 33, 1836–1846.

Mutlu, E.A., Gillevet, P.M., Rangwala, H., Sikaroodi, M., Naqvi, A., Engen, P.A., Kwasny, M., Lau, C.K., Keshavarzian, A., 2012. Colonic microbiome is altered in alcoholism. Am. J. Physiol. Gastrointest. Liver Physiol. 302 (9), G966–G978.

Nanji, A.A., Khettry, U., Sadrzadeh, S.M., 1994. Lactobacillus feeding reduces endotoxemia and severity of experimental alcoholic liver (disease). Proc. Soc. Exp. Biol. Med. 205, 243–247.

Nanji, A.A., Khettry, U., Sadrzadeh, S.M., Yamanaka, T., 1993. Severity of liver injury in experimental alcoholic liver disease. Correlation with plasma endotoxin, prostaglandin E2, leukotriene B4, and thromboxane B2. Am. J. Pathol. 142, 367–373.

Naseribafrouei, A., Hestad, K., Avershina, E., Sekelja, M., Linløkken, A., Wilson, R., Rudi, K., 2014. Correlation between the human fecal microbiota and depression. Neurogastroenterol. Motil. 26 (8), 1155–1162.

Nicholson, J.K., Holmes, E., Kinross, J., Burcelin, R., Gibson, G., Jia, W., Pettersson, S., 2012. Host-gut microbiota metabolic interactions. Science 336, 1262–1267.

Noel, X., Van der Linden, M., Schmidt, N., Sferrazza, R., Hanak, C., Le Bon, O., De Mol, J., Kornreich, C., Pelc, I., Verbanck, P., 2001. Supervisory attentional system in nonamnesic alcoholic men. Arch. Gen. Psychiatry 58, 1152–1158.

Nutt, D.J., King, L.A., Phillips, L.D., Independent Scientific Committee on Drugs, 2010. Drug harms in the UK: a multicriteria decision analysis. Lancet 376, 1558–1565.

Okvist, A., Johansson, S., Kuzmin, A., Bazov, I., Merino-Martinez, R., Ponomarev, I., Mayfield, R.D., Harris, R.A., Sheedy, D., Garrick, T., Harper, C., Hurd, Y.L., Terenius, L., Ekström, T.J., Bakalkin, G., Yakovleva, T., 2007. Neuroadaptations in human chronic alcoholics: dysregulation of the NF-kappaB system. PLoS One 2 (9), e930.

Osterndorff-Kahanek, E.A., Becker, H.C., Lopez, M.F., Farris, S.P., Tiwari, G.R., Nunez, Y.O., Harris, R.A., Mayfield, R.D., 2015. Chronic ethanol exposure produces time- and brain region-dependent changes in gene coexpression networks. PLoS One 10 (3), e0121522.

Osterndorff-Kahanek, E., Ponomarev, I., Blednov, Y.A., Harris, R.A., 2013. Gene expression in brain and liver produced by three different regimens of alcohol consumption in mice: comparison with immune activation. PLoS One 8 (3), e59870.

Parlesak, A., Schäfer, C., Schütz, T., Bode, J.C., Bode, C., 2000. Increased intestinal permeability to macromolecules and endotoxemia in patients with chronic alcohol abuse in different stages of alcohol-induced liver disease. J. Hepatol. 32, 742–747.

Pascual, M., Baliño, P., Aragón, C.M., Guerri, C., 2015. Cytokines and chemokines as biomarkers of ethanol-induced neuroinflammation and anxiety-related behavior: role of TLR4 and TLR2. Neuropharmacology 89, 352–359.

Pascual, M., Balino, P., Alfonso-Loeches, S., Aragon, C.M., Guerri, C., 2011. Impact of TLR4 on behavioral and cognitive dysfunctions associated with alcohol-induced neuroinflammatory damage. Brain Behav. Immun. 25 (Suppl. 1), S80–S91.

Qin, X., Deitch, E.A., 2015. Dissolution of lipids from mucus: a possible mechanism for prompt disruption of gut barrier function by alcohol. Toxicol. Lett. 232 (2), 356–362.

Rao, R.K., 2008. Acetaldehyde-induced barrier disruption and paracellular permeability in caco-2 cell monolayer. Methods Mol. Biol. 447, 171–183.

Rao, R., 2009. Endotoxemia and gut barrier dysfunction in alcoholic liver disease. Hepatology 50 (2), 638–644.

Robinson, G., Most, D., Ferguson, L.B., Mayfield, J., Harris, R.A., Blednov, Y.A., 2014. Neuroimmune pathways in alcohol consumption: evidence from behavioral and genetic studies in rodents and humans. Int. Rev. Neurobiol. 118, 13–39.

Rehm, J., Shield, K.D., Gmel, G., Rehm, M.X., Frick, U., 2013. Modeling the impact of alcohol dependence on mortality burden and the effect of available treatment interventions in the European Union. Eur. Neuropsychopharmacol. J. Eur. Coll. Neuropsychopharmacol. 23, 89–97.

Reichenberg, A., Yirmiya, R., Schuld, A., Kraus, T., Haack, M., Morag, A., Pollmächer, T., 2001. Cytokine-associated emotional and cognitive disturbances in humans. Arch. Gen. Psychiatry 58 (5), 445–452.

Samak, G., Aggarwal, S., Rao, R.K., 2011. ERK is involved in EGF-mediated protection of tight junctions, but not adherens junctions, in acetaldehyde-treated caco-2 cell monolayers. Am. J. Physiol. Gastrointest. Liver Physiol. 301, G50–G59.

Sandor, F., Buc, M., 2005. Toll-like receptors. I. Structure, function and their ligands. Folia Biol. (Praha) 51 (5), 148–157.

Saunders, P.R., Santos, J., Hanssen, N.P., Yates, D., Groot, J.A., Perdue, M.H., 2002. Physical and psychological stress in rats enhances colonic epithelial permeability via peripheral CRH. Dig. Dis. Sci. 47, 208–215.

Saunders, S.M., Zygowicz, K.M., D'Angelo, B.R., 2006. Person-related and treatment related barriers to alcohol treatment. J. Subst. Abuse Treat. 30, 261–270.

Schedlowski, M., Engler, H., Grigoleit, J.-S., 2014. Endotoxin-induced experimental systemic inflammation in humans: a model to disentangle immune-to-brain communication. Brain Behav. Immun. 35, 1–8.

Schomerus, G., Lucht, M., Holzinger, A., Matschinger, H., Carta, M.G., Angermeyer, M.C., 2011. The stigma of alcohol dependence compared with other mental disorders: a review of population studies. Alcohol Alcohol. 46, 105–112.

Schuckit, M.A., 2000. Genetics of the risk for alcoholism. Am. J. Addict./Am. Acad. Psychiat. Alcohol. Addict. 9, 103–112.

Shenkin, A., 2006. Serum prealbumin: Is it a marker of nutritional status or of risk of malnutrition? Clin. Chem. 52, 2177–2179.

Silhavy, T.J., Kahne, D., Walker, S., 2010. The bacterial cell envelope. Cold Spring Harb. Perspect. Biol. 2 (5), a000414.

Smith, R.S., 1991. The macrophage theory of depression. Med. Hypotheses 35 (4), 298–306.

Söderholm, J.D., Yates, D.A., Gareau, M.G., Yang, P.C., MacQueen, G., Perdue, M.H., 2002. Neonatal maternal separation predisposes adult rats to colonic barrier dysfunction in response to mild stress. Am. J. Physiol-Gastrointest. Liver Physiol. 283, G1257–G1263.

Sokol, H., Pigneur, B., Watterlot, L., Lakhdari, O., Bermúdez-Humarán, L.G., Gratadoux, J.J., Blugeon, S., Bridonneau, C., Furet, J.P., Corthier, G., Grangette, C., Vasquez, N., Pochart, P., Trugnan, G., Thomas, G., Blottière, H.M., Doré, J., Marteau, P., Seksik, P., Langella, P., 2008. *Faecalibacterium prausnitzii* is an anti-inflammatory commensal bacterium identified by gut microbiota analysis of Crohn disease patients. Proc. Natl. Acad. Sci. U.S.A. 105, 16731–16736.

Summa, K.C., Voigt, R.M., Forsyth, C.B., Shaikh, M., Cavanaugh, K., Tang, Y., Vitaterna, M.H., Song, S., Turek, F.W., Keshavarzian, A., 2013. Disruption of the circadian clock in mice increases intestinal permeability and promotes alcohol-induced hepatic pathology and inflammation. PLoS One 8, e67102.

Suzuki, T., Seth, A., Rao, R., 2008. Role of phospholipase Cgamma-induced activation of protein kinase Cepsilon (PKCepsilon) and PKCbetaI in epidermal growth factor-mediated protection of tight junctions from acetaldehyde in caco-2 cell monolayers. J. Biol. Chem. 283, 3574–3583.

Swanson, G., Forsyth, C.B., Tang, Y., Shaikh, M., Zhang, L., Turek, F.W., Keshavarzian, A., 2011. Role of intestinal circadian genes in alcohol-induced gut leakiness. Alcohol. Clin. Exp. Res. 35, 1305–1314.

Szabo, G., Lippai, D., 2014. Converging actions of alcohol on liver and brain immune signaling. Int. Rev. Neurobiol. 118, 359–380.

Szabo, G., Mandrekar, P., Petrasek, J., Catalano, D., 2011. The unfolding web of innate immune dysregulation in alcoholic liver injury. Alcohol. Clin. Exp. Res. 35 (5), 782–786.

Takeuchi, O., Hoshino, K., Kawai, T., Sanjo, H., Takada, H., Ogawa, T., Takeda, K., Akira, S., 1999. Differential roles of TLR2 and TLR4 in recognition of gram-negative and gram-positive bacterial cell wall components. Immunity 11 (4), 443–451.

Tang, Y., Forsyth, C.B., Farhadi, A., Rangan, J., Jakate, S., Shaikh, M., Banan, A., Fields, J.Z., Keshavarzian, A., 2009. Nitric oxide-mediated intestinal injury is required for alcohol-induced gut leakiness and liver damage. Alcohol. Clin. Exp. Res. 33 (7), 1220–1230.

Teitelbaum, A.A., Gareau, M.G., Jury, J., Yang, P.C., Perdue, M.H., 2008. Chronic peripheral administration of corticotropin-releasing factor causes colonic barrier dysfunction similar to psychological stress. AJP Gastrointest. Liver Physiol. 295, G452–G459.

de Timary, P., Cani, P.D., Duchemin, J., Neyrinck, A.M., Gihousse, D., Laterre, P.F., Badaoui, A., Leclercq, S., Delzenne, N.M., Stärkel, P., 2012. The loss of metabolic control on alcohol drinking in heavy drinking alcohol-dependent subjects. PLoS One 7, e38682.

de Timary, P., Cordovil de Sousa Uva, M., Denoel, C., Hebborn, L., Derely, M., Desseilles, M., Luminet, O., 2013. The associations between self-consciousness, depressive state and craving to drink among alcohol dependent patients undergoing protracted withdrawal. PLoS One 8, e71560.

de Timary, P., Luts, A., Hers, D., Luminet, O., 2008. Absolute and relative stability of alexithymia in alcoholic inpatients undergoing alcohol withdrawal: relationship to depression and anxiety. Psychiatry Res. 157, 105–113.

Tong, J., Wang, Y., Chang, B., Zhang, D., Liu, P., Wang, B., 2013a. Activation of RhoA in alcohol-induced intestinal barrier dysfunction. Inflammation 36 (3), 750–758.

Tong, J., Wang, Y., Chang, B., Zhang, D., Wang, B., 2013b. Evidence for the involvement of RhoA signaling in the ethanol-induced increase in intestinal epithelial barrier permeability. Int. J. Mol. Sci. 14 (2), 3946–3960.

Uekermann, J., Daum, I., 2008. Social cognition in alcoholism: a link to prefrontal cortex dysfunction? Addiction 103, 726–735.

Uekermann, J., Channon, S., Winkel, K., Schlebusch, P., Daum, I., 2007. Theory of mind, humour processing and executive functioning in alcoholism. Addiction 102, 232–240.

Van Eck, M., Berkhof, H., Nicolson, N., Sulon, J., 1996. The effects of perceived stress, traits, mood states, and stressful daily events on salivary cortisol. Psychosom. Med. 58, 447–458.

Venkatesh, M., Mukherjee, S., Wang, H., Li, H., Sun, K., Benechet, A.P., Qiu, Z., Maher, L., Redinbo, M.R., Phillips, R.S., Fleet, J.C., Kortagere, S., Mukherjee, P., Fasano, A., Le Ven, J., Nicholson, J.K., Dumas, M.E., Khanna, K.M., Mani, S., 2014. Symbiotic bacterial metabolites regulate gastrointestinal barrier function via the xenobiotic sensor PXR and toll-like receptor 4. Immunity 41 (2), 296–310.

Vetreno, R.P., Qin, L., Crews, F.T., 2013. Increased receptor for advanced glycation end product expression in the human alcoholic prefrontal cortex is linked to adolescent drinking. Neurobiol. Dis. 59, 52–62.

Voigt, R.M., Forsyth, C.B., Keshavarzian, A., 2013. Circadian disruption: potential implications in inflammatory and metabolic diseases associated with alcohol. Alcohol. Res. Curr. Rev. 35, 87.

Volkow, N.D., Li, T.K., 2004. Drug addiction: the neurobiology of behaviour gone awry. Nat. Rev. Neurosci. 5, 963–970.

Wang, H., Li, X., Wang, C., Zhu, D., Xu, Y., 2014a. Abnormal ultrastructure of intestinal epithelial barrier in mice with alcoholic steatohepatitis. Alcohol 48 (8), 787–793.

Wang, Y., Tong, J., Chang, B., Wang, B., Zhang, D., Wang, B., 2014b. Effects of alcohol on intestinal epithelial barrier permeability and expression of tight junction-associated proteins. Mol. Med. Rep. 9 (6), 2352–2356.

Ward, L.A., Johnson, K.A., Robinson, I.M., Yokoyama, M.T., 1987. Isolation from swine feces of a bacterium which decarboxylates p-hydroxyphenylacetic acid to 4-methylphenol (p-cresol). Appl. Environ. Microbiol. 53, 189–192.

Whitman, B.A., Knapp, D.J., Werner, D.F., Crews, F.T., Breese, G.R., 2013. The cytokine mRNA increase induced by withdrawal from chronic ethanol in the sterile environment of brain is mediated by CRF and HMGB1 release. Alcoholism. Clin. Exp. Res. 37 (12), 2086–2097.

Worthington, B.S., Meserole, L., Syrotuck, J.A., 1978. Effect of daily ethanol ingestion on intestinal permeability to macromolecules. Am. J. Dig. Dis. 23 (1), 23–32.

Wright, C.E., Strike, P.C., Brydon, L., Steptoe, A., 2005. Acute inflammation and negative mood: mediation by cytokine activation. Brain Behav. Immun. 19 (4), 345–350.

Wu, Y., Lousberg, E.L., Moldenhauer, L.M., Hayball, J.D., Coller, J.K., Rice, K.C., Watkins, L.R., Somogyi, A.A., Hutchinson, M.R., 2012. Inhibiting the TLR4-MyD88 signalling cascade by genetic or pharmacological strategies reduces acute alcohol- induced sedation and motor impairment in mice. Br. J. Pharmacol. 165 (5), 1319–1329.

Xie, G., Zhong, W., Zheng, X., Li, Q., Qiu, Y., Li, H., Chen, H., Zhou, Z., Jia, W., 2013. Chronic ethanol consumption alters mammalian gastrointestinal content metabolites. J. Proteome Res. 12, 3297–3306.

Yan, A.W., Fouts, D.E., Brandl, J., Stärkel, P., Torralba, M., Schott, E., Tsukamoto, H., Nelson, K.E., Brenner, D.A., Schnabl, B., 2011. Enteric dysbiosis associated with a mouse model of alcoholic liver disease. Hepatology 53 (1), 96–105.

Yirmiya, R., 1996. Endotoxin produces a depressive-like episode in rats. Brain Res. 711 (1–2), 163–174.

Yirmiya, R., Weidenfeld, J., Pollak, Y., Morag, M., Morag, A., Avitsur, R., Barak, O., Reichenberg, A., Cohen, E., Shavit, Y., Ovadia, H., 1999. Cytokines, "depression due to a general medical condition," and antidepressant drugs. Adv. Exp. Med. Biol. 461, 283–316.

Yokoyama, M.T., Carlson, J.R., 1979. Microbial metabolites of tryptophan in the intestinal tract with special reference to skatole. Am. J. Clin. Nutr. 32, 173–178.

Zheng, X., Xie, G., Zhao, A., Zhao, L., Yao, C., Chiu, N.H., Zhou, Z., Bao, Y., Jia, W., Nicholson, J.K., Jia, W., 2011. The footprints of gut microbial-mammalian co-metabolism. J. Proteome Res. 10, 5512–5522.

Zhong, W., Zhao, Y., McClain, C.J., Kang, Y.J., Zhou, Z., 2010. Inactivation of hepatocyte nuclear factor-4{alpha} mediates alcohol-induced downregulation of intestinal tight junction proteins. Am. J. Physiol. Gastrointest. Liver Physiol. 299 (3), G643–G651.

Zimmermann, U.S., Blomeyer, D., Laucht, M., Mann, K.F., 2007. How gene–stress–behavior interactions can promote adolescent alcohol use: the roles of predrinking allostatic load and childhood behavior disorders. Pharmacol. Biochem. Behav. 86, 246–262.

Zolotarevsky, Y., Hecht, G., Koutsouris, A., Gonzalez, D.E., Quan, C., Tom, J., Mrsny, R.J., Turner, J.R., 2002. A membrane-permeant peptide that inhibits MLC kinase restores barrier function in in vitro models of intestinal disease. Gastroenterology 123 (1), 163–172.

Zhou, J., Crews, F., 2010. Induction of innate immune gene expression cascades in brain slice cultures by ethanol: key role of NF-kappaB and proinflammatory cytokines. Alcohol. Clin. Exp. Res. 34 (5), 777–789.

Zywiak, W.H., Westerberg, V.S., Connors, G.J., Maisto, S.A., 2003. Exploratory findings from the reasons for drinking questionnaire. J. Subst. Abuse Treat. 25, 287–292.

Gut Microbiota and Metabolism

18

P.M. Ryan

Teagasc Food Research Centre, Fermoy, Cork, Ireland; University College Cork, School of Microbiology, Cork, Ireland; University College Cork, APC Microbiome Institute, Cork, Ireland

N.M. Delzenne

Catholic University of Louvain, Louvain Drug Research Institute, Metabolism and Nutrition Research Group, Brussels, Belgium

INTRODUCTION

Obesity is typically characterized molecularly by a low-grade systemic inflammation and is associated with a wide cluster of metabolic alterations, including glucose homeostasis disorders (eg, glucose intolerance, insulin resistance, and type II diabetes), cardiovascular diseases or risk factors (eg, hypertension, dyslipidemia, and fibrinolysis disorders), and nonalcoholic fatty liver disease (Ogden et al., 2007). Although the pathogenesis of obesity is recognized to be at least in part genetic, the impact of environmental stresses on human metabolism must not be understated. The gut microbiota may be a key exteriorized organ and can be considered an important environmental factor that can contribute to the onset of these metabolic dysregulations (for reviews see Cani and Delzenne, 2009; Cani et al., 2012; Delzenne et al., 2011; Ryan et al., 2015). The gut microbiota is involved in the regulation of numerous physiological pathways by affecting different functions of the host (Cani, 2014). Among these regulations, the influence of gut microbes on energy metabolism is of particular interest because it has been suggested to be a driving force in the pathogenesis of obesity.

Although the sheer numbers of bacteria that reside on each epithelial ecosystem of our body is in itself intriguing, it is the fact that the collective genes expressed by these organisms outnumber our own by a factor of more than 100 that is most staggering and relevant to our metabolic health (Qin et al., 2010). An elegant series of animal studies from the groups of Gordon (Ridaura et al., 2013) and Blaser (Cho et al., 2012) have previously demonstrated without doubt the central role that the gut microbiota play in health and obesity onset and the pressures that modern antibiotic exposures (including subtherapeutic levels) can put on the composition and functionality of this microbial organ.

In this chapter we discuss recent evidence supporting the hypothesis that the gut microbiota can influence host metabolism using various mechanisms and that changes in microbiota composition trigger modifications of metabolic behavior. Among the tools available to modulate the gut microbiota, with interesting effects on host health, probiotic and prebiotic approaches appear as particularly interesting. Those concepts have been revisited, taking into account the fact that the administration of live bacteria or prebiotic nutrients exerts more global metabolic effects as opposed to simply targeting a limited number of bacterial species involved in host metabolism.

GUT MICROBIOTA COMPOSITION AND METABOLIC DISORDERS

The importance of our intestinal bacteria has long been overlooked, in part because of the dearth of tools available to analyze the complex diversity of species in any comprehensive manner. Since the introduction of high-throughput sequencing technologies to microbiome research, several papers and subsequent reviews have supported the idea that a dysbiosis (ie, altered gut microbiota composition and/or activity related to host disease) characterizes overweight, obese, or diabetic individuals (Everard and Cani, 2013; Petschow et al., 2013). Regarding the inadequate composition of the gut microbiota, obese and overweight people were initially characterized by a change in the Firmicutes/Bacteroidetes ratio. However, several studies, including human cohorts, reported no variations in this ratio between diabetic or obese patients and controls. Thus this ratio would appear an unimportant or overly crude metric, and the extended concept of dysbiosis to other bacterial phyla, genera or species seems more appropriate to characterize obesity and associated disorders (reviewed in Zhao, 2013). In addition and more recently, the concept of "enterotypes" has been proposed: the analysis of the microbial composition of human fecal samples revealed that the bacterial population can be stratified into three robust clusters. Abundance is a measure of the relative proportion of each bacterial phyla inside of an ecosystem whereas diversity takes into account the number of bacterial phyla identified (richness) in addition to their relative abundance. Despite being very useful descriptors of the bacterial ecosystem in general, neither of those seems to be reliable or reproducible indicators of the diabetic status of the host (Zhang et al., 2013). Animal experiments suggest a clear separation between diabetic and nondiabetic subjects based on their microbiota profiles, but the interpersonal variability in human subjects most likely masks these wide-scale differences. Therefore it appears that in addition to these quantitative modifications of microbial phyla, obesity and some related metabolic diseases might be associated with modifications of microbial gene expression and therefore with the modulation of metabolic functions of the gut microbiota. It is interesting to note that in this regard metabolic dysfunction in type II diabetic patients has previously been characterized by a reduced microbiome gene count (Le Chatelier et al., 2013).

The microbiome is now considered as a new therapeutic target against obesity and its linked diseases (Cani and Delzenne, 2011). In fact, changes in dietary habits and especially an enrichment in some bioactive food components present in whole-grain cereals are able to modify the composition of the gut microbiota and could be helpful in prevention of chronic diseases, including obesity and related disorders, such as type II diabetes (Gil et al., 2011). Human studies have shown the importance of diet in relation to the microbiota (Claesson et al., 2012; Lynch et al., 2015), and this remains the most reproducible method of altering the composition of our microbiota (David et al., 2014). Wu et al. (2011) have shown that microbiome composition may change 24h after initiating a high-fat/low-fiber or a high-fiber/low-fat diet, but that enterotype identity remained stable during a 10-day nutritional intervention. They suggest that food ingredients such as dietary fibers, which are not digested by host enzymes but are fermented by gut bacteria, could modulate the gut microbiome in a relatively short period of time, independent of the effect of changes in transit time.

DYSBIOSIS ASSOCIATED WITH METABOLIC DISORDERS

Several studies have identified individual taxa as important markers for the onset of obesity and diabetes, although the exact roles of some of these species are not currently known. The genera *Bacteroides*, *Roseburia*, and *Akkermansia*, as well as *Faecalibacterium prausnitzii*, were depleted in type II diabetic Chinese subjects, whereas *Dorea*, *Prevotella*, and *Collinsella* had relatively higher abundance (Zhang et al., 2013). In humans and mice, *Prevotella*, *Akkermansia*, and enterobacteria have previously been shown to significantly vary between obese and lean subjects (reviewed in Cani et al., 2014). A reduction in a cluster of genes belonging to *Roseburia* and *F. prausnitzii* was identified as a discriminant marker for the prediction of diabetic status in European women (Karlsson et al., 2013). In an obese French cohort, *F. prausnitzii* was lower than in control subjects, and an increase of this bacterium was correlated with improved inflammatory status (Furet et al., 2010). However, this bacterium was increased in obese Indian children compared with lean controls, highlighting once again the specificity of the population, age, and diet in phenotype–taxonomy associations (Balamurugan et al., 2010). A proportion of these taxa mentioned above are known short-chain fatty acid (SCFA; ie, butyrate, propionate and acetate) producers, which are metabolites of bacterial fermentation recognized to interact with host metabolism and barrier function, whereas the pathways through which many of the other altered taxa impact host health remain largely yet to be elucidated. However, recent research has indicated indole—a metabolite of tryptophan catabolism—as a potential modulator of insulin secretion and sensitivity, as well as gut barrier function through stimulation of glucagon-like peptide (GLP)-1 and two secretions, respectively (Chimerel et al., 2014). The proposed pathways through which these metabolites act on host metabolism will be further discussed later in this chapter.

PREBIOTIC AND PROBIOTIC AS TOOLS TO MODULATE DYSBIOSIS IN METABOLIC DISEASES

Manipulation of the gut microbiota composition and functionality offers a promising means of managing or treating metabolic disorders. In this respect, probiotics and prebiotics offer the most robust and safe methods of achieving such an alteration. Probiotics are "live microorganisms that, when administered in adequate amounts, confer a health benefit to the host (ie, in humans; Hill et al., 2014). Put differently, probiotic interventions aim to introduce a bacterial strain or cocktail of strains, which express a desirable set of genes, at levels that may result in a beneficial host physiological effect. A list of intervention studies with probiotics in animal models of obesity and in humans has previously been reported (Druart et al., 2014). Animal studies suggest that regulation of lipid and glucose metabolism, reduction of adipose cell size, inflammation in adipose tissue, and reduction of inflammation in the liver could be at least in part implicated in the antiobesity effects of probiotics. Human trials have been performed, and some probiotic interventions have resulted in improvements of metabolic disorders related to obesity. However, the mechanisms of action and relevant effects on adiposity have not been sufficiently elucidated to prove true causative effects. Furthermore, regarding probiotics, a clarification of the strain and the dose required to counteract obesity and related disorders is necessary before the generalization of the use of these microorganisms. Very interesting developments in the production of bacterial strains able to produce bioactive metabolites such as conjugated linoleic acid (CLA) or conjugated linolenic acids have been reported (Druart et al., 2014; Hennessy et al., 2012). Both of these bioactive lipids are known to favorably affect host lipid and glucose metabolism (Miranda et al., 2009) as well as adipose weight management (Koba et al., 2002), and although there are major technological challenges (Gorissen et al., 2015), the development of such probiotics could be promising in the management of metabolic disorders related to obesity.

By analogy, the concept of prebiotics was born in 1995, referring to some fermentable carbohydrates that, through their metabolism by gut microorganisms, selectively modulate the composition and/or activity of the gut microbiota, thus conferring a beneficial physiological effect on the host (Bindels et al., 2015). It is interesting to note that carbohydrates with prebiotic properties are able to promote bacteria that are less present in obese or diabetic individuals, such as bifidobacteria, *F. prausnitzii*, *Akkermansia muciniphila*, or *Roseburia* (Zhang et al., 2013). Highly fermentable carbohydrates, such as inulin-type fructans, arabinoxylans, or glucans, are able to counteract several metabolic alterations linked to obesity, including hyperglycemia, inflammation, and hepatic steatosis, at least in animal models (Delzenne et al., 2015). The mechanistic studies suggest that the changes in the gut microbiota occurring upon prebiotic consumption can be related to an improvement of gut bacterial functions implicated in the regulation of host energy homeostasis. The promotion of gut hormone release, changes in the gut barrier integrity, and/or the release of bacterial-derived metabolites (such as SCFAs, CLA, and bile acids) could all participate in the improvement of host health in the particular context of overfeeding and obesity

(Hennessy et al., 2012). Appropriate human intervention studies with dietary fiber allowing to selectively promote beneficial bacteria, or with food containing colonic nutrients, are essential to confirm the relevance of these food ingredients in the nutritional management of overweight and obesity.

GUT MICROBIOTA, OBESITY, AND BEHAVIOR: THE MODULATION OF THE GUT ENDOCRINE FUNCTION AS A KEY TARGET

We have previously shown that the beneficial effects of nutrients that are prone to control obesity upon fermentation in the gut (prebiotics) require a functional GLP-1 receptor and affect obesity by increasing the release of gut hormones, such as GLP-1 and GLP-2 (Cani et al., 2006, 2009; Delzenne et al., 2013). These endocrine peptides represent an interesting pathway involved in the cross-talk between gut microbes and the host cell. More importantly, they are considered as potential targets to regulate endocrine peptides through the gut microbiota. Using complementary approaches involving specific modulation of the gut microbiota (antibiotics, probiotics, prebiotics) and pharmacological inhibition or activation of the GLP-2 receptor, we discovered that gut microbiota participate in the modulation of gut barrier function and the consequent systemic inflammatory phenotype (for review see Cani et al., 2014; Geurts et al., 2014). Although the enteroendocrine function of the gut is an important mechanism in regulating appetite through the release of key satietogenic or orexigenic hormones, molecular links between the gut microbiota and enteroendocrine function of the gut remain largely unknown.

As previously introduced, bacterial metabolites termed SCFAs issued from the fermentation of polysaccharides are capable of modulating the levels of several gut hormones involved in glucose and energy homeostasis, such as GLP-1 and ghrelin. In addition, these metabolites can circulate in the blood and thus act on peripheral targets to modulate insulin sensitivity and whole host energy metabolism. Experimental studies demonstrated that butyrate and acetate suppress weight gain in mice with high-fat diet-induced obesity, and propionate was shown to reduce food intake (Bindels et al., 2013). Once in circulation, these fatty acids have even been shown to act on organs as foreign as the kidneys, in which they promote hypotension through vasodilation (Pluznick et al., 2013). Those effects could be linked to the members of a recently identified G-protein–coupled receptor (GPR) family that includes GPR-43 and GPR-41 (Cani et al., 2013). Studies have shown that SCFAs binding to GPR-43 and GPR-41 increase plasma levels of GLP-1 and peptide YY (PYY), leading to improved glucose homeostasis and reduced appetite (for review see Everard and Cani, 2014). It is interesting to note that studies in animals have shown that butyrate activates the expression of genes involved in intestinal gluconeogenesis through a cyclic adenosine monophosphate–dependent mechanism whereas propionate promotes intestinal gluconeogenic gene expression via a gut–brain neural circuit involving GPR-41. The subsequent release of glucose in the portal vein contributes to the regulation of glycemia and insulin sensitivity (De Vadder et al., 2014).

Recent data have shown that the production of indole, a bacterial metabolite of tryptophan catabolism (Yokoyama and Carlson, 1979), also influences the secretion of GLP-1 by intestinal enteroendocrine cells. Chimerel et al. (2014) discovered that indole inhibited voltage-gated potassium (K^+) channels, thereby changing the action potential of L cells, and led to enhanced calcium ion (Ca^{2+}) entry, which acutely triggers GLP-1 secretion. More importantly, they found that over a longer period of stimulation, indole acts as an inhibitor of mitochondrial metabolism, resulting in a lowered intracellular adenosine triphosphate (ATP) concentration, which induces the opening of ATP-sensitive K^+ channels, thereby hyperpolarizing the plasma membrane and slowing GLP-1 release.

Over the last 10 years, studies have demonstrated that bile acids are not only important in the digestion of dietary lipids, but they also act as signaling molecules in the context of energy, glucose, and lipid metabolism (Nie et al., 2015). A recent paper has shown that the pretreatment of diet-induced obese mice with antibiotics (vancomycin and bacitracin), which reduces the levels of the major bacterial phyla (Bacteroidetes and Firmicutes) in the gut and changes the production of bacterial metabolites, improves glucose intolerance and insulin resistance without affecting obesity by increasing active GLP-1 secretion. The authors pointed out the increase of primary conjugated bile acids (taurocholic acid) as a potential key driver of GLP-1 secretion and as a key regulator of host glucose homeostasis (Hwang et al., 2015). Certain members of the gut microbiota are capable of expressing enzymes, termed bile salt hydrolases (BSHs), which act on conjugated bile acids and cleave away the glycine or taurine amino group, leaving unconjugated bile acids. Unconjugated secondary bile acids (eg, lithocholic and deoxycholic acids) have been demonstrated to have significant signaling potential and can activate TGR-5, a GPR mainly located on intestinal enteroendocrine cells that has been shown to improve liver function and glucose tolerance in obese mice by regulating intestinal GLP-1 production (Prawitt et al., 2011). It is interesting to note that hydrogen sulfide (H_2S), which can be produced by bacteria expressing sulfate-reducing enzymes, may counteract TGR-5 activation and has an inhibitory effect on GLP-1 (and PYY release) (Thomas et al., 2009). The BSH reaction also renders these unconjugated bile acids exposed to further degradation by enzymes produced by other members of the microbiota, ultimately reducing their reabsorption in the ileum. We now know that the deconjugation and excretion of bile acids in turn suppresses the enterohepatic farnesoid X receptor (FXR)-fibroblast growth factor-15 axis in mice (Degirolamo et al., 2014). This suppression acts to promote de novo synthesis of bile acids in the liver, in turn decreasing circulating and liver triglycerides and plasma non-high-density lipoprotein particles (Kumar et al., 2011; Joyce et al., 2014). In addition, FXR is recognized as an important receptor in the pathogenesis of metabolic dysfunction, the expression of which is found to be downregulated in type II diabetic mice (Duran-Sandoval et al., 2004). Joyce et al. (2014) have shown that promoting BSH activity in the gut microbiota, through the introduction of a recombinant *Escherichia coli* expressing a BSH homolog, can directly control body weight, blood cholesterol, hepatic lipids, and fat mass gain through modification of the bile pool size and profile.

CONCLUSIONS

The gut microbiota has evolved to function as a central metabolic organ with implications for seemingly every biological system of its human host. This bacterial ecosystem demonstrates great plasticity; thus it can be substantially modified by environmental stresses such as the nutrients and pharmaceuticals that we consume on a regular basis. These modifications or perturbations can leave the host exposed to the development of a range of noncommunicable metabolic dysfunctions. Conversely, the manipulation of these bacteria may offer a potential therapeutic target in metabolic disease prevention. In this chapter we have discussed the manner in which metabolic health is shaped by our gut microbiota, and we have introduced the potential scope and limitations of probiotics and prebiotics as nonintrusive therapies for metabolic diseases. Fig. 18.1 summarizes the way by which the gut microbiota creates a dialog with host tissues, thereby influencing host physiology. The production of bioactive metabolites that are absorbed (ie, CLA, bile acids, etc.), the translocation of bacterial elements (ie, lipopolysaccharide) in situations of gut barrier alterations, or the interaction of metabolites with host intestinal cells that release hormones, or cytokines able to act at a "distance" (namely on brain) are all occurring and participate

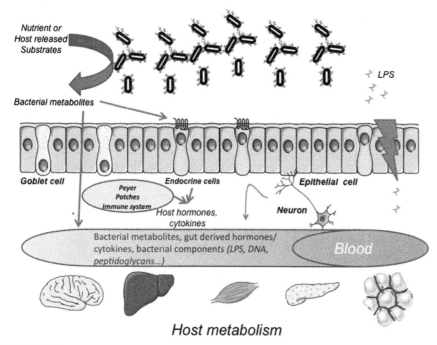

FIGURE 18.1

Pathways through which the gut microbiota can affect host metabolic function and behavior. *LPS*, lipopolysaccharide.

in eubiosis and/or dysbiosis. Although research to date implies that these therapies are entirely promising, and we recognize that there is interaction with a range of host systems (from immune to endocrine functions), it is clear that significant efforts targeted toward elucidating mechanisms of action are necessary for successful treatment of these chronic diseases. In addition to these mechanistic studies, convincing clinical evidence of efficacy is of utmost importance and is now becoming overdue.

REFERENCES

Balamurugan, R., George, G., Kabeerdoss, J., Hepsiba, J., Chandragunasekaran, A.M., Ramakrishna, B.S., 2010. Quantitative differences in intestinal *Faecalibacterium prausnitzii* in obese Indian children. Br. J. Nutr. 103 (3), 335–338.

Bindels, L.B., Delzenne, N.M., Cani, P.D., Walter, J., 2015. Towards a more comprehensive concept for prebiotics. Nat. Rev. Gastroenterol. Hepatol. 12 (5), 303–310.

Bindels, L.B., Dewulf, E.M., Delzenne, N.M., 2013. GPR43/FFA2: physiopathological relevance and therapeutic prospects. Trends Pharmacol. Sci. 34 (4), 226–232.

Cani, P.D., Delzenne, N.M., 2009. The role of the gut microbiota in energy metabolism and metabolic disease. Curr. Pharm. Des. 15 (13), 1546–1558.

Cani, P.D., Osto, M., Geurts, L., Everard, A., 2012. Involvement of gut microbiota in the development of low-grade inflammation and type 2 diabetes associated with obesity. Gut Microbes 3 (4).

Cani, P.D., 2014. Metabolism in 2013: the gut microbiota manages host metabolism. Nat. Rev. Endocrinol. 10 (2), 74–76.

Cho, I., Yamanishi, S., Cox, L., Methe, B.A., Zavadil, J., Li, K., Gao, Z., Mahana, D., Raju, K., Teitler, I., et al., 2012. Antibiotics in early life alter the murine colonic microbiome and adiposity. Nature 488 (7413), 621–626.

Cani, P.D., Delzenne, N.M., 2011. The gut microbiome as therapeutic target. Pharmacol. Ther. 130 (2), 202–212.

Claesson, M.J., Jeffery, I.B., Conde, S., Power, S.E., O'Connor, E.M., Cusack, S., Harris, H.M.B., Coakley, M., Lakshminarayanan, B., O'Sullivan, O., et al., 2012. Gut microbiota composition correlates with diet and health in the elderly. Nature 488 (7410), 178–184.

Cani, P.D., Geurts, L., Matamoros, S., Plovier, H., Duparc, T., 2014. Glucose metabolism: focus on gut microbiota, the endocannabinoid system and beyond. Diabete. Metab. 40 (4), 246–257.

Chimerel, C., Emery, E., Summers David, K., Keyser, U., Gribble Fiona, M., Reimann, F., 2014. Bacterial metabolite indole modulates incretin secretion from intestinal enteroendocrine L cells. Cell Rep. 9 (4), 1202–1208.

Cani, P.D., Knauf, C., Iglesias, M.A., Drucker, D.J., Delzenne, N.M., Burcelin, R., 2006. Improvement of glucose tolerance and hepatic insulin sensitivity by oligofructose requires a functional glucagon-like peptide 1 receptor. Diabetes 55 (5), 1484–1490.

Cani, P.D., Possemiers, S., Van de, W.T., Guiot, Y., Everard, A., Rottier, O., Geurts, L., Naslain, D., Neyrinck, A.M., Lambert, D.M., et al., 2009. Changes in gut microbiota control inflammation in obese mice through a mechanism involving GLP-2-driven improvement of gut permeability. Gut 58, 1091–1103.

Cani, P.D., Everard, A., Duparc, T., 2013. Gut microbiota, enteroendocrine functions and metabolism. Curr. Opin. Pharmacol. 13 (6), 935–940.

Delzenne, N.M., Neyrinck, A.M., Backhed, F., Cani, P.D., 2011. Targeting gut microbiota in obesity: effects of prebiotics and probiotics. Nat. Rev. Endocrinol. 7 (11), 639–646.

David, L.A., Maurice, C.F., Carmody, R.N., Gootenberg, D.B., Button, J.E., Wolfe, B.E., Ling, A.V., Devlin, A.S., Varma, Y., Fischbach, M.A., et al., 2014. Diet rapidly and reproducibly alters the human gut microbiome. Nature 505 (7484), 559–563.

Druart, C., Alligier, M., Salazar, N., Neyrinck, A.M., Delzenne, N.M., 2014. Modulation of the gut microbiota by nutrients with prebiotic and probiotic properties. Adv. Nutr. 5 (5), 624s–633s.

Delzenne, N.M., Cani, P.D., Everard, A., Neyrinck, A.M., Bindels, L.B., 2015. Gut microorganisms as promising targets for the management of type 2 diabetes. Diabetologia 58 (10), 2206–2217.

Delzenne, N.M., Neyrinck, A.M., Cani, P.D., 2013. Gut microbiota and metabolic disorders: how prebiotic can work. Br. J. Nutr. 109 (Suppl. 2), S81–S85.

Degirolamo, C., Rainaldi, S., Bovenga, F., Murzilli, S., Moschetta, A., 2014. Microbiota modification with probiotics induces hepatic bile acid synthesis via down regulation of the Fxr-Fgf15 axis in mice. Cell Rep. 7 (1), 12–18.

De Vadder, F., Kovatcheva-Datchary, P., Goncalves, D., Vinera, J., Zitoun, C., Duchampt, A., Bäckhed, F., Mithieux, G., 2014. Microbiota-generated metabolites promote metabolic benefits via gut-brain neural circuits. Cell 156 (1), 84–96.

Duran-Sandoval, D., Mautino, G., Martin, G., Percevault, F., Barbier, O., Fruchart, J.C., Kuipers, F., Staels, B., 2004. Glucose regulates the expression of the farnesoid X receptor in liver. Diabetes 53 (4), 890–898.

Everard, A., Cani, P.D., 2013. Diabetes, obesity and gut microbiota. Best Pract. Res. Clin. Gastroenterol. 27 (1), 73–83.

Everard, A., Cani, P.D., 2014. Gut microbiota and GLP-1. Rev. Endocr. Metab. Disord. 15 (3), 189–196.

Furet, J.P., Kong, L.C., Tap, J., Poitou, C., Basdevant, A., Bouillot, J.L., Mariat, D., Corthier, G., Dore, J., Henegar, C., et al., 2010. Differential adaptation of human gut microbiota to bariatric surgery-induced weight loss: links with metabolic and low-grade inflammation markers. Diabetes 59 (12), 3049–3057.

Gil, A., Ortega, R.M., Maldonado, J., 2011. Wholegrain cereals and bread: a duet of the Mediterranean diet for the prevention of chronic diseases. Public Health Nutr. 14 (12A), 2316–2322.

Gorissen, L., Leroy, F., De Vuyst, L., De Smet, S., Raes, K., 2015. Bacterial production of conjugated linoleic and linolenic acid in foods: a technological challenge. Crit. Rev. Food Sci. Nutr. 55 (11), 1561–1574.

Geurts, L., Neyrinck, A.M., Delzenne, N.M., Knauf, C., Cani, P.D., 2014. Gut microbiota controls adipose tissue expansion, gut barrier and glucose metabolism: novel insights into molecular targets and interventions using prebiotics. Benefic. Microbes 5 (1), 3–17.

Hill, C., Guarner, F., Reid, G., Gibson, G.R., Merenstein, D.J., Pot, B., Morelli, L., Canani, R.B., Flint, H.J., Salminen, S., et al., 2014. Expert consensus document: the International Scientific Association for Probiotics and Prebiotics consensus statement on the scope and appropriate use of the term probiotic. Nat. Rev. Gastroenterol. Hepatol. 11 (8), 506–514.

Hennessy, A.A., Barrett, E., Paul Ross, R., Fitzgerald, G.F., Devery, R., Stanton, C., 2012. The production of conjugated alpha-linolenic, gamma-linolenic and stearidonic acids by strains of bifidobacteria and propionibacteria. Lipids 47 (3), 313–327.

Hwang, I., Park, Y.J., Kim, Y.R., Kim, Y.N., Ka, S., Lee, H.Y., Seong, J.K., Seok, Y.J., Kim, J.B., 2015. Alteration of gut microbiota by vancomycin and bacitracin improves insulin resistance via glucagon-like peptide 1 in diet-induced obesity. Faseb J. 29 (6), 2397–2411.

Joyce, S.A., MacSharry, J., Casey, P.G., Kinsella, M., Murphy, E.F., Shanahan, F., Hill, C., Gahan, C.G.M., 2014. Regulation of host weight gain and lipid metabolism by bacterial bile acid modification in the gut. Proc. Natl. Acad. Sci. 111 (20), 7421–7426.

Karlsson, F.H., Tremaroli, V., Nookaew, I., Bergstrom, G., Behre, C.J., Fagerberg, B., Nielsen, J., Backhed, F., 2013. Gut metagenome in European women with normal, impaired and diabetic glucose control. Nature 498 (7452), 99–103.

Koba, K., Akahoshi, A., Yamasaki, M., Tanaka, K., Yamada, K., Iwata, T., Kamegai, T., Tsutsumi, K., Sugano, M., 2002. Dietary conjugated linolenic acid in relation to CLA differently modifies body fat mass and serum and liver lipid levels in rats. Lipids 37 (4), 343–350.

Kumar, R., Grover, S., Batish, V.K., 2011. Hypocholesterolaemic effect of dietary inclusion of two putative probiotic bile salt hydrolase-producing *Lactobacillus plantarum* strains in Sprague-Dawley rats. Br. J. Nutr. 105 (4), 561–573.

Le Chatelier, E., Nielsen, T., Qin, J., Prifti, E., Hildebrand, F., Falony, G., Almeida, M., Arumugam, M., Batto, J.-M., Kennedy, S., et al., 2013. Richness of human gut microbiome correlates with metabolic markers. Nature 500 (7464), 541–546.

Lynch, D.B., Jeffery, I.B., Cusack, S., O'Connor, E.M., O'Toole, P.W., 2015. Diet-microbiota-health interactions in older subjects: implications for healthy aging. Interdiscip. Top. Gerontol. 40, 141–154.

Miranda, J., Fernandez-Quintela, A., Macarulla, M.T., Churruca, I., Garcia, C., Rodriguez, V.M., Simon, E., Portillo, M.P., 2009. A comparison between CLNA and CLA effects on body fat, serum parameters and liver composition. J. Physiol. Biochem. 65 (1), 25–32.

Nie, Y.-F., Hu, J., Yan, X.-H., 2015. Cross-talk between bile acids and intestinal microbiota in host metabolism and health. J. Zhejiang Univ. Sci. B 16 (6), 436–446.

Ogden, C.L., Yanovski, S.Z., Carroll, M.D., Flegal, K.M., 2007. The epidemiology of obesity. Gastroenterology 132 (6), 2087–2102.

Petschow, B., Dore, J., Hibberd, P., Dinan, T., Reid, G., Blaser, M., Cani, P.D., Degnan, F.H., Foster, J., Gibson, G., et al., 2013. Probiotics, prebiotics, and the host microbiome: the science of translation. Ann. N. Y. Acad. Sci. 22 (10), 12303.

Pluznick, J.L., Protzko, R.J., Gevorgyan, H., Peterlin, Z., Sipos, A., Han, J., Brunet, I., Wan, L.X., Rey, F., Wang, T., et al., 2013. Olfactory receptor responding to gut microbiota-derived signals plays a role in renin secretion and blood pressure regulation. Proc. Natl. Acad. Sci. USA 110 (11), 4410–4415.

Prawitt, J., Caron, S., Staels, B., 2011. Bile acid metabolism and the pathogenesis of type 2 diabetes. Curr. Diab. Rep. 11 (3), 160–166.

Qin, J.J., Li, R.Q., Raes, J., Arumugam, M., Burgdorf, K.S., Manichanh, C., Nielsen, T., Pons, N., Levenez, F., Yamada, T., et al., 2010. A human gut microbial gene catalogue established by metagenomic sequencing. Nature 464 (7285), U59–U70.

Ryan, P.M., Ross, R.P., Fitzgerald, G.F., Caplice, N.M., Stanton, C., 2015. Functional food addressing heart health: do we have to target the gut microbiota? Curr. Opin. Clin. Nutr. Metab. Care 18 (6), 566–571.

Ridaura, V.K., Faith, J.J., Rey, F.E., Cheng, J., Duncan, A.E., Kau, A.L., Griffin, N.W., Lombard, V., Henrissat, B., Bain, J.R., et al., 2013. Gut microbiota from twins discordant for obesity modulate metabolism in mice. Science 341 (6150).

Thomas, C., Gioiello, A., Noriega, L., Strehle, A., Oury, J., Rizzo, G., Macchiarulo, A., Yamamoto, H., Mataki, C., Pruzanski, M., et al., 2009. TGR5-mediated bile acid sensing controls glucose homeostasis. Cell Metab. 10 (3), 167–177.

Wu, G.D., Chen, J., Hoffmann, C., Bittinger, K., Chen, Y.Y., Keilbaugh, S.A., Bewtra, M., Knights, D., Walters, W.A., Knight, R., et al., 2011. Linking long-term dietary patterns with gut microbial enterotypes. Science 334 (6052), 105–108.

Yokoyama, M.T., Carlson, J.R., 1979. Microbial metabolites of tryptophan in the intestinal tract with special reference to skatole. Am. J. Clin. Nutr. 32 (1), 173–178.

Zhao, L., 2013. The gut microbiota and obesity: from correlation to causality. Nat. Rev. Microbiol. 11 (9), 639–647.

Zhang, X., Shen, D., Fang, Z., Jie, Z., Qiu, X., Zhang, C., Chen, Y., Ji, L., 2013. Human gut microbiota changes reveal the progression of glucose intolerance. PLoS One 8 (8), e71108.

Influence of the Microbiota on the Development and Function of the "Second Brain"— The Enteric Nervous System

19

K. Mungovan, E.M. Ratcliffe

McMaster University, Farncombe Family Digestive Health Research Institute, Department of Pediatrics, Hamilton, ON, Canada

INTRODUCTION

There has been increasing recognition of the role of microbiota in influencing key physiological processes, including the gastrointestinal (GI) function. Not only has the gut flora been shown to influence key components of the intestinal mucosa such as epithelial cell maturation, innate immunity, and angiogenesis (Bry, 1996; Hooper et al., 2003; Stappenbeck et al., 2002), but it has also been demonstrated to be important in the normal development of the enteric nervous system (ENS) (Anitha et al., 2012; Collins et al., 2014).

In this chapter, we review of the normal development of the ENS and the establishment of the intestinal microflora. We discuss how microbiota might influence the development and function of the ENS and highlight proposed mechanisms for interaction. Finally, we frame these findings in the context of potential clinical relevance.

DEVELOPMENT OF THE ENTERIC NERVOUS SYSTEM

The ENS is a network of neurons and supporting glial cells that supply the entire length of the digestive tract, including the gallbladder and pancreas. The term *enteric nervous system* was coined in 1921 by British physiologist John Langley, who classified it as a branch of the autonomic nervous system, alongside the sympathetic and parasympathetic branches (Langley, 1921). Although the classification has withstood the test of time, research on the ENS has since revealed an unanticipated degree of complexity that far surpasses that of the other branches of the autonomic nervous system (Furness and Costa, 1987). Unlike the rest of the autonomic nervous system, in which every postganglionic neuron communicates with the CNS via a

The Gut-Brain Axis. http://dx.doi.org/10.1016/B978-0-12-802304-4.00019-0

preganglionic neuron, most neurons of the ENS are not directly innervated by neurons of the spinal cord (Furness and Costa, 1987). Such functional independence is unique among peripheral organs and is mediated by complex microcircuits of intrinsic primary afferent neurons, interneurons, and motor neurons found in the gut wall (Furness et al., 1998).

The ENS is also distinguished by its size, comprising a greater number of neurons than the entire spinal cord (Gershon, 1999b). Unlike the postganglionic neurons of the sympathetic and parasympathetic nervous systems, which are almost exclusively noradrenergic and cholinergic, respectively, the ENS comprises at least 25 distinct neurotransmitters (McConalogue and Furness, 1994). Given its unique ability to function independently from the CNS, its considerable size, and its remarkable neurochemical diversity, the ENS has been referred to as the body's "second brain" (Gershon, 1999b).

The major functions of the ENS include coordinating motility reflexes, controlling water and electrolyte exchange across the mucosal epithelium, regulating local blood flow, and modulating immune processes (Costa et al., 2000). Neurons of the ENS are arranged into two major plexuses that line the length of the GI tract: the myenteric plexus and the submucosal plexus. Neuronal cell bodies in each plexus are grouped into small, regularly spaced ganglia connected to one another by bundles of nerve fibers called internodal strands. The myenteric plexus, located between the longitudinal and circular muscle layers, is primarily responsible for controlling digestive motility. The submucosal plexus, embedded within connective tissue between the circular muscle and muscularis mucosa, coordinates absorption and secretion reflexes in response to changes in the luminal environment (Furness and Costa, 1987; Gershon, 1999b).

In addition to these intrinsic networks, the GI tract is also innervated by extrinsic fibers from the sympathetic and parasympathetic nervous systems (Ratcliffe, 2011). Afferent sensory fibers ascend to the CNS via the nodose and dorsal root ganglia (Blackshaw et al., 2007). Through these connections, the CNS is able to sense the intestinal contents and modulate the activity of the ENS. Therefore the ENS, although capable of functioning independently of the CNS, normally works in concert with the other branches of the autonomic nervous system to coordinate digestive functions.

PRENATAL DEVELOPMENT OF THE ENTERIC NERVOUS SYSTEM

The ENS, including both enteric neurons and glia, derives from the neural crest (Le Douarin and Kalcheim, 1999). The neural crest-derived precursors that migrate to the gut come from three regions of the neural crest. Most crest-derived cells come from the vagal crest and colonize the entire bowel (Le Douarin and Teillet, 1973). A smaller set migrates from the sacral crest and only colonizes the postumbilical gut (Le Douarin and Teillet, 1973; Pomeranz and Gershon, 1990; Pomeranz et al., 1991; Serbedzija et al., 1991). The truncal crest contributes to the colonization of the esophagus (Durbec et al., 1996). The crest-derived cells that migrate to the bowel constitute a heterogeneous population that changes progressively as a function of developmental age while precursor cells are migrating and after they have reached the gut (Gershon, 1999a; Henion and Weston, 1997; Newgreen and Young, 2002a,b; Weston, 1991). Some premigratory cells are fate restricted, others are pluripotent, and some continue to be pluripotent after they have reached the bowel. Enteric neural crest-derived precursors are sorted into lineages, which can be identified by a combination of the transcription factors and growth factors on which they depend. Furthermore, this sorting is mediated, in part, by the interactions of enteric neural crest-derived cells with the enteric microenvironment. Depending on the combination of lineage and interaction with the microenvironment, enteric neural crest-derived cells may become either enteric neurons that can be characterized by their chemical coding or enteric glia. Therefore the fates of enteric neuronal/glial precursors are determined by intrinsic and extrinsic factors, ultimately giving rise to the full range of cell types present in the mature ENS.

Although advances have been made in understanding highly visible genetic defects of the ENS, such as in Hirschsprung's disease, in which the ENS is missing in a whole segment of bowel, little is known about more subtle defects that could potentially occur in subsets of enteric neurons, ENS synapses, or in the development of enteric glia (Gershon and Ratcliffe, 2004; Young, 2008). It is possible that these more subtle defects can be mediated by changes in the enteric microenvironment. Early in vitro experiments showed that different types of neuronal cells could be differentiated from isolated neural crest-derived cells by altering the tissue culture medium in which they were grown, supporting the concept that the microenvironment can play a role in modulating neuronal phenotypic expression (Ziller et al., 1987). More recent studies have focused on identifying the factors responsible for inducing specific cellular phenotypes. For example, growth factors of the bone morphogenetic protein family appear to increase the proportion of late-arising neurons in the ENS, including dopaminergic neurons (Chalazonitis et al., 2008). Loss of neuronal serotonin has been associated with a decrease in the proportion of dopaminergic and gamma-aminobutyric acid neurons, suggesting that serotonin is also part of the microenvironment that can influence the fate of late-born neurons (Li et al., 2011). Finally, glial cells appear to play a role in programming of the ENS, as suggested by the significant changes in neurochemical coding of the mouse enteric plexuses after selective ablation of glial cells (Aube et al., 2006).

Although the framework of the ENS is largely established by the time of birth, an increasing body of research is demonstrating that fine-tuning continues into the postnatal period when microenvironmental factors have the potential to play a more prominent role.

POSTNATAL DEVELOPMENT OF THE ENTERIC NERVOUS SYSTEM

The development of the ENS does not stop at birth. Although the potential for postnatal development has been known for some time, it is only recently that the extent of postnatal maturation of enteric neurons is being appreciated, especially in the context of early life influences (Gershon, 2012). In morphological studies, terminal differentiation of enteric neurons has been demonstrated to occur after birth, with terminally differentiated neurons coexisting with dividing neural precursor cells (Pham et al., 1991). The grouping of enteric neurons into mature ganglia has also been shown to persist in early life (Faure et al., 2007), with ongoing adaptation of the three-dimensional architecture of the enteric innervation during postnatal development in mice (Schafer et al., 1999) and humans (Wester et al., 1999). These structural observations have been complimented by protein studies that have demonstrated altered protein expression in the rat myenteric plexus across the first 2 weeks of life (Hagl et al., 2005).

In earlier functional studies, intestinal motility patterns have been described as immature in early postnatal life in mice (Roberts et al., 2007) and humans (Burns et al., 2009). The postnatal maturation and function of enteric neurons is potentially related to fine-tuning of chemical coding. In studies of colonic motility in rats beginning at 2 weeks of life, increased colonic motility was found to correspond with an increasing proportion of cholinergic excitatory motor neurons in the myenteric plexus (de Vries et al., 2010). More recent detailed functional studies have demonstrated that although functional synapses and the two main classes of enteric neurons (Dogiel type I and II) can be distinguished electrophysiologically and morphologically at birth, major changes in electrophysiological properties and morphology are ongoing within the first 2 weeks of life and between 2 weeks of life and adulthood (Foong et al., 2012).

The fact that the ENS is still developing during the postnatal period suggests that it is still plastic and therefore sensitive to changes in the enteric microenvironment (Gershon, 2012). One important change that coincides with this timeframe is the colonization of the GI tract by a complex array of microbial species (Hooper, 2004; Mackie et al., 1999).

MICROBIAL COLONIZATION OF THE GASTROINTESTINAL TRACT

The fetus has traditionally been considered to exist in a sterile environment in utero, with birth representing the first exposure of the infant to microbial species (Fanaro et al., 2003). In fact, the presence of any bacteria in utero was thought to be pathologic and linked to preterm labor (Goldenberg et al., 2000). However, more recently, not only has the maternal microbial environment been shown to be dynamic in normal pregnancy (Collado et al., 2008; Koren et al., 2012) but emerging evidence is supporting the concept that exposure to microbiota might begin in utero under non-pathological conditions. Bacterial DNA has been detected in the amniotic fluid of healthy term infants (Bearfield et al., 2002; Rautava et al., 2012), and several strains have been cultured from umbilical cord blood of healthy neonates (Jimenez et al., 2005). Not only are bacteria being found in fetal fluids, but studies are suggesting that bacterial colonization of the GI tract might even begin before birth. The first bowel movements passed by infants, referred to as meconium, have been found to contain several bacterial species (Jimenez et al., 2008). Because this finding was contrary to the general belief that meconium is sterile, the investigators used an animal model to control for the possibility for postnatal contamination of meconium. To do so, pregnant mice were fed a milk formula containing genetically labeled *Enterococcus faecium*, and the meconium of the offspring was analyzed after a sterile Caesarean delivery. The investigators found that the genetically labeled bacteria could indeed be cultured from the meconium of the offspring of treated dams, thus supporting a model of prenatal vertical transmission of microbiota in mammals (Jimenez et al., 2008). The concept of prenatal colonization of the GI tract has been further supported by research demonstrating that the composition of meconium microbiota is substantially different from that of the microbial colonies that would be potential contaminants, such as the vaginal, rectal, and skin flora of the mother (Gosalbes et al., 2013), and that bacterial 16S rRNA can be isolated from the meconium of preterm and from full-term infants (Ardissone et al., 2014).

Although the colonization of the GI tract might begin during the prenatal period, the time of birth and early postnatal period remain the most significant opportunities for bacterial colonization. Multiple factors have been found to influence the composition of the intestinal microbiota in early life (Fig. 19.1), including gestational age, mode of delivery, maternal contact, administration of antibiotics, and type of infant feeding (Azad et al., 2013; Fak et al., 2008; Fanaro et al., 2003; Lamouse-Smith et al., 2011; Penders et al., 2006). For example, the initial colonizing flora of an infant can depend on whether the infant is born by vaginal delivery or by Caesarean section.

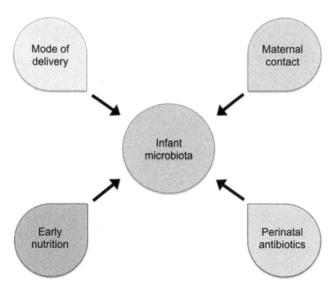

FIGURE 19.1 Multiple factors influence the establishment of the infant microbiome.

These factors include mode of delivery, maternal contact, exposure to perinatal antibiotics, and choice of early nutrition.

When born by vaginal delivery, the early colonizing microbiota of the infant, including that found in meconium, has been found to more closely resemble the mother's vaginal flora and be dominated by *Lactobacillus* species (Dominguez-Bello et al., 2010). On the other hand, infants born by Caesarean section acquire an early microbiota that more closely resembles that of their mother's skin, dominated by the common but potentially pathogenic bacterial species *Staphylococcus* and *Acinetobacter* (Dominguez-Bello et al., 2010). By 1 month of age, the intestinal microbiota of Caesarean section delivered infants differs most from that of vaginally delivered infants by a significant decrease in their levels of *Bacteroides fragilis* (Penders et al., 2006). This difference persists up to 6 months of age, highlighting the effect of the early colonization period on the development of the intestinal flora (Gronlund et al., 1999).

The intestinal environment of neonates is oxygen-rich, providing ideal conditions for invading facultative aerobes to proliferate. As the oxygen becomes gradually depleted by around 1 week of age, the initial aerobic colonies give way to facultative and obligate anaerobic species characteristic of the adult gut flora (Guaraldi and Salvatori, 2012). *Bifidobacteria*, *Clostridia*, and *Bacteroides* are the first anaerobic species to colonize the gut (Adlerberth, 2008). After delivery, the major source of bacteria becomes the mother's skin, via modes of transfer such as holding, caressing, and breastfeeding (Morelli, 2008). Breast milk contains up to 10^9 microbes/L, originating from the nipple and surrounding skin as well as the milk ducts of the breast (West et al., 1979). Formula-fed infants acquire bacteria from the equipment used to prepare the formula and the water used for suspension of the solution (Mackie et al., 1999). Feeding also indirectly influences intestinal microbiota composition by providing substrates that favor the expansion of certain colonies and by altering the physiology of the developing intestinal mucosa (Le Huerou-Luron et al., 2010). Although the bacterial species found in the digestive tracts of breast- and formula-fed infants appear to be largely the same, their relative proportions significantly differ (Mackie et al., 1999). Using molecular techniques, several studies have confirmed that purely breast-fed infants have a significantly greater proportion of *Bifidobacteria* and decreased proportion of *Bacteroides* compared with formula-fed infants (Bezirtzoglou et al., 2011; Fallani et al., 2010; Harmsen et al., 2000). Therefore early-life introduction of either breast milk or formula can have a significant impact on the composition of the intestinal microbiota.

By the end of the first year of life, when most children are being weaned from breast milk and/or infant formula with more exclusive intake of solid foods, the intestinal microbiota begins to resemble that of the adult GI tract (Palmer et al., 2007; Stark and Lee, 1982). A mature microflora comprises between 500 and 3000 unique bacterial species (Pfeiffer and Sonnenburg, 2011), reaching concentrations of 10^{11}–10^{12} microbes/mL of luminal content (Whitman et al., 1998). Although there is substantial interindividual variability (Lozupone et al., 2012), most microbial species in the adult GI tract belong to a limited number of broad taxonomic divisions, namely the phyla Bacteroidetes and Firmicutes, represented by the anaerobes *Bacteroides*, *Eubacterium*, and *Clostridium* (Palmer et al., 2007). In healthy humans the concentration of microbiota increases progressively from the stomach to the large intestine, with the highest concentrations of bacteria found in the distal ileum and colon (Blaut and Clavel, 2007).

Overall, the microbial colonization of the GI tract has been shown to be critical for normal host physiology and to play a role in the developmental programming of adaptive immunity (Hooper et al., 2012), epithelial barrier function (Bry et al., 1996), and intestinal angiogenesis (Hooper et al., 2003; Stappenbeck et al., 2002). Given that the ENS is still developing throughout the initial period of colonization, it is also potentially subject to influences from colonizing bacteria.

INFLUENCE OF MICROBIOTA ON THE DEVELOPMENT OF THE ENTERIC NERVOUS SYSTEM

The germ-free (GF) mouse, which exists in a sterile environment completely devoid of microorganisms, has proven to be an important tool in understanding the complex relationship between a host and its microbial residents. GF mice are often compared to specific pathogen-free (SPF) mice, which comprise a complex commensal flora that is free of major pathogenic species and thus can serve as a control. Observations in neonatal GF mice have provided support for the hypothesis that intestinal microbiota affect the development of the ENS (Fig. 19.2). At postnatal day 3, the ENS of GF mice was found to be structurally abnormal compared with that of SPF mice. The repeating lattice-like arrangement of the SPF myenteric plexus stood in contrast with that of GF mice, which was less ordered with thinner internodal strands in the jejunum and ileum and a reduction in total nerve density and number of neurons per ganglia (Collins et al., 2014). Colonization of GF dams with altered Shaedler flora, a simplified flora comprising only eight bacterial strains, was sufficient to restore the normal patterning of the ENS in their offspring (Collins et al., 2014). These structural observations are complimented by functional data showing impaired GI motility in corresponding regions of early postnatal GF mice. Specifically, the frequency and amplitude of intestinal contractions were significantly reduced in the jejunum and ileum of GF mice (Collins et al., 2014).

More recently, studies in GF mice have also shown a reduction in a population of enteric glial cells, which, similar to enteric neurons, are also derived from the neural crest-derived precursors that colonize the gut. In this work the average number and density of mucosal enteric glial cells were found to be significantly reduced in GF mice compared with conventionally raised mice at 8 weeks of age whereas the enteric glial networks within the myenteric and submucosal plexi were unaffected (Kabouridis et al., 2015). If the GF mice were conventionalized at 4 weeks of age, then the network of mucosal enteric glial cells was found to be restored (Kabouridis et al., 2015). Therefore the postnatal ability of mucosal enteric glia to invade the intestinal mucosa and form a normal network seems to depend on the presence of intestinal microbiota.

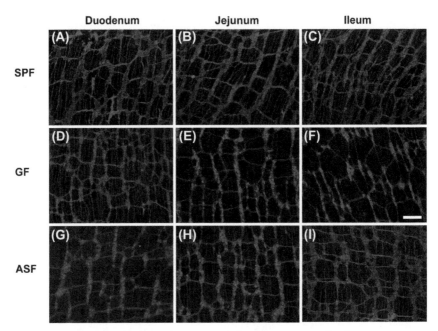

FIGURE 19.2 The myenteric plexus is hypoplastic in early postnatal GF mice.

Myenteric nerves were visualized by immunolabeling with antibodies to PGP9.5 (red (gray in print versions)). (A–C) The myenteric plexus in the SPF duodenum, jejunum, and ileum appear organized in a lattice-like network, with even spacing between ganglia and uniform thickness of connective nerve fibers. (D) The myenteric plexus in the GF duodenum resembles that of the SPF duodenum. (E, F) In GF mice, the myenteric plexus of the jejunum and ileum appears unorganized, with fewer ganglia and thinner connecting nerve fibers. (G–I) In ASF colonized mice, the structure appears similar to that observed in SPF-colonized animals. Bar = 120 μm. *SPF*, specific pathogen-free; *GF*, germ-free; *ASF*, altered Shaedler flora.

From Collins, J., Borojevic, R., Verdu, E.F., Huizinga, J.D., Ratcliffe, E.M., 2014. Intestinal microbiota influence the early postnatal development of the enteric nervous system. Neurogastroenterol. Motil. 26, 98–107; permission for reproduction to be obtained.

These early-life abnormalities in the ENS of GF animals have been shown to persist to adulthood. Irregularities in the patterning of the myenteric plexus of the adult GF rat cecum were already described in the 1960s (Dupont et al., 1965). More recently, GF mice at 4 weeks of age were found to have a significant reduction in neuronal numbers in the myenteric plexus of the colon (Anitha et al., 2012). Furthermore, these persistent changes to the ENS in adult GF animals can manifest with functional deficits. The excitability of intrinsic primary afferent neurons has been found to be significantly reduced in adult GF mice compared with SPF controls, suggesting that commensal microbiota are necessary for the development of normal electrophysiological profiles in enteric neurons (McVey Neufeld et al., 2013).

PROPOSED MECHANISMS FOR MICROBIAL–ENTERIC NERVOUS SYSTEM INTERACTIONS

The potential mechanisms underlying the ability of intestinal microbiota to interact with the ENS is becoming a subject of intense research (Fig. 19.3). One way to gain insight into mechanisms has been to identify the specific neuronal populations most affected when the intestinal microbiota are missing. Thus far, nitrergic neurons, which are involved in GI motility, have been identified as being the most affected in GF mice, with a proportional increase in nitrergic neurons found in the myenteric plexus of the small intestine at postnatal day 3 (Collins et al., 2014) and a decrease in nitrergic neurons found in the myenteric plexus of the colon at 4 weeks (Anitha et al., 2012). Within a similar timeline, dopaminergic neurons have also been found to be decreased in the myenteric plexus of the GF mouse ileum, with a significant decrease noted at postnatal day 7 and persisting to 4 weeks of age (Mungovan et al., 2013).

Until recently it might have been presumed that bacterial interactions with the nervous system would be indirect via the immune system, but emerging work is

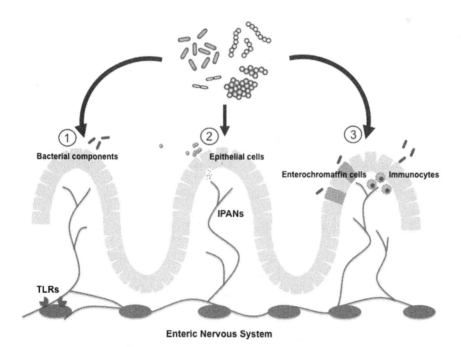

FIGURE 19.3 Potential mechanisms for microbial-ENS interactions.

(1) Bacterial components (such as LPS) are sensed by TLRs present on enteric neurons. (2) Bacterial interactions with IPANs are mediated through epithelial cells. (3) Bacterial interactions with the ENS might be indirect through enterochromaffin cells or through immunocytes. *ENS*, enteric nervous system; *LPS*, lipopolysaccharide; *TLRs*, toll-like receptors; *IPANs*, intrinsic primary neurons.

demonstrating that bacteria are not only able to interact directly with the nervous system (Chiu et al., 2013) but specifically with the ENS (Khoshdel et al., 2013; Mao et al., 2013). Given the integrity of the intestinal mucosal barrier, it is more likely that bacterial components, rather than intact bacteria themselves, are interacting with enteric nerves (Kamada and Kao, 2013).

Most emerging research has been identifying toll-like receptors (TLRs), specifically TLR4 and TLR2, in mediating microbial-ENS interactions. TLRs are able to sense microbial structures and thus trigger immune responses to invading pathogens (Akira and Takeda, 2004). Although classically expressed by immune cells, TLRs are now known to be expressed by a wide diversity of cell populations, including neurons (van Noort and Bsibsi, 2009). In fact, TLR3, TLR4, and TLR7 have all been demonstrated to be present in the human ENS (Barajon et al., 2009). However, the most detailed studies so far have focused on TLR4 and TLR2. TLR4 is able to detect lipopolysaccharide (LPS), a component of the outer membrane of gram-negative bacteria, and signal through the nuclear factor-κB (NF-κB) pathway. TLR4 has been identified on neural stem/progenitor cells isolated from the ENS (Schuster et al., 2014). Our laboratory has found that TLR4 is present in early postnatal enteric neurons (unpublished data), and other laboratories have found that enteric TLR4 expression is maintained until adult life (Anitha et al., 2012; Rumio et al., 2006). Mice lacking TLR4 expression demonstrate abnormalities in the ENS, including a reduction in enteric neurons and specifically in nitrergic neurons, with delayed GI motility (Anitha et al., 2012). Exposure to LPS can stimulate myenteric neurons in vivo (Rumio et al., 2006), enhance proliferation, and modify differentiation of enteric neural stem/progenitor cells (Schuster et al., 2014). It can lead to increased neuronal cell survival (Anitha et al., 2012) but also to the loss of rat myenteric neurons in vitro depending on concentration (Voss and Ekblad, 2014). Furthermore, NF-κB has been shown to promote the survival of enteric neurons (Anitha et al., 2012). NF-κB activation has also been shown to favor neuronal differentiation in primary cortical neurons (Bonini et al., 2011), which is of interest in the context of the previously described changes in chemical coding in early postnatal GF mice (Collins et al., 2014; Mungovan et al., 2013).

Likewise, TLR2, which mediates immune responses to pathogens and regulates epithelial barrier function, has also recently been identified in the ENS (Brun et al., 2013). Not only was TLR2 identified in the enteric neurons of the adult mouse ileum, but it was also found to be expressed by enteric glia and intestinal smooth muscle cells (Brun et al., 2013). Furthermore, *Tlr2*$^{-/-}$ mice had alterations in ENS structure, chemical coding, and motility. These defects seem to be mediated by glial cell-line–derived neurotrophic factor (GDNF), a factor required in the enteric microenvironment for survival and proliferation (Gianino et al., 2003), because GDNF was found to be decreased in *Tlr2*$^{-/-}$ mice and in mice depleted of intestinal microbiota (Brun et al., 2013). Furthermore, administration of GDNF to the *Tlr2*$^{-/-}$ mice completely restored the observed abnormalities in ENS structure and function (Brun et al., 2013). The possibility that GDNF is mediating the response of the ENS to changes in the intestinal microbial environment is also supported by our observations that GDNF is decreased in postnatal intestine of GF mice (Mungovan et al., 2015).

Research has also been emerging demonstrating that epithelium neuron signaling might be key in mediating microbial-ENS interactions. This concept was initially supported by the observation that intestinal microbiota are necessary for the normal excitability of the intrinsic primary afferent neurons that innervate the intestinal mucosa (McVey Neufeld et al., 2013). In a follow-up study aimed to discern the role of the epithelium in microbial-ENS communication, microvesicles were formed from the probiotic *Lactobacillus rhamnosus* JB-1 and enriched for heat shock protein components. These microvesicles only produced functional effects on enteric neurons, as measured by patch clamping, when applied to the epithelium with no effect when directly applied to enteric neurons (Al-Nedawi et al., 2015). In other work, it has been suggested that interactions between bacteria and enteric neurons could be indirect and mediated through enterochromaffin cells (Rhee et al., 2009) or through immune cells such as macrophages in the muscularis externa (Muller et al., 2014).

Lastly, although investigations involving TLRs implicate bacterial components as being a major influence on the postnatal ENS, it is certainly possible that other common bacterial factors or metabolites may be equally or more critical. For example, butyrate, a short-chain fatty acid end product of bacterial fermentation, has been demonstrated to induce neuroplastic changes in enteric neurons (Suply et al., 2012). Ultimately, microbiota might directly or indirectly interact with the ENS through non-neuronal cells or conceivably through a combination of the two.

POTENTIAL FOR PROBIOTIC THERAPY TO INFLUENCE THE ENS

A limited number of studies have investigated the potential for probiotic therapy to specifically influence the ENS. In adult animal models, administration for 2 weeks with the probiotic *L. rhamnosus* JB-1 has been shown to downregulate intrinsic primary afferent neurons (Wang et al., 2010a). Further detailed physiological experiments have shown that the action of *L. rhamnosus* JB-1 can be mimicked by a calcium-dependent potassium channel blocker, suggesting that probiotic therapy can alter the electrophysiology of enteric neurons (Wang et al., 2010b). In younger animal models, an increased density of galanin- and calcitonin gene-related peptide- immunoreactive neurons has been reported in the ileum of piglets treated with the probiotic *Pediococcus acidilactici*, supporting the concept that early-life exposure to probiotic therapy has the potential to influence the development of the ENS (di Giancamillo et al., 2010).

Clinical studies have already documented the treatment potential of probiotics in humans. For example, preterm newborns, after receiving a 1-month course of *Lactobacillus reuteri*, were found to have a significant decrease in regurgitation and a significant increase in the rate of gastric emptying as compared with preterm newborns who had been randomly assigned to receive a placebo (Indrio et al., 2008). Infants receiving *L. reuteri* for treatment of constipation were found to have a significantly higher frequency of bowel movements than infants receiving a placebo (Coccorullo et al., 2010).

CLINICAL RELEVANCE

Disorders of GI motility, such as gastroesophageal reflux disease, abdominal pain, and constipation, are among the most common diagnoses for which children require medical attention (Chitkara et al., 2007). These disorders are not only common but they also bring about significant morbidity, including respiratory compromise, malnutrition, recurrent vomiting, discomfort, pain, and reduced quality of life (Gariepy and Mousa, 2009). Although the pathophysiologies of many GI motility disorders are largely unknown, there has been increasing recognition that alterations in the microbiota might play a role. In population studies, children exposed to antibiotics in early life have an increased incidence of abdominal pain (Uusijarvi et al., 2012). Furthermore, altered stool microbiota profiles have been documented in children with irritable bowel syndrome and with constipation (Rigsbee et al., 2012; Zoppi et al., 1998).

Increasing evidence is suggesting that the initial pattern of colonization of the gut sets the foundation for a microbial composition that lasts a lifetime (Yatsunenko et al., 2012). What is unknown is the extent to which disrupting the normal pattern of colonization in early life, such as through antibiotics, has lasting effects throughout childhood to adulthood (Nicholson et al., 2012). One of the most common reasons that infants might be exposed to antibiotics in early life is through the maternal administration of broad-spectrum intravenous antibiotics during labor as prophylactic management of pregnant women that test positive for group B *Streptococcus* (GBS) (Verani et al., 2010). In North America, 30% of infants are exposed to intrapartum antibiotics because of maternal GBS status (Spaetgens et al., 2002; Van Dyke et al., 2009). The implementation of routine GBS screening has led to positive outcomes with a 30-fold decrease in early-onset GBS sepsis in neonates (Schrag et al., 2000). However, the success has potentially led to complacency with regard to possible negative consequences of such large-scale use of antibiotics during a critical period during which the neonate is in the process of adapting to the outside world (Bedford Russell and Murch, 2006). This critical period is becoming increasingly recognized through animal studies, which demonstrate that maternal administration of intrapartum antibiotics can result in decreased stomach growth, increased intestinal permeability (Fak et al., 2008), and altered immune responses (Lamouse-Smith et al., 2011) in the offspring. The clinical relevance is highlighted by human studies that are beginning to detect changes in the stool microbiota profile of infants exposed to intrapartum antibiotics (Azad et al., 2013).

CONCLUSIONS

The potential for microbiota to influence the development of the ENS can be both exciting and daunting. Although microbiota or their products might emerge as potential therapies to prevent or mitigate diseases that involve the ENS, caution is also suggested when proposing an early-life intervention that disrupts the normal colonization of the GI tract because the long-term consequences are as yet unknown. Fortunately, there is growing interest in the field with an emphasis on mechanistic studies. It is hoped the future will hold a deeper understanding as to how the microbiota can communicate with the ENS and ultimately serve as the foundation for the development of new therapeutic agents.

REFERENCES

Adlerberth, I., 2008. Factors influencing the establishment of the intestinal microbiota in infancy. Nestle Nutr. Workshop Ser. Paediatr. Program. 62, 13–29, discussion 29–33.

Akira, S., Takeda, K., 2004. Toll-like receptor signalling. Nat. Rev. Immunol. 4, 499–511.

Al-Nedawi, K., Mian, M.F., Hossain, N., Karimi, K., Mao, Y.K., Forsythe, P., Min, K.K., Stanisz, A.M., Kunze, W.A., Bienenstock, J., 2015. Gut commensal microvesicles reproduce parent bacterial signals to host immune and enteric nervous systems. FASEB J. 29, 684–695.

Anitha, M., Vijay-Kumar, M., Sitaraman, S.V., Gewirtz, A.T., Srinivasan, S., 2012. Gut microbial products regulate murine gastrointestinal motility via Toll-like receptor 4 signaling. Gastroenterology 143, 1006–1016, e1004.

Ardissone, A.N., de la Cruz, D.M., Davis-Richardson, A.G., Rechcigl, K.T., Li, N., Drew, J.C., Murgas-Torrazza, R., Sharma, R., Hudak, M.L., Triplett, E.W., et al., 2014. Meconium microbiome analysis identifies bacteria correlated with premature birth. PloS One 9, e90784.

Aube, A.C., Cabarrocas, J., Bauer, J., Philippe, D., Aubert, P., Doulay, F., Liblau, R., Galmiche, J.P., Neunlist, M., 2006. Changes in enteric neurone phenotype and intestinal functions in a transgenic mouse model of enteric glia disruption. Gut 55, 630–637.

Azad, M.B., Konya, T., Maughan, H., Guttman, D.S., Field, C.J., Chari, R.S., Sears, M.R., Becker, A.B., Scott, J.A., Kozyrskyj, A.L., et al., 2013. Gut microbiota of healthy Canadian infants: profiles by mode of delivery and infant diet at 4 months. CMAJ 185, 385–394.

Barajon, I., Serrao, G., Arnaboldi, F., Opizzi, E., Ripamonti, G., Balsari, A., Rumio, C., 2009. Toll-like receptors 3, 4, and 7 are expressed in the enteric nervous system and dorsal root ganglia. J. Histochem. Cytochem. 57, 1013–1023.

Bearfield, C., Davenport, E.S., Sivapathasundaram, V., Allaker, R.P., 2002. Possible association between amniotic fluid micro-organism infection and microflora in the mouth. BJOG 109, 527–533.

Bedford Russell, A.R., Murch, S.H., 2006. Could peripartum antibiotics have delayed health consequences for the infant? BJOG 113, 758–765.

Bezirtzoglou, E., Tsiotsias, A., Welling, G.W., 2011. Microbiota profile in feces of breast- and formula-fed newborns by using fluorescence in situ hybridization (FISH). Anaerobe 17, 478–482.

Blackshaw, L.A., Brookes, S.J., Grundy, D., Schemann, M., 2007. Sensory transmission in the gastrointestinal tract. Neurogastroenterol. Motil. 19, 1–19.

Blaut, M., Clavel, T., 2007. Metabolic diversity of the intestinal microbiota: implications for health and disease. J. Nutr. 137, 751S–755S.

Bonini, S.A., Ferrari-Toninelli, G., Uberti, D., Montinaro, M., Buizza, L., Lanni, C., Grilli, M., Memo, M., 2011. Nuclear factor kappaB-dependent neurite remodeling is mediated by Notch pathway. J. Neurosci. 31, 11697–11705.

Brun, P., Giron, M.C., Qesari, M., Porzionato, A., Caputi, V., Zoppellaro, C., Banzato, S., Grillo, A.R., Spagnol, L., De Caro, R., et al., 2013. Toll-like receptor 2 regulates intestinal inflammation by controlling integrity of the enteric nervous system. Gastroenterology 145, 1323–1333.

Bry, L., Falk, P.G., Midtvedt, T., Gordon, J.I., 1996. A model of host-microbial interactions in an open mammalian ecosystem. Science (New York, N.Y.) 273, 1380–1383.

Burns, A.J., Roberts, R.R., Bornstein, J.C., Young, H.M., 2009. Development of the enteric nervous system and its role in intestinal motility during fetal and early postnatal stages. Semin. Pediatr. Surg. 18, 196–205.

Chalazonitis, A., Pham, T.D., Li, Z., Roman, D., Guha, U., Gomes, W., Kan, L., Kessler, J.A., Gershon, M.D., 2008. Bone morphogenetic protein regulation of enteric neuronal phenotypic diversity: relationship to timing of cell cycle exit. J. Comp. Neurol. 509, 474–492.

Chitkara, D.K., Talley, N.J., Weaver, A.L., Katusic, S.K., De Schepper, H., Rucker, M.J., Locke 3rd, G.R., 2007. Incidence of presentation of common functional gastrointestinal disorders in children from birth to 5 years: a cohort study. Clin. Gastroenterol. Hepatol. 5, 186–191.

Chiu, I.M., Heesters, B.A., Ghasemlou, N., Von Hehn, C.A., Zhao, F., Tran, J., Wainger, B., Strominger, A., Muralidharan, S., Horswill, A.R., et al., 2013. Bacteria activate sensory neurons that modulate pain and inflammation. Nature 501, 52–57.

Coccorullo, P., Strisciuglio, C., Martinelli, M., Miele, E., Greco, L., Staiano, A., 2010. *Lactobacillus reuteri* (DSM 17938) in infants with functional chronic constipation: a double-blind, randomized, placebo-controlled study. J. Pediatr. 157, 598–602.

Collado, M.C., Isolauri, E., Laitinen, K., Salminen, S., 2008. Distinct composition of gut microbiota during pregnancy in overweight and normal-weight women. Am. J. Clin. Nutr. 88, 894–899.

Collins, J., Borojevic, R., Verdu, E.F., Huizinga, J.D., Ratcliffe, E.M., 2014. Intestinal microbiota influence the early postnatal development of the enteric nervous system. Neurogastroenterol. Motil. 26, 98–107.

Costa, M., Brookes, S.J., Hennig, G.W., 2000. Anatomy and physiology of the enteric nervous system. Gut 47 (Suppl. 4), iv15–iv19, discussion iv26.

Dominguez-Bello, M.G., Costello, E.K., Contreras, M., Magris, M., Hidalgo, G., Fierer, N., Knight, R., 2010. Delivery mode shapes the acquisition and structure of the initial microbiota across multiple body habitats in newborns. Proc. Natl. Acad. Sci. U. S. A. 107, 11971–11975.

Dupont, J.R., Jervis, H.R., Sprinz, H., 1965. Auerbach's plexus of the rat cecum in relation to the germfree state. J. Comp. Neurol. 125, 11–18.

Durbec, P.L., Larsson-Blomberg, L.B., Schuchardt, A., Costantini, F., Pachnis, V., 1996. Common origin and developmental dependence on *c-ret* of subsets of enteric and sympathetic neuroblasts. Development (Cambridge, England) 122, 349–358.

Fak, F., Ahrne, S., Molin, G., Jeppsson, B., Westrom, B., 2008. Microbial manipulation of the rat dam changes bacterial colonization and alters properties of the gut in her offspring. Am. J. Physiol. 294, G148–G154.

Fallani, M., Young, D., Scott, J., Norin, E., Amarri, S., Adam, R., Aguilera, M., Khanna, S., Gil, A., Edwards, C.A., et al., 2010. Intestinal microbiota of 6-week-old infants across Europe: geographic influence beyond delivery mode, breast-feeding, and antibiotics. J. Pediatr. Gastroenterol. Nutr. 51, 77–84.

Fanaro, S., Chierici, R., Guerrini, P., Vigi, V., 2003. Intestinal microflora in early infancy: composition and development. Acta Paediatr. Suppl. 91, 48–55.

Faure, C., Chalazonitis, A., Rheaume, C., Bouchard, G., Sampathkumar, S.G., Yarema, K.J., Gershon, M.D., 2007. Gangliogenesis in the enteric nervous system: roles of the polysialylation of the neural cell adhesion molecule and its regulation by bone morphogenetic protein-4. Dev. Dyn. 236, 44–59.

Foong, J.P., Nguyen, T.V., Furness, J.B., Bornstein, J.C., Young, H.M., 2012. Myenteric neurons of the mouse small intestine undergo significant electrophysiological and morphological changes during postnatal development. J. Physiol. 590, 2375–2390.

Furness, J.B., Costa, M., 1987. The Enteric Nervous System. Churchill Livingstone, New York.

Furness, J.B., Kunze, W.A., Bertrand, P.P., Clerc, N., Bornstein, J.C., 1998. Intrinsic primary afferent neurons of the intestine. Prog. Neurobiol. 54, 1–18.

Gariepy, C.E., Mousa, H., 2009. Clinical management of motility disorders in children. Semin. Pediatr. Surg. 18, 224–238.

Gershon, M.D., 1999a. Disorders of enteric neuronal development: insights from transgenic mice. Am. J. Physiol. 40, G262–G267.

Gershon, M.D., 1999b. The enteric nervous system: a second brain. Hosp. Pract. 34, 31–32 35-38, 41-32 passim.

Gershon, M.D., 2012. The play is still being written on opening day: postnatal maturation of enteric neurons may provide an opening for early life mischief. J. Physiol. 590, 2185–2186.

Gershon, M.D., Ratcliffe, E.M., 2004. Developmental biology of the enteric nervous system: pathogenesis of Hirschsprung's disease and other congenital dysmotilities. Semin. Pediatr. Surg. 13, 224–235.

di Giancamillo, A., Vitari, F., Bosi, G., Savoini, G., Domeneghini, C., 2010. The chemical code of porcine enteric neurons and the number of enteric glial cells are altered by dietary probiotics. Neurogastroenterol. Motil. 22, e271–e278.

Gianino, S., Grider, J.R., Cresswell, J., Enomoto, H., Heuckeroth, R.O., 2003. GDNF availability determines enteric neuron number by controlling precursor proliferation. Development (Cambridge, England) 130, 2187–2198.

Goldenberg, R.L., Hauth, J.C., Andrews, W.W., 2000. Intrauterine infection and preterm delivery. N. Engl. J. Med. 342, 1500–1507.

Gosalbes, M.J., Llop, S., Valles, Y., Moya, A., Ballester, F., Francino, M.P., 2013. Meconium microbiota types dominated by lactic acid or enteric bacteria are differentially associated with maternal eczema and respiratory problems in infants. Clin. Exp. Allergy 43, 198–211.

Gronlund, M.M., Lehtonen, O.P., Eerola, E., Kero, P., 1999. Fecal microflora in healthy infants born by different methods of delivery: permanent changes in intestinal flora after cesarean delivery. J. Pediatr. Gastroenterol. Nutr. 28, 19–25.

Guaraldi, F., Salvatori, G., 2012. Effect of breast and formula feeding on gut microbiota shaping in newborns. Front. Cell. Infect. Microbiol. 2, 94.

Hagl, C.I., Thil, O., Holland-Cunz, S., Faissner, R., Wandschneider, S., Schnolzer, M., Lohr, M., Schafer, K.H., 2005. Proteome analysis of isolated myenteric plexus reveals significant changes in protein expression during postnatal development. Auton. Neurosci. 122, 1–8.

Harmsen, H.J., Wildeboer-Veloo, A.C., Raangs, G.C., Wagendorp, A.A., Klijn, N., Bindels, J.G., Welling, G.W., 2000. Analysis of intestinal flora development in breast-fed and formula-fed infants by using molecular identification and detection methods. J. Pediatr. Gastroenterol. Nutr. 30, 61–67.

Henion, P.D., Weston, J.A., 1997. Timing and pattern of cell fate restrictions in the neural crest lineage. Development (Cambridge, England) 124, 4351–4359.

Hooper, L.V., 2004. Bacterial contributions to mammalian gut development. Trends Microbiol. 12, 129–134.

Hooper, L.V., Littman, D.R., Macpherson, A.J., 2012. Interactions between the microbiota and the immune system. Science (New York, N.Y.) 336, 1268–1273.

Hooper, L.V., Stappenbeck, T.S., Hong, C.V., Gordon, J.I., 2003. Angiogenins: a new class of microbicidal proteins involved in innate immunity. Nat. Immunol. 4, 269–273.

Indrio, F., Riezzo, G., Raimondi, F., Bisceglia, M., Cavallo, L., Francavilla, R., 2008. The effects of probiotics on feeding tolerance, bowel habits, and gastrointestinal motility in preterm newborns. J. Pediatr. 152, 801–806.

Jimenez, E., Fernandez, L., Marin, M.L., Martin, R., Odriozola, J.M., Nueno-Palop, C., Narbad, A., Olivares, M., Xaus, J., Rodriguez, J.M., 2005. Isolation of commensal bacteria from umbilical cord blood of healthy neonates born by cesarean section. Curr. Microbiol. 51, 270–274.

Jimenez, E., Marin, M.L., Martin, R., Odriozola, J.M., Olivares, M., Xaus, J., Fernandez, L., Rodriguez, J.M., 2008. Is meconium from healthy newborns actually sterile? Res. Microbiol. 159, 187–193.

Kabouridis, P.S., Lasrado, R., McCallum, S., Chng, S.H., Snippert, H.J., Clevers, H., Pettersson, S., Pachnis, V., 2015. Microbiota controls the homeostasis of glial cells in the gut lamina propria. Neuron 85, 289–295.

Kamada, N., Kao, J.Y., 2013. The tuning of the gut nervous system by commensal microbiota. Gastroenterology 145, 1193–1196.

Khoshdel, A., Verdu, E.F., Kunze, W., McLean, P., Bergonzelli, G., Huizinga, J.D., 2013. *Bifidobacterium longum* NCC3001 inhibits AH neuron excitability. Neurogastroenterol. Motil. 25, e478–484.

Koren, O., Goodrich, J.K., Cullender, T.C., Spor, A., Laitinen, K., Backhed, H.K., Gonzalez, A., Werner, J.J., Angenent, L.T., Knight, R., et al., 2012. Host remodeling of the gut microbiome and metabolic changes during pregnancy. Cell 150, 470–480.

Lamouse-Smith, E.S., Tzeng, A., Starnbach, M.N., 2011. The intestinal flora is required to support antibody responses to systemic immunization in infant and germ free mice. PloS One 6, e27662.

Langley, J.N., 1921. The Autonomic Nervous System, Part 1. Heffer, W. Cambridge.

Le Douarin, N.M., Kalcheim, C., 1999. The Neural Crest, second ed. Cambridge University Press, Cambridge, UK.

Le Douarin, N.M., Teillet, M.A., 1973. The migration of neural crest cells to the wall of the digestive tract in avian embryo. J. Embryol. Exp. Morphol. 30, 31–48.

Le Huerou-Luron, I., Blat, S., Boudry, G., 2010. Breast- v. formula-feeding: impacts on the digestive tract and immediate and long-term health effects. Nutr. Res. Rev. 23, 23–36.

Li, Z., Chalazonitis, A., Huang, Y.Y., Mann, J.J., Margolis, K.G., Yang, Q.M., Kim, D.O., Cote, F., Mallet, J., Gershon, M.D., 2011. Essential roles of enteric neuronal serotonin in gastrointestinal motility and the development/survival of enteric dopaminergic neurons. J. Neurosci. 31, 8998–9009.

Lozupone, C.A., Stombaugh, J.I., Gordon, J.I., Jansson, J.K., Knight, R., 2012. Diversity, stability and resilience of the human gut microbiota. Nature 489, 220–230.

Mackie, R.I., Sghir, A., Gaskins, H.R., 1999. Developmental microbial ecology of the neonatal gastrointestinal tract. Am. J. Clin. Nutr. 69, 1035S–1045S.

Mao, Y.K., Kasper, D.L., Wang, B., Forsythe, P., Bienenstock, J., Kunze, W.A., 2013. Bacteroides fragilis polysaccharide A is necessary and sufficient for acute activation of intestinal sensory neurons. Nat. Commun. 4, 1465.

McConalogue, K., Furness, J.B., 1994. Gastrointestinal neurotransmitters. Bailliere's Clin. Endocrinol. Metab. 8, 51–76.

McVey Neufeld, K.A., Mao, Y.K., Bienenstock, J., Foster, J.A., Kunze, W.A., 2013. The microbiome is essential for normal gut intrinsic primary afferent neuron excitability in the mouse. Neurogastroenterol. Motil. 25, e183–e188.

Morelli, L., 2008. Postnatal development of intestinal microflora as influenced by infant nutrition. J. Nutr. 138, 1791S–1795S.

Muller, P.A., Koscso, B., Rajani, G.M., Stevanovic, K., Berres, M.L., Hashimoto, D., Mortha, A., Leboeuf, M., Li, X.M., Mucida, D., et al., 2014. Crosstalk between muscularis macrophages and enteric neurons regulates gastrointestinal motility. Cell 158, 300–313.

Mungovan, K., Borojevic, R., Ratcliffe, E.M., 2013. Influence of intestinal microbiota on the postnatal development of dopaminergic enteric neurons. J. Pediatr. Gastroenterol. Nutr. 57, E149–E150.

Mungovan, K., Borojevic, R., Ratcliffe, E.M., 2015. Influence of the intestinal microbiota on the expression of GDNF in postnatal mouse intestine. Can. J. Gastroenterol. Hepatol. 29, A319.

Newgreen, D., Young, H.M., 2002a. Enteric nervous system: development and developmental disturbances–part 1. Pediatr. Dev. Pathol. 5, 224–247.

Newgreen, D., Young, H.M., 2002b. Enteric nervous system: development and developmental disturbances–part 2. Pediatr. Dev. Pathol. 5, 329–349.

Nicholson, J.K., Holmes, E., Kinross, J., Burcelin, R., Gibson, G., Jia, W., Pettersson, S., 2012. Host-gut microbiota metabolic interactions. Science (New York, N.Y.) 336, 1262–1267.

Palmer, C., Bik, E.M., DiGiulio, D.B., Relman, D.A., Brown, P.O., 2007. Development of the human infant intestinal microbiota. PLoS Biol. 5, e177.

Penders, J., Thijs, C., Vink, C., Stelma, F.F., Snijders, B., Kummeling, I., van den Brandt, P.A., Stobberingh, E.E., 2006. Factors influencing the composition of the intestinal microbiota in early infancy. Pediatrics 118, 511–521.

Pfeiffer, J.K., Sonnenburg, J.L., 2011. The intestinal microbiota and viral susceptibility. Front. Microbiol. 2, 92.

Pham, T.D., Gershon, M.D., Rothman, T.P., 1991. Time of origin of neurons in the murine enteric nervous system. J. Comp. Neurol. 314, 789–798.

Pomeranz, H.D., Gershon, M.D., 1990. Colonization of the avian hindgut by cells derived from the sacral neural crest. Dev. Biol. 137, 378–394.

Pomeranz, H.D., Rothman, T.P., Gershon, M.D., 1991. Colonization of the post-umbilical bowel by cells derived from the sacral neural crest: direct tracing of cell migration using an intercalating probe and a replication-deficient retrovirus. Development (Cambridge, England) 111, 647–655.

Ratcliffe, E.M., 2011. Molecular development of the extrinsic sensory innervation of the gastrointestinal tract. Auton. Neurosci. 161, 1–5.

Rautava, S., Collado, M.C., Salminen, S., Isolauri, E., 2012. Probiotics modulate host-microbe interaction in the placenta and fetal gut: a randomized, double-blind, placebo-controlled trial. Neonatology 102, 178–184.

Rhee, S.H., Pothoulakis, C., Mayer, E.A., 2009. Principles and clinical implications of the brain-gut-enteric microbiota axis. Nature reviews. Gastroenterol. Hepatol. 6, 306–314.

Rigsbee, L., Agans, R., Shankar, V., Kenche, H., Khamis, H.J., Michail, S., Paliy, O., 2012. Quantitative profiling of gut microbiota of children with diarrhea-predominant irritable bowel syndrome. Am. J. Gastroenterol. 107, 1740–1751.

Roberts, R.R., Murphy, J.F., Young, H.M., Bornstein, J.C., 2007. Development of colonic motility in the neonatal mouse-studies using spatiotemporal maps. Am. J. Physiol. 292, G930–G938.

Rumio, C., Besusso, D., Arnaboldi, F., Palazzo, M., Selleri, S., Gariboldi, S., Akira, S., Uematsu, S., Bignami, P., Ceriani, V., et al., 2006. Activation of smooth muscle and myenteric plexus cells of jejunum via Toll-like receptor 4. J. Cell. Physiol. 208, 47–54.

Schafer, K.H., Hansgen, A., Mestres, P., 1999. Morphological changes of the myenteric plexus during early postnatal development of the rat. Anat. Rec. 256, 20–28.

Schrag, S.J., Zywicki, S., Farley, M.M., Reingold, A.L., Harrison, L.H., Lefkowitz, L.B., Hadler, J.L., Danila, R., Cieslak, P.R., Schuchat, A., 2000. Group B streptococcal disease in the era of intrapartum antibiotic prophylaxis. N. Engl. J. Med. 342, 15–20.

Schuster, A., Klotz, M., Schwab, T., Di Liddo, R., Bertalot, T., Schrenk, S., Martin, M., Nguyen, T.D., Nguyen, T.N., Gries, M., et al., 2014. Maintenance of the enteric stem cell niche by bacterial lipopolysaccharides? Evidence and perspectives. J. Cell. Mol. Med. 18, 1429–1443.

Serbedzija, G.N., Burgan, S., Fraser, S.E., Bronner-Fraser, M., 1991. Vital dye labeling demonstrates a sacral neural crest contribution to the enteric nervous system of chick and mouse embryos. Development (Cambridge, England) 111, 857–866.

Spaetgens, R., DeBella, K., Ma, D., Robertson, S., Mucenski, M., Davies, H.D., 2002. Perinatal antibiotic usage and changes in colonization and resistance rates of group B streptococcus and other pathogens. Obstet. Gynecol. 100, 525–533.

Stappenbeck, T.S., Hooper, L.V., Gordon, J.I., 2002. Developmental regulation of intestinal angiogenesis by indigenous microbes via Paneth cells. Proc. Natl. Acad. Sci. U. S. A. 99, 15451–15455.

Stark, P.L., Lee, A., 1982. The microbial ecology of the large bowel of breast-fed and formula-fed infants during the first year of life. J. Med. Microbiol. 15, 189–203.

Suply, E., de Vries, P., Soret, R., Cossais, F., Neunlist, M., 2012. Butyrate enemas enhance both cholinergic and nitrergic phenotype of myenteric neurons and neuromuscular transmission in newborn rat colon. Am. J. Physiol. 302, G1373–G1380.

Uusijarvi, A., Simren, M., Ludvigsson, J.F., Wickman, M., Kull, I., Alm, J.S., Olen, O., 2012. Use of antibiotics during infancy and childhood and risk of recurrent abdominal pain. Gastroenterology 142, S-158.

Van Dyke, M.K., Phares, C.R., Lynfield, R., Thomas, A.R., Arnold, K.E., Craig, A.S., Mohle-Boetani, J., Gershman, K., Schaffner, W., Petit, S., et al., 2009. Evaluation of universal antenatal screening for group B streptococcus. N. Engl. J. Med. 360, 2626–2636.

van Noort, J.M., Bsibsi, M., 2009. Toll-like receptors in the CNS: implications for neurodegeneration and repair. Prog. Brain Res. 175, 139–148.

Verani, J.R., McGee, L., Schrag, S.J., 2010. Prevention of perinatal group B streptococcal disease–revised guidelines from CDC, 2010. MMWR Recomm. Rep. 59, 1–36.

Voss, U., Ekblad, E., 2014. Lipopolysaccharide-induced loss of cultured rat myenteric neurons – role of AMP-activated protein kinase. PloS One 9, e114044.

de Vries, P., Soret, R., Suply, E., Heloury, Y., Neunlist, M., 2010. Postnatal development of myenteric neurochemical phenotype and impact on neuromuscular transmission in the rat colon. Am. J. Physiol. 299, G539–G547.

Wang, B., Mao, Y.K., Diorio, C., Pasyk, M., Wu, R.Y., Bienenstock, J., Kunze, W.A., 2010a. Luminal administration ex vivo of a live *Lactobacillus* species moderates mouse jejunal motility within minutes. Faseb J. 24 (10), 4078–4088.

Wang, B., Mao, Y.K., Diorio, C., Wang, L., Huizinga, J.D., Bienenstock, J., Kunze, W., 2010b. *Lactobacillus reuteri* ingestion and IK(Ca) channel blockade have similar effects on rat colon motility and myenteric neurones. Neurogastroenterol. Motil. 22, 98–107, e133.

West, P.A., Hewitt, J.H., Murphy, O.M., 1979. Influence of methods of collection and storage on the bacteriology of human milk. J. Appl. Bacteriol. 46, 269–277.

Wester, T., O'Briain, D.S., Puri, P., 1999. Notable postnatal alterations in the myenteric plexus of normal human bowel. Gut 44, 666–674.

Weston, J.A., 1991. Sequential segregation and fate of developmentally restricted intermediate cell populations in the neural crest lineage. Curr. Top. Dev. Biol. 25, 133–153.

Whitman, W.B., Coleman, D.C., Wiebe, W.J., 1998. Prokaryotes: the unseen majority. Proc. Natl. Acad. Sci. U. S. A. 95, 6578–6583.

Yatsunenko, T., Rey, F.E., Manary, M.J., Trehan, I., Dominguez-Bello, M.G., Contreras, M., Magris, M., Hidalgo, G., Baldassano, R.N., Anokhin, A.P., et al., 2012. Human gut microbiome viewed across age and geography. Nature 486, 222–227.

Young, H.M., 2008. Functional development of the enteric nervous system–from migration to motility. Neurogastroenterol. Motil. 20 (Suppl. 1), 20–31.

Ziller, C., Fauquet, M., Kalcheim, C., Smith, J., Le Douarin, N.M., 1987. Cell lineages in peripheral nervous system ontogeny: medium-induced modulation of neuronal phenotypic expression in neural crest cell cultures. Dev. Biol. 120, 101–111.

Zoppi, G., Cinquetti, M., Luciano, A., Benini, A., Muner, A., Bertazzoni Minelli, E., 1998. The intestinal ecosystem in chronic functional constipation. Acta Paediatr. 87, 836–841.

Dietary Interventions and Irritable Bowel Syndrome

20

A. Thomas

Houston Methodist Hospital and Weill Cornell Medical College, Department of Medicine, Houston, TX, United States

E.M.M. Quigley

Houston Methodist Hospital and Weill Cornell Medical College, Division of Gastroenterology and Hepatology, Houston, TX, United States

INTRODUCTION

The notion that the gut could in some way interact with the brain or even modulate its function has probably been prevalent since antiquity and was highly popular in Victorian times ("vile humors," etc.). A scientific basis to such interactions began to emerge in the last century through pioneering work on hepatic encephalopathy (providing a formal basis for the microbiota-gut-brain axis) (Phillips et al., 1952; Martini et al., 1957; Phear et al., 1956) as well as on the impact of stress on the gastrointestinal tract (Almy and Tulin, 1947). Since then a host of clinical scenarios have come to be seen as representing interactions between the "big brain" in the cranium and the "little brain" in the gut. For example, the gastrointestinal symptoms that are so common among those who suffer from Parkinson's disease (PD) are now understood to represent not only the impact of the involvement of brain stem nuclei that regulate certain gut functions by this neurodegenerative disorder but also the direct participation of autonomic and enteric neurons in the PD disease process. However, over the past several decades the concept of a bidirectional gut-brain axis has become central to considerations of the pathophysiology and management of a challenging gastrointestinal disorder—irritable bowel syndrome (IBS). This entity will serve as the model for our discussion of the brain-gut axis.

IBS is a chronic functional gastrointestinal disorder characterized by abdominal pain or discomfort associated with abnormal bowel habit in the absence of any currently detectable structural, physiological, or biochemical abnormalities of the gastrointestinal tract. In the absence of such markers of organic disease, IBS continues to be recognized and defined on the basis of symptom clusters, in the absence, of course, of any organic explanation for these same symptoms. Of the various symptom-based definitions that have been advanced, those developed by the Rome foundation have gained the most traction and have been widely adopted by those who

The Gut-Brain Axis. http://dx.doi.org/10.1016/B978-0-12-802304-4.00020-7

design clinical trials in IBS. According to Rome III, the latest iteration of the Rome process, IBS is defined by the presence of "recurrent abdominal pain or discomfort for at least three days per month in the past three months, associated with two or more of the following: improvement with defecation, onset associated with a change in the frequency of stool or onset associated with a change in the form or appearance of stool" (Longstreth et al., 2006).

IBS is responsible for imparting considerable morbidity and a significant economic burden throughout the world and in Western society in particular (Canavan et al., 2014; Huang et al., 2014; Buono et al., 2014; Hou et al., 2014). Despite these costs to society and the individual coupled with decades of clinical and laboratory investigations into the pathophysiology of IBS, our understanding of IBS remains incomplete; therefore its treatment is somewhat unsatisfactory (Bellini et al., 2014). Nevertheless, the concept of the gut-brain axis has served as a useful framework for understanding IBS, and the various manifestations and/or presentations of IBS can be seen to locate themselves on one or another point along this axis in any given individual (Al Omran and Aziz, 2014) (Fig. 20.1). Thus such symptoms as pain and bloating may arise primarily from disturbances in gut muscle or the enteric nervous system in one IBS sufferer and be predominantly generated by central input in another.

The latter circumstance is exemplified by the IBS patient with significant psychiatric co-morbidity. These co-morbidities provide another rationale for the use of treatment strategies that modulate the gut-brain axis in IBS. There is the suggestion that the gut microbiome may play a role in the pathogenesis of depression and anxiety per se (Dinan and Cryan, 2013). Moreover, IBS and such psychiatric disorders as depression and schizophrenia (Dinan, 2009; Dennison et al., 2012) may share a proinflammatory phenotype; antiinflammatory actions of some probiotics (vide infra) could be relevant to all of these entities.

Abnormalities in the gut microbiome, the host immune response, the epithelial barrier, intestinal secretion, and systemic immune mediators (Simrén et al., 2013; Lee and Lee, 2014; Hyland et al., 2014; Camilleri, 2012; Piche, 2014; Buckley et al., 2014) have been variably identified in IBS subjects and experimental models of IBS (Fig. 20.1). Novel therapeutic strategies have begun to target these putative abnormalities. In particular, as the role of the microbiota in IBS has come to be explored, changes in microbial composition have been described (Lee and Lee, 2014) and enthusiasm for therapeutic interventions that could beneficially modulate the microbiota has increased (Quigley and Shanahan, 2014; Shanahan and Quigley, 2014). Among these, diets and the food supplements probiotics and prebiotics are of particular interest.

DIET, THE MICROBIOME, AND IRRITABLE BOWEL SYNDROME

Dietary fiber (≥25 g/day) has been traditionally recommended for patients with constipation-predominant IBS (C-IBS; American Gastroenterological Association Medical Position Statement, 2002). Fiber supplementation increases fecal mass and may accelerate transit (Spiller et al., 2007). It must be remembered that a major

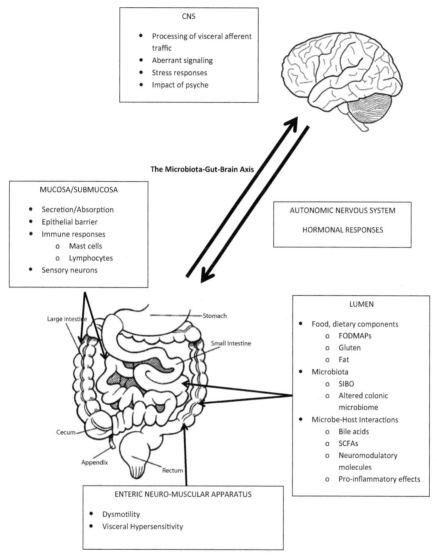

FIGURE 20.1

Factors involved in the pathophysiology of irritable bowel syndrome. *SFCA*s, short-chain fatty acid; *FODMAP*s, fermentable oligo-, di-, and monosaccharides and polyols; *SIBO*, small intestinal bacterial overgrowth.

contributor to the increase in fecal mass that occurs with fiber is bacterial mass resulting from the "prebiotic" effects of various fibers. Fruits and vegetables contain both soluble (pectins, hemicellulose) and insoluble (cellulose, lignin) fiber, whereas cereals and bran contain mainly insoluble fiber. Although the usual recommendation is to increase dietary fiber, particularly cereal bran, in C-IBS recent rigorous appraisals of various forms of fiber in IBS have shown that insoluble fiber makes symptoms worse in 55% whereas only 11% report benefit. Soluble fiber may be better tolerated and fiber supplements such psyllium and ipsaghula, which are not only soluble but poorly fermented, may be especially suitable (American Gastroenterological Association Medical Position Statement, 2002). The main drawbacks to the use of fiber are flatulence and bloating (Brandt et al., 2009; Ford et al., 2008). Indeed, for those with predominant bloating and/or distension, reducing dietary fiber and particularly wheat bran has been recommended in nonconstipated IBS. Although the effects of fiber, in general, on the colonic microbiome have been well studied, there are few data on relationships among particular fiber sources, changes in the microbiome, and clinical outcomes in IBS.

Aware that food is a major precipitant of their symptoms, IBS sufferers have experimented with various exclusion diets on the assumption that they have a hypersensitivity or intolerance to one or more food constituents (Hayes et al., 2014). Although there is little evidence to support a role for classical food allergy in IBS, a considerable volume of data suggests that food intolerance may be an issue (Quigley et al., 2009). Initially the focus, in this regard, was on lactose, sucrose, and sorbitol; agents that can certainly cause diarrhea and bloating on acute exposure but may not be very relevant to more long-term problems in IBS. More recently the focus has been on two, more broadly based diets: gluten-free and diets low in **f**ermentable **o**ligo-, **d**i-, and **m**onosaccherides, **a**nd **p**olyols (FODMAPs).

Interactions between IBS and celiac disease are complex. Firstly, celiac disease nowadays tends to present with vague IBS-like symptoms; thus there is the possibility of diagnostic confusion. Secondly, celiac patients (similar to individuals with inflammatory bowel disease) may continue to have IBS-like symptoms when in apparent remission (O'Leary et al., 2002). Thirdly, there is some, but by no means consistent, evidence that subtle gluten sensitivity may be detectable in some IBS patients. The term non-celiac gluten sensitivity (or intolerance) has emerged to describe those individuals who seem intolerant of gluten (or of wheat-containing diets) yet do not satisfy criteria for celiac disease (Kabbani et al., 2014). This concept is supported by studies demonstrating the precipitation of global IBS symptoms on exposure to gluten (Biesiekierski et al., 2011; Brottveit et al., 2013; Carroccio et al., 2012; Vazquez-Roque et al., 2013; Biesiekierski et al., 2013) and their improvement with gluten restriction (Vazquez-Roque et al., 2013; Biesiekierski et al., 2013).

Another novel dietary approach also based on reducing fermentable substances in the diet has been the low-FODMAPs diet. Although this diet is complex and rather restrictive, it has led to improvements in individual and global symptoms in IBS (Biesiekierski et al., 2013; Shepherd et al., 2013; Staudacher et al., 2011; Halmos et al., 2014), most recently in a small randomized controlled trial (Halmos et al., 2014). These same authors have also demonstrated that the benefits of gluten-free diet in IBS lie not in avoidance of hypersensitivity to gluten per se but, rather in the removal of a major FODMAP from the diet—fructans (Biesiekierski et al., 2013).

Again, these diets have implications for the microbiome; a low FODMAP diet reduces microbiota abundance and the absolute abundance of butyrate-producing bacteria, *Bifidobacteria* spp., and the mucus-associated bacterium *Akkermansia muciniphila* (Halmos et al., 2015). The long-term consequences of such diet-induced changes are unknown.

PROBIOTICS IN IRRITABLE BOWEL SYNDROME
A SCIENTIFIC BASIS FOR THE USE OF PROBIOTICS IN IRRITABLE BOWEL SYNDROME

Although some may feel that it is too restrictive by excluding the biological and potentially beneficial effects of dead organisms, bacterial components, and products—the most widely used definition continues to assert that probiotics are "live microorganisms that, when administered in adequate amounts confer a health benefit on the host" (Hill et al., 2014).

Data from animal models, and clinical research in humans, have revealed several properties of probiotics that exert effects along the gut-brain (or microbiome-gut-brain) axis that could be of value in the management of IBS (Fig. 20.2). These include antibacterial and antiinflammatory effects, modulation of gut motility and visceral hypersensitivity, restoration of epithelial integrity, and directly altering the microbiome and its metabolic activity. As one travels along the microbiome-gut-brain axis one can garner data supporting effects of probiotics on the various stages of this journey: from the gut microbiome itself, through the epithelial barrier, to the intrinsic neuromuscular apparatus of the gut, and all of the way to the CNS.

Stimulated by the observation that IBS can develop de novo after an episode of gastroenteritis (Thabane et al., 2007); post-infectious IBS (PI-IBS), researchers have, of late, been engaged in exploring the hypothesis that IBS may result from a disturbed microbiota (Jeffrey et al., 2012; Quigley, 2011).

Several lines of evidence support the idea that IBS might be associated with alterations in the gut microbiota and include descriptions of differences in the colonic microbiota between IBS subjects and age- and gender-matched controls (Codling et al., 2010; Carroll et al., 2011; Durbán et al., 2012; Parkes et al., 2012; Kassinen et al., 2007; Krogius-Kurikka et al., 2009; Rajilić-Stojanović et al., 2011; Saulnier et al., 2011; Rigsbee et al., 2012; Carroll et al., 2012; Duboc et al., 2012; Chassard et al., 2012; Jeffery et al., 2012; Jalanka-Tuovinen et al., 2014; Durbán et al., 2013), the somewhat controversial suggestion that small intestinal bacterial overgrowth may be more prevalent in IBS (Pimentel et al., 2000, 2003; Quigley, 2007; Quigley and Abu-Shanab, 2009; Ford et al., 2009), and the possibility that the state of low-level immune activation described in IBS might be triggered or sustained by the microbiota (Quigley, 2012). More tangible illustrations of the potential role of the microbiota are provided by the aforementioned impact of changes in two fundamental functions of microbiota; bile acid deconjugation and fermentation; on stool and

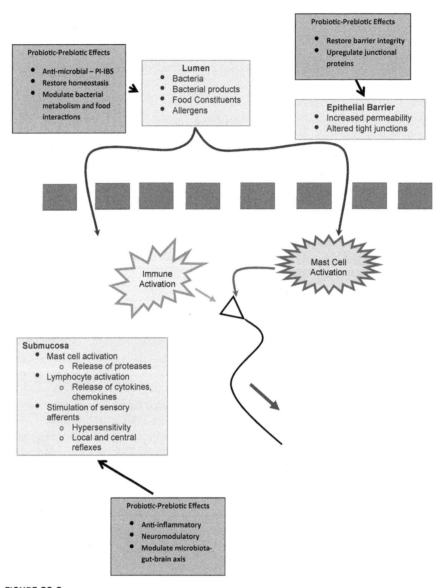

FIGURE 20.2

Luminal, mucosal, and submucosal factors that may contribute to irritable bowel syndrome (IBS) and how probiotics may beneficially affect IBS. *PI-IBS*, Post-infectious IBS.

gas volumes; and, perhaps more convincingly, by the clinical benefits observed in response to selected interventions that are likely to modify the gut microbiota in IBS and related disorders—antibiotics, prebiotics, and probiotics (Quigley, 2011). Among the former are studies demonstrating a consistent, albeit modest, effect of the poorly absorbable antibiotic rifaximin on IBS symptoms and bloating among subjects with diarrhea-predominant IBS (Pimentel et al., 2011).

However, it must be conceded that relationships between clinical benefits from these interventions and changes in the microbiota have yet to be firmly established. There are, as yet, no data on the impact of rifaximin on the microbiota in IBS, and limited data indicate that some changes may occur in relation to the administration of a probiotic but that they are transient and persist only as long as the probiotic is consumed (Ng et al., 2013; Charbonneau et al., 2013).

There is indeed some evidence that probiotic administration may diminish visceral hypersensitivity in animal models (Kamiya et al., 2006; Verdu et al., 2006; Ait-Belgnaoui et al., 2006; Eutamene et al., 2007; Johnson et al., 2011). Furthermore, effects on motility and perception could also go some way toward explaining the beneficial effects of probiotics on bloating given current concepts on the roles of altered gas transit and visceral hypersensitivity in the pathogenesis of this symptom (Quigley, 2002, 2003; Serra et al., 2001). Indeed, one probiotic organism, *Bifidobacterium lactis* DN-173-010, has been shown to accelerate colonic transit, reduce abdominal girth, and alleviate bloating in subjects with C-IBS (Agrawal et al., 2009). In a model relevant to postinfectious IBS, the probiotic bacterium *Lactobacillus paracasei* has been shown to reverse changes in intestinal muscle function consequent upon infection of an animal model with *Trichinella spiralis* (Verdu et al., 2004). This latter finding indicates that a luminally administered probiotic can influence inflammatory processes beyond the mucosal surface. By reducing mucosal inflammation (vide infra), probiotics could decrease immune-mediated activation of enteric motor and sensory neurons and modify neural traffic between the gut and the CNS.

Alterations in gut permeability, in IBS, first described in postinfectious IBS (Spiller et al., 2000), have subsequently been reported among subjects with IBS in general and especially among those with diarrhea-predominant IBS (Camilleri, 2012; Piche, 2014). Whether, such changes in permeability are a cause or a consequence of mucosal immune responses or reflect injury inflicted by an altered microbiome remains to be defined (Piche, 2014). What is clear is that probiotic/commensal organisms can, in experimental models, restore barrier integrity through positive effects on very fundamental aspects of tight-junction physiology and biochemistry (Hyland et al., 2014; Ait-Belgnaoui et al., 2006; Madsen et al., 2001; Laval et al., 2014). Some of these effects have been replicated in man (Persborn et al., 2013).

Hints to suggest efficacy for probiotics in disorders beyond the gut accumulate and include evidence of their ability to modulate systemic immune responses (Sheil et al., 2004; Groeger et al., 2013). Of relevance to IBS are very recent and exciting data on the ability of orally administered probiotics and other modifications of the microbiota to influence behavior, mood, cerebral function and morphology, and especially stress responses in experimental animals (Collins et al., 2012; Bravo et al., 2011; Cryan and O'Mahony, 2011; Cryan and Dinan, 2012; Desbonnet et al., 2014). Given the proinflammatory phenotype associated with such psychiatric disorders as depression, a disorder that is commonly co-morbid with IBS, the antiinflammatory actions of some probiotics may also be relevant to IBS. Ongoing studies of the microbiome-gut-brain axis may reveal not only more objective targets for intervention but also identify those bacterial components or products that may have optimal biological activity; initial studies do, indeed, suggest that subtle changes in the microbiome can influence brain function in man (Tillisch et al., 2013).

CLINICAL EVIDENCE OF EFFICACY OF PROBIOTICS IN IRRITABLE BOWEL SYNDROME

There have been numerous systematic reviews and meta-analyses of probiotics in IBS. In interpreting such aggregate data one must be mindful of how unique probiotic strains are and how different combinations, formulations, and doses may exert very different effects yet they all tend to be lumped together in these papers. Nevertheless, the most recent, and arguably complete, meta-analysis concluded that there was an overall beneficial effect for probiotics in adult IBS and for combinations and bifidobacteria but not lactobacilli (Ford et al., 2014). A similar exercise performed on studies conducted among children and teenagers concluded that *Lactobacillus* GG, *Lactobacillus reuteri* DSM17938, and the probiotic cocktail VSL#3 (which contains *Lactobacillus acidophilus*, *Lactobacillus plantarum*, *Lactobacillus casei*, *Lactobacillus bulgaricus*, *Bifidobacterium breve*, *Bifidobacterium longum*, *Bifidobacterium infantis*, and *Streptococcus thermophiles*) improved IBS symptomatology (Korterink et al., 2014). Of note, *L. reuteri* DSM17938 seemed to result in a reduction in abdominal pain that persisted well after probiotic ingestion had ceased (Korterink et al., 2014).

At this time it is not clear which IBS patient is most likely to respond to a particular probiotic. In some studies, benefits were limited to those with prominent bloating or flatulence; in others involving specific strain effects were more global (O'Mahony and McCarthy et al., 2005; Whorwell et al., 2006). Likewise, in a study in children involving VSL#3 significant improvements in abdominal pain, bloating, and global IBS symptoms were noted but there was no effect on diarrhea or constipation (Guandalini et al., 2010). In their study Kruis et al. (2012) noted that the best symptomatic response to *Escherichia coli* nissle was obtained among those who were likely to harbor a disturbed microbiome; those who had developed IBS after a bout of gastroenterocolitis and/or a course of treatment with an antibiotic. Are probiotic combinations/cocktails superior to single organism preparations? Although meta-analyses suggest that these combination products are effective, there have been few head-to-head comparisons of any formulations. In one such study a bifidobacterium was found to be superior to a *Lactobacillus* (O'Mahony and McCarthy et al., 2005), but there have been no comparisons of single strains versus combinations. Likewise, there are few data on optimal dose with only one dose ranging study to date that suggested that a dose of 10^8 was superior to 10^6 with the latter faring no better than placebo (Whorwell et al., 2006).

PREBIOTICS

Prebiotics are carbohydrates that transit undigested through the small intestine and eventually reach the colon where they increase stool bulk, enhance calcium absorption, and stimulate the growth and/or the activity of beneficial bacteria, specifically bifidobacteria and lactobacilli (Roberfroid, 1993; Roberfroid et al., 2010; Novak and Vetvicka, 2008). Well-studied prebiotics include galactooligosaccharides (GOS), fructooligosaccharides (FOS), inulin, and β-glucan (Roberfroid, 1993; Roberfroid et al., 2010; Novak and Vetvicka, 2008; Hunter et al., 1999). In addition, a few of these carbohydrates, namely mannanoligosaccharides, inulin, and β-glucan, also referred to as immunosaccharides, can serve as direct stimulators of innate immunity (Hunter et al., 1999).

Although a very time-honored strategy that has been used in IBS for decades, dietary fiber, may owe some of its efficacy to a prebiotic effect, there have been relatively few formal studies of prebiotics in IBS. In a randomized control cross-over study, Hunter and colleagues treated 21 patients with an FOS in a dose of 6 g/day (Olesen and Gudmand-Hoyer, 2000). They concluded that there were no significant differences in symptom responses between patients in treatment and placebo arms of the study. In a larger study Olesen and Gudmand-Hoyer randomized 96 patients to receive either 20 g/day of FOS or placebo for 12 weeks and found that FOS, in this higher dose, actually increased symptoms (Paineau et al., 2008). In contrast, Paineau and colleagues using a much lower dose of 5 g/day of FOS noted some improvements in global symptoms and bloating (Guandalini, 2014). Silk et al. (2009) addressed the dose issue further by comparing the effects of 3.5 g/day of GOS, 7 g/day of GOS, and placebo in a randomized fashion in 44 IBS patients over 4 weeks. GOS, at both doses, increased the numbers of bifidobacteria in fecal samples. Although GOS at the lower dose resulted in a global relief of bloating and flatulence, at higher doses it worsened these symptoms, again emphasizing the critical importance of dose. Negative effects of prebiotics at higher doses may relate to excessive production of intra-luminal gases by fermentation of undigested carbohydrates and related changes in colonic volume (Major et al., 2014; Ong et al., 2010).

CONCLUSION

Strategies ranging from diet to prebiotics, probiotics, and antibiotics that modulate the microbiota have emerged as potentially valuable approaches to the management of IBS. Several issues need to be resolved. Firstly, the primacy of changes in the microbiota in the genesis of IBS symptomatology needs to be established. Secondly, the biological impact of these therapies on the microbiome-gut-brain axis, in human subjects with IBS, needs to be defined and the beneficial effects that have been so well and repeatedly demonstrated in animal models need to be confirmed. Finally, and, perhaps most importantly, we need more high-quality clinical trials of prebiotics, probiotics, and antibiotics in IBS—trials that will define the most responsive target population(s) as well as optimal strain(s), dose, formulation, and duration of therapy. Only then will the true role of this promising strategy be fully appreciated.

REFERENCES

Agrawal, A., Houghton, L.A., Morris, J., Reilly, B., Guyonnet, D., Goupil Feuillerat, N., Schlumberger, A., Jakob, S., Whorwell, P.J., 2009. Clinical trial: the effects of a fermented milk product containing *Bifidobacterium lactis* DN-173-010 on abdominal distension and gastrointestinal transit in irritable bowel syndrome with constipation. Aliment. Pharmacol. Ther. 29, 104–114.

Ait-Belgnaoui, A., Han, W., Lamine, F., Eutamene, H., Fioramonti, J., Bueno, L., Theodorou, V., 2006. *Lactobacillus farciminis* treatment suppresses stress-induced visceral hypersensitivity: a possible action through interaction with epithelial cells cytoskeleton contraction. Gut 55, 1090–1094.

Al Omran, Y., Aziz, Q., 2014. The brain-gut axis in health and disease. Adv. Exp. Med. Biol. 817, 135–153.

Almy, T.P., Tulin, M., 1947. Alterations in colonic function in man under stress; experimental production of changes simulating the irritable colon. Gastroenterology 8, 616–626.

American Gastroenterological Association, 2002. American Gastroenterological Association medical position statement: irritable bowel syndrome. Gastroenterology 123, 2105–2107.

Bellini, M., Gambaccini, D., Stasi, C., Urbano, M.T., Marchi, S., Usai-Satta, P., 2014. Irritable bowel syndrome: a disease still searching for pathogenesis, diagnosis and therapy. World J. Gastroenterol. 20, 8807–8820.

Biesiekierski, J.R., Newnham, E.D., Irving, P.M., Barrett, J.S., Haines, M., Doecke, J.D., Shepherd, S.J., Muir, J.G., Gibson, P.R., 2011. Gluten causes gastrointestinal symptoms in subjects without celiac disease: a double-blind randomized placebo-controlled trial. Am. J. Gastroenterol. 106, 508–514.

Biesiekierski, J.R., Peter, S.L., Newnham, E.D., Rosella, O., Muir, J.G., Gibson, P.R., 2013. No effects of gluten in patients with self-reported non-celiac gluten sensitivity after dietary reduction of low-fermentable, poorly absorbed, short-chain fatty acids. Gastroenterology 145, 320–328.

Brandt, L.J., Chey, W.D., Foxx-Orenstein, A.E., Schiller, L.R., Schoenfeld, P.S., Spiegel, B.M., Talley, N.J., Quigley, E.M., Moayyedi, P., 2009. American College of Gastroenterology Task Force on IBS. Am. J. Gastroenterol. 104, S1–S35.

Bravo, J.A., Forsythe, P., Chew, M.V., Escaravage, E., Savignac, H.M., Dinan, T.G., Bienenstock, J., Cryan, J.F., 2011. Ingestion of *Lactobacillus* strain regulates emotional behavior and central GABA receptor expression in a mouse via the vagus nerve. Proc. Natl. Acad. Sci. U S A 108, 16050–16055.

Brottveit, M., Beitnes, A.C., Tollefsen, S., Bratlie, J.E., Jahnsen, F.L., Johansen, F.E., Sollid, L.M., Lundin, K.E., 2013. Mucosal cytokine response after short-term gluten challenge in celiac disease and non-celiac gluten sensitivity. Am. J. Gastroenterol. 108, 842–850.

Buckley, M.M., O'Halloran, K.D., Rae, M.G., Dinan, T.G., O'Malley, D., 2014. Modulation of enteric neurons by interleukin-6 and corticotropin-releasing factor contributes to visceral hypersensitivity and altered colonic motility in a rat model of irritable bowel syndrome. J. Physiol. 592 (Pt 23), 5235–5250 [Epub ahead of print].

Buono, J.L., Tourkodimitris, S., Sarocco, P., Johnston, J.M., Carson, R.T., 2014. Impact of linaclotide treatment on work productivity and activity impairment in adults with irritable bowel syndrome with constipation: results from 2 randomized, double-blind, placebo-controlled phase 3 trials. Am. Health Drug Benefits 7, 289–297.

Camilleri, M., 2012. Peripheral mechanisms in irritable bowel syndrome. N. Engl. J. Med. 367, 1626–1635.

Canavan, C., West, J., Card, T., 2014. Review article: the economic impact of the irritable bowel syndrome. Aliment. Pharmacol. Ther. 40, 1023–1034.

Carroccio, A., Mansueto, P., Iacono, G., Soresi, M., D'Alcamo, A., Cavataio, F., Brusca, I., Florena, A.M., Ambrosiano, G., Seidita, A., Pirrone, G., Rini, G.B., 2012. Non-celiac wheat sensitivity diagnosed by double-blind placebo-controlled challenge: exploring a new clinical entity. Am. J. Gastroenterol. 107, 1898–1906.

Carroll, I.M., Ringel-Kulka, T., Keku, T.O., Chang, Y.H., Packey, C.D., Sartor, R.B., Ringel, Y., 2011. Molecular analysis of the luminal- and mucosal-associated intestinal microbiota in diarrhea-predominant irritable bowel syndrome. Am. J. Physiol. Gastrointest. Liver Physiol. 301, G799–G807.

Carroll, I.M., Ringel-Kulka, T., Siddle, J.P., Ringel, Y., 2012. Alterations in composition and diversity of the intestinal microbiota in patients with diarrhea-predominant irritable bowel syndrome. Neurogastroenterol. Motil. 24, 521–530.

Charbonneau, D., Gibb, R.D., Quigley, E.M., 2013. Fecal excretion of *Bifidobacterium infantis* 35624 and changes in fecal microbiota after eight weeks of oral supplementation with encapsulated probiotic. Gut Microbes 4, 201–211.

Chassard, C., Dapoigny, M., Scott, K.P., Crouzet, L., Del'homme, C., Marquet, P., Martin, J.C., Pickering, G., Ardid, D., Eschalier, A., Dubray, C., Flint, H.J., Bernalier-Donadille, A., 2012. Functional dysbiosis within the gut microbiota of patients with constipated-irritable bowel syndrome. Aliment. Pharmacol. Ther. 35, 828–838.

Codling, C., O'Mahony, L., Shanahan, F., Quigley, E.M., Marchesi, J.R., 2010. A molecular analysis of fecal and mucosal bacterial communities in irritable bowel syndrome. Dig. Dis. Sci. 55, 392–397.

Collins, S.M., Surette, M., Bercik, P., 2012. The interplay between the intestinal microbiota and the brain. Nat. Rev. Microbiol. 10, 735–742.

Cryan, J.F., Dinan, T.G., 2012. Mind-altering microorganisms: the impact of the gut microbiota on brain and behaviour. Nat. Rev. Neurosci. 13, 701–712.

Cryan, J.F., O'Mahony, S.M., 2011. The microbiome-gut-brain axis: from bowel to behavior. Neurogastroenterol. Motil. 23, 187–192.

Dennison, U., McKernan, D., Cryan, J., Dinan, T., 2012. Schizophrenia patients with a history of childhood trauma have a pro-inflammatory phenotype. Psychol. Med. 42, 1865–1871.

Desbonnet, L., Clarke, G., Shanahan, F., Dinan, T.G., Cryan, J.F., 2014. Microbiota is essential for social development in the mouse. Mol. Psychiatry 19, 146–148.

Dinan, T.G., Cryan, J.F., 2013. Melancholic microbes: a link between gut microbiota and depression? Neurogastroenterol. Motil. 25, 713–719.

Dinan, T.G., 2009. Inflammatory markers in depression. Curr. Opin. Psychiatry 22, 32–36.

Duboc, H., Rainteau, D., Rajca, S., Humbert, L., Farabos, D., Maubert, M., Grondin, V., Jouet, P., Bouhassira, D., Seksik, P., Sokol, H., Coffin, B., Sabaté, J.M., 2012. Increase in fecal primary bile acids and dysbiosis in patients with diarrhea-predominant irritable bowel syndrome. Neurogastroenterol. Motil. 24, 513–520.

Durbán, A., Abellán, J.J., Jiménez-Hernández, N., Salgado, P., Ponce, M., Ponce, J., Garrigues, V., Latorre, A., Moya, A., 2012. Structural alterations of faecal and mucosa-associated bacterial communities in irritable bowel syndrome. Environ. Microbiol. Rep. 4, 242–247.

Durbán, A., Abellán, J.J., Jiménez-Hernández, N., Artacho, A., Garrigues, V., Ortiz, V., Ponce, J., Latorre, A., Moya, A., 2013. Instability of the faecal microbiota in diarrhoea-predominant irritable bowel syndrome. FEMS Microbiol. Ecol. 86, 581–589.

Eutamene, H., Lamine, F., Chabo, C., Theodorou, V., Rochat, F., Bergonzelli, G.E., Corthésy-Theulaz, I., Fioramonti, J., Bueno, L., 2007. Synergy between *Lactobacillus paracasei* and its bacterial products to counteract stress-induced gut permeability and sensitivity increase in rats. J. Nutr. 137, 1901–1907.

Ford, A.C., Talley, N.J., Spiegel, B.M., Foxx-Orenstein, A.E., Schiller, L., Quigley, E.M., Moayyedi, P., 2008. Effect of fibre, antispasmodics, and peppermint oil in the treatment of irritable bowel syndrome: systematic review and meta-analysis. BMJ 337, a2313.

Ford, A.C., Spiegel, B.M., Talley, N.J., Moayyedi, P., 2009. Small intestinal bacterial overgrowth in irritable bowel syndrome: systematic review and meta-analysis. Clin. Gastroenterol. Hepatol. 7, 1279–1286.

Ford, A.C., Quigley, E.M., Lacy, B.E., Lembo, A.J., Saito, Y.A., Schiller, L.R., Soffer, E.E., Spiegel, B.M., Moayyedi, P., 2014. Efficacy of prebiotics, probiotics, and synbiotics in irritable bowel syndrome and chronic idiopathic constipation: systematic review and meta-analysis. Am. J. Gastroenterol. 109, 1547–1561.

Groeger, D., O'Mahony, L., Murphy, E.F., Bourke, J.F., Dinan, T.G., Kiely, B., Shanahan, F., Quigley, E.M., 2013. *Bifidobacterium infantis* 35624 modulates host inflammatory processes beyond the gut. Gut Microbes 4, 325–339.

Guandalini, S., Magazzù, G., Chiaro, A., La Balestra, V., Di Nardo, G., Gopalan, S., et al., 2010. VSL#3 improves symptoms in children with irritable bowel syndrome: a multicenter, randomized, placebo-controlled, double-blind, crossover study. J. Pediatr. Gastroenterol. Nutr. 51, 24–30.

Guandalini, S., August 28, 2014. Are probiotics or prebiotics useful in pediatric irritable bowel syndrome or inflammatory bowel disease? Front. Med. (Lausanne) 1, 23.

Halmos, E.P., Power, V.A., Shepherd, S.J., Gibson, P.R., Muir, J.G., 2014. A diet low in FODMAPs reduces symptoms of irritable bowel syndrome. Gastroenterology 146, 67–75.

Halmos, E.P., Christophersen, C.T., Bird, A.R., Shepherd, S.J., Gibson, P.R., Muir, J.G., 2015. Diets that differ in their FODMAP content alter the colonic luminal microenvironment. Gut 64, 93–100.

Hayes, P., Corish, C., O'Mahony, E., Quigley, E.M.M., 2014. A dietary survey of patients with irritable bowel syndrome. J. Hum. Nut. Diet 27 (Suppl.), 36–47.

Hill, C., Guarner, F., Reid, G., Gibson, G.R., Merenstein, D.J., Pot, B., et al., 2014. Expert consensus document: the International Scientific Association for Probiotics and Prebiotics consensus statement on the scope and appropriate use of the term probiotic. Nat. Rev. Gastroenterol. Hepatol. 11, 506–514.

Hou, X., Chen, S., Zhang, Y., Sha, W., Yu, X., Elsawah, H., Afifi, A.F., El-Khayat, H.R., Nouh, A., Hassan, M.F., Fatah, A.A., Rucker Joerg, I., Sánchez Núñez, J.M., Osthoff Rueda, R., Jurkowska, G., Walczak, M., Malecka-Panas, E., Linke, K., Hartleb, M., Janssen-van Solingen, G., 2014. Quality of life in patients with irritable bowel syndrome (IBS), assessed using the IBS-quality of life (IBS-QOL) measure after 4 and 8 weeks of treatment with mebeverine hydrochloride or pinaverium bromide: results of an international prospective observational cohort study in Poland, Egypt, Mexico and China. Clin. Drug Investig. 34, 783–793.

Huang, H., Taylor, D.C., Carson, R.T., Sarocco, P., Friedman, M., Munsell, M., Blum, S.I., Menzin, J., 2014. Economic evaluation of linaclotide for the treatment of adult patients with irritable bowel syndrome with constipation in the United States. J. Med. Econ. 1–31.

Hunter, J.O., Tuffnell, Q., Lee, A.J., 1999. Controlled trial of oligofructose in the management of irritable bowel syndrome. J. Nutr. 129 (Suppl. 7), 1451S–1453S.

Hyland, N.P., Quigley, E.M., Brint, E., 2014. Microbiota-host interactions in irritable bowel syndrome: epithelial barrier, immune regulation and brain-gut interactions. World J. Gastroenterol. 20, 8859–8866.

Jalanka-Tuovinen, J., Salojärvi, J., Salonen, A., Immonen, O., Garsed, K., Kelly, F.M., Zaitoun, A., Palva, A., Spiller, R.C., de Vos, W.M., 2014. Faecal microbiota composition and host-microbe cross-talk following gastroenteritis and in postinfectious irritable bowel syndrome. Gut 63, 1737–1745.

Jeffery, I.B., O'Toole, P.W., Öhman, L., Claesson, M.J., Deane, J., Quigley, E.M., Simrén, M., 2012. An irritable bowel syndrome subtype defined by species-specific alterations in faecal microbiota. Gut 61, 997–1006.

Jeffrey, I.B., Quigley, E.M., Öhman, L., Simrén, M., O'Toole, P.W., 2012. The microbiota link to irritable bowel syndrome: an emerging story. Gut Microbes 3, 572–576.

Johnson, A.C., Greenwood-Van Meerveld, B., McRorie, J., 2011. Effects of *Bifidobacterium infantis* 35624 on post-inflammatory visceral hypersensitivity in the rat. Dig. Dis. Sci. 56, 3179–3186.

Kabbani, T.A., Vanga, R.R., Leffler, D.A., Villafuerte-Galvez, J., Pallav, K., Hansen, J., Mukherjee, R., Dennis, M., Kelly, C.P., 2014. Celiac disease or non-celiac gluten sensitivity? An approach to clinical differential diagnosis. Am. J. Gastroenterol. 109 (5), 741–746 [Epub ahead of print].

Kamiya, T., Wang, L., Forsythe, P., Goettsche, G., Mao, Y., Wang, Y., Tougas, G., Bienenstock, J., 2006. Inhibitory effects of *Lactobacillus reuteri* on visceral pain induced by colorectal distension in Sprague-Dawley rats. Gut 55, 191–196.

Kassinen, A., Krogius-Kurikka, L., Mäkivuokko, H., Rinttilä, T., Paulin, L., Corander, J., Malinen, E., Apajalahti, J., Palva, A., 2007. The fecal microbiota of irritable bowel syndrome patients differs significantly from that of healthy subjects. Gastroenterology 133, 24–33.

Korterink, J.J., Ockeloen, L., Benninga, M.A., Tabbers, M.M., Hilbink, M., Deckers Kocken, J.M., 2014. Probiotics for childhood functional gastrointestinal disorders: a systematic review and meta-analysis. Acta Paediatr. 103, 365–372.

Krogius-Kurikka, L., Lyra, A., Malinen, E., Aarnikunnas, J., Tuimala, J., Paulin, L., Mäkivuokko, H., Kajander, K., Palva, A., 2009. Microbial community analysis reveals high level phylogenetic alterations in the overall gastrointestinal microbiota of diarrhoea-predominant irritable bowel syndrome sufferers. BMC Gastroenterol. 9, 95.

Kruis, W., Chrubasik, S., Boehm, S., Stange, C., Schulze, J., 2012. A double-blind placebo controlled trial to study therapeutic effects of probiotic *Escherichia coli* Nissle 1917 in subgroups of patients with irritable bowel syndrome. Int. J. Colorectal Dis. 27, 467–474.

Laval, L., Martin, R., Natividad, J., Chain, F., Miquel, S., de Maredsous, C.D., Capronnier, S., Sokol, H., Verdu, E., van Hylckama Vlieg, J., Bermúdez-Humarán, L., Smokvina, T., Langella, P., 2014. *Lactobacillus rhamnosus* CNCM I-3690 and the commensal bacterium *Faecalibacterium prausnitzii* A2-165 exhibit similar protective effects to induced barrier hyper-permeability in mice. Gut Microbes 6 (1), 1–9 [Epub ahead of print].

Lee, K.N., Lee, O.Y., 2014. Intestinal microbiota in pathophysiology and management of irritable bowel syndrome. World J. Gastroenterol. 20, 8886–8897.

Longstreth, G.F., Thompson, W.G., Chey, W.D., Houghton, L.A., Mearin, F., Spiller, R.C., 2006. Functional bowel disorders. Gastroenterology 130, 1480–1491.

Madsen, K., Cornish, A., Soper, P., McKaigney, C., Jijon, H., Yachimel, C., Doyle, J., Jewell, L., De Simone, C., 2001. Probiotic bacteria enhance murine and human intestinal epithelial barrier function. Gastroenterology 121, 580–591.

Major, G., Teale, A., Pritchard, S., Marciani, L., Whelan, K., Gowland, P., et al., 2014. OC070 dietary supplementation with FODMAPS increases fasting colonic volume and breath hydrogen in healthy volunteers: a mechanistic study using MRI. Gut 63 (Suppl. 1) A35.

Martini, G.A., Phear, E.A., Ruebner, B., Sherlock, S., 1957. The bacterial content of the small intestine in normal and cirrhotic subjects: relation to methionine toxicity. Clin. Sci. 16, 35–51.

Ng, S.C., Lam, E.F., Lam, T.T., Chan, Y., Law, W., Tse, P.C., Kamm, M.A., Sung, J.J., Chan, F.K., Wu, J.C., 2013. Effect of probiotic bacteria on the intestinal microbiota in irritable bowel syndrome. J. Gastroenterol. Hepatol. 28, 1624–1631.

Novak, M., Vetvicka, V., 2008. Beta-glucans, history, and the present: immunomodulatory aspects and mechanisms of action. J. Immunotoxicol. 5, 47–57.

O'Leary, C., Wieneke, P., Buckley, S., O'Regan, P., Cronin, C.C., Quigley, E.M.M., Shanahan, F., 2002. Coeliac disease and irritable bowel-type symptoms. Am. J. Gastroenterol. 97, 1463–1467.

O'Mahony, L., McCarthy, J., Kelly, P., Hurley, G., Luo, F., Chen, K., O'Sullivan, G.C., Kiely, B., Collins, J.K., Shanahan, F., Quigley, E.M., 2005. *Lactobacillus* and *Bifidobacterium* in irritable bowel syndrome: symptom responses and relationship to cytokine profiles. Gastroenterology 128, 541–551.

Olesen, M., Gudmand-Hoyer, E., 2000. Efficacy, safety, and tolerability of fructooligosaccharides in the treatment of irritable bowel syndrome. Am. J. Clin. Nutr. 2, 1570–1575.

Ong, D.K., Mitchell, S.B., Barrett, J.S., Shepherd, S.J., Irving, P.M., Biesiekierski, J.R., et al., 2010. Manipulation of dietary short chain carbohydrates alters the pattern of gas production and genesis of symptoms in irritable bowel syndrome. J. Gastroenterol. Hepatol. 25, 1366–1373.

Paineau, D., Payen, F., Panserieu, S., Coulombier, G., Sobaszek, A., Lartigau, I., et al., 2008. The effects of regular consumption of short-chain fructo-oligosaccharides on digestive comfort of subjects with minor functional bowel disorders. Br. J. Nutr. 99, 311–318.

Parkes, G.C., Rayment, N.B., Hudspith, B.N., Petrovska, L., Lomer, M.C., Brostoff, J., Whelan, K., Sanderson, J.D., 2012. Distinct microbial populations exist in the mucosa-associated microbiota of sub-groups of irritable bowel syndrome. Neurogastroenterol. Motil. 24, 31–39.

Persborn, M., Gerritsen, J., Wallon, C., Carlsson, A., Akkermans, L.M., Söderholm, J.D., 2013. The effects of probiotics on barrier function and mucosal pouch microbiota during maintenance treatment for severe pouchitis in patients with ulcerative colitis. Aliment. Pharmacol. Ther. 38, 772–783.

Phear, E.A., Ruebner, B., Sherlock, S., Summerskill, W.H., 1956. Methionine toxicity in liver disease and its prevention by chlortetracycline. Clin. Sci. 15, 93–117.

Phillips, G.B., Schwartz, R., Gabuzda Jr., G.J., Davidson, C.S., 1952. The syndrome of impending hepatic coma in patients with cirrhosis of the liver given certain nitrogenous substances. N. Engl. J. Med. 247, 239–246.

Piche, T., 2014. Tight junctions and IBS–the link between epithelial permeability, low-grade inflammation, and symptom generation? Neurogastroenterol. Motil. 26, 296–302.

Pimentel, M., Chow, E.J., Lin, H.C., 2000. Eradication of small intestinal bacterial overgrowth reduces symptoms of irritable bowel syndrome. Am. J. Gastroenterol. 95, 3503–3506.

Pimentel, M., Chow, E.J., Lin, H.C., 2003. Normalization of lactulose breath testing correlates with symptom improvement in irritable bowel syndrome: a double-blind, randomized, placebo-controlled study. Am. J. Gastroenterol. 98, 412–419.

Pimentel, M., Lembo, A., Chey, W.D., Zakko, S., Ringel, Y., Yu, J., Mareya, S.M., Shaw, A.L., Bortey, E., Forbes, W.P., for the TARGET Study Group, 2011. Rifaximin therapy for patients with irritable bowel syndrome without constipation. N. Engl. J. Med. 364, 22–32.

Quigley, E.M.M., Abu-Shanab, A., 2009. The diagnosis of small intestinal bacterial overgrowth: the challenges persist! Expert Rev. Gastroenterol. Hepatol. 3, 77–87.

Quigley, E.M., Shanahan, F., 2014. The future of probiotics for disorders of the brain-gut axis. Adv. Exp. Med. Biol. 817, 417–432.

Quigley, E.M.M., Morcos, A., Dinan, T., 2009. Irritable bowel syndrome – role of food in pathogenesis and management. J. Dig. Dis. 10, 237–246.

Quigley, E.M.M., 2002. The role of gas in IBS. In: Camilleri, M., Spiller, R.C. (Eds.), Irritable Bowel Syndrome. Diagnosis and Treatment. WB Saunders Co, Philadelphia, pp. 77–84.

Quigley, E.M.M., 2003. From comic relief to real understanding; how intestinal gas causes symptoms. Gut 52, 1659–1661.

Quigley, E.M.M., 2007. A 51-year old with IBS. Test or treat for bacterial overgrowth? Clin. Gastroenterol. Hepatol. 5, 114–1143.

Quigley, E.M.M., 2011. Therapies aimed at the gut microbiota and inflammation. Antibiotics, probiotics/prebiotics/synbiotics, anti-inflammatory therapies. Gastroenterol. Clin. North Am. 40, 207–222.

Quigley, E.M., 2012. Bugs on the brain; brain in the gut-seeking explanations for common gastrointestinal symptoms. Ir. J. Med. Sci. 182, 1–6.

Rajilić-Stojanović, M., Biagi, E., Heilig, H.G., Kajander, K., Kekkonen, R.A., Tims, S., de Vos, W.M., 2011. Global and deep molecular analysis of microbiota signatures in fecal samples from patients with irritable bowel syndrome. Gastroenterology 141, 1792–1801.

Rigsbee, L., Agans, R., Shankar, V., Kenche, H., Khamis, H.J., Michail, S., Paliy, O., 2012. Quantitative profiling of gut microbiota of children with diarrhea-predominant irritable bowel syndrome. Am. J. Gastroenterol. 107, 1740–1751.

Roberfroid, M., et al., 2010. Prebiotic effects: metabolic and health benefits. Br. J. Nutr. 104 (Suppl. 2), S1–S63.

Roberfroid, M., 1993. Dietary fiber, inulin, and oligofructose: a review comparing their physiological effects. Crit. Rev. Food Sci. Nutr. 33, 103–148.

Saulnier, D.M., Riehle, K., Mistretta, T.A., Diaz, M.A., Mandal, D., Raza, S., Weidler, E.M., Qin, X., Coarfa, C., Milosavljevic, A., Petrosino, J.F., Highlander, S., Gibbs, R., Lynch, S.V., Shulman, R.J., Versalovic, J., 2011. Gastrointestinal microbiome signatures of pediatric patients with irritable bowel syndrome. Gastroenterology 141, 1782–1791.

Serra, J., Azpiroz, F., Malagelada, J.R., 2001. Impaired transit and tolerance of gas in the irritable bowel syndrome. Gut 48, 14–19.

Shanahan, F., Quigley, E.M., 2014. Manipulation of the microbiota for treatment of IBS and IBD-challenges and controversies. Gastroenterology 146, 1554–1563.

Sheil, B., McCarthy, J., O'Mahony, L., Bennett, M.W., Ryan, P., Fitzgibbon, J.J., Kiely, B., Collins, J.K., Shanahan, F., 2004. Is the mucosal route of administration essential for probiotic function? Subcutaneous administration is associated with attenuation of murine colitis and arthritis. Gut 53, 694–700.

Shepherd, S.J., Lomer, M.C., Gibson, P.R., 2013. Short-chain carbohydrates and functional gastrointestinal disorders. Am. J. Gastroenterol. 108, 707–717.

Silk, D.B., Davis, A., Vulevic, J., Tzortzis, G., Gibson, G.R., 2009. Clinical trial: the effects of a trans-galactooligosaccharide prebiotic on faecal microbiota and symptoms in irritable bowel syndrome. Aliment. Pharmacol. Ther. 29 (5), 508–518. http://dx.doi.org/10.1111/j.1365-2036.2008.03911.x.

Simrén, M., Barbara, G., Flint, H.J., Spiegel, B.M., Spiller, R.C., Vanner, S., Verdu, E.F., Whorwell, P.J., Zoetendal, E.G., 2013. Intestinal microbiota in functional bowel disorders: a Rome Foundation report. Gut 62, 159–176.

Spiller, R.C., Jenkins, D., Thornley, J.P., Hebden, J.M., Wright, T., Skinner, M., Neal, K.R., 2000. Increased rectal mucosal enteroendocrine cells, T lymphocytes, and increased gut permeability following acute Campylobacter enteritis and in post-dysenteric irritable bowel syndrome. Gut 47, 804–811.

Spiller, R., Aziz, Q., Creed, F., Emmanuel, A., Houghton, L., Hungin, P., Jones, R., Kumar, D., Rubin, G., Trudgill, N., Whorwell, P., 2007. Guidelines on the irritable bowel syndrome: mechanisms and practical management. Gut 56, 1770–1798.

Staudacher, H.M., Whelan, K., Irving, P.M., Lomer, M.C., 2011. Comparison of symptom response following advice for a diet low in fermentable carbohydrates (FODMAPs) versus standard dietary advice in patients with irritable bowel syndrome. J. Hum. Nutr. Diet 24, 487–495.

Thabane, M., Kottachchi, D.T., Marshall, J.K., 2007. Systematic review and meta-analysis: the incidence and prognosis of post-infectious irritable bowel syndrome. Aliment. Pharmacol. Ther. 26, 535–544.

Tillisch, K., Labus, J., Kilpatrick, L., Jiang, Z., Stains, J., Ebrat, B., Guyonnet, D., Legrain-Raspaud, S., Trotin, B., Naliboff, B., Mayer, E.A., 2013. Consumption of fermented milk product with probiotic modulates brain activity. Gastroenterology 144, 1394–1401.

Vazquez-Roque, M.I., Camilleri, M., Smyrk, T., Murray, J.A., Marietta, E., O'Neill, J., Carlson, P., Lamsam, J., Janzow, D., Eckert, D., Burton, D., Zinsmeister, A.R., 2013. A controlled trial of gluten-free diet in patients with irritable bowel syndrome-diarrhea: effects on bowel frequency and intestinal function. Gastroenterology 144, 903–911.

Verdu, E.F., Bercik, P., Bergonzelli, G.E., Huang, X.X., Blennerhasset, P., Rochat, F., Fiaux, M., Mansourian, R., Corthesy-Theulaz, I., Collins, S.M., 2004. *Lactobacillus paracasei* normalizes muscle hypercontractility in a murine model of postinfective gut dysfunction. Gastroenterology 127, 826–837.

Verdu, E.F., Bercik, P., Verma-Gandhu, M., Huang, X.-X., Blenerhasset, P., Jackson, W., Mao, Y., Wang, L., Rochat, F., Collins, S.M., 2006. Specific probiotic therapy attenuates antibiotic induced visceral hypersensitivity in mice. Gut 55, 182–190.

Whorwell, P.J., Altringer, L., Morel, J., Bond, Y., Charbonneau, D., O'Mahony, L., Kiely, B., Shanahan, F., Quigley, E.M., 2006. Efficacy of an encapsulated probiotic *Bifidobacterium infantis* 35624 in women with irritable bowel syndrome. Am. J. Gastroenterol. 101, 1581–1590.

The Role of the Microbiota and Potential for Dietary Intervention in Chronic Fatigue Syndrome

A. Kirchgessner

Seton Hall University, School of Health and Medical Sciences, Department of Interprofessional Health Sciences and Health Administration, South Orange, NJ, United States

INTRODUCTION

Chronic fatigue syndrome (CFS) is a disabling disorder characterized by unexplained, relapsing fatigue that significantly impairs daily activity and diminishes quality of life (Alfari and Buchwald, 2003; Prinis et al., 2006). CFS is accompanied by substantial symptoms related to cognitive, immune, and autonomic dysfunction. Disease mechanisms are complex (White, 2004), with no single causal factor identified. According to the Centers for Disease Control (CDC), the overall prevalence of CFS in the United States is as many as 4 million people (Reyes et al., 2003; Engel and Neurath, 2010); up to 80% of those affected are women (Jason et al., 1999). Because of its disabling and long-term nature, and because it often affects individuals in the most productive parts of their lives, CFS represents a considerable burden to people affected (Dancey and Friend, 2008) and an economic burden for society and healthcare institutions (Bombardier and Buchwald, 1995; Reynolds et al., 2004).

The diagnosis of CFS has been debated for many years (see Brurberg et al., 2014; for review). Holmes et al. (1988) coined the term *chronic fatigue syndrome* in 1988 as an alternative to *chronic Epstein–Barr virus syndrome* . In 1994 the CDC published a revised and more inclusive case definition (CDC-1994/Fukuda) that defines CFS on the fulfillment of two major criteria: (1) chronic fatigue (CF) of at least 6-month duration that (2) is accompanied by at least four additional symptoms (neurocognitive disorders, sore throat, tender lymph nodes, muscle pain, multiple joint pain, headache, nonrefreshing sleep, or postexertional malaise lasting more than 24 h; Fukuda et al., 1994).

The term myalgic encephalomyelitis (ME) is often used interchangeably with CFS or in combination (ME/CFS). The term ME had been used prior to the term CFS (Acheson, 1959). It was applied as a descriptive diagnosis for a series of outbreaks of a contagious condition, causing symptoms such as extreme fatigue, weakness, pain, dizziness, and neurocognitive problems. However, some investigators argue that CFS

The Gut-Brain Axis. http://dx.doi.org/10.1016/B978-0-12-802304-4.00021-9

and ME are qualitatively distinct diagnostic classes with regard to clinical symptoms, severity of illness, and biomarkers (Jason et al., 2012; Maes et al., 2012).

According to Jason et al. (2012), the ME criteria appear to select a group of patients with more functional impairments as well as more severe postexertional malaise symptoms than those meeting the CDC-1994/Fukuda criteria. Consequently, Maes and colleagues proposed that ME/CFS patients should be subdivided into those with (lasting more than 24 h) and those without postexertional malaise into CFS and ME, respectively (Maes et al., 2012). Nevertheless, the assertion that CFS and ME are different clinical entities is still disputed. Recent reports suggest that the diagnostic reliability and validity of CFS and ME might be affected by how postexertional malaise is defined and assessed in self-report surveys (Jason et al., 2015). Because the CDC-1994/Fukuda case definition of CFS remains the most frequently cited and is also the most extensively validated one in adult and pediatric studies (Brurberg et al., 2014; Werker et al., 2013), the term CFS is pragmatically used in the present review. According to this case definition, the population prevalence of adult CFS is estimated to be less than 1% (Bruberg et al., 2014). It is interesting to note that the prevalence for self-reporting assessment of CFS was higher (3.3%) compared with clinical assessment (0.8%).

In addition to disabling fatigue, sleep disturbances, headaches, and cognitive dysfunction that are extensively described in the literature, CFS is characterized by mood changes, such as anxiety and depression (Wessely et al., 1998). It is well documented that people with chronic illness have higher levels of depression and that people with CF tend to be more depressed than many other illness groups (Skapinakis et al., 2003). Nevertheless, CFS and depression are distinct diagnostic categories (Maes and Twisk, 2010). Moreover, a considerable percentage of CFS patients experience gastrointestinal (GI) symptoms, including abdominal pain or discomfort and an alteration in bowel habit (Maes et al., 2014). In fact, 35%–92% of CFS patients have been diagnosed with irritable bowel syndrome (IBS; Wessely et al., 1999; Whitehead et al., 2002; Aaron and Buchwald, 2001; Korszun et al., 1998; Gomborone et al., 1996; Endicott, 1998; Morriss et al., 1999; Aaron et al., 2001), the most prevalent functional disorder of the gut with a high psychiatric co-morbidity (Hausteiner-Wiehle and Henningsen, 2014). Approximately 14% of IBS patients have CFS (Jones et al., 2001; Whorwell et al., 1986). Co-occurrence of CFS and IBS is associated with increased plasma levels of proinflammatory cytokines such as interleukin (IL)-6, IL-8, IL-1β, and tumor necrosis factor (TNF)-α (Scully et al., 2010). Several underlying mechanisms that require further investigation could serve as potential explanatory hypotheses for the appearance of IBS-like symptoms in CFS. These include alterations of the gut microbiota, the genes of which represent the intestinal microbiome, and modulation of the brain-gut axis, a bidirectional communication system that includes the CNS and the enteric nervous system (ENS), the intrinsic innervation of the gut. The brain-gut axis monitors and mediates the effects of emotions on gut function, which may be reflected by changes in gut physiology and gut symptoms.

The human gut harbors a diverse population of bacterial species, which is symbiotic and important for well-being. Gut microbiota can exert numerous effects on the intestinal neuroimmune system and influence various host functions such as the immune response, metabolic activity, and physiological function (O'Hara and Shanahan, 2007). Several diseases have been associated with alterations of the normal composition of the gut microbiota, which is referred to as dysbiosis, ranging from systemic disorders such as obesity and diabetes (Fallucca et al., 2014), to GI disorders such as inflammatory bowel disease (IBD; Frank et al., 2007), functional constipation (Kim et al., 2015), and IBS (see Mayer et al., 2014; for review). There is now evidence to suggest that dysbiosis may play a role in the pathogenesis of CFS (Logan et al., 2003; Sheedy et al., 2009).

Dysbiosis of the gut microbiota has been implicated in CFS pathophysiology in terms of enhanced gut permeability, immune activation, and altered intestinal motility. In addition, a growing body of animal research supports an important influence of the gut microbiota on CNS function, influencing emotional behaviors (Lyte et al., 1998; Goehler et al., 2007). A recent study has demonstrated that a similar relationship might exist in humans. Consumption of a fermented milk product with probiotic bacteria for 4 weeks by healthy women influenced brain activity in regions that control central processing of emotion and sensation (Tillisch et al., 2013). The Food and Agricultural Organization and the World Health Organization define probiotics as "live microorganisms which when administered in adequate amounts, confer a health benefit on the host" (FAO/WHO, 2001; Guarner and Schaafsma, 1998). Thus modulation of the gut microbiota with probiotics could affect emotional behavior in humans. In addition, probiotics have the potential to decrease mood-regulating systemic proinflammatory cytokines, decrease oxidative stress, and improve nutritional status (Logan et al., 2003). For example, orally consumed lactic acid producing–bacteria have been shown to prevent and/or alleviate GI disturbances and to normalize the cytokine profile, which might benefit CFS patients that have a cytokine imbalance (Sullivan et al., 2009). These findings lend further support to the presence of a gut–brain interface, one that may be modulated by gut microbiota and play a role in CFS.

Although considerable progress has been made in recent years, a major gap in the knowledge of the pathogenesis of CFS remains and has precluded the discovery of effective forms of treatment for this disabling disorder. This review will provide a brief overview of the current understanding of the role of the gut microbiota in CFS and the potential for dietary intervention by probiotics in alleviating its debilitating symptoms.

HUMAN GUT MICROBIOTA
COMPOSITION

The human gut microbiota is composed of an enormous number of microbes, generally regarded as commensal bacteria. Collectively, the gut microbiota contain a total of 10^{13}–10^{14} microbes, outnumbering cells of the body by 10-fold

(Savage, 1977; Salonen et al., 2009). The number and diversity of these microbial populations differs in regions of gut, with the majority (predominantly anaerobes) hosted within the colon (Turnbaugh et al., 2007; Khanna and Tosh, 2014). It has been estimated that 60% of the fecal mass is composed of bacteria (Zoetendal et al., 2006).

Initial studies on gut microbiota composition were limited by the difficulty to culture all intestinal microbes (Zoetendal et al., 2006). Using bacterial genome sequencing and metagenome analysis, researchers have now begun to demonstrate the diversity of the human gut microbiota, which contains more than 1000 phylotypes at the species level (Andoh et al., 2009). The application of these molecular techniques has also revealed that species inhabiting the GI tract are dominated by anaerobic bacteria that belong to only three bacterial phyla: the gram-positive Firmicutes and Actinobacteria, and the gram-negative Bacteriodetes. In adults, greater than 90% of the microbiota in the normal distal gut is represented by the Firmicutes and Bacteriodetes phyla, followed by Actinobacteria, Proteobacteria, Verrucomicrobia, Fusobacteria, and Cyanobacteria (Zoetendal et al., 2006). The Firmicutes, which is the largest bacterial phylum, consists of more than 200 genera, including *Lactobacillus*, *Mycoplasma*, *Bacillus*, and *Clostridium* species. The Bacteriodetes phylum (including ~20 genera) is composed of three large classes of gram-negative bacteria: *Cytophaga*, *Flavobacterium*, and *Bacteroidales*. The Actinobacteria phylum consists of gram-positive bacteria and includes the genus *Bifidobacterium*.

Humans are born essentially devoid of a gut microbiota. The gut microbiota has fully matured by the first 1–2 years of life, and it generally reflects the microbiota of the parents and even those of extended relatives. *Faecalibacterium prausnitzii*, *Roseburia intestinalis*, *Bacteroides uniformis*, and species of *Bifidobacterium* and *Lactobacillus* are present in most people (Luzupone et al., 2012). Once established, the composition of the gut microbiota remains fairly stable throughout the individual's life; however, in the long term, it can be affected by external factors, such as dietary intake. For example, consumption of red meat and the so-called "Western diet" (ie, high in fat and sugar and low in fiber) seems to favor the growth of bacteria belonging to the Firmicutes phylum including *Clostridium*, *Eubacterium*, and *Enterococcus* species and a decrease of several *Bacteroides* species. In contrast, the Bacteriodetes bacteria, similar to the *Prevotella* species, dominate in vegetarians with preferential expression of genes involved in starch breakdown. In fact, a recent study in mice suggests that dietary intake appears to be more important than host genetics in shaping individual variations in host-associated microbial communities (Carmody et al., 2015). In animal and human studies, a high-fat, high-sugar Western diet promotes the same changes in gut microbiota found in obesity, such as a 50% reduction of Bacteroidetes and proportional division-wide increase in Firmicutes (Ley et al., 2005). It is important to note that these changes in microbial composition and its metabolic effects were totally reversed after a shift back to a standard diet. In humans, after randomization to either carbohydrate-restricted or fat-restricted diets for 52 weeks, the proportion of Bacteroidetes increased over time, mirroring reductions in body weight (Ley et al., 2006).

The intestinal microbiota consists of two distinct ecosystems: luminal bacteria, which are dispersed in liquid feces, and mucosa-associated bacteria, which are bound to the mucus layer adjacent to the intestinal epithelium. In healthy and diseased individuals, the mucosa-associated microbiota differs in composition from those in feces (Kerckhoffs et al., 2011). Luminal microbiota constitute the majority of the gut microbiota. The mucosa-associated microbiota, although fewer, differ from one region of the gut to the other. Therefore the stool sample may provide a more representative view of the global microbiota than a single mucosal punch biopsy, which is also more difficult to obtain in humans. However, differences in microbiota associated with the mucosa may be more critical to understanding the relationship between gut microbiota and epithelial barrier function.

The gut microbiota regulates various functions. It provides nutrients and energy for the host through the fermentation of nondigestible dietary components in the colon, and without this inherent microbial community we would be unable to digest plant polysaccharides and would have trouble extracting lipids from our diet. In fact, the gut microbiota exert a great variety of functional properties affecting human physiology and pathology, including maintenance of intestinal epithelial homeostasis, development of the host immune system, protection against foodborne pathogens, and drug metabolism (Fukuda and Ohno, 2014; Hooper et al., 2012; Jia et al., 2008). In healthy individuals, the gut microbiota is balanced; however, this balance can be altered by several factors. An alteration of the composition of the gut microbiota (ie, dysbiosis) is associated with several GI diseases and other extraintestinal disorders and can act as a source of infection or chronic low-grade inflammation (Jimenez, 2009).

DYSBIOSIS OF THE GUT MICROBIOTA

Dysbiosis of the gut microbiota has been implicated in IBD, such as Crohn's disease and ulcerative colitis, leading to chronic inflammation and mucosal damage in genetically predisposed hosts (Matricon et al., 2010; Koboziev et al., 2014). In a human model analysis using 16S rRNA sequencing, the gut microbiota of IBD patients differed from that of healthy controls. IBD was associated with lower Bacteroidetes and Firmicutes, especially in regions of active inflammation (Frank et al., 2007). These groups of bacteria are particularly important because they produce short-chain fatty-acid metabolites, which have potent antiinflammatory properties and may enhance epithelial barrier integrity. Changes in gut microbiota composition in IBD also include a higher proportion of Proteobacteria, such as Enterobacteriaceae (Fava and Danese, 2011), which has consistently been associated with colorectal cancer (Leung et al., 2015). An excessive abundance of *Desulfovibrio* species has been described in ulcerative colitis (Rowan et al., 2010), which has the ability to generate sulfides.

Dysbiosis of the gut microbiota is also found in IBS (Kerckhoffs et al., 2011; Parkes et al., 2012; Pimentel et al., 2013). On the basis of the analysis of fecal samples, Rajilić-Stojanović et al. (2011) reported decreased abundance of *Bifidobacterium* and *Lactobacillus* and an increased Firmicutes:Bacteroidetes ratio at the phylum level in IBS patients. Parkes et al. (2012) performed an analysis of frozen rectal biopsies using bacterial group-specific oligonucleotide probes and found an expansion of mucosa-associated microbiota in IBS patients, mainly *Bacteroides* and *Clostridia*. In addition, they found that the mucosal *Bifidobacterium* were lower in IBS patients than in controls, together with a negative correlation between the mucosal *Bifidobacterium* and the number of days patients experienced pain or discomfort.

Bifidobacterium and *Lactobacillus* have also been shown to be less abundant components of the gut microbiota of adult patients with functional constipation (Khalif et al., 2005; Kim et al., 2015) or constipation predominant-IBS (Chassard et al., 2012). *Bifidobacterium* are clearly associated with beneficial effects on gut motility because probiotic supplementation (*Bifidobacterium animalis* DN-173 010) shortened colonic transit time in healthy women (Marteau et al., 2002). In addition, *Bifidobacterium lactis* HN019 decreased whole gut transit in adults with functional GI symptoms (Waller et al., 2011). *Bifidobacterium* have also been shown to reduce intestinal lipopolysaccharide (LPS) levels and decrease proinflammatory cytokine concentrations (Riedel et al., 2006.) Thus *Bifidobacterium* improve gut motility and can dampen an inflammatory state.

Dysbiosis of the gut microbiota is also observed in stress. Psychological stress also alters the gut microbiota toward a reduction of *Bifidobacterium* and *Lactobacillus* (Bailey et al., 2004). Stress in neonatal Rhesus monkeys was reported to reduce the numbers of *Lactobacilli* in the fecal flora in association with increased susceptibility for opportunistic infections (Bailey and Coe, 1999). Restraint conditions, acoustic stress, and food deprivation have all been shown to promote dysbiosis of the gut microbiota in various animal studies (Tannock and Savage, 1974; Suzuki et al., 1983). It is interesting to note that stress (eg, psychological, physical exhaustion) is a well-established trigger factor for CFS (Maes et al., 2007).

DYSBIOSIS IN CHRONIC FATIGUE SYNDROME

Several studies have reported changes in gut microbiota composition in CFS. Investigations have shown that there is a reduction in beneficial bacteria, such as *Bifidobacterium*, and an increase in the abundance of aerobic bacteria (Evengard et al., 2007; Lorusso et al., 2009; Butt et al., 1998; Sheedy et al., 2009; Logan et al., 2003). As previously discussed, a reduction in *Bifidobacterium* has been reported in patients with IBS (Malinen et al., 2005), IBD (Favier et al., 1997; Gueimonde et al., 2007), and in animal models of stress (Bailey et al., 2004).

Logan et al. (2003) proposed that low levels of *Bifidobacterium* and small intestinal bacterial overgrowth (SIBO), due to the expansion of colonic bacteria into the small intestine, could result in immune dysfunction in CFS patients. Symptoms of SIBO resemble those of IBS (bloating, diarrhea, abdominal pain, and constipation) and symptoms commonly observed in CFS (Logan and Beaulne, 2002). Successful eradication of bacteria by the administration of antibiotics was accompanied with a reduction of GI complaints and led to significant improvements in memory, pain, and depression. Various strains of *Bifidobacterium* have been used to successfully treat SIBO (Kanamori et al., 2001), supporting the idea that functional bowel symptoms are due to alterations in the gut microbiota and emphasizing the importance of restoring the normal gut microbiota in disease management.

Butt et al. (1998) presented evidence of altered fecal microbiota in CFS patients compared with normal, healthy controls. The mean distribution of the gram-negative *Escherichia coli* as a percentage of the total aerobic flora of control subjects was 92% compared with 49% in CFS patients. Among aerobes, the D-lactic acid producing *Enterococcus* and *Streptococcus* species were strongly overrepresented in CFS patients. Moreover, it was shown that the higher the aerobic enterococcal count, the more severe the neurological and cognitive deficits, including nervousness, memory loss, forgetfulness, and confusion (Butt et al., 1998). Sheedy et al. (2009) later confirmed these findings in fecal samples of CFS patients with GI symptoms. Using culture-based assays, Sheedy et al. (2009) observed that the total count for *Enterococcus* and *Streptococcus* species for the CFS group was 52% of the total aerobic intestinal flora, which is significantly higher than the 12% seen in control subjects.

Patients with D-lactic acidosis present with similar symptoms (headaches, weakness, cognitive impairment, fatigue, pain, and severe lethargy) to patients with CFS (Calderini et al., 2003; Stolberg et al., 1982). Thus increased intestinal colonization of D-lactic acid producing bacteria may result in cognitive and neurological responses in CFS patients as reported in patients with D-lactic acidosis. The link between gut microbiota and cognitive problems is further supported by a study reporting a positive effect of probiotic supplementation (*Lactobacillus casei*) on emotional and anxiety symptoms in CFS patients (Gaab et al., 2005). In another study, administration of probiotic strains (*Lactobacillus paracasei*, *Lactobacillus acidophilus*, *B. lactis*) also resulted in a significant improvement of neurocognitive functions but not of fatigue and physical activity scores (Raber et al., 1998).

Frémont et al. (2013) used high-throughput 16S rRNA gene sequencing to investigate the microbiota composition of stool samples from Belgian and Norwegian CFS patients. By sequence analysis, they found that the composition of gut microbiota differed in CFS patients (diagnosed according to the CDC/Fukuda criteria) compared with matched healthy controls. Most sequences found in the subjects (controls and patients) belonged to one of the four phyla Actinobacteria, Bacteroidetes, Firmicutes, or Proteobacteria, which is in agreement with previous reports from human gut microbiota studies (Rajilić-Stojanović et al., 2007). However, the relative proportions of these major phyla differed from one individual to another. In fact, the geographical origin of the sample had an influence on the Firmicutes:Bacteriodetes ratio, which was significantly higher in Norwegian samples than in Belgium samples.

The study also revealed alterations of gut microbiota composition in CFS patients. Norwegian CFS patients differed from their matched controls by showing decreased percentages of several Firmicutes subpopulations (*Roseburia*, *Syntrophococcus*, *Holdemania*, *Dialister*), a 20-fold increase of *Lactonifactor*, and a 3.8-fold increase of the Bacteroidetes genus *Alistipes*. It is interesting to note that higher levels of *Alistipes* taxa are associated with greater frequency of abdominal pain in IBS (Saulnier et al., 2011). Changes in gut microbiota were less pronounced in the Belgian CFS patients. Nevertheless, in both Norwegian and Belgian CFS patients, there was a significant increase of the Firmicute *Lactonifactor*, known to be involved in the bacterial conversion of plant lignans into the bioactive enterolignans enterooldiol and enterolactone and to have antiestrogenic and anticancer effects (Webb and McCullough, 2005).

In Belgian patients the increase of *Lactonifactor* was paralleled by a decrease of the Actinobacteria *Asaccharobacter* (Frémont et al., 2013). *Asaccharobacter* is involved in the metabolism of phytoestrogens, which have the capacity to regulate vitamin D receptor (VDR) activity and vitamin D synthesis. The vitamin D system is critical for maintenance of gut mucosal immunity, and several reports have shown a link between VDR insufficiency and colitis development in humans and in experimental colitis animal models (Lim et al., 2005; Cross et al., 2011; Li et al., 2015). Approximately 70% of IBS sufferers reported that high-dose vitamin D3 supplementation improved their IBS symptoms (Sprake et al., 2012); however, a randomized control trial is needed to confirm this finding. VDR function may also be altered in CFS (Hoeck and Pall, 2011). Thus, as proposed by Proal et al. (2013), the regulation of the VDR could be a useful therapeutic target in the management of CFS symptoms.

PROBIOTICS IN CHRONIC FATIGUE SYNDROME

As has been highlighted in previous sections, dysbiosis of the gut microbiota has been reported in CFS. Thus modulation of the gut microbiota by probiotics could offer a potential target for disease intervention.

The most commonly used probiotics are members of the *Lactobacilli*, *Enterococci*, and *Bifidobacterium* groups (Ouwehand et al., 2002); however, others include nonpathogenic bacilli such as *E. coli* Nisle 1917 and yeasts such as *Saccharomyces boulardii*. The *Bifidobacterium* strains are the most extensively studied and used in probiotic products. An aberrant *Bifidobacterium* number or composition is the most frequently reported alteration observed in several disease states. Probiotics have been shown to be well tolerated with few side effects, making them a potential attractive treatment option for the management of CFS.

The idea that probiotics may improve quality of life is not a new one. Dr. George Porter Phillips first reported in 1910 that although *Lactobacillus* tablets and powder were ineffective, a gelatin-whey formula with live lactic acid–producing bacteria improved depressive symptoms in adults with melancholia. It is well known that stress exposure during early life in rats disrupts the microbiota profile and leads to increased stress reactivity in adulthood. Treatment of rat pups with the probiotic *Lactobacillus* sp. normalized stress hormone levels (Rao et al., 2009). Early-life stress also leads to increased depressive-like behavior in adult rats. Treatment of rats exposed to stress during early life with the probiotic *Bifidobacterium infantis* reduced the depressive-like symptoms in adulthood (Desbonnet et al., 2010).

A few studies have shown that probiotics may have antidepressant or anxiety-reducing effects in humans. In one study the positive effects of the probiotics *Lactobacillus helveticus* R0052 and *Bifidobacterium longum* R0175 in an animal model were confirmed in adult volunteers in a randomized, double-blind trial (Messaoudi et al., 2011). The probiotics, given to healthy subjects for 30 days, reduced psychological distress, measured by the Hopkins Symptom Checklist and the Hospital Anxiety and Depression Scale (Messaoudi et al., 2011). A reduction of urinary cortisol was also observed. Furthermore, in a clinical study on individuals with CFS, administration of probiotics over a 2-month trial resulted in fewer anxiety-related symptoms (Rao et al., 2009). Administration of the *L. casei* strain Shirota (LcS; 24 billion cfu/day) to adult patients meeting the CDC-1994/Fukuda criteria was found at 8 weeks to cause a significant increase in both *Lactobacillus* and *Bifidobacterium* in those taking the LcS and there was also a significant decrease in anxiety symptoms (Rao et al., 2009). The elevation of Bifidobacteria levels is a positive finding because *Bifidobacterium* levels may be low in CFS (Logan et al., 2003).

Evidence has grown to support the efficacy of probiotics, especially the *Lactobacillus* and *Bifidobacterium* species in the management of GI disturbances, which are prominent in CFS. Mice fed *B. infantis* 35,624 or *Lactobacillus salivarius* UCC118 displayed significantly reduced small intestinal transit in vivo (Lomasney et al., 2014). In humans *B. animalis* DN-173 010 shortened colonic transit time in healthy women (Marteau et al., 2002) and *B. lactis* HN019 decreased whole gut transit in adults with functional GI symptoms (Waller et al., 2011).

On the basis of several meta-analyses, probiotics appear to have some benefit in treating IBS (for review, see Aragon et al., 2010; Mayer et al., 2014; Guyonnet et al., 2007). Ortiz-Lucas et al. (2013) evaluated 10 studies with a focus on the specific organisms that are potentially effective. A significant benefit on pain relief was found for *Bifidobacterium breve*, *B. longum*, and *L. acidophilus*. Horvath et al. (2011) reviewed three studies of *Lactobacillus rhamnosus* in children with IBS and reported a significant benefit for pain improvement.

In the gut, probiotics can have a beneficial effect via several mechanisms. First, probiotics can improve intestinal barrier function. An increase in Bifidobacteria in *ob/ob* mice was associated with a significant improvement of gut permeability measured in vivo; this improvement was linked to an increase in tight-junction (TJ) mRNA expression and protein distribution (Cani et al., 2009). In addition, the increase in Bifidobacteria was correlated with a decrease in plasma LPS concentrations (Cani et al., 2009). Enhancement of barrier function by probiotic bacteria has been observed in both in vitro models and in vivo animal models (Ohland and Wallace, 2010). A probiotic mixture VSL#3, a proprietary preparation consisting of a high concentration of eight different probiotic strains, improved intestinal epithelial integrity and reduced its permeability, conferring protection against inflammatory luminal constituents coming from bacteria or diet (Madsen et al., 2001). Madsen et al. also showed that VSL#3 conferred resistance to *Salmonella* invasion by reducing intestinal permeability. In addition, some strains of probiotics alter the immune activity of the host (Sierra et al., 2010). Furthermore, they may also inhibit the mucosal adhesion of pathogens and thus reduce infection severity (Sherman et al., 2005).

Using culture-based assays, Sheedy et al. (2009) observed significantly increased proportions of D-lactic acid–producing *Enterococcus* and *Streptococcus* spp. in fecal samples of CFS patients. Excess D-lactic acid production could contribute to mitochondrial dysfunction and lead to neurocognitive impairments in patients because D-lactic acidosis is known to affect CNS function. The link between gut microbiota and cognitive problems was further supported by a study reporting a positive effect of probiotic supplementation (*L. casei*) on emotional and anxiety symptoms in CFS patients (Gaab et al., 2005). In another study administration of probiotic strains (*L. paracasei*, *L. acidophilus*, *B. lactis*) also resulted in a significant improvement of neurocognitive functions, but not of fatigue and physical activity scores (Raber et al., 1998).

Probiotics have also been shown to decrease levels of C-reactive protein (CRP) and levels of proinflammatory cytokines in CFS patients. CRP is an acute phase protein synthesized by hepatocytes and adipocytes in response to peripheral proinflammatory cytokines. An elevated serum or plasma level of CRP is a clinically reliable indicator of a systemic proinflammatory state. Elevated levels of CRP are found in CFS (Groeger et al., 2013; Spence et al., 2008; Raison et al., 2009), along with a higher baseline level of TNF-α. After 8 weeks of oral administration of *B. infantis* 35,624, a significant reduction of plasma CRP and TNF-α levels was observed in CFS patients whereas it attenuated the levels of IL-6. No such effect was noted in the placebo control group. In general, a reduction of these inflammatory markers would be regarded as indicative of clinical remission and of a lower risk of relapse. TNF-α and IL-6 are proinflammatory cytokines that are elevated in various conditions and are involved in the transcriptional regulation of CRP.

It should be kept in mind that to achieve beneficial effects, probiotics have to reach their site of action in sufficient numbers. Studies have shown that numbers of viable probiotic cells tend to decline in probiotic supplemented food products and during GI transit. To improve the viability in both of these cases, microencapsulation is one of the techniques used to protect bacteria against adverse conditions during manufacture and storage and its transit in the GI tract. Singh et al. (2012) reported that *Lactobacillus acidophilus*–loaded floating beads (LAB FBs) attenuated the symptoms associated with CFS in an animal model of CFS. In addition, animals treated with LAB FBs exhibited lower TNF-α levels in serum (Singh et al., 2012).

DYSBIOSIS IN CHRONIC FATIGUE SYNDROME: POSSIBLE CAUSES AND CONSEQUENCES

Bacterial and Viral Infections

Early conceptualizations of CFS focused on the role of bacterial and viral infection because upper respiratory system and flu-like infections often precede the onset of CFS, and CFS often occurs in epidemics. Bacterial and viral infections, including

Epstein–Barr virus (EBV), *Coxiella burnetii*, Parvo B19, and *Mycoplasma*, are well-known trigger factors associated with the onset of CFS. Moreover, infections also function as maintaining factors.

EBV infection has been shown to cause extreme fatigue during the acute illness and to be a risk factor for developing CFS, with a prevalence rate of 8% observed at 6 months (White et al., 1998; Moss and Spence, 2006). However, EBV was found in only 15%–30% of all biopsies (Frémont et al., 2009). Thus the involvement of EBV has not been conclusively proven. Other infections that are associated with CFS are human herpes virus (HHV)-6 and HHV-7, cytomegalovirus, enteroviruses, Borna disease, *Chlamydia pneumonia*, and *Borrelia burgdorferi* (Morris et al., 2014).

Lomardi et al. (2011) reported finding a gamma retrovirus in peripheral blood mononuclear cell DNA from approximately 67% of CFS patients compared with only 3.6% of healthy persons using polymerase chain reaction (PCR) testing. The agent was named xenotropic murine leukemia virus (MLV)-related virus (XMRV) because its *env* gene was nearly identical to that of xenotropic MLV, an infectious endogenous MLV that preferentially infects cells from foreign species, including humans. Almost half of the CFS patients in this study described the onset of their symptoms as related to an acute viral disease. In addition, virus isolation and antibody detection were reported in some CFS patients. However, two studies from the United Kingdom using PCR testing alone or together with serologic testing reported negative XMRV results in CFS patients (Erlwein et al., 2010; Groom et al., 2010). XMRV was also not detected by PCR testing in CFS patients from the Netherlands (van Kupperveld et al., 2010), China (Hong et al., 2010), or the United States (Switzer et al., 2010), questioning the association of XMRV with CFS.

Impaired Mucosal Barrier Function and a "Leaky Gut"

Dysbiosis of the gut microbiota could play a role in the etiology of CFS by impairing mucosal barrier function, resulting in increased permeability, endotoxemia, and chronic low-grade inflammation. The intestinal mucosa, which consists of a single layer of columnar epithelial cells, is one of the most important components of the innate immune system and all that separates the inside of the body from a very "dirty" outside environment. To protect itself from uncontrolled inflammatory responses, the intestinal mucosa has developed mechanisms to restrain bacterial growth, limit direct contact with the bacteria, and prevent bacterial dissemination into the underlying tissue.

Mucosal barrier function is maintained by several interrelated systems, including mucous secretion, chloride and water secretion, and the binding together of epithelial cells at their apical junctions by TJ proteins. Together, they act as the "gatekeeper" of the mucosal barrier. Studies have shown that the gut microbiota change the expression and distribution of TJ proteins and thereby regulate intestinal barrier function (Ulluwishewa et al., 2011). Colonization of the gut microbiota is normally limited to an outer "loose" mucus layer, whereas an "inner" adherent mucus layer is largely devoid of bacteria. In IBS and other chronic inflammatory diseases of the gut, the mucus layer becomes more permeable to bacteria, resulting in a "leaky gut" and leakage of water and protein into the gut lumen, and to the translocation of intraluminal solutes into the circulation (Johansson et al., 2014).

Commensal bacteria and probiotics have been shown to promote mucosal barrier function in vitro and in vivo. Probiotics preserve the mucosal barrier in mouse models of colitis (Madsen et al., 2001) and reduce intestinal permeability in human patients with Crohn's disease (Gupta et al., 2000). Probiotic treatment also reduces mucosal barrier dysfunction after psychological stress in rats (Zareie et al., 2006). Similarly, treating isolated epithelial cells with *E. coli* Nissle 1917 (Zyrek et al., 2007; Ukena et al., 2007), metabolites secreted by *B. infantis* (Ewaschuk et al., 2008), or *Lactobacillus plantarum* MB452 (Anderson et al., 2010) results in increased expression of proteins important to maintaining mucosal barrier integrity. Furthermore, commensal microbiota and probiotics are also known to decrease mucosal barrier dysfunction caused by cytokines (Resta-Lenert and Barrett, 2006).

Recent work has shown that a leaky gut can play a role in the etiology of CFS by initiating an inflammatory state through an immune response to the LPS-containing membranes of gram-negative bacteria, referred to as endotoxin. Under normal physiological conditions, endotoxin is continuously released into the intestinal lumen, but it does not exhibit any pathogenic effects. However, when the body suffers severe trauma, systemic infections, or intestinal ischemia, a large amount of the endotoxin will translocate into the blood causing intestinal endotoxemia (Cani et al., 2008). LPS can trigger the inflammatory process by binding to the CD14 toll-like receptor (TLR)-4 complex at the surface of innate immune cells. Activation of TLR4 causes the secretion of proinflammatory cytokines, such as TNF-α (Cani et al., 2008), which usually enhances the epithelial defect by increasing the rate of cell shedding from the villus tip. Under these conditions a gap is created in the intestinal mucosa that is too large to be plugged by the redistribution of TJ proteins.

Cani et al. (2007) elegantly demonstrated that after 1 month of high-fat feeding, mice exhibited an obese phenotype accompanied by a change in gut microbiota composition (reduction of *Bifidobacterium* and *Eubacteria* spp.) and a 2- to 3-fold increase in circulating LPS levels, which they called "metabolic endotoxemia." The role of LPS in triggering systemic inflammation was subsequently studied in healthy human subjects. A high-fat, high-carbohydrate meal induced a significant increase in postprandial plasma LPS, accompanied by an increased expression of TLR4, TNF-α, and IL-6. These increases were absent after consuming a meal rich in fiber and fruit (Anderson et al., 2007). Furthermore, high-fat feeding reduced the expression of TJ proteins, leading to increased gut permeability (Ghanim et al., 2009). Thus diet-induced dysbiosis of gut microbiota could have a significant impact on microbial LPS production; therefore avoidance of excessive dietary fat intake may ensure a more "healthy" gut microbiota.

Increased translocation of endotoxin through the gut wall is found in CFS, as demonstrated by increased levels of serum immunoglobulin (Ig)-A and IgM to LPS of gram-negative bacteria (ie, *Hafnia alvei, Pseudomonas aeruginosa, Morganella morganii, Proteus mirabillis, Pseudomonas putida, Citrobacter koseri, Klebsiella pneumonia*; Maes et al., 2007; Cani et al., 2007; de La Serre et al., 2010; Amar et al., 2011a,b). The prevalence and median values for serum IgA against the LPS of enterobacteria were significantly greater in patients with CFS than in normal volunteers and patients with partial CFS. Increased translocation of endotoxins was accompanied by inflammation, as shown by increased plasma levels of IL-1 and TNF-α and activation of cell-mediated immunity (CMI). In this study serum IgA levels were also significantly correlated with the severity of CFS symptoms, as measured by the FibroFatigue scale (Maes et al., 2007), a reliable and valid measuring instrument that is used to monitor symptom severity and change during treatment of CFS patients (Zachrisson et al., 2002).

In a subsequent study Maes et al. (2012) measured the IgA and IgM responses to the LPS of six different enterobacteria, serum IL-1, TNF-α, neopterin, and elastase levels and examined the relationship to symptom severity in patients with CFS and CF. The Fibromyalgia and Chronic Fatigue Syndrome Rating Scale assessed the severity of symptoms. The study confirmed previous findings (Maes et al., 2007) and demonstrated that increased IgA responses in CFS are associated with inflammation and CMI activation. In addition, patients with an abnormally high IgA response showed higher ratings indicative of IBS than subjects with a normal IgA response. Using cluster analysis performed on GI symptoms, Maes et al. (2014) reported that abdominal discomfort, strongly associated with the diagnosis of IBS, was significantly higher in subjects with CFS (~60%) than in patients with CF (~18%). Patients with both CFS and IBS had poorer appetite; increased abdominal pain; and increased severity of loose stools, diarrhea, nausea, and gastric reflux. In fact, patients with CFS could be divided into two subgroups based on the presence or absence of gut dysfunction. Both the IgA and IgM responses to LPS of enterobacteria were significantly higher in CFS patients with GI symptoms than those without. Dysbiosis of gut microbiota; increased gut permeability; and chronic, low-grade inflammation are found in patients with IBS (Zhou et al., 2009; Lee and Tack, 2010). Thus, similar to IBS, impaired mucosal barrier function and increased translocation of enterobacteria may be responsible for the gut dysfunction and chronic, low-grade inflammation observed in CFS patients.

A leaky gut could also play a role in the etiology of CFS symptoms outside of the gut. For example, Butt and colleagues reported that fatigue presentation in CFS patients with symptoms of IBS was more severe than in CFS patients without IBS (Butt et al., 2001). This is not surprising because the gut microbiota influences the sensory, motor, and immune system of the gut and interacts with higher brain centers even at extremely low levels (Lee and Tack, 2010). Therefore an aberrant gut microbiota and mucosal barrier dysfunction may actually be creating an "irritable" bowel by modulating the activity of the brain-gut axis.

Psychological stress has been shown to be an important contributing factor in the development of CFS (Oka et al., 2013; Borsini et al., 2014) and IBS (for review, see Qin et al., 2014). Although further studies are needed to identify the mechanisms underlying this association, dysbiosis and disruption of the mucosal barrier appear to play a role. For example, chronic water avoidance stress in rats can induce dysbiosis of the gut microbiota and enhance bacterial wall adherence, which in turn is expected to stimulate hyperactive responses in the mucosal immune system (Chen et al., 2003). Vanuytsel et al. (2014) have shown that psychological stress (public speech) and a single intravenous bolus of corticotropin-releasing factor increased small intestinal permeability in healthy humans. Consequently, enhanced gut permeability could contribute to the symptom generation observed during stress. This may at least partially explain the link between psychological stress and both CFS and IBS (Qin et al., 2014). The strong linkage probably originates from the brain-gut axis. It is well known that the brain communicates with the gut (ENS); however, gut symptoms can aggravate psychological disorders (eg, depression and anxiety). Thus stress directly or indirectly affects the composition and growth of the microbiota, which modulate the bidirectional communication between the brain and gut axis.

Intestinal Barrier Dysfunction and Chronic Inflammation

Intestinal barrier dysfunction has been found to play a pathogenic role not only in CFS, but also in IBS and other functional gut-related disorders. Moreover, there is now evidence that increased gut permeability is associated with chronic low-grade inflammation, characterized by increased levels of proinflammatory cytokines, such as IL-6, IL-1, or TNF-α.

In a study designed to examine the cytokine profile among a group of IBS patients with and without CFS, all patients with IBS were shown to have increased plasma levels of IL-6 and IL-8 (Scully et al., 2010). In addition, patients with IBS and CFS were found to have increased levels of two other proinflammatory cytokines, TNF-α and IL-1β (Scully et al., 2010). TNF-α plays a central role in the pathogenesis of IBD. In fact, anti-TNF antibodies (infliximab, etanercept) are used to diminish the increased levels of TNF-α during inflammation associated with IBD. Increased TNF-α has been demonstrated to increase epithelial permeability and produce colonic motility dysfunction. Enteric neurons express both TNF and IL-1β receptors (O'Malley et al., 2011). Because gut function is primarily regulated by the ENS, a component of the autonomic nervous system with the unique ability to function independently from the CNS (for review, see Furness, 2008), the cytokine-induced modulation of enteric neurons can alter GI motility, absorption, secretion, and blood flow. Thus the frequent association between CFS and IBS (Maes et al., 2014) could be governed by elevated circulating proinflammatory cytokines acting either locally or on the brain-gut axis.

Several studies have demonstrated ENS structural changes associated with gut inflammation. For example, damage to axons has been observed in the inflamed human intestine in episodes of IBD (Geboes and Collins, 1998; Villanacci et al., 2008; Dvorak et al., 1993). In fact, consequences of intestinal inflammation, even if mild, persist for weeks beyond the point at which detectable inflammation has subsided (for review see Lakhan and Kirchgessner, 2010). Thus persistent changes in GI nerve function, resulting in dysmotility, pain, and gut dysfunction long after the resolution of the initiating inflammatory event, could also contribute to the GI disorders observed in CFS.

CONCLUSION

Recent studies have shown that dysbiosis of the gut microbiota is associated with symptoms of CFS. A question that remains to be explored is the causal relationship between dysbiosis and disease onset. Is an aberrant gut microbiota a preexisting, causative, or at least predisposing factor for the disease? Or does dysbiosis occur as a consequence of the disease, triggered by stress, immune dysfunctions, or pathogen infections in the intestine? Amar et al. (2011a,b) found that in patients without diabetes or obesity at baseline, pathogens in the microbiome led to 16S rDNA blood serum concentrations significantly elevated in those who went on to develop diabetes. Further studies will have to clarify if the observed alterations in gut microbiota in CFS are a primary abnormality responsible for CFS symptoms or if the observed changes are secondary to CFS-related alterations in various gut functions. Perhaps both of these mechanisms could contribute to the persistence of altered bidirectional brain-gut interactions.

On the basis of several studies, probiotics appear to provide some benefit in CFS. However, despite reports showing the potential of the specific probiotic strains to improve the balance of the gut microbiota that is altered in CFS, there is not enough clinical evidence recommending their therapeutic use for CFS at this time. Several of the studies in the existing literature have limitations, such as inadequate sample size, poor study design, heterogeneity of CFS patients (eg, with and without gut symptoms), and the use of multiple probiotic strains and doses across studies. In addition, knowledge of their long-term efficacy is still lacking. Moreover, randomized control trials on the use of probiotics in CFS are lacking. In light of the heterogeneity of mechanisms contributing to CFS symptoms, subsets of patients with specific microbiota alterations may benefit from specific interventions aimed at normalizing a particular dysbiotic state. However, the identification of subsets of CFS patients with distinct patterns of dysbiosis will require large-scale studies in well phenotyped patients. It is clear that additional studies, including investigations examining the efficacy of prebiotics and/or synbiotics and fecal microbial transplantation in CFS, are needed. A direct evaluation of the impact of these various therapies on the gut microbiota would be of interest and could complement the rather subjective data derived from questionnaires, which may also be subject to recall bias. These studies would open up a new therapeutic horizon for CFS and are very important before the medical community will accept the addition of a probiotic as a supplement for CFS therapy.

REFERENCES

Aaron, L.A., Buchwald, D., 2001. A review of the evidence for overlap among unexplained clinical conditions. Ann. Intern. Med. 134, 868–881.

Aaron, L.A., Herrell, R., Ashton, S., Belcourt, M., Schmaling, K., Goldberg, J., Buchwald, D., 2001. Comorbid clinical conditions in chronic fatigue, a co-twin control study. J. Gen. Intern. Med. 16, 24–31.

Acheson, E.D., 1959. The clinical syndrome variously called benign myalgic encephalomyelitis, Iceland disease and epidemic neuromyasthenia. Am. J. Med. 26, 569–595.

Afari, N., Buchwald, D., 2003. Chronic fatigue syndrome: a review. Am. J. Psychiatry 160, 221–236.

Amar, J., Chabo, C., Waget, A., Klopp, P., Vachoux, C., Bermudez-Humaran, L.G., Smirnova, N., Berge, M., Sulpice, T., Lahtinen, S., Ouwehand, A., Langella, P., Rautonen, N., Sansonetti, P.J., Burcelin, R., 2011a. Intestinal mucosal adherence and translocation of commensal bacteria at the early onset of type 2 diabetes, molecular mechanisms and probiotic treatment. EMBO Mol. Med. 3, 559–572.

Amar, J., Serino, M., Lange, C., Chabo, C., Iacovoni, J., Mondot, S., Lepage, P., Klopp, C., Mariette, J., Bouchez, O., Perez, L., Courtney, M., Marre, M., Klopp, P., Lantieri, O., Dore, J., Charles, M.A., Balkau, B., Burcelin, R., 2011b. Involvement of tissue bacteria in the onset of diabetes in humans: evidence for a concept. Diabetologia 54, 3055–3061.

Anderson, P.D., Mehta, N.N., Wolfe, M.L., Hinkle, C.C., Pruscino, L., Comiskey, L.L., Tabita-Martinez, J., Sellers, K.F., Rickels, M.R., Ahima, R.S., Reilly, M.P., 2007. Innate immunity modulates adipokines in humans. J. Clin. Endocrinol. Metab. 92, 2272–2279.

Anderson, R.C., Cookson, A.L., McNabb, W.C., Park, Z., McCann, M.J., Kelly, W.J., Roy, N.C., 2010. *Lactobacillus plantarum* MB452 enhances the function of the intestinal barrier by increasing the expression levels of genes involved in tight junction formation. BMC Microbiol. 10, 316.

Andoh, A., Benno, Y., Kanauchi, O., Fujiyama, Y., 2009. Recent advances in molecular approaches to gut microbiota in inflammatory bowel disease. Curr. Pharm. Des. 15, 1066–2073.

Aragon, G., Aragon, D., Borum, M., Doman, D.B., 2010. Probiotic therapy for irritable bowel syndrome. Gastroenterol. Hepatol. 6, 39–44.

Bailey, M.T., Coe, C., 1999. Maternal separation disrupts the integrity of the intestinal microflora in infant rhesus monkeys. Dev. Psychobiol. 35, 146–155.

Bailey, M.T., Lubach, G., Coe, C.L., 2004. Prenatal stress alters bacterial colonization of the gut in infant monkeys. J. Pediatr. Gastroenterol. Nutr. 38, 414–421.

Bombardier, C., Buchwald, D., 1995. Chronic fatigue, chronic fatigue syndrome, and fibromyalgia. Disability and health-care use. Med. Care 34, 924–930.

Borsini, A., Hepgul, N., Mondelli, V., Chalder, T., Pariante, C.M., 2014. Childhood stressors in the development of fatigue syndromes, a review of the past 20 years of research. Psychol. Med. 44, 1809–1823.

Brurberg, K.G., Fonhus, M.S., Larun, L., Flottorp, S., Malterud, K., 2014. Case definitions for chronic fatigue syndrome/myalgic encephalomyelitis (CFS/ME), a systematic review. BMJ Open 4, e003973.

Butt, H.L., Dunstain, R.H., McGregor, N.R., Roberts, T.K., Zerbes, M., Klineberg, U., 1998. Alteration of the Bacterial Microbial Flora in Chronic Fatigue/Pain Patients. From myth towards management. Many Australia.

Butt, H.L., Dunstan, R., McGregor, N.R., Roberts, T.K., 2001. Bacterial colonosis in patients with persistent fatigue. Proceedings of the AHMF International Clinical and Scientific Conference Sydney, Australia.

Caldarini, M.I., Pons, S., D'Agostino, D., DePaula, J.A., Greco, G., Negri, G., Ascione, A., Bustos, D., 2003. Fecal flora in a patient with short bowel syndrome. An in vitro study on effect of pH on D-lactic acid production. Dig. Dis. Sci. 41, 1649–1652.

Cani, P.D., Bibiloni, R., Knauf, C., Waget, A., Neyrinck, A.M., Delzenne, N.M., Burcelin, R., 2008. Changes in gut microbiota control metabolic endotoxemia-induced inflammation in high-fat diet induced obesity and diabetes in mice. Diabetes 57, 1470–1481.

Cani, P.D., Possemiers, S., Van De Wiele, T., Guiot, Y., Everard, A., Rottier, O., Geurts, L., Naslain, D., Neyrinck, A., Lambert, D.M., Muccioli, G.G., Delzenne, N.M., 2009. Changes in gut microbiota control inflammation in obese mice through a mechanism involving GLP-2-drive improvement of gut permeability. Gut 58, 1091–1103.

Cani, P.D., Amar, J., Iglesias, M.A., Poggi, M., Knauf, C., Bastelica, D., Neyrinck, A.M., Fava, F., Tuohy, K.M., Chabo, C., Waget, A., Delmee, E., Cousin, B., Sulpice, T., Chamontin, B., Ferrieres, J., Tanti, J.F., Gibson, G.R., Casteilla, L., Delzenne, N.M., Alessi, M.C., Burcelin, R., 2007. Metabolic endotoxemia initiates obesity and insulin resistance. Diabetes 56, 1761–1772.

Carmody, R.N., Gerber, G.K., Luevano Jr., J.M., Gatti, D.M., Somes, L., Svenson, K.L., Turnbaugh, P.J., 2015. Diet dominates host genotype in shaping the murine gut microbiota. Cell Host Microbe 17, 72–84.

Chassard, C., Dapoigny, M., Scott, K.P., Crouzet, L., Del'homme, C., Marquet, P., Martin, J.C., Pickering, G., Ardid, D., Eschalier, A., Dubray, C., Flint, H.J., Bernalier-Donadille, A., 2012. Functional dysbiosis with the gut microbiota of patients with constipated-irritable bowel syndrome. Aliment. Pharmacol. Ther. 35, 828–838.

Chen, C., Brown, D.R., Xie, Y., Green, B.T., Lyte, M., 2003. Catecholamines modulate *Escherichia coli* O157:H7 adherence to murine cecal mucosa. Shock 20, 183–188.

Cross, H.S., Nittke, T., Kallay, E., 2011. Colonic vitamin D metabolism, implications for the pathogenesis of inflammatory bowel disease and colorectal cancer. Mol. Cell Endocrinol. 347, 70–79.

Dancey, C.P., Friend, J., 2008. Symptoms, impairment and illness intrusiveness- their relationship with depression in women with ME/CFS. Psychol. Health 23, 983–999.

de La Serre, C.B., Ellis, C.L., Lee, J., Hartman, A.L., Rutledge, J.C., Raybould, H.E., 2010. Propensity to high-fat diet induced obesity in rats is associated with changes in the gut microbiota and gut inflammation. Am. J. Physiol. Gastrointest. Liver Physiol. 299, G440–G448.

Desbonnet, L., Garrett, L., Clarke, G., Kiely, B., Cryan, J.F., Dinan, T.G., 2010. Effects of the probiotic *Bifidobacterium infantis* in the maternal separation model of depression. Neuroscience 170, 1179–1188.

Dvorak, A.M., Onderdonk, A.B., McLeod, R.S., Monahan-Earley, R.A., Cullen, J., Antonioli, D.A., Blair, J.E., Morgan, E.S., Cisneros, R.L., Estrella, P., 1993. Axonal necrosis of enteric autonomic nerves in continent ileal pouches. Possible implications pathogenesis Crohn's disease. Ann. Surg. 217, 260–271.

Endicott, N.A., 1998. Chronic fatigue syndrome in psychiatric patients, lifetime and premorbid personal history of physical health. Psychosom. Med. 60, 744–751.

Engel, M.A., Neurath, M.F., 2010. New pathophysiological insights and modern treatment of IBD. J. Gastroenterol. 45, 571–583.

Erlwein, O., Kaye, S., McClure, M.O., Weber, J., Wills, G., Collier, D., Wessely, S., Cleare, A., 2010. Failure to detect the novel retrovirus XMRV in chronic fatigue syndrome. PLoS One 5, e8519.

Evengard, B., Nord, C.E., Sullivan, A., 2007. Patients with chronic fatigue syndrome have higher numbers of anaerobic bacteria in the intestine compared to healthy subjects. Eur. Soc. Clin. Microbiol. Infect. Dis. 17, S340.

Ewaschuk, J.B., Diaz, H., Meddings, L., Diederichs, B., Dmytrash, A., Backer, J., Looijer-van Langen, M., Madsen, K.L., 2008. Secreted bioactive factors from *Bifidobacterium infantis* enhance epithelial cell barrier function. Am. J. Physiol. Gastrointest. Liver Physiol. 295, G1025–G1034.

Falluca, F., Porrata, C., Fallucca, S., Pianesi, M., 2014. Influence of diet on gut microbiota, inflammation and type 2 diabetes mellitus. First experience with macrobiotic Ma-Pi 2 diet. Diabetes Metab. Res. Suppl. 1, 48–54.

FAO/WHO, 2001. Health and Nutritional Properties of Probiotics in Food Including Powder Milk With Live Lactic Acid Bacteria Report.

Fava, F., Danese, S., 2011. Intestinal microbiota in inflammatory bowel disease: friend or foe? World J. Gastroenterol. 17, 557–566.

Favier, C., Neur, C., Mizon, C., Cortot, A., Colombel, J.F., Mizon, J., 1997. Fecal beta-D-galactosidase production and *Bifidobacteria* are decreased in Crohn's disease. Dig. Dis. Sci. 42, 817–822.

Frank, D.N., St Amand, A.L., Feldman, R.A., Boedeker, E.C., Harpaz, N., Pace, N.R., 2007. Molecular-phylogenetic characterization of microbial community imbalances in human inflammatory bowel diseases. Proc. Natl. Acad. Sci. USA 104, 13780–13785.

Frémont, M., Metzger, K., Rady, H., Hulstaert, J., De Meirleir, K., 2009. Detection of herpesviruses and parvovirus B19 in gastric and intestinal mucosa of chronic fatigue syndrome patients. In Vivo 23, 209–213.

Frémont, M., Coomans, D., Massart, S., De Meirleir, K., 2013. High-throughput 16S rRNA gene sequencing reveals alterations of intestinal microbiota in myalgic encephalomyelitis/chronic fatigue syndrome patients. Anaerobe 22, 50–56.

Fukuda, K., Straus, S.E., Hickie, I., Sharpe, M.C., Dobbins, J.G., Komaroff, A., 1994. The chronic fatigue syndrome, a comprehensive approach to its definition and study. International Chronic Fatigue Syndrome Study Group. Ann. Intern. Med. 121, 953–959.

Fukuda, S., Ohno, H., 2014. Gut microbiome and metabolic diseases. Semin. Immunopathol. 36, 103–114.

Furness, J.B., 2008. The enteric nervous system, normal functions and enteric neuropathies. Neurogastroenterol. Motil. 20, 32–38.

Gaab, J., Rohleder, N., Heitz, V., Engert, V., Schad, T., Schurmeyer, T.H., Ehlert, U., 2005. Stress-induced changes in LPS-induced pro-inflammatory cytokine production in chronic fatigue syndrome. Psychoneuroendocrinology 30, 188–198.

Geboes, K., Collins, S., 1998. Structural abnormalities of the nervous system in Crohn's disease and ulcerative colitis. Neurogastroenterol. Motil. 10, 189–202.

Ghanim, H., Abuaysheh, S., Sia, C.L., Korzeniewski, K., Chaudhuri, A., Fernandez-Real, J.M., Dandona, P., 2009. Increase in plasma endotoxin concentrations and the expression of toll-like receptors and suppressor of cytokine signaling-3 in mononuclear cells after a high-fat, high-carbohydrate meal: implications for insulin resistance. Diabetes Care 32, 2281–2287.

Goehler, L.F., Lyte, M., Gaykema, R.P., 2007. Infection-induced viscerosensory signals from the gut enhance anxiety: implications for psychoneuroimmunology. Brain Behav. Immun. 21, 721–726.

Gomborone, J.E., Gorard, D.A., Dewsnap, P.A., Libby, G.W., Farthing, M.J., 1996. Prevalence of irritable bowel syndrome in chronic fatigue. J. R. Coll. Physicians London 30, 512–513.

Groeger, D., O'Mahoney, L., Murphy, E.F., Bourke, J.F., Dinan, T.G., Kiely, B., Shanahan, F., Quigley, E.M., 2013. *Bifidobacterium infantis* 35624 modulates host inflammatory processes beyond the gut. Gut Microbe 4, 325–339.

Groom, H.C., Boucherit, V.C., Makinson, K., Randal, E., Baptista, S., Hagan, S., Gow, J.W., Mattes, F.M., Breuer, J., Kerr, J.R., Stoye, J.P., Bishop, K.N., 2010. Absence of xenotropic murine leukemia virus-related virus in UK patients with chronic fatigue syndrome. Retrovirology 7, 10.

Guarner, F., Schaafsma, G.J., 1998. Probiotics. Int. J. Food Microbiol. 39, 237–238.

Gueimonde, M., Ouwehand, A., Huhtinen, H., Salminen, E., Salminen, S., 2007. Qualitative and quantitative analyses of the bifidobacterial microbiota in the colonic mucosa of patients with colorectal cancer, diverticulitis and inflammatory bowel disease. World J. Gastroenterol. 13, 3985–3989.

Gupta, P., Andrew, H., Kirschner, B.S., Guandalini, S., 2000. Is lactobacillus GG helpful in children with Crohn's disease? Results of a preliminary, open-label study. J. Pediatr. Gastroenterol. Nutr. 31, 453–457.

Guyonnet, D., Chassany, O., Ducrotte, P., Picard, C., Mouret, M., Mercier, C.H., Matuchansky, C., 2007. Effect of a fermented milk containing *Bifidobacterium animalis* DN-173 010 on the health-related quality of life and symptoms in irritable bowel syndrome in adults in primary care: a mulicentre, randomized, double-blind, controlled trial. Aliment. Pharmacol. Ther. 26, 475–486.

Hausteiner-Wiehle, C., Henningsen, P., 2014. Irritable bowel syndrome, relations with functional, mental, and somatoform disorders. World Gastroenterol. 20, 6024–6030.

Hoeck, A.D., Pall, M.L., 2011. Will vitamin D supplementation ameliorate diseases characterized by chronic inflammation and disease? Med. Hypotheses 76, 208–213.

Holmes, G.P., Kaplan, J.E., Gantz, N.M., Komaroff, A.L., Schonberger, L.B., Straus, S.E., Jones, J.F., Dubois, R.E., Cunninghan-Rundles, C., Pahwa, S., Tosato, G., Zegans, L.S., Purtilo, D.T., Brown, N., Schooley, R.T., Brus, I., 1988. Chronic fatigue syndrome, a working case definition. Ann. Intern. Med. 108, 387–389.

Hong, P., Li, J., Li, Y., 2010. Failure to detect xenotropic murine leukaemia virus-related virus in Chinese patients with chronic fatigue syndrome. Virol. J. 7, 224.

Hooper, L.V., Littman, D.R., Macpherson, A.J., 2012. Interactions between the microbiota and the immune system. Science 336, 1268–1273.

Horvath, A., Dziechciarz, P., Szajewska, H., 2011. Meta-analysis, *Lactobacillus rhamnosus* GG for abdominal pain-related functional gastrointestinal disorders in childhood. Aliment. Pharmacol. Ther. 33, 1302–1310.

Jason, L.A., Richman, J.A., Rademaker, A.W., Jordan, K.M., Plioplys, A.V., Taylor, R.R., McCready, W., Huang, C.F., Plioplys, S., 1999. A community-based study of chronic fatigue syndrome. Arch. Intern. Med. 159, 2129–2137.

Jason, L.A., Evans, M., So, S., Scott, J., Brown, A., 2015. Problems in defining post-exertional malaise. J. Prev. Interv. Community 43, 20–31.

Jason, L.A., Brown, A., Clyne, E., Bartgis, L., Evans, M., Brown, M., 2012. Contrasting case definitions for chronic fatigue syndrome, myalgic encephalomyelitis/chronic fatigue syndrome and myalgic encephalomyelitis. Eval. Health Prof. 35, 280–304.

Jia, W., Li, H., Zhao, L., Nicholson, J.K., 2008. Gut microbiota, a potential new territory for drug targeting. Nat. Rev. Drug Discov. 7, 123–129.

Jimenez, M., 2009. Treatment of irritable bowel syndrome with probiotics. An etiopathogenic approach at last? Rev. Esp. Enferm. Dig. (Madrid) 101, 553–564.

Johansson, M.E., Gustafsson, J.K., Holmen-Larsson, J., Jabbar, K.S., Xia, L., Xu, H., Ghishan, F.K., Carvalho, F.A., Gewirtz, A.T., Sjovall, H., Hansson, G.C., 2014. Bacteria penetrate the normally impenetrable inner colon mucus layer in both murine colitis models and patients with ulcerative colitis. Gut 63, 281–291.

Jones, K.R., Palsson, O.S., Levy, R.L., Feld, A.D., Longstreth, G.F., Bradshaw, B.H., Drossman, D.A., Whitehead, W.E., 2001. Comorbid disorders and symptoms in irritable bowel syndrome compared to other gastroenterology patients. Gastroenterology 120, A66.

Kanamori, Y., Hashizume, K., Sugiyama, M., Morotomi, M., Yuki, N., 2001. Combination therapy with *Bifidobacterium breve*, *Lactobacillus casei*, and galactooligasaccharides dramatically improved the intestinal function in a girl with short bowel syndrome: a novel synbiotics therapy for intestinal failure. Dig. Dis. Sci. 45, 2010–2016.

Kerckhoffs, A.P., Ben-Amor, K., Samsom, M., van der Rest, M.E., de Vogel, J., Knol, J., Akkermans, L.M., 2011. Molecular analysis of fecal and duodenal samples reveals significantly higher prevalence and numbers of *Psuedomonas aeruginosa* in irritable bowel syndrome. J. Med. Microbiol. 60, 236–245.

Khalif, I.L., Quigley, E.M., Konovitch, E.A., Maximova, I.D., 2005. Alterations in the colonic flora and intestinal permeability and evidence of immune activation in chronic constipation. Dig. Liver Dis. 37, 838–849.

Khanna, S., Tosh, P.K., 2014. A clinician's primer on the role of the microbiome in human health and disease. Mayo Clinic Proc. 89, 107–114.

Kim, S.E., Choi, S.C., Park, K.S., Park, M.I., Shin, J.E., Lee, T.H., Jung, K.W., Koo, H.S., Myung, S.J., 2015. Change of fecal floral and effectiveness of the short-term VSL#3 probiotic treatment in patients with functional constipation. J. Neurogastroenterol. Motil. 21, 111–120.

Koboziev, I., Reinoso Webb, C., Furr, K.L., Grisham, M.B., 2014. Role of the enteric microbiota in intestinal homeostasis and inflammation. Free Radic. Biol. Med. 68, 122–133.

Korszun, A., Papadopoulos, E., Demitrack, M., Engleberg, C., Crofford, L., 1998. The relationship between temporomandibular disorders and stress-associated syndromes. Oral Surg. Oral Med. Oral Pathol. Oral Radiol. Endod. 86, 416–420.

Lakhan, S.E., Kirchgessner, A., 2010. Neuroinflammation in inflammatory bowel disease. J. Neuroinflam. 7, 37.

Lee, K.J., Tack, J., 2010. Altered intestinal microbiota in irritable bowel syndrome. Neurgastroenterol. Motil. 22, 493–498.

Leung, A., Tsoi, H., Yu, J., 2015. *Fusobacterium* and *Escherichia*: models of colorectal cancer driver by microbiota and the utility of microbiota in colorectal cancer screening. Expert Rev. Gastroenterol. Hepatol. 12, 1–7.

Ley, R.E., Backhed, F., Turnbaugh, P., Lozupone, C.A., Knight, R.D., Gordon, J.L., 2005. Obesity alters gut microbial ecology. Proc. Natl. Acad. Sci. 102, 11070–11075.

Ley, R.E., Turnbaugh, P.J., Klein, S., Gordon, J.I., 2006. Microbial ecology: human gut microbes associated with obesity. Nature 444, 1022–1023.

Li, Y.C., Chen, Y., Du, J., 2015. Critical roles of intestinal epithelial vitamin D receptor signaling in controlling gut mucosal inflammation. J. Steroid. Biochem. Mol. Biol. Jan 17.

Lim, W.C., Hanauer, S.B., Li, Y.C., 2005. Mechanisms of disease, vitamin D and inflammatory bowel disease. Nat. Clin. Pract. Gastroenterol. Hepatol. 2, 308–315.

Lombardi, V.C., Hagen, K.S., Hunter, K.W., Diamond, J.W., Smith-Gagen, J., Yang, W., Milkovits, J.A., 2011. Xenotropic murine leukemia virus-related virus-associated chronic fatigue syndrome reveals a distinct inflammatory signature. In Vivo 25, 307–314.

Logan, A., Rao, V., Irani, D., 2003. Chronic fatigue syndrome, lactic acid bacteria may be of therapeutic value. Med. Hypothesis 60, 915–923.

Logan, A.C., Beaulne, T.M., 2002. The treatment of small intestinal bacterial overgrowth with enteric-coated peppermint oil: a case report. Altern. Med. Rev. 7, 410–417.

Lomasney, K.W., Cryan, J.F., Hyland, N.P., 2014. Converging effects of a *Bifidobacterium* and *Lactobacillus* probiotic strain on mouse intestinal physiology. Am. J. Physiol. Gastrointest. Liver Physiol. 307, G241–G247.

Lorusso, L., Mikhaylova, S.V., Capelli, E., Ferrari, D., Ngonga, G.K., Ricevuti, G., 2009. Immunological aspects of chronic fatigue syndrome. Autoimmun. Rev. 8, 287–291.

Luzupone, C.A., Stombaugh, J.I., Gordon, J.I., Jansson, J.K., Knight, R., 2012. Diversity, stability and resilience of the human gut microbiota. Nature 489, 220–230.

Lyte, M., Varcoe, J.J., Bailey, M.T., 1998. Anxiogenic effect of subclinical bacterial infection in mice in the absence of overt immune activation. Physiol. Behav. 65, 63–68.

Madsen, K., Cornish, A., Soper, P., McKaigney, C., Jijon, H., Yachimec, C., Doyle, J., Jewell, L., De Simone, C., 2001. Probiotic bacteria enhance murine and human intestinal epithelial barrier function. Gastroenterology 121, 580–591.

Maes, M., Leunis, J.C., Geffard, M., Berk, M., 2014. Evidence for the existence of Myalgic Encephalomyelitis/Chronic Fatigue Syndrome with and without abdominal discomfort (irritable bowel) syndrome. Neuro Endocrinol. Lett. 35, 445–453.

Maes, M., Mihaylova, I., Leunis, J.C., 2007. Increased serum IgA and IgM against LPS enterobacteria in chronic fatigue syndrome (CFS), indication for the involvement of gram-negative enterobacteria in the etiology of CFS and for the presence of an increased gut-intestinal permeability. J. Affect. Dis. 99, 237–240.

Maes, M., Twisk, F.N., 2010. Chronic fatigue syndrome, Harvey and Wessely's (bio) psychosocial model versus a bio(psychosocial) model based on inflammatory and oxidative and nitrosative stress pathways. BMC Med. 8, 35.

Maes, M., Twisk, F.N., Johnson, C., 2012. Myalgic Encephalomyelitis (ME), Chronic Fatigue Syndrome (CFS), and Chronic Fatigue (CF) are distinguished accurately: results of supervised learning techniques applied on clinical and inflammatory data. Psychiatry Res. 200, 754–760.

Malinen, E., Rinttila, T., Kajander, K., Matto, J., Kassinen, A., Krogius, L., Saarela, M., Korpela, R., Palva, A., 2005. Analysis of the fecal microbiota of irritable bowel syndrome patients and healthy controls with real-time PCR. Am. J. Gastroenterol. 100, 373–382.

Marteau, P., Cuillerier, E., Meance, S., Gerhardt, M.F., Myara, A., Bouvier, M., Bouley, C., Tondu, F., Bommelaer, G., Grimaud, J.C., 2002. *Bifidobacterium animalis* strain DN-173 010 shortens the colonic transit time in healthy women: a double-blind, randomized controlled study. Aliment. Pharmacol. Ther. 16, 587–593.

Matricon, J., Barnich, N., Ardid, D., 2010. Immunopathogenesis of inflammatory bowel disease. Self Nonself 1, 299–309.

Mayer, E.A., Savidge, T., Shulman, R.J., 2014. Brain-gut microbiome interactions and functional bowel disorders. Gastroenterology 146, 1500–1512.

Messaoudi, M., Violle, N., Bisson, J.F., Desor, D., Javelot, H., Rougeot, C., 2011. Beneficial psychological effects of a probiotic formulation (*Lactobacillus helveticus* R0052 and *Bifidobacterium longum* R0175) in healthy human volunteers. Gut Microbe 2, 256–261.

Morris, G., Berk, M., Galecki, P., Maes, M., 2014. The emerging role of autoimmunity in myalgic encephalomyelitis/chronic fatigue syndrome (ME/CFS). Mol. Neurobiol. 49, 741–756.

Morriss, R.K., Ahmed, M., Wearden, A.J., Mullis, R., Strickland, P., Appleby, L., Campbell, I.T., Pearson, D., 1999. The role of depression in pain, psychophysiological syndromes and chronic fatigue syndrome. J. Affect. Disord. 55, 143–148.

Moss-Morris, R., Spence, M., 2006. To "lump" or to "split" the functional somatic syndrome, can infectious and emotional risk factors differentiate between the onset of chronic fatigue syndrome and irritable bowel syndrome? Psychol. Med. 68, 463–469.

O'Hara, A.M., Shanahan, F., 2007. Gut microbiota, mining for the therapeutic potential. Clin. Gastroenterol. Hepatol. 5, 274–284.

O'Malley, D., Liston, M., Hyland, N.P., Dinan, T.G., Cryan, J.F., 2011. Colonic soluble mediators from the maternal separation model of irritable bowel syndrome activate submucosal neurons via an interleukin-6-dependent mechanism. Am. J. Physiol. 300, G241–G252.

Ohland, C.L., Wallace, K.M., 2010. Probiotic bacteria and intestinal epithelial barrier function. Am. J. Physiol. Gastrointest. Liver Physiol. 298, G807–G819.

Oka, T., Kanemitsu, Y., Sudo, N., Hayashi, H., Oka, K., 2013. Psychological stress contributed to the development of low-grade fever in a patient with chronic fatigue syndrome, a case report. Biopsychosoc. Med. 7, 7.

Ortiz-Lucas, M., Tobias, A., Saz, P., Sebastian, J.J., 2013. Effect of probiotic species on irritable bowel syndrome symptoms: a bring up to date meta-analysis. Rev. Esp. Enferm. Dig. 105, 19–36.

Ouwehand, A.C., Salminen, S., Isolauri, E., 2002. Probiotics, an overview of beneficial effects. Antonie Van Leeuwenhoek 82, 279–289.

Parkes, G.C., Rayment, N.B., Hudspith, B.N., Petrovska, L., Lomer, M.C., Brostoff, J., Whelan, K., Sanderson, J.D., 2012. Distinct microbial populations exist in the mucosa-associated microbiota of sub-groups of irritable bowel syndrome. Neurogastroenterol. Motil. 24, 31–39.

Phillips, J., 1910. The treatment of melancholia by the lactic acid bacillus. J. Ment. Sci. 56, 422–431.

Pimentel, M., Talley, N.J., Quigley, E.M., Hani, A., Sharara, A., Mahachai, V., 2013. Report from the multinational irritable bowel syndrome initiative 2012. Gastroenterology 144, e1–e5.

Prinis, J.B., van der Meer, J.W., Bleijenberg, G., 2006. Chronic fatigue syndrome. Lancet 367, 346–355.

Proal, A.D., Albert, P.J., Marshall, T.G., Blaney, G.P., Lindseth, I.A., 2013. Immunostimulation in the treatment of chronic fatigue syndrome/myalgic encephalomyelitis. Immunol. Res. 56, 398–412.

Qin, H.-Y., Cheng, C.-W., Tang, X.-D., Bian, Z.-X., 2014. Impact of psychological stress on irritable bowel syndrome. World J. Gastroenterol. 20, 14126–14131.

Raber, J., Sorg, O., Horn, T.F., Yu, N., Koob, G.F., Campbell, I.L., Bloom, F.E., 1998. Inflammatory cytokines, putative regulators of neuronal and neuroendocrine function. Brain Res. Brain Res. Rev. 26, 320–326.

Raison, C.L., Lin, J.M., Reeves, W.C., 2009. Association of peripheral inflammatory markers with chronic fatigue in a population-based sample. Brain Behav. Immun. 23, 327–337.

Rajilić-Stojanović, M., Smidt, H., de Vos, W.M., 2007. Diversity of the human gastrointestinal tract microbiota revisited. Environ. Microbiol. 9, 2125–2136.

Rajilić-Stojanović, M., Biagi, E., Heilig, H.G., Kajander, K., Kekkonen, R.A., Tims, S., de Vos, W.M., 2011. Global and deep molecular analysis of microbiota signatures in fecal samples from patients with irritable bowel syndrome. Gastroenterology 141, 1792–1801.

Rao, A.V., Bested, A.C., Beaulne, T.M., Katzman, M.A., Iorio, C., Berardi, J.M., Logan, A.C., 2009. A randomized double-blind, placebo-controlled pilot study of a probiotic in emotional symptoms of chronic fatigue syndrome. Gut Pathog. 6.

Resta-Lenert, S., Barrett, K.E., 2006. Probiotics and commensals reverse TNF-alpha and IFN-gamma-induced dysfunction in human intestinal epithelial cells. Gastroenterology 130, 731–746.

Reyes, M., Nisenbaum, R., Hoaglin, D.C., Unger, E.R., Emmons, C., Randall, B., Stewart, J.A., Abbey, S., Jones, J.F., Gantz, N., Minden, S., Reeves, W.C., 2003. Prevalence and incidence of chronic fatigue syndrome in Wichita, Kansas. Arch. Intern. Med. 163, 1530–1536.

Reynolds, K.J., Vernon, S.D., Bouchery, E., Reeves, W.C., 2004. The economic impact of chronic fatigue syndrome. Cost Eff. Resour. Alloc. 2, 4.

Riedel, C.U., Foata, F., Phillippe, D., Adolfsson, O., Eikmanns, B.J., Blum, S., 2006. Anti-inflammatory effects of bifidobacteria by inhibition of LPS-induced NFkappaB activation. World J. Gastroenterol. 12, 3729–3735.

Rowan, F., Docherty, N.G., Murphy, M., Murphy, B., Calvin Coffey, J., O-Connell, P.R., 2010. Disulfovibrio bacterial species are increased in ulcerative colitis. Dis. Colon Rectum 53, 1530–1536.

Salonen, A., Palva, A., de Vos, W.M., 2009. Microbial functionality in the human intestinal tract. Front. Biosci. 14, 3074–3084.

Saulnier, D.M., Riehle, K., Mistretta, T.A., Diaz, M.A., Mandal, D., Raza, S., Weidler, E.M., Qin, S., Coarfa, C., Milosavljevic, A., Petrosino, J.F., Highlander, S., Gibbs, R., Lynch, S.V., Shulman, R.J., Versalovic, J., 2011. Gastrointestinal microbiome signatures of pediatric patients with irritable bowel syndrome. Gastroenterology 141, 1782–1791.

Savage, D.C., 1977. Microbial ecology of the gastrointestinal tract. Annu. Rev. Microbiol. 31, 107–133.

Scully, P., McKernan, D.P., Keohane, J., Groeger, D., Shanahan, F., Dinan, T.G., Quigley, E.M., 2010. Plasma cytokine profiles in females with irritable bowel syndrome and extra-intestinal co-morbidity. Am. J. Gastroenterol. 105, 2235–2243.

Skapinakis, P., Lewis, G., Meltzer, H., 2003. Clarifying the relationship between unexplained chronic fatigue and psychiatric morbidity, results from a community survey in Great Britain. Int. Rev. Psychiatry 15, 57–64.

Sherman, P.M., Johnson-Henry, K.C., Yeung, H.P., Ngo, P.S., Goulet, J., Tompkins, T.A., 2005. Probiotics reduce enterohemorrhagic *Escherichia coli* O157:H7- and enteropathogenic *E. coli* O127:H6-induced changes in polarized T84 epithelial cell monolayers by reducing bacterial adhesion and cytoskeletal rearrangements. Infect Immun. 73, 5183–5188.

Sheedy, J.R., Wettenhall, R.E., Scanlon, D., Gooley, P.R., Lewis, D.P., McGregor, N., Stapleton, D.I., Butt, H.L., DeMeirleir, K.L., 2009. Increased D-lactic acid intestinal bacteria in patients with chronic fatigue syndrome. In Vivo 23, 621–628.

Sierra, S., Lara-Villoslada, F., Sempere, L., Olivares, M., Boza, J., Xaus, J., 2010. Intestinal and immunological effects of daily oral administration of *Lactobacillus salivarius* CECT5713 to healthy adults. Anaerobe 16, 195–200.

Singh, P.K., Chopra, K., Kuhad, K., Kaur, I.P., 2012. Role of *Lactobacillus acidophilus* loaded floated beads in chronic fatigue syndrome, behavioral and biochemical evidences. Neurogastroenterol. Motil. 24, 366–370.

Sprake, E.F., Grant, V.A., Corfe, B.M., December 13, 2012. Vitamin D3 as a novel treatment for irritable bowel syndrome, single case leads to critical analysis of patient centered data. BMJ Case Rep.

Spence, V.A., Kennedy, G., Belch, J.J., Hill, A., Khan, F., 2008. Low-grade inflammation and arterial wave reflection in patients with chronic fatigue syndrome. Clin. Sci. (Lond) 114, 561–566.

Stolberg, L., Rolfe, R., Gitlin, N., Merritt, J., Mann Jr., L., Linder, J., Finegold, S., 1982. D-lactic acidosis due to abnormal gut flora. N. Engl. J. Med. 306, 1344–1348.

Sullivan, A., Nord, C.E., Evengard, B., 2009. Effect of supplement with lactic-acid producing bacteria on fatigue and physical activity in patients with chronic fatigue syndrome. Nutr. J. 8, 4.

Suzuki, K., Harasawa, R., Yoshitake, Y., Mitsuoka, T., 1983. Effects of crowding and heat stress on intestinal flora, body weight gain, and feed efficiency of growing rats and chicks. Nippon Jujigaku Zasshi 45, 331–338.

Switzer, W.M., Jia, H., Hohn, O., Zheng, H.-Q., Tang, S., Shankar, A., Bannert, N., Simmons, G., Hendry, R.M., Falkenberg, V.R., Reeves, W.C., Heneine, W., 2010. Absence of evidence of xenotropic murine leukemia virus-related virus infection in persons with chronic fatigue syndrome and healthy controls in the United States. Retrovirology 7, 57.

Tannock, G.W., Savage, D., 1974. Influences of dietary and environmental stress on microbial populations in the murine gastrointestinal tract. Infect. Immun. 9, 591–598.

Tillisch, K., Labus, J., Kilpatrick, L., Jiang, Z., Stains, J., Ebrat, B., Guyonnet, D., Legrain-Raspaud, S., Trotin, B., Naliboff, B., Mayer, E.A., 2013. Consumption of fermented milk product with probiotic modulates brain activity. Gastroenterology 144, 1392–1401.

Turnbaugh, P.J., Ley, R.E., Hamady, M., Fraser-Liggett, C.M., Knight, R., Gordon, J.I., 2007. The human microbiome project. Nature 449, 804–810.

Ukena, S.N., Singh, A., Dringenberg, U., Engelhardt, R., Seidler, U., Hansen, W., Bleich, A., Bruder, D., Franzke, A., Rogler, G., Suerbaum, S., Buer, J., Gunzer, F., Westendorf, A.M., 2007. Probiotic *Escherichi coli* Nissle 1917 inhibits leaky gut by enhancing mucosal integrity. PLoS One 2, e1318.

Ulluwishewq, D., Anderson, R.C., McNabb, W.C., Moughan, P.J., Wells, J.M., Roy, N.C., 2011. Regulation of tight junction permeability by intestinal bacteria and dietary components. J. Nutr. 141, 769–776.

van Kuppeveld, F.J., Jong, A.S., Lanke, K.H., Verhaegh, G.W., Melchers, W.J., Swanink, C.M., Bleijenberg, G., Netea, M.G., Galama, J.M., van der Meer, J.W., 2010. Prevalence of xenotropic murine leukemia virus-related virus in patients with chronic fatigue syndrome in the Netherlands: retrospective analysis of samples from an established cohort. BMJ 340, c1018.

Vanuytsel, T., van Wanrooy, S., Vanheel, H., Vanormelingen, C., Verschueren, S., Houben, E., Salim Rasoel, S., Toth, J., Holvoet, L., Farre, R., Van Oudenhove, L., Boeckxstaens, G., Verbeke, K., Tack, J., 2014. Psychological stress and corticotropin-releasing hormone increase intestinal permeability in humans by a mast cell-dependent mechanism. Gut 63, 1293–1299.

Villanacci, V., Bassotti, G., Nascimbeni, R., Antonelli, E., Cadei, M., Fisogni, S., Salerni, B., Geboes, K., 2008. Enteric nervous system abnormalities in inflammatory bowel disease. Neurogastroenterol. Motil. 20, 1009–1016.

Waller, P.A., Gopal, P.K., Leyer, G.J., Ouwehand, A.C., Reifer, C., Stewart, M.E., Miller, L.E., 2011. Dose-response effect of *Bifidobacterium lactis* HN019 on whole gut transit time and functional gastrointestinal symptoms in adults. Scand. J. Gastroenterol. 46, 1057–1064.

Webb, A.L., McCullough, M.L., 2005. Dietary lignans: potential role in cancer prevention. Nutr. Cancer 51, 117–131.

Werker, C.L., Nijhif, S.L., van de Putte, E.M., 2013. Clinical practice, chronic fatigue syndrome. Eur. J. Pediatr. 172, 1293–1298.

Wessely, S., Hotopf, M., Sharpe, M., 1998. Chronic Fatigue and Its Syndromes. Oxford University Press, New York.

Wessely, S., Nimnuan, C., Sharpe, M., 1999. Functional somatic syndrome, one or many? Lancet 354, 936–939.

White, P.D., Thomas, J.M., Amess, J., Crawford, D.H., Grover, S.A., Kangro, H.O., Clare, A.W., 1998. Incidence, risk and prognosis of acute and chronic fatigue syndromes and psychiatric disorders after glandular fever. Br. J. Psychiatry 173, 475–481.

White, P.D., 2004. What causes chronic fatigue syndrome? BMJ 329, 928–929.

Whitehead, W.E., Palsson, O., Jones, K.R., 2002. Systematic review of the comorbidity of irritable bowel syndrome with other disorders, what are the causes and implications? Gastroenterology 122, 1140–1156.

Whorwell, P.J., McCallum, M., Creed, F.H., Roberts, C.T., 1986. Noncolonic features of irritable bowel syndrome. Gut 27, 37–40.

Zachrisson, O., Regland, B., Jahreskog, M., Kron, M., Gottfries, C.G., 2002. A rating scale for fibromyalgia and chronic fatigue syndrome (the FibroFatigue scale). J. Psychosom. Res. 52, 501–509.

Zareie, M., Johnson-Henry, K., Jury, J., Yang, P.C., Ngan, B.Y., McKay, D.M., Soderholm, J.D., Perdue, M.H., Sherman, P.M., 2006. Probiotics prevent bacterial translocation and improve intestinal barrier function in rats following chronic psychological stress. Gut 55, 1553–1560.

Zhou, Q., Zhang, B., Verne, G.N., 2009. Intestinal membrane permeability and hypersensitivity in the irritable bowel syndrome. Pain 146, 41–46.

Zoetendal, E.G., Vaughan, E.E., de Vos, W.M., 2006. A microbial world within us. Mol. Microbiol. 59, 1639–1650.

Zyrek, A.A., Cichon, C., Helms, S., Enders, C., Sonnenborn, U., Schmidt, M.A., 2007. Cellular mechanisms underlying the probiotic effects of *Escherichia coli* Nissle 1917 involve ZO-2 and PKCzeta redistribution resulting in tight junction epithelial barrier repair. Cell Microbiol. 9, 804–816.

Translating Microbiome Science to Society— What's Next?

22

F. Shanahan

University College Cork, APC Microbiome Institute, Cork, Ireland; University College Cork, Department of Medicine, Cork, Ireland; University College Cork, School of Medicine, Cork, Ireland

G. Fitzgerald

University College Cork, APC Microbiome Institute, Cork, Ireland; University College Cork, Department of Medicine and School of Microbiology, Cork, Ireland

INTRODUCTION

Predicting the future is fraught with hazard and generally unwise. Predicting change and identifying what should change is more productive. More than a decade ago, the former US Secretary of State for Defense, Donald Rumsfeld, was pilloried for humorously distinguishing between the "knowns" and "unknowns," each of which may either be known or unknown (Graham, 2014). However, when uncoupled from its context, there was a curious wisdom in his words. Identifying the known unknowns is relatively simple and forms the basis of the research questions we should set. However, it is the unknown unknowns that excite, occasionally embarrass, and motivate us to do science.

In science, as in all areas of human endeavor, there are self-evident problems and changes waiting to happen. Indeed, the best way of appreciating what might happen in the future is to learn from what has already happened. Here we identify some of the problems in microbiome science and its translation to seemingly disparate branches of research, such as the gut-brain-microbiome axis. As with the former US Secretary of State, our views are heartfelt and personal, but we reserve the right to change our minds when the facts change.

WHAT SHOULD CHANGE—OBSTACLES TO LINKING SCIENCE AND SOCIETY

It is commonplace to hear scientists call for more funding for more research to do bigger and better clinical trials to enhance our understanding of the microbiota and host–microbiome interactions. Yes, of course, but such calls are redundant, lack incisiveness, and border on the inane. In Table 22.1, we draw attention to some of the problems that impede effective translation of microbiome science to society. Most of these are political or educational but are no less important than those that relate solely to science.

The Gut-Brain Axis. http://dx.doi.org/10.1016/B978-0-12-802304-4.00022-0

Table 22.1 Barriers to Translating Microbiome Science to Society

Sectors of Society	Problem
The media	• Misportrayal of probiotics as all being the same • Emphasis on sensation over truth
The regulators	• Lack of clarity • Lagging behind the science • Insufficient policing of false claims
Public health officialdom	• Ineffective messages to the public • Excessive focus on antibiotic resistance rather than risk of collateral damage to microbiota in promoting judicious use of antibiotics • Poor communication of role of diet on microbiota
Product suppliers	• Poor labeling of probiotic/prebiotic products • Poor oversight of quality control and shelf life
The scientists	• Excessive use of hyperbole • Poor language • Failure to standardize terminology and methodology
Consumers	• Poor understanding of risk and benefit • Limited evidence of critical thinking in appraising product and scientific claims

FLAWED CONCEPTS AND BAD LANGUAGE

Similar to politicians, scientists would benefit from continual reminders of George Orwell's wonderful refrain (Orwell, 1946): "…the slovenliness of our language makes it easier…to have foolish thoughts." To appreciate the problems that may arise because of bad language in the area of microbiome science, one need look no further than to the difficulties surrounding the word *probiotic*. Some enthusiasts actually impeded their own cause because of their counterproductive claims that a probiotic must always be linked with beneficial effects; therefore any agent linked with unwanted side effects cannot be referred to as a probiotic. This self-defining health benefit with its circular logic, easily reduced to the absurd, naturally created a problem for regulatory agencies and led to rejection of the unqualified use of the term *probiotic*.

A more insidious problem is the loose, almost frivolous, misuse of the word *dysbiosis*, including by several contributors to this book! Familiarity with an oft-repeated word or concept does not make it correct. Those who persist in using the word usually wish to portray in some vague sense that there is a change in the microbiota. The word is not only unnecessary, it is imprecise, implies an understanding where none may exist, and generally reflects lazy thinking. Furthermore, the word gives a vague sense that the changed microbiota is in some way a bad thing, whereas it might actually be an appropriate response to some insult. Failure to appreciate this might lead inappropriate treatments aimed at restoring the microbiota to some presumed standard of normality. In addition, widespread use of the term *dysbiosis* has, in part, been

Table 22.2 Bad Language: Terms and Concepts That Should be Retired

Word/Concept	Comment
"Unculturable"	More correctly termed: "not yet" cultured.
"Good" and "bad" bacteria	The distinction between friend and foe depends on context—including the age and genetic status of the host. Any bacterium in the wrong place at the wrong time may be a bad thing.
"Boosting" the immune system	Other than the use of vaccination to boost specific acquired immune responses, the notion of non-specific stimulation of the immune system is probably more likely to be dangerous than beneficial.
"Autoimmune" diseases	Most so-called autoimmune disorders involve tissue damage that is immune mediated with collateral damage to the host but not due to immune responses directed at self.
"Leaky gut" syndrome	Not a true syndrome. Needs refinement with specific data concerning changes in permeability and barrier function and reconciliation with the apparent lack of systemic sequelae in humans with known barrier breaks.
Dysbiosis	An unnecessary and harmful term as discussed in text.

responsible for accusations of overstatement of results (Hanage, 2014; Shanahan, 2015); claims that a disease is linked with dysbiosis sounds more sensational than a more precise, simple statement that the microbiota is altered. The most compelling argument against the use of this odious word is that it creates a distancing effect from the truth; such is the antithesis of science.

Other outdated or unhelpful terms in need of retirement are included in Table 22.2. In addition, a proposed standardized vocabulary for microbiome research is welcome (Marchesi and Ravel, 2015), as are proposals for standardized methodology and analysis of microbiome studies, including higher quality metadata (Goodrich et al., 2014; Huttenhower et al., 2014).

UNREALISTIC EXPECTATIONS AND EXTRAPOLATIONS FROM EXPERIMENTAL ANIMALS

It is noteworthy that the greatest success story in microbiome science to date—the discovery of the causative role of *Helicobacter pylori* in peptic ulcer disease and gastric cancer—was based on observations in humans, not experimental animals. The same can be said of advances in understanding *Clostridium difficile*–associated disease. Despite this, most studies on the mechanisms of host–microbe interaction are conducted using murine models. Few will dispute the value of experimental animal models for establishing preliminary hypotheses to be tested and for exploring plausible disease mechanisms. However, the degree to which results from studies of the microbiome in murine models can be extrapolated to humans has been questioned by many investigators.

Elsewhere, we have highlighted some of the disparities in research findings from animal and human studies (Shanahan and Quigley, 2014). Firstly, the human microbiome is more complex and diverse than that of rodents, particularly laboratory-housed animals. Secondly, the human diet is more diverse than that of captive animals. Thirdly, humans have markedly more robust coping and stress responses than those of an inbred laboratory animal in captivity. Fourthly, murine models of inflammatory disease tend to be monophasic and do not reflect the relapsing and remitting nature of its human counterpart. Finally, results of therapeutic manipulation of the microbiome with pro- and prebiotics in animals have been a poor predictor of responses in humans. This has contributed to unrealistic or exaggerated claims and expectations for such agents in human disorders, particularly inflammatory conditions (Shanahan and Quigley, 2014).

The risk of relying on data obtained primarily from murine studies may be particularly evident in investigations of what is now popularly referred to as the brain-gut-microbe axis. Although the existence of such an intercellular axis of communication undoubtedly exists, its significance may be prone to overstatement in the absence of confirmatory studies in humans. Claims that microbes might influence human mood, behavior, and psychiatric disease are sensational and likely to receive widespread representation and misrepresentation in the lay press. That microbial metabolites from the gut can affect the brain is well known from clinical observations of humans with liver failure. However, the uptake of microbial metabolites under normal circumstances is unlikely to have a profound influence on human brain function. The Darwinian success of our species runs counter to such a notion. In addition, as alluded to already, there is a multiplicity of confounding variables in human lifestyle and behavior that are not addressed in studies of captive laboratory animals. The challenge for researchers in this field is to confirm the relevance and scope of their observations in humans. The temptation to repeat the same experiment or vary the experimental conditions in animals will not satisfy what is required for progress.

CHALLENGES AND OPPORTUNITIES

Until recently, the pharmaceutical industry has been slow to enter the field of microbiome science, unsure as to how it might be exploited and unfamiliar with live organisms as biotherapeutics. However, since the first comparative studies of germ-free and colonized animals were performed in the last century, it has been clear that the microbiota is a source of positive and negative regulatory signals for several organ systems in the host. The prospect of mining these microbial-derived signals for new drug discovery is likely to attract greater pharmaceutical interest (Shanahan, 2010).

Likewise, the food industry has been uncertain in its approach to the microbiome, generally restricting its interest to probiotics and prebiotic supplements. However, the

Table 22.3 Current Challenges for the Pharmaceutical and Food Sectors

Changing Course of Big Pharma	Changing Course of Agrifood Industry
Decline in discovery of new molecular entities	Enhanced public awareness of relationship between food and health
Emphasis on biologics over small molecules	Increasing interest in medical foods
Genotyping exceeds phenotyping	Risk averse society
Fragmentation of the market	Niche markets
Decline of the "blockbuster" drug	Increasing interest in functional foods
Partnerships and alliances	Regulatory constraints over health claims
Open innovation	

modest health benefits from such supplements imply that large numbers of study subjects are required for controlled trials to demonstrate statistically significant benefits. The food industry has traditionally been reluctant to bear the cost of such controlled trials, contending that in comparison with pharmaceuticals, the margins of profit for foods are narrow. However, the food industry cannot continue to hide behind such arguments, nor will it be able to favor clever marketing as a substitute for rigorous science. The pharma and food sectors face a changing commercial landscape with many hurdles, including an uncertain regulatory environment (Table 22.3).

For both commercial sectors, the exploration of live biotherapeutic agents should no longer be limited to lactic acid bacteria, and a new generation of probiotic or beneficial microbes is a real prospect. Indeed, the success of fecal microbial transplantation in *Clostridium difficile*–associated disease and its widespread use in other conditions raises the specter of developing artificial or designer stool as a future therapeutic or preventive strategy. The pharmaceutical sector will continue to address disease treatment, but for the food industry, there is the opportunity to expand its market to the prevention of disease, particularly as new microbial biomarkers emerge that may identify those at greatest risk of disease. Finally, because diet represents one of the strongest lifestyle influences on the composition, diversity, and metabolic behavior of the microbiota, the food industry needs to place the microbiome at the center of its strategies for the design of future foods. Consumers and regulators will increasingly expect that the food industry address the impact of diet on the microbiota and on its role in chronic metabolic and immunologic disorders.

CONCLUSION—BOLD PREDICTIONS

Notwithstanding our caution regarding the hazards of predictions, we will risk the following bold pronouncements in the spirit of provoking scientific rebuttal. First, research on the microbiome will eclipse that of the human genome in the next decade for impact on human health. Second, the search for new biomarkers and early diagnostics will be fulfilled in many cases by the discovery and application of microbial biomarkers to predict risk and resistance to disease. For example, current biomarkers of colorectal cancer are actually markers of early established disease whereas microbial biomarkers offer the prospect of predicting risk of development of disease. Third, an increasing list of drugs will be shown to be metabolized by the gut microbiome, and potential impact on the microbiome will be a requirement for new drug discovery. Whether the same is true for topical therapies, cosmetics, and the skin microbiome is a provocative notion. Fourth, age-dependent effects of the microbiome on the maturation and homeostasis of the immune and other systems will focus attention toward the extremes of life. Thus examining the microbiome in midlife after the development of immune and metabolic disorders may be too late, outside of the early window during which the microbiome is becoming established and during which its imprint on immune and metabolic development is maximal. Finally, the design of future foods will have to take into consideration not only the impact on host nutrition in terms of quantity and quality of nutrients but also diversity. Thus the diversity of nutritional intake is likely to relate to the diversity of the composition of the microbiota.

ACKNOWLEDGMENTS

The authors are supported in part by Science Foundation Ireland in the form of a research center grant (SFI/12/RC/2273) to the APC Microbiome Institute, which receives grants from the following industry partners: Alimentary Health, Ltd.; Cremo; Danone; Friesland Campina; GE; General Mills; Janssen; Kerry Foods; Mead Johnson Nutrition; Nutricia; Second Genome; Sigmoid Pharma; Suntory; and 4D Pharma. This has neither influenced nor constrained the content of this manuscript.

REFERENCES

Goodrich, J.K., Di Rienzi, S.C., Poole, A.C., Koren, O., Walters, W.A., Caporaso, J.G., Knight, R., Ley, R.E., 2014. Conducting a microbiome study. Cell 158, 250–262.

Graham, D.A., March 27, 2014. Rumsfeld's knowns and unknowns: the intellectual history of a quip. The Atlantic. http://www.theatlantic.com/politics/archive/2014/03/rumsfelds-knowns-and-unknowns-the-intellectual-history-of-a-quip/359719/ (accessed 07.11.15.).

Hanage, W.P., 2014. Microbiome science needs a healthy dose of scepticism. Nature 512, 247–248.

Huttenhower, C., Knight, R., Brown, C.T., Caporaso, J.G., Clemente, J.C., Gevers, D., Franzosa, E.A., et al., 2014. Advancing the microbiome research community. Cell 159, 227–230.

Marchesi, J.R., Ravel, J., 2015. The vocabulary of microbiome research: a proposal. Microbiome 3, 31.

Orwell, G., 1946. Politics of the English Language. Available at: http://www.npr.org/blogs/ombudsman/Politics_and_the_English_Language-1.pdf (accessed 17.12.13.).

Shanahan, F., 2010. Gut microbes: from bugs to drugs. Am. J. Gastroenterol. 105, 275–279.

Shanahan, F., Quigley, E.M., 2014. Manipulation of the microbiota for treatment of IBS and IBD – challenges and controversies. Gastroenterology 146, 1554–1563.

Shanahan, F., 2015. Separating the microbiome from the hyperbolome. Genome Med. 7, 17.

Index

Note: Page numbers followed by "f" indicate figures and "t" indicate tables.